S0-DSP-700

Parent-Youth Relations: Cultural and Cross-Cultural Perspectives

Parent-Youth Relations: Cultural and Cross-Cultural Perspectives has been previously published as *Marriage & Family Review*, Volume 35, Numbers 3/4 2003, and Volume 36, Numbers 1/2/3/4 2004.

The *Marriage & Family Review* Monographic "Separates"

Below is a list of "separates," which in serials librarianship means a special issue simultaneously published as a special journal issue or double-issue *and* as a "separate" hardbound monograph. (This is a format which we also call a "DocuSerial.")

"Separates" are published because specialized libraries or professionals may wish to purchase a specific thematic issue by itself in a format which can be separately cataloged and shelved, as opposed to purchasing the journal on an on-going basis. Faculty members may also more easily consider a "separate" for classroom adoption.

"Separates" are carefully classified separately with the major book jobbers so that the journal tie-in can be noted on new book order slips to avoid duplicate purchasing.

You may wish to visit Haworth's website at . . .

http://www.HaworthPress.com

. . . to search our online catalog for complete tables of contents of these separates and related publications.

You may also call 1-800-HAWORTH (outside US/Canada: 607-722-5857), or Fax 1-800-895-0582 (outside US/Canada: 607-771-0012), or e-mail at:

docdelivery@haworthpress.com

Parent-Youth Relations: Cultural and Cross-Cultural Perspectives, edited by Gary W. Peterson, Suzanne K. Steinmetz, and Stephan M. Wilson (Vol. 35, No. 3/4, 2003; Vol. 36, No. 1/2/3/4, 2004). *A comprehensive examination of how culture interconnects with parent-child relationships.*

Emotions and the Family, edited by Richard A. Fabes, PhD (Vol. 34, No. 1/2/3/4, 2002). *"An exciting collection. The contributors insightfully unfold the nature of emotions as relational processes in marriage and parenting, and illuminate how emotional communication, competence, and regulation color family life. Chapters on siblings, stepfamilies, economic stress, and family therapy add richness to the collective portrayal of how emotions infuse marital and parent-child relationships. Scholars of marital and family life will find this a valuable resource." (Ross A. Thompson, PhD, Carl A. Happold Distinguished Professor of Psychology, University of Nebraska)*

Gene-Environment Processes in Social Behaviors and Relationships, edited by Kirby Deater-Deckard, PhD, and Stephen A. Petrill, PhD (Vol. 33, No. 1/2/3, 2002). *"During recent years there have been somewhat fruitless battles on whether family influences or peer influences are more important in children's psychological development. This book is both innovative and helpful in seeking to bring the two sets of influences together through a range of studies using twin, adoptee, and stepfamily designs to assess how genetic and environmental influences may work together in bringing about individual differences in children's emotions, behavior and especially social relationships. The different research approaches provide some new ways of thinking about, and investigating, how interpersonal relationships develop and have their effects." (Michael Rutter, MD, FRS, Professor of Developmental Psychopathology, Institute of Psychiatry, King's College, London)*

Pioneering Paths in the Study of Families: The Lives and Careers of Family Scholars, edited by Suzanne K. Steinmetz, PhD, MSW, and Gary W. Peterson, PhD (Vol. 30, No. 3, 2000; Vol. 30, No. 4, 2001; Vol. 31, No. 1/2/3/4, 2001; Vol. 32, No. 1/2, 2001). *The fascinating autobiographies of 40 leading scholars in sociology, family studies, psychology, and child development.*

FATHERHOOD: Research, Interventions and Policies, edited by H. Elizabeth Peters, PhD, Gary W. Peterson, PhD, Suzanne K. Steinmetz, PhD, MSW, and Randal D. Day, PhD (Vol. 29, No. 2/3/4, 2000). *Brings together the latest facts to help researchers explore the father-child relationship and determine what factors lead fathers to be more or less involved in the lives of their children, including human social behavior, not living with a child, being denied visiting privileges, and social norms regarding gender differences versus work responsibilities.*

Concepts and Definitions of Family for the 21st Century, edited by Barbara H. Settles, PhD, Suzanne K. Steinmetz, PhD, MSW, Gary W. Peterson, PhD, and Marvin B. Sussman, PhD (Vol. 28, No. 3/4, 1999). *Views family from a U.S. perspective and from many different cultures and societies. The controversial question "What is family?" is thoroughly examined as it has become an increasingly important social policy concern in recent years as the traditional family has changed.*

The Role of the Hospitality Industry in the Lives of Individuals and Families, edited by Pamela R. Cummings, PhD, Francis A. Kwansa, PhD, and Marvin B. Sussman, PhD (Vol. 28, No. 1/2, 1998). *"A must for human resource directors and hospitality educators." (Dr. Lynn Huffman, Director, Restaurant, Hotel, and Institutional Management, Texas Tech University, Lubbock, Texas)*

Stepfamilies: History, Research, and Policy, edited by Irene Levin, PhD, and Marvin B. Sussman, PhD (Vol. 26, No. 1/2/3/4, 1997). *"A wide range of individually valuable and stimulating chapters that form a wonderfully rich menu from which readers of many different kinds will find exciting and satisfying selections." (Jon Bernardes, PhD, Principal Lecturer in Sociology, University of Wolverhampton, Castle View Dudley, United Kingdom)*

Families and Adoption, edited by Harriet E. Gross, PhD, and Marvin B. Sussman, PhD (Vol. 25, No. 1/2/3/4, 1997). *"Written in a lucid and easy-to-read style, this volume will make an invaluable contribution to the adoption literature." (Paul Sachdev, PhD, Professor, School of Social Work, Memorial University of Newfoundland, St. John's, Newfoundland, Canada)*

The Methods and Methodologies of Qualitative Family Research, edited by Jane F. Gilgun, PhD, LICSW, and Marvin B. Sussman, PhD (Vol 24, No. 1/2/3/4, 1997). *"An authoritative look at the usefulness of qualitative research methods to the family scholar." (Family Relations)*

Intercultural Variation in Family Research and Theory: Implications for Cross-National Studies, Volumes I and II, edited by Marvin B. Sussman, PhD, and Roma S. Hanks, PhD (Vol. 22, No. 1/2/3/4, and Vol. 23, No. 1/2/3/4, 1997). *Documents the development of family research in theory in societies around the world and inspires continued cross-national collaboration on current research topics.*

Families and Law, edited by Lisa J. McIntyre, PhD, and Marvin B. Sussman, PhD (Vol. 21, No. 3/4, 1995). *With this new volume, family practitioners and scholars can begin to increase the family's position in relation to the law and legal system.*

Exemplary Social Intervention Programs for Members and Their Families, edited by David Guttmann, DSW, and Marvin B. Sussman, PhD (Vol. 21, No. 1/2, 1995). *An eye-opening look at organizations and individuals who have created model family programs that bring desired results.*

Single Parent Families: Diversity, Myths and Realities, edited by Shirley M. H. Hanson, RN, PhD, Marsha L. Heims, RN, EdD, Doris J. Julian, RN, EdD, and Marvin B. Sussman, PhD (Vol. 20, No. 1/2/3/4, 1994). *"Remarkable! . . . A significant work and is important reading for multidisciplinary family professionals including sociologists, educators, health care professionals, and policymakers." (Maureen Leahey, RN, PhD, Director, Outpatient Mental Health Program, Director, Family Therapy Training Program, Calgary District Hospital Group)*

Families on the Move: Immigration, Migration, and Mobility, edited by Barbara H. Settles, PhD, Daniel E. Hanks III, MS, and Marvin B. Sussman, PhD (Vol 19, No 1/2/3/4, 1993). *Examines the current research on family mobility, migration, and immigration and discovers new directions for understanding the relationship between mobility and family life.*

American Families and the Future: Analyses of Possible Destinies, edited by Barbara H. Settles, PhD, Roma S. Hanks, PhD, and Marvin B. Sussman, PhD (Vol. 18, No. 3/4, 1993). *This book discusses a variety of issues that face and will continue to face families in coming years and describes various strategies families can use in their decision-making processes.*

Publishing in Journals on the Family: Essays on Publishing, edited by Roma S. Hanks, PhD, Linda Matocha, PhD, RN, and Marvin B. Sussman, PhD (Vol. 18, No. 1/2, 1993). *This helpful book contains varied perspectives from scholars at different career stages and from editors of* *major publication outlets, providing readers with important information necessary to help them systematically plan a productive scholarly career.*

Publishing in Journals on the Family: A Survey and Guide for Scholars, Practitioners, and Students, edited by Roma S. Hanks, PhD, Linda Matocha, PhD, RN, and Marvin B. Sussman, PhD (Vol. 17, No. 3/4, 1992). *"Comprehensive. . . . Includes listings for some 200 social science journals whose editors have expressed an interest in publishing empirical research and theoretical articles about the family." (Reference & Research Book News)*

Wider Families: New Traditional Family Forms, edited by Teresa D. Marciano, PhD, and Marvin B. Sussman, PhD (Vol. 17, No. 1/2, 1992). *"An insightful and informative compilation of essays on the subject of wider families." (Journal of Marriage and the Family)*

Families: Intergenerational and Generational Connections, edited by Susan K. Pfeifer, PhD, and Marvin B. Sussman, PhD (Vol. 16, No. 1/2/3/4, 1991). *"The contributors challenge and move dramatically from outdated myths and stereotypes concerning who and what is family, what its members do, and how they continue its traditions to contemporary views of families and their relationships." (Contemporary Psychology)*

Corporations, Businesses, and Families, edited by Roma S. Hanks, PhD, and Marvin B. Sussman, PhD (Vol. 15, No. 3/4, 1991). *"Examines the changing relationship between family systems and work organizations." (Economic Books)*

Families in Community Settings: Interdisciplinary Perspectives, edited by Donald G. Unger, PhD, and Marvin B. Sussman, PhD (Vol. 15, No. 1/2, 1990). *"An excellent introduction in which to frame and understand the central issues." (Abraham Wandersman, PhD, Professor, Department of Psychology, University of South Carolina)*

Homosexuality and Family Relations, edited by Frederick W. Bozett, RN, DNS, and Marvin B. Sussman, PhD (Vol. 14, No. 3/4, 1990). *"Offers a smorgasbord of familial topics. . . . Provides references for those seeking more information." (Lesbian News)*

Cross-Cultural Perspectives on Families, Work, and Change, edited by Katja Boh, PhD, Giovanni Sgritta, PhD, and Marvin B. Sussman, PhD (Vol. 14, No. 1/2, 1990). *"On the cutting edge of this new perspective that sees a modern society as a set of influences that affect human beings and not just a collection of individual orphans." (John Mogey, DSc, Adjunct Professor of Sociology, Arizona State University)*

Museum Visits and Activities for Family Life Enrichment, edited by Barbara H. Butler, PhD, and Marvin B. Sussman, PhD (Vol. 13, No. 3/4, 1989). *"Very interesting reading . . . a fine synthesis of current thinking concerning families in museums." (Jane R. Glaser, Special Assistant, Office of the Assistant Secretary for Museums, Smithsonian Institution, Washington, DC)*

AIDS and Families, edited by Eleanor D. Macklin, PhD (Vol. 13, No. 1/2, 1989). *"A highly recommended book. Will provide family professionals, policymakers, and researchers with a foundation for further exploration on the largely unresearched topic of AIDS and the family." (Family Relations)*

Transitions to Parenthood, edited by Rob Palkovitz, PhD, and Marvin B. Sussman, PhD (Vol. 12, No. 3/4, 1989). *In this insightful volume, experts discuss the issues, changes, and problems involved in becoming a parent.*

Deviance and the Family, edited by Frank E. Hagan, PhD, and Marvin B. Sussman, PhD (Vol. 12, No. 1/2, 1988). *Leading experts in the fields of criminal justice, sociology, and family services explain the causes of deviance as well as the role of the family.*

Alternative Health Maintenance and Healing Systems for Families, edited by Doris Y. Wilkinson, PhD, and Marvin B. Sussman, PhD (Vol. 11, No. 3/4, 1988). *This important book offers timely discussions of current approaches and treatments in modern medicine that have had great impact upon family health care.*

'Til Death Do Us Part: How Couples Stay Together, edited by Jeanette C. Lauer and Robert C. Lauer (Supp. #1, 1987). *"A landmark study that will serve as a classic for the emerging ethic of commitment to marriage, family, and community." (Gregory W. Brock, PhD, Professor of Family Science and Marriage and Family Therapy, University of Wisconsin)*

Childhood Disability and Family Systems, edited by Michael Ferrari, PhD, and Marvin B. Sussman, PhD (Vol. 11, No. 1/2, 1987). *A motivating book that offers new and enlightening perspectives for professionals working with disabled children and their families.*

Family Medicine: The Maturing of a Discipline, edited by William J. Doherty, PhD, Charles E. Christianson, MD, ScM, and Marvin B. Sussman, PhD (Vol. 10, No. 3/4, 1987). *"Well-written essays and a superb introduction concerning various aspects of the field of family medicine (or as it is sometimes called, family practice)." (The American Journal of Family Therapy)*

Families and the Prospect of Nuclear Attack/Holocaust, edited by Teresa D. Marciano, PhD, and Marvin B. Sussman, PhD (Vol. 10, No. 2, 1986). *Experts address the issues and effects of the continuing threat of nuclear holocaust on the behavior of families.*

The Charybdis Complex: Redemption of Rejected Marriage and Family Journal Articles, edited by Marvin B. Sussman, PhD (Vol. 10, No. 1, 1986). *An examination of the "publish-or-perish" syndrome of academic publishing, with a frank look at peer review.*

Men's Changing Roles in the Family, edited by Robert A. Lewis, PhD, and Marvin B. Sussman, PhD (Vol. 9, No. 3/4, 1986). *"Brings together a wealth of findings on men's family role enactment . . . provides a well-integrated, carefully documented summary of the literature on men's roles in the family that should be useful to both family scholars (in their own work and the classroom) and practitioners." (Contemporary Sociology)*

Families and the Energy Transition, edited by John Byrne, David A. Schulz, and Marvin B. Sussman, PhD (Vol. 9, No. 1/2, 1985). *An important appraisal of the future of energy consumption by families and the family's adaptations to decreasing energy availability.*

Pets and the Family, edited by Marvin B. Sussman, PhD (Vol. 8, No. 3/4, 1985). *"Informative and thorough coverage of what is currently known about the animal/human bond." (Canada's Mental Health)*

Personal Computers and the Family, edited by Marvin B. Sussman, PhD (Vol 8, No. 1/2, 1985). *A pioneering volume that explores the impact of the personal computer on the modern family.*

Women and the Family: Two Decades of Change, edited by Beth B. Hess, PhD, and Marvin B. Sussman, PhD (Vol. 7, No. 3/4, 1984). *"A scholarly, thorough, readable, informative, well-integrated, current overview of social science research on women and the family." (Journal of Gerontology)*

Obesity and the Family, edited by David J. Kallen, PhD, and Marvin B. Sussman, PhD (Vol. 7, No. 1/2, 1984). *"Should be required reading for all persons touched by the problem of obesity–the teachers, the practitioners of every discipline, and the obese themselves." (Journal of Nutrition Education)*

Human Sexuality and the Family, edited by James W. Maddock, PhD, Gerhard Neubeck, EdD, and Marvin B. Sussman, PhD (Vol. 6, No. 3/4, 1984). *"Twelve chapters that not only add some new ideas about the place of sexuality in the family but also go beyond this to show how widely sexuality influences human behavior and thought . . . excellent." (Siecus Report)*

Social Stress and the Family: Advances and Developments in Family Stress Theory and Research, edited by Hamilton I. McCubbin, Marvin B. Sussman, PhD, and Joan M. Patterson (Vol. 6, No. 1/2, 1983). *An informative anthology of recent theory and research developments pertinent to family stress.*

The Ties That Bind: Men's and Women's Social Networks, edited by Laura Lein, PhD, and Marvin B. Sussman, PhD (Vol. 5, No. 4, 1983). *An examination of the networks for men and women in a variety of social contexts.*

Monographs "Separates" list continued at the back

ALL HAWORTH BOOKS AND JOURNALS
ARE PRINTED ON CERTIFIED
ACID-FREE PAPER

Parent-Youth Relations: Cultural and Cross-Cultural Perspectives

Gary W. Peterson
Suzanne K. Steinmetz
Stephan M. Wilson
Editors

Parent-Youth Relations: Cultural and Cross-Cultural Perspectives has been previously published as *Marriage & Family Review*, Volume 35, Numbers 3/4 2003, and Volume 36, Numbers 1/2/3/4 2004.

HQ
799.15
.P34
2005
West

The Haworth Press, Inc.

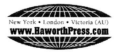

New York • London • Victoria (AU)
www.HaworthPress.com

Parent-Youth Relations: Cultural and Cross-Cultural Perspectives
has been previously published as *Marriage & Family Review*, Volume
35, Numbers 3/4 2003, and Volume 36, Numbers 1/2/3/4 2004.

© 2005 by The Haworth Press, Inc. All rights reserved. No part of this work may be reproduced or utilized in any form or by any means, electronic or mechanical, including photocopying, microfilm and re-
cording, or by any information storage and retrieval system, without permission in writing from the
publisher. Printed in the United States of America.

The development, preparation, and publication of this work has been undertaken with great care. However, the publisher, employees, editors, and agents of The Haworth Press and all imprints of The
Haworth Press, Inc., including The Haworth Medical Press® and Pharmaceutical Products Press®, are
not responsible for any errors contained herein or for consequences that may ensue from use of materials or information contained in this work. Opinions expressed by the author(s) are not necessarily those
of The Haworth Press, Inc. With regard to case studies, identities and circumstances of individuals discussed herein have been changed to protect confidentiality. Any resemblance to actual persons, living
or dead, is entirely coincidental.

Cover design by Kerry E. Mack

Library of Congress Cataloging-in-Publication Data

Parent-youth relations : cultural and cross-cultural perspectives / Gary W. Peterson, Suzanne K.
Steinmetz, Stephan M. Wilson, editors.
     p. cm.
    "Previously published as Marriage & family review, volume 35, numbers 3/4 2003, and
volume 36, numbers 1/2/3/4 2004."
    Includes bibliographical references and index.
    ISBN-13: 978-0-7890-2482-4 (hard cover : alk. paper)
    ISBN-10: 0-7890-2482-9 (hard cover : alk. paper)
    ISBN-13: 978-0-7890-2483-1 (soft cover : alk. paper)
    ISBN-10: 0-7890-2483-7 (soft cover : alk. paper)
    1. Parent and teenager–Cross-cultural studies. I. Peterson, Gary W. II. Steinmetz, Suzanne K.
III. Wilson, Stephan M. IV. Marriage & family review.
  HQ799.15.P34 2005
  306.874'089–dc22
                                         20050057

Indexing, Abstracting & Website/Internet Coverage

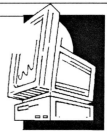

Marriage & Family Review

This section provides you with a list of major indexing & abstracting services and other tools for bibliographic access. That is to say, each service began covering this periodical during the year noted in the right column. Most Websites which are listed below have indicated that they will either post, disseminate, compile, archive, cite or alert their own Website users with research-based content from this work. (This list is as current as the copyright date of this publication.)

Abstracting, Website/Indexing Coverage . . . . Year When Coverage Began

- *Abstracts in Social Gerontology: Current Literature on Aging* 1993
- *Academic Abstracts/CD-ROM* 1993
- *Academic ASAP <http://www.galegroup.com>* 1989
- *Academic Search: Database of 2,000 selected academic serials, updated monthly: EBSCO Publishing* 1996
- *Academic Search Elite (EBSCO)* 1993
- *Academic Search Premier (EBSCO) <http://www.epnet.com/academic/acasearchprem.asp>* 1993
- *AgeLine Database <http://research.aarp.org/ageline>* 1991
- *AGRICOLA Database: a bibliographic database of citations to the agricultural literature created by the National Agricultural Library and its cooperators <http://www.natl.usda.gov/ag98>* . . . 1992
- *AGRIS <http://www.fao.org/agris/>* 1992
- *Applied Social Sciences Index & Abstracts (ASSIA) (Online: ASSI via Data-Star) (CDRom: ASSIA Plus) <http://www.csa.com>* 1993
- *AURSI African Urban & Regional Science Index. A scholarly & research index which synthesises & compiles all publications on urbanization & regional science in Africa within the world. Published annually* 2004

(continued)

(continued)

(continued)

- *Psychological Abstracts (PsycINFO) <http://www.apa.org>* 1978

- *RESEARCH ALERT/ISI Alerting Services*
  <http://www.isinet.com> 1992

- *Sage Family Studies Abstracts (SFSA)* 1992

- *ScienceDirect Navigator (Elsevier)*
  <http://www.info.sciencedirect.com> 2002

- *Scopus (Elsevier) <http://www.info.scopus.com>* 2002

- *Social Science Source: Coverage of 400 journals in the social*
  sciences area; updated monthly; EBSCO Publishing 1996

- *Social Scisearch <http://www.isinet.com>* 1992

- *Social Services Abstracts <http://www.csa.com>* 1990

- *Social Work Abstracts*
  <http://www.silverplatter.com/catalog/swab.htm> 1992

- *SocioAbs <http://www.csa.com>* 1990

- *Sociological Abstracts (SA) <http://www.csa.com>* 1990

- *Special Educational Needs Abstracts* 1992

- *Studies on Women and Gender Abstracts*
  <http://www.tandf.co.uk/swa> 1992

- *SwetsWise <http://www.swets.com>* 2001

- *Violence and Abuse Abstracts: A Review of Current Literature*
  on Interpersonal Violence (VAA) 1995

   *Exact start date to come.

(continued)

Special Bibliographic Notes related to special journal issues
(separates) and indexing/abstracting:

- indexing/abstracting services in this list will also cover material in any "separate" that is co-published simultaneously with Haworth's special thematic journal issue or DocuSerial. Indexing/abstracting usually covers material at the article/chapter level.
- monographic co-editions are intended for either non-subscribers or libraries which intend to purchase a second copy for their circulating collections.
- monographic co-editions are reported to all jobbers/wholesalers/approval plans. The source journal is listed as the "series" to assist the prevention of duplicate purchasing in the same manner utilized for books-in-series.
- to facilitate user/access services all indexing/abstracting services are encouraged to utilize the co-indexing entry note indicated at the bottom of the first page of each article/chapter/contribution.
- this is intended to assist a library user of any reference tool (whether print, electronic, online, or CD-ROM) to locate the monographic version if the library has purchased this version but not a subscription to the source journal.
- individual articles/chapters in any Haworth publication are also available through the Haworth Document Delivery Service (HDDS).

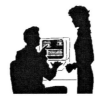

Parent-Youth Relations: Cultural and Cross-Cultural Perspectives

CONTENTS

ABOUT THE EDITORS

Gary W. Peterson, PhD, is Head and Professor of Family Studies and Social Work, Miami University, Oxford, Ohio. Previously, he was head and Professor, Department of Child and Family Studies, College of Human Ecology, University of Tennessee, Knoxville. He is former Chair and Professor, Department of Human Development, Washington State University, Pullman, Washington, and is former Professor and Chair of the Department of Sociology at Arizona State University. He is also former Chair of the Department of Family Resources and Human Development at Arizona State University. Dr. Peterson's general area of research and scholarly expertise is adolescent development within the context of family and parent-child relationships. Currently, he is analyzing the impact of ethnic and cultural issues in samples of adolescents from the People's Republic of China, Russia, India, Mexico, Chile, and the U.S. Previous research using samples from the U.S. examined health issued in Mexican-American populations of adolescents and young adults as well as influences on the life plans of low-income, rural youth from Appalachian areas of the United States. Peterson's research papers have appeared in such publications as *Journal of Marriage and the Family, Family Relations, Journal of Adolescent Research, Youth and Society, Family Science Review, Family Process*, and *Family Issues.* He was co-editor of *Handbook of Marriage and the Family* (2nd ed.) and *Adolescents in Families.* Major review articles on parent-child and parent-adolescent relationships have appeared in several books including *Advances in Adolescent Development, Handbook for Family Diversity, Handbook of Marriage and the Family* (1st and 2nd editions), and *Families Across Time: A Life Course Perspective.* Dr. Peterson has been a guest editor for special issues of several research journals and has been a member of the Board of Directors for the National Council on Family Relations.

Suzanne K. Steinmetz, PhD, MSW, DAPA, is Professor and former Chair of Sociology at Indiana University-Purdue University at Indianapolis (IUPUI). She is certified as a civil and family mediator and, with her husband, mediates neighborhood disputes for Indianapolis Superior Courts. Dr. Steinmetz does pro bono therapy with a focus on individuals with a diagnosis of Dissociative Identity Disorder. Credited as being one of the founders of the field of family violence, she was the first scholar to bring the problems of battered husbands and elder abuse into the public arena as a result of her Congressional testimony in 1978. She has served on the Board of Directors of the Society for the Study for Social Problems and was President of both the University of Delaware's and Indiana University's chapters of Sigma Xi, the National Science Society. Steinmetz has authored two research monographs, *Duty Bound: Elder Abuse and Family Care* and *Cycle of Violence: Assertive, Aggressive and Abusive Family Interaction*; co-authored *Behind Closed Doors: Violence in American Families* and *Marriage and Family Reality: Historical and Contemporary Analysis*; and co-edited *Family Support Systems Across the Life Span, Violence in the Family, Concepts and Definitions of Family for the 21st Century, Fatherhood: Research, Interventions and Policies,* and *Pioneering Paths in the Study of Families: The Lives and Careers of Family Scholars.* She also co-edited *Handbook of Marriage and the Family* (1st and 2nd editions) and *Sourcebook of Family Theory and Methods: A Contextual Approach,* two major reference books in the discipline. Steinmetz has also authored over 75 additional publications and is currently working on annotating a text written by Tongo Takebe, an early 20th century Japanese theorist.

Stephan M. Wilson, PhD, is Professor and Chair of the Department of Human Development and Family Studies at the University of Nevada in Reno. His research and scholarly articles have appeared in numerous edited collections. He is on the editorial boards of *Family Relations* and *Marriage & Family Review.* Dr. Wilson also serves as an occasional reviewer for many journals, including the *Journal of Social and Personal Relationships, The Sociological Quarterly,* the *Journal of Adolescent Research,* and the *Journal of Family Issues.*

PART I

PARENTING STYLES
IN DIVERSE PERSPECTIVES

Introduction:
Parenting Styles in Diverse Perspectives

Gary W. Peterson
Suzanne K. Steinmetz
Stephan M. Wilson

A common thread in this first group of articles is the examination of parenting styles both within a culture and cross-culturally. There are several questions posited. First, how can one best capture parenting styles with and between countries? Second, can one successfully 'transport and test' an instrument across cultures? Third, how can one best reflect intra-cultural diversity as well as inter-cultural diversity when studying parenting styles? And finally, does a particular parenting style, e.g., authoritarian, mean the same thing in different cultures?

The opening article of this section, "Cultural and Cross-Cultural Perspectives on Parent-Youth Relations," by Peterson, Steinmetz, and Wilson, provides an overview of the diverse approaches to studying parent- child relations both culturally and cross-culturally. The authors examine the advantages and limitations when researchers use similar concepts and instruments with different cultures as well as different ethnic groups with a culture. They also address the differences in interpretation of concepts and youth outcomes between western and non-western cultures/ethnic groups.

Baumrind's (1971; 1991) typology of parenting styles: authoritarian, authoritative, permissive, and neglecting parenting had found that authoritative parents are high in responsiveness whereas authoritarian parents are low in this attribute. It appears than authoritative parenting results in favorable developmental outcome for western societies. However, this has been widely debated when applied to Chinese population in diverse cultures. The dichotomy of authoritarian versus authoritative parenting differs by culture, ethnicity, social class and immigrant status. The first three articles in this collection specif-

http://www.haworthpress.com/store/product.asp?sku=J002
© 2003 by The Haworth Press, Inc. All rights reserved.
10.1300/J002v35n03_01

ically examine the differences in parenting styles between Chinese and western cultures as well cultural differences within a given ethnic group.

Lim and Lim emphasize that we should avoid the wholesale acceptance of western concepts and instruments noting that western "authoritarian" parents are not the same as Chinese authoritarian parents. In their article, "Parenting Style and Child Outcomes in Chinese and Immigrant Chinese Families–Current Findings and Cross-Cultural Considerations in Conceptualization and Research," the authors open this collection with a review of extant research on parenting styles across cultures. They provide a discussion of theoretical and philosophical perspective on childrearing styles and the problems when attempting to apply them to non-western cultures.

Using observational methods and questionnaire data, Tam and Lam in their article, "A Cultural Exploration Based on Structured Observational Methods in Hong Kong," expanded the understanding of parenting in a Chinese context by identifying culture- and domain-specific patterns of parenting behaviors and examining their impact on children's school- related performance. They discovered the four styles of parenting noted by Baumrind. However, authoritative parenting that was task-oriented, rather than permissive parenting, appeared to be the most prevalent style of parenting reflecting the importance of education as a major channel of upward social mobility.

"Ethnicity and Parenting Styles Among Singapore Families," by Quah, utilized the systemic-ecological, symbolic interaction, and developmental perspective to expand the concept of ethnic identity. She demonstrates the pervasiveness of ethnic identity and its ability to shape a person's self-identity. Quah believes that although the tendency has been to explore difference between ethnic groups, one needs also to explore the diversity within ethnic groups. Examining her sample in terms of four ethnic groups within Singapore: Chinese, Malay, Indian, and "Other" (which constitutes only 1.4% of the population), Quah analyzed eight parenting styles. Variations within ethnic groups were noted. For example, although Chinese were least likely to openly demonstrate affection, religious affiliation provided additional influence. Buddhist or Taoist parents were considerably less likely to show open affection, but more likely to be active in the performance of parenting roles when compared within other Chinese parents. Quah further notes that although education diminishes the cultural differences in parenting styles among Chinese, Malay, and Indian Singaporeans, there is considerably cultural diversity.

The next four articles examine parenting styles cross-culturally. In a manner similar to the "transport and test" approach used by Bradford and colleagues discussed below, Rohner, Khaleque and Cournoyer analyzed data using PARTheory, specifically the personality sub-theory to test parental acceptance/rejection. In their article, "Cross-National Perspectives on Parental

Acceptance-Rejection Theory," they examine the components of this personality sub-theory across a number of countries and various ethnic groups within the United States. Using a large body of research collected over four decades based on the PARTheory personality sub-theory instruments, the authors arrive at two overarching findings. First, there is a class of behaviors that universally appear to convey the symbolic message that a parent or attachment figure loves or does not love me. Second, variables such as nationality, ethnicity, social class, race or gender do not appear to override the universal tendency to respond in a similar way to perceived acceptance or rejection.

In their article, "A Multi-National Study of Interparental Conflict, Parenting and Adolescent Functioning; South Africa, Bangladesh, China, India, Bosnia, Germany, Palestine, Colombia and the United States," Bradford and colleagues used a "transport and test" approach as an initial step in systematic comparative research. They compared nine countries for cross-cultural variation and three ethnic groups for cultural comparisons within South Africa. Although substantially different, both overt and covert Interparental Conflict (IPC) was positively correlated with depression and antisocial behavior. The authors note that the sample was composed of youth, ages 14-17, who were currently attending school. Although limiting any study to those youth still attending school since many nations set 16 as the age for mandatory attendance, this is particularly problematic for third-world countries.

"The Relationship Between Parenting Behaviors and Adolescent Achievement and Self-Efficacy in Chile and Ecuador," by Ingoldsby, Schvaneveldt, Supple and Bush, examines parenting styles across different cultures. They hypothesized that youth would experience higher levels of achievement orientation (educational effort) and greater self-efficacy (a sense of competence and initiative) when their parents would interact with them using strategies of positive induction (reasoning and support), monitoring (keeping track of the child's activities), and autonomy (freedom granting). They found that parents use of positive induction predicted greater achievement orientation for Ecuadorian youth, whereas mothers' and fathers' monitoring of behaviors predicted achievement orientation and self-efficacy among Chilean youth. In both cultures, female students exhibited higher levels of achievement orientation than did males; other pathways to achieving outcomes varied by culture.

The final article in this section is "Parent-Adolescent Relations and Problem Behaviors: Hungary, the Netherlands, Switzerland, and the United States," by Vazsonyi. In this article, the predictive strength of three of the most commonly used measures of parent-child relations (parental closeness, support and monitoring) and adolescent low self- control were used in identifying adolescent problem behaviors. These finding were supported in the four samples. The findings provide still additional support for the idea of universal developmental processes.

On the one hand, this set of articles, and those that follow in the other parts of this collection, challenge some widely held views about "universal" processes or outcomes of parent-child relations cross-culturally. On the other hand, the collection does reveal some widespread phenomena that may provide clues to (human) species-wide developmental processes between parents and children. It has been our intent to draw scholars from a wide variety of disciplines, settings, perspectives, and cultures to provide new and sometimes exigent scholarship on cross-national and cross-cultural parent-child relations. We believe that this set of articles that examine diversity in parenting styles easily meets these goals.

REFERENCES

Baumrind, D. (1971). Current patterns of parental authority. *Developmental Psychology Monographs, 4,* 1-102.

Baumrind, D. (1991). Effective parenting during the early adolescent transition. In P. A. Cowan & M. Hetherington (Eds.), *Family transitions* (pp. 111-163). Hillsdale, NJ: Lawrence Erlbaum.

Cultural and Cross-Cultural Perspectives on Parent-Youth Relations

Gary W. Peterson
Suzanne K. Steinmetz
Stephan M. Wilson

ABSTRACT. The primary topic addressed in this paper is 'how cultures and parent-youth relationships are interdependent.' An initial objective is to describe what is meant by a cultural and cross-cultural perspective on parent-youth relationships. Subsequently, the nature and connections between the concepts 'socialization' and 'culture' are explored as they apply to parent-youth relations. Finally, the benefits of a cultural and cross-cultural perspective are examined, with particular attention devoted to diminishing ethnocentric viewpoints and building more comprehensive theories of parent-youth socialization. *[Article copies available for a fee from The Haworth Document Delivery Service: 1-800-HAWORTH. E-mail address: <docdelivery@haworthpress.com> Website: <http://www.HaworthPress.com> © 2003 by The Haworth Press, Inc. All rights reserved.]*

KEYWORDS. Cross-cultural perspectives, ethnocentrism, culture, cultural perspectives, parent-youth relationships, socialization, youth

---

Gary W. Peterson is Head and Professor, Department of Family Studies and Social Work, 451 McGuffey Hall, Miami University, Oxford, OH 45056. Suzanne K. Steinmetz is Professor, Department of Sociology, Indiana University-Purdue University at Indianapolis, 425 University Blvd., Indianapolis, IN 46202. Stephan M. Wilson is affiliated with the Department of Human Development and Family Studies, College of Human and Community Sciences, University of Nevada, Reno, 1664 North Virginia St., Reno, NV 89557-0131, Mail Stop #140.

http://www.haworthpress.com/store/product.asp?sku=J002
© 2003 by The Haworth Press, Inc. All rights reserved.
10.1300/J002v35n03_02

7

PARENT-YOUTH RELATIONSHIPS:
CULTURAL AND CROSS-CULTURAL PERSPECTIVES

The primary topic addressed in this and the following four issues of Marriage & Family Review is 'how cultures and parent-youth relationships are interdependent.' The means chosen to address this topic and related ideas is the impressive collection of papers on parent-youth relations from around the globe that follow this introductory article. Written from diverse perspectives, these papers provide us with insight into parent-youth relationships within a variety of cultures, societies, and nations. Some are comparative across societies, nations, or subgroups and seek to identify similarities and differences. Others explore one culture or social group and seek to understand particular nuances of meaning and unique relationship patterns existing in one cultural or societal context.

An initial objective of this introductory article, therefore, is to describe a cultural and cross-cultural perspective for parent-youth relationships. This topic also requires that we explore the nature of and connections between the concepts 'socialization' and 'culture' as they apply to parent-youth relations. Finally, we will describe why a cultural and cross- cultural perspective can make substantial contributions to our understanding of parent-youth relationships.

A Cultural and Cross-Cultural Perspective
on Parent-Youth Relations

We have initiated this project to advance our understanding of parent-youth relations from the standpoint of cultural and cross-cultural family science/family sociology. Such a perspective guides us to focus primarily, not on psychological phenomena at the individual level of analysis (though some of this is done), but on aspects of relationships within families and the implications they have for the development of parents and children. Even more important is the belief underscored here that family relationships, and more specifically, parent-youth relationships, must always be examined from a culturally sensitive perspective, an approach that much of western social science has neglected (Berry, Poortinga, Segall, & Dasen, 2002; Kagitcibasi, 1996). Our assumption in sponsoring this project is to promote the idea that the parent-youth relationship, a fundamental aspect of family life, is shaped in formative ways by culture (see Ingoldsby, Schvaneveldt, Supple, & Bush; and Bradford, Barber, Olsen, Maughan, Erikson, Ward, & Stolz in this volume). At the same time, however, we recognize that the parent-youth relationship, as perhaps the primary human association, not only socializes the young both for membership in their particular culture, but also serves as an interpersonal arena for cultural change.

Examining parent-youth relations from a cultural and cross-cultural perspective means that our object of study should be scrutinized both for unique nuances provided by each culture (i.e., a perspective referred to as *cultural relativism*) as well as for patterns shared across cultures that approach universality (i.e., a perspective referred to as *universalism*). Considerable controversy exists between the perspective of cultural universalism versus the perspective of cultural relativity for studying both the human experience in general and parent-youth relations in particular.

This debate is represented, in part, by contrasting the *emic* and *etic* traditions in cultural and cross-cultural research (Berry, 1969; Pike, 1967). An emic approach, to begin with, develops constituent constructs, and examines parent-youth relationships from the standpoint of one cultural community. Thus, an *emic* or 'relativist' approach investigates parent-youth relations from an 'insider's' perspective, making sure that the meanings, values, and norms from the chosen culture guide the resulting interpretations. A strict emic approach focuses on parent-youth patterns and meanings within one culture and promotes the view that making comparisons across cultures is analogous to comparing apples to oranges. In contrast, an *etic* approach makes use of constructs and examines parent-youth relationships based on the presumption that at least some invariant patterns exist across social groups. Consequently, an etic strategy takes an 'outsider's' viewpoint, using comparative strategies, with the intent being to identify commonalities, some of which may be universal across cultures (Berry, 1969; 1999).

Although these strategies are often posed as antagonistic, we believe that studies of emic, or indigenous relationship patterns within one culture, and etic, or comparative quests for universal patterns, are not opposites but are compatible and complementary (Kagitcibasi, 1996; Sinha, 1997; Yang, 2000). This balanced view of cultural and cross-cultural family science is analogous to the search for common patterns in individual behavior within the discipline of psychology, which also recognizes that sophisticated individual differences exist. Much like an array of individuals who demonstrate both commonly held and idiosyncratic behaviors, emic and etic approaches are necessary to identify both what can be generalized and what is unique about parent-youth relationships across cultures.

We believe, of course, that many shades of gray exist between finding cultural universals and complete cultural originality in the various strategies that parents from diverse contexts use to guide their young into mature discourse within their societies. Efforts to portray these approaches as being fundamentally at odds with each other strikes us as an exercise in creating false dichotomies, much like the endless wranglings concerning the fundamental incompatibility between qualitative and quantitative research. From our viewpoint, such debates are exercises in categorical thinking, when, in fact, continuities are prevalent, shades of gray exist, and complementary linkages exist between the dueling approaches. Much like clear social expectations coexist along with aspects of ambiguity in our social lives, it is not difficult for us to conceive how etic and emic approaches can work hand in hand.

Parent-youth relationship patterns identified by studying one culture, for example, can subsequently be explored for generality in other cultures (Enriquez, 1993). Moreover, relationship patterns found to generalize across cultures should be examined carefully for cultural nuances and unique meanings before concluding that surface level similarity constitutes universality (Rogoff, 2003). We are strong advocates of constantly trying to identify similarities and differences across cultures (see Barrea; Bush, Supple & Lash; and Stolz, Barber, Olsen, Ericksen, Bradford, & Maughan in later issues of this collection), but also believe in caution about asserting that identified patterns have the same meanings and consequences across cultures (e.g., see Esteinou; and Peterson, Cobas, Bush, Supple, & Wilson, see later parts of this collection).

Socialization and the Parent-Youth Relationship

Substantial attention is devoted in the articles composing this collection to the application of the concept *'socialization'* to the parent-youth relationship–or the process through which the young are provided the capacities and meanings that compose membership in a particular culture. Although a culture is a complex set of symbols and ideas that provide meaning or definitions for a way of life, socialization refers to a set of interpersonal processes through which cultural meaning is passed on and changed. Becoming a member of a culture occurs through seemingly mundane dynamics of everyday life, which are, in fact, a truly remarkable set of processes. Through these complicated dynamics, the young develop abilities to function successfully as sophisticated human beings within society. The young are encouraged to take on the particular values, beliefs, and practices of their social group as a means of developing the cognitive skills and social competencies for adapting to a particular way of life (Peterson & Hann, 1999; Peterson & Leigh, 1990; Wilson & Peterson, 2000). At the same time, however, socialization is a reciprocal process, with parents being shaped by these dynamics as well as children (Kaltenborn; Lu & Kao; and Yang & Rettig in later parts of this collection). Moreover, socialization does not ensure cultural transmission to the next generation, because parenting skills, specific cultural influences, and the values of the larger society often fail to be realized in the outcomes of the young (Steinmetz, 1999; see Vazsonyi in this issue; Noack & Buhl; McClellan, Heaton, Forste, & Barber; and Yoon, in later parts of this collection).

Socialization is the process through which a person becomes capable of participating in society, but is also the means through which a society or culture reproduces itself (Elkin & Handel, 1989). Central components of this process are behaviors and practices that encourage individuals to participate effectively in a society's major institutions and to inhibit the development of undesirable behavior. Socialization is a complex, multidirectional process involving all the major institutions and social settings in which individuals have direct or indirect experiences, including religious institutions, work settings, schools, the mass media, political and governmental institutions, neighborhoods, and families (Bronfenbrenner, 1979). For reasonable continuity to exist, therefore, the socialization process must result in a sufficient degree of shared meanings so that social life can continue and each person gets a sense of where they fit (Mead, 1934).

Traditional conceptions of socialization within the parent-youth relationship are restricted to the obvious notion that, to become sufficiently socialized, the young are influenced by parents to internalize one's cultural context as a means of adapting to society (Inkeles, 1968; Parsons & Bales, 1955). Although certainly true, in part, too much emphasis has been placed on how young children are shaped and guided by parents (or other social agents) to become enculturated members of society. Referred to as '*deterministic*' or '*social mold*' conceptions of socialization (Steinmetz, 1979; Peterson & Hann, 1999), the young are often conceptualized as passive recipients of parental influence. From this perspective, children and adolescents often are viewed as posing unsocialized threats to cultural continuity, especially when they are viewed as insufficiently initiated into the life-ways of the larger social group (Parsons & Bales, 1955).

A more accurate view of socialization, however, recognizes that children must be initiated into society to some degree by parents, but also that children are active participants in this social discourse. Instead of being unidirectional in nature, socialization within the parent-youth relationship is conceptualized as being at least a bidirectional process, if not even more complex in character (Corsaro, 1997; Kuczynski, 2003; Peterson & Hann, 1999; Steinmetz, 1979). Through this dynamic, transactional process, children increasingly develop social identities defined in terms of their cultural context and use these self-conceptions as a means to assign meaning, define goals that guide their behavior, and act back upon society in a creative, individualistic manner (Kuczynski, 2003; Peterson & Hann, 1999; Stryker, 2001).

The socialized person, therefore, emerges from social interaction, not simply by internalizing norms and conforming to society, but in terms of responses shaped by meanings, individual interpretations, negotiations with others, and shared experiences (Cooley, 1902; Stryker, 2001). Socialization within the parent-youth relationship, therefore, is a dialectical process in which continuity, creativity, and change are complementary components of a larger whole (Kuczynski, 2003; Peterson, 1995). The parent-youth relationship is a continuous process of continuity and change in which both partners increasingly share meanings, but are always changing in respect to each other. The result is a long-term relationship involving countless social exchanges through which parents jointly co-construct outcomes that have meaning and consequence within their cultural circumstance (Peterson, 1995).

Culture and the Parent-Youth Relationship

Another fundamental idea conveyed in this collection is the pervasive integration of culture and the parent-youth relationship or, more precisely, how across social groups, parent-youth relationships will be different, demonstrate common patterns, contribute to cultural transmission, and act as a catalyst for cultural change. Most observers would agree that *'culture,'* as a construct, is one of the most difficult ideas for social scientists to describe and clearly define. Although characterized many ways, one of the earliest anthropological definition of culture was offered by Tylor (1871:42) who proposed that culture was a 'complex whole which includes knowledge, belief, art, morals, laws, customs and any other capabilities acquired by man as a member of society.' Certainly, culture refers to the comprehensive social heritage or man-made totality that distinguishes members of one group from another (Herskovits, 1948; Hofstede, 1980). Included within this broad conception of culture, for example, are the ecological setting, the social structure, and the value orientations that provide the context for parent-youth relations (Trommsdorf & Kornadt, 2003).

A culture includes both the beliefs that constitute a culture's symbolic inheritance and the norms and moral standards that arise from these beliefs. A culture's symbolic inheritance provides the basis, in part, for the roles individuals should perform, the shared rituals and processes for life transitions (e.g., Dunham, Kidwell, & Wilson, 1986; Wilson, Ngige, & Trolinger, in press), the ultimate meaning of things, and the place of the individual's life in the vast scheme of things. A central component of culture is the capacity to structure group behavior through normative definitions that govern the activities of individuals, such as those occurring within parent-youth relations. Consequently, culture refers to the knowledge, norms, rules, symbols, language, attitudes, values, habits, and motivations that members of a group often share. These integrated components of culture are combined in complex ways to provide a common conception of reality within the parent-youth relationship.

Many cultural influences are powerful and virtually unconscious, often functioning as unquestioned aspects of everyday life that provide daily common sense to parents and children. Whether explicit or implicit, cultural traditions and values are pervasive influences on the informal interactions that occur between parents and children, other societal relationships, and the formal institutions of society. Cultural habits become regarded as routine or natural, much like background noise.

Culture can be viewed, therefore, as a shared symbolic system that develops through interaction processes (Boesch, 1991; Bruner, 1996). From this perspective, parent-youth relations are shaped, in part, from interactions that occur in a given cultural context, and at the same time, contribute to the complex process of transmitting and transforming cultural meaning (Trommsdorf & Kornadt, 2003).

The existence and pervasive qualities of cultures do not, however, provide precise templates for behavior nor guarantee exact transmission from one generation to another. Cultural life is patterned and repetitive, for sure, but this does not eliminate uncertainty, particularly because cultures are both malleable and subject to substantial intra-cultural variation. Cultural patterns change over time, sometimes slowly, but other times quite rapidly, due to major historic events such as wars, civil conflicts, or major socioeconomic forces like modernization and globalization (see Peterson, Cobas, Bush, Supple, & Wilson; Wejnert & Djumabaeva; Steinmetz; and Walper, Noack, Schwarz, & Kruse in later parts of this collection).

Within cultures, at the individual, regional, and community levels of analysis, variations on a theme coexist along with unifying practices and principles (e.g., Wilson & Peterson, 2000). Consequently, we can view humans as being shaped by and as products of culture, but, at the same time, a particular culture owes its very existence and continuity to relationships like those existing between parents and children. Culture is most accurately portrayed as a phenomenon 'in process,' with people (e.g., parents and children) acting to perpetuate and create their cultural life-ways as they socialize each other (Berger & Luckmann, 1966; Mead, 1934).

Complete transmission of the existing culture at any one time would not allow for novelty, change, and responses to new situations, whereas the complete failure of transmission would not permit continuity across generations. Neither of these extremes characterizes how culture functions in a general manner, nor how cultural influences become manifest within parent-youth relations. Instead of such extremes, a balanced and more accurate view is that members of a group are not passive recipients of culture, but often find creative ways to act independently and provide creative twists on established patterns. An important awareness, in part, is to understand how culture is conveyed through the parent-youth relationship, but also how actions and interactions within the parent-youth relationship may contribute to cultural change.

An important contribution of a cultural perspective is to increase our understanding of beliefs that serve as the basis for developmental goals that shape the behavior of parents and children. Should children be taught that members of their culture must 'be their own persons' and 'take care of themselves'–or should they be ensured that 'one's personal welfare is largely determined by making contributions to the overall welfare of their group'? Should the young be taught that the 'interests of their family' must come before their own personal ambitions? Moreover, is it important to emphasize self-expression and demonstrations of emotion, or is the focus on maintaining a more subdued expression of the self that requires some distance and evokes respect? Once positions are taken on these issues, such culturally defined goals can provide social expectations that shape how parenting is supposed to be conducted and what particular outcomes are used to define the meaning of socially competent qualities for children (Peterson & Hann, 1999).

From the parents' perspectives, for example, parental ethnotheories, are the culturally defined beliefs, values, and practices of parents (or other caregivers) regarding the proper way to raise the young within a particular cultural community (Harkness & Super, 1995; Sigel, McGillicudy-Delisi, & Goodnow, 1992). The practices prescribed by such beliefs include social expectations for such things as how warmth is expressed, whether physical punishment is tolerated, when toilet training is initiated, and the degree to which school work is monitored by parents (e.g., Bean, Bush, McKenry, & Wilson, in press).

Although we should be cautious about over-generalizing child-rearing patterns, cultures that emphasize socializing the young for autonomy from parents may place greater emphasis on the use of rational control attempts from parents, frequent discussion, mutuality, and democratic decision-making processes. In contrast, cultures that focus primarily on socializing the young for responsiveness to one's family or community interests may emphasize more restrictive forms of control aimed at maintaining parental (elder) influences within many aspects of children's lives (see Stolz et al.; Xia, Xie, Zhou, DeFrain, Meredith, & Combs; and Peterson, Cobas, Bush, Supple, & Wilson in later issues of this collection). The overall idea, therefore, is that cultural beliefs shape both the attributes of the young that are valued in a culture, the parental beliefs about how to attain these desired goals, and the resulting socialization strategies used to foster the valued outcomes in the young (Peterson & Hann, 1999).

Diminishing Ethnocentrism:
A Benefit of Cultural and Cross-Cultural Perspectives

Perhaps the most important benefit of examining parent-youth relations from cultural and cross-cultural perspectives is the role these viewpoints can play in preventing the worst manifestations of ethnocentrism. The concept 'ethnocentrism' refers to the practice of using one's own cultural standards as the baseline against which all other groups are evaluated, with the result being that other cultural practices are judged to be peculiar, inferior, immoral, or unwise (Levine & Campbell, 1972; Rogoff, 2003). Conclusions are drawn without considering the particular origins, meanings, values, and functions characteristic of the other culture. Instead, it is simply taken for granted, based on insufficient knowledge, that one's own culture is superior.

In varying degrees, everyone is probably a victim of this form of cultural myopia, simply because it is very difficult, if not impossible, to free oneself from our daily symbolic constructions about what is reality and what is not–or what is normal and what is not (Berger & Luckman, 1966). One of the challenges for cultural and cross-cultural scholars who study families, however, is to help individuals recognize that one's culture is not the normative standard by which other cultural communities are judged.

In some of its worst forms, ethnocentrism underlies many examples of Western comparative studies, driven by implied 'deficit models,' in which European American child-rearing practices are reified as "normal" compared to "deficient" approaches of other cultures (Rogoff, 2003). Moreover, the extensive dominance of middle-class European American life-ways in an increasingly globalized world often inhibits members of this group from even recognizing that their own life-ways constitute a distinctive culture. Instead, it is simply assumed that 'culture' is something that other groups have, or the degree to which 'foreign' practices deviate from the 'true reality' of local norms.

Effective challenges to ethnocentric thinking will require that cultural and cross-cultural scholarship be pursued so that our own community's assumptions about the parent-youth relationship are confronted. For example, becoming sensitized to the functionality of different cultural practices requires that we challenge common western assumptions and recognize that parents in some cultures may have solid reasons to de-emphasize such things as demonstrative expressions of warmth (affection) in favor of greater detachment from the young (see Quah; Rohner, Khaleque, & Cournoyer, this section). Moreover, the American assumption that an authoritative parental style, consisting of firm, rational control, high levels of supportiveness, and reluctance to use physical punishment, may not be the most successful means to foster youthful social competence within all cultures. Several observers suggest that this may be the case, certainly to the degree of efficacy demonstrated for authoritative styled with western, middle-class youth. Instead, other forms of parental control exist in other contexts, rooted in distinctive cultural traditions that convey the particular meanings of the specific culture at issue (Chao, 2001; see Lim & Lim; Tam & Lam; and Quah in this issue; Zhan in later parts of the collection).

Physical punishment, a common parenting practice around the world, is also likely to have different meanings and consequences across cultures (Hale-Benson, 1986). American mothers, for example, appear to encourage the development of aggression toward peers by young children when they make frequent use of physical punishment. This finding, however, has not been replicated in African American samples (Deater-Deckard, Dodge, Bates, & Pettit, 1996), possibly because European American, but not African-American parents, believe that physical punishment is an approach of last resort, indicating that parents have lost control. In contrast, African American parents may view their neighborhoods and societal circumstances as more threatening environments requiring different childrearing strategies (i.e., due to criminal activity, discrimination, racism, and police violence in their neighborhoods). The result is that African American parents and children may view physical punishment as a direct, 'no nonsense' means of preparing their young for the hostile circumstances they are likely to face.

Another 'sacred' European American parenting practice, indepen- dence training, may be more context-bound than is frequently acknowledged in the culturally insensitive scholarship on this topic from the West (Rogoff, 2003). For example, the American preoccupation with fostering autonomy, beginning very early through the urgency of American parents to have their newborns sleep in separate bedrooms, has been viewed frequently as a cultural oddity by others around the globe (Super, 1981; Trevathan & McKenna, 1994).

Child-rearing in many cultures around the globe contrasts significantly with the European American focus on fostering autonomy in the young, which is designed to prepare the young for a society that emphasizes individual attainment and individualism (Peterson, 1995; Rogoff, 2003). Instead of focusing on developing a 'separated self,' children in many cultures are encouraged, through a variety of strategies, to become interdependent, or respond to and coordinate with group interests, while simultaneously making progress toward autonomy. As a number of observers have concluded, the young can be socialized to coordinate, conform to, and be connected to others, while pursuing their own self-will, taking action, and making their own decisions (Kagitcibasi, 1996; Peterson, 1995). In short, children in some cultures are simply not socialized to treat autonomy and connectedness as incompatible opposites, but as complementary traits that can be balanced (Peterson, 1995).

An overall assessment, therefore, is that being faced with viable cultural alternatives is an effective way to diminish ethnocentrism by decentering and assuming the cultural perspectives of others. This requires us to question the infallibility of our own socialization experiences and to experience the cultural diversity provided within a variety of communities. Culturally sensitive research can make us aware of the 'encultured' nature of everyday life. Consequences of cultural decentering may include enhanced understanding of other life-ways, growing awareness of functional options, greater tolerance for differences, and more willingness to make cultural changes.

More Comprehensive Theory:
A Benefit of Cultural and Cross-Cultural Perspectives

The best way of increasing our knowledge is to build more comprehensive theories that provide generalizable principles about parent-youth relationships. This is accomplished most effectively by developing constructs rooted in systematic theory, formalizing constructs into testable hypotheses, and applying empirical tests to the hypotheses (Burr, 1973). Social scientists engage in theory testing processes as an established means to (1) identify phenomena worth investigating, (2) accumulate and organize knowledge, (3) develop and test predictions, (4) interpret how relationships operate, and (5) provide explanations in a precise manner that broadens our subsequent understanding (White & Klein, 2002). In short, we want our theories to provide interpretations of the widest possible array of parent-youth phenomena and to demonstrate greater depth and breadth in the explanations that are provided.

A logical conclusion, therefore, is that conducting research within the widest array of cultures, nations, and societies is necessary to build the most comprehensive and insightful theories about parent-youth relationships. This can help us overcome, what continues to be, a domination of the social science industry (and our theoretical explanations) by western family scholars and the imposition of an indigenous, European American view of parent-youth socialization (Kagitcibasi, 1996). Consequently, testing our theoretical constructs in diverse cultural circumstances becomes imperative, especially since a primary goal of science is to build the most comprehensive and externally valid theoretical knowledge from observations acquired in a variety of contexts (Bronfenbrenner, 1979). Cross-cultural tests of theory maximize the range of variation in a relationship pattern compared to research within one setting. An important goal, therefore, is to minimize critiques that our theories about parent-youth relationships are parochial constructions, based on observations almost exclusively from dominant cultural communities, which are prominent but circumscribed in their generality. Although a theory can receive increased support and never be proven in an absolute sense, confirming evidence from diverse cultural contexts provides more compelling evidence that patterns based in theory at least approximate universality.

A major point of these introductory comments, therefore, is that understanding the parent-youth relationship and one's own culture are inseparable processes. Both are interdependent and partially shape the other in fundamental ways. Moreover, gaining a thorough understanding of parent-youth relationships and one's own cultural heritage requires that scholars examine how childrearing is conducted within the cultural nuances of other social contexts. This also suggests that immigrant families often face the complicated challenge of raising their children to fit into the new culture, while attempting to retain the values, attitudes, and behaviors of the culture of origin.

REFERENCES

Baumrind, D. (1991). Effective parenting during the early adolescent transition. In P. A. Cowan & M. Hetherington (Eds.). *Family transitions* (pp. 111-163). Hillsdale, NJ: Lawrence Erlbaum.

Bean, R. A., Bush, K. R., McKenry, P. C., & Wilson, S. M. (in press). The impact of parental support, behavioral control, and psychological control on the academic achievement and self-esteem of African-American and European-American adolescents. *Journal of Adolescent Research.*

Berger, P. L., & Luckman, T. (1966). *The social construction of reality.* New York: Doubleday.

Berry, J. W. (1969). On cross-cultural comparability. *International Journal of Psychology, 4,* 119-128.

Berry, J. W. (1999). Emics and etics: A symbiotic relationship. *Culture and Psychology, 5,* 165-171.

Berry, J. W., Poortinga, Y. H., Segall, M. H., & Dasen, P. R. (2002). *Cross-cultural psychology: Research and applications.* Cambridge, MA: Cambridge University Press.

Boesch, E. E. (1991). *Symbolic action theory and cultural psychology.* Berlin: Springer-Verlag.

Bronfenbrenner, U. (1979). *The ecology of human development: Experiments by nature and design.* Cambridge, MA: Harvard University Press.

Bruner, J. S. (1996). *Acts of meaning.* Cambridge, MA: Harvard University Press.

Burr, W. R. (1973). *Theory construction and the sociology of the family.* New York: John Wiley.

Chao, R. K. (2001). Extending research on the consequences of parenting style for Chinese Americans and European Americans. *Child Development, 72,* 1832-1843.

Cooley, C. H. (1902). *Human nature and the social order.* New York: Scribner's.

Corsaro, W. A. (1997). *The sociology of childhood.* Thousand Oaks, CA: Pine Forge Press.

Deater-Deckard, K., Dodge, K. A., Bates, J. E., & Pettit, G. S. (1996). Physical discipline among African American and European American mothers: Links to children's externalizing behaviors. *Developmental Psychology, 32,* 1065-1072.

Dunham, R., Kidwell, J. S., & Wilson, S. M. (1986). Rites of passage at adolescence: A ritual process paradigm. *Journal of Adolescent Research, 1*(2), 139-154.

Elkin, F., & Handel, G. (1988). *The child and society: The process of socialization.* New York: McGraw Hill.

Enriquez, V. G. (1993). Developing a Filipino psychology. In U. Kim & J. W. Berry (Eds.). Indigenous psychologies: *Research and experience in cultural context* (pp. 152-169). Newbury Park, CA: Sage Publications.

Harkness, S., & Super, C. H. (Eds.) (1995). *Parents' cultural belief systems: Their origins, expressions, and consequences.* New York: Guilford.

Herskovits, M. J. (1948). *Man and his works: The science of cultural anthropology.* New York: Knopf.

Hofstede, G. (1980). *Culture's consequences: International differences in work related values.* Beverly Hills, CA: Sage Publications.

Inkeles, A. (1968). Society, social structure, and child socialization. In J.A. Clausen (Ed.). *Socialization and society* (pp. 73-129). Boston, MA: Little Brown.

Kagitcibasi, C. (1996). *Family and human development across cultures: A view from the other side.* Mahwah, NJ: Lawrence Erlbaum Associated.

Kuczynski, L. (2003). Beyond bidirectionality: Bilateral conceptual frameworks for understanding dynamics in parent-youth relations. In L. Kuczynski (Ed.). *Handbook of dynamics in parent-youth relations* (pp. 3-24). Thousand Oaks, CA: Sage Publications.

Levine, R. A., & Campbell, D. T. (1972). *Ethnocentrism.* New York: Wiley.

Mead, G. H. (1934). *Mind, self, & society.* Chicago: The University of Chicago Press.

Medora, N. P., Wilson, S. M., & Larson, J. H. (1996). Parenting strategies of low-income African-American, Latino-American, Anglo-American, and Asian-American mothers. *Family Science Review, 9,* 107-122.

Parsons, T., & Bales, R. (1955). *Family socialization and interaction process.* New York: Free Press.

Peterson, G. W., & Hann, D. (1999). Socializing parents and children in families. In M. B. Sussman, S. K. Steinmetz, & G. W. Peterson (Eds.). *Handbook of marriage and the family* (pp. 327-370). New York: Plenum Press.

Peterson, G. W. (1995). Autonomy and connectedness. In R. D. Day, K. R. Gilbert, B. H. Settles, & W. R. Burr (Eds.). *Research and theory in family science.* Pacific Grove, CA: Brooks/Cole.

Peterson, G. W., & Leigh, G. K. (1990). The family and social competence in adolescence. In T. P. Gullotta, G. R. Adams, & R. Montemayor (Eds.). *Developing social competency in adolescence: Advances in adolescent development, Vol. 3* (pp. 97-138). Newbury Park, CA: Sage.

Pike, K. L. (1967). *Language in relation to a unified theory of the structure of human behavior*. The Hague: Mouton.

Rogoff, B. (2003). *The cultural nature of human development*. Oxford: Oxford University Press.

Rohner, R. P., Khaleque, A., & Cournoyer, D. E. (in press). Cross-national perspectives on parental acceptance-rejection theory. *Marriage and Family Review*.

Sigel, I. E., McGillicuddy-De Lisi, A., & Goodnow, J. J. (Eds.) (1992). *Parental belief systems: The psychological consequences for children* (2nd Ed.). Hillsdale, NJ: Erlbaum.

Sinha, D. (1997). Indigenizing psychology. In J. W. Berry, Y. H. Poortinga, & J. Pandey (Eds.). Theory and method. *Handbook of cross-cultural psychology, Vol. 1* (2nd ed., pp. 129-169). Boston, MA: Allyn and Bacon.

Steinmetz, S. K. (1979). Disciplinary techniques and their relationship to aggressiveness, dependency and conscience. In W. R. Burr, R. Hill, F. I. Nye, & I. L. Reiss (Eds.). *Contemporary theories about the family-Vol. 1* (pp. 405-438). New York: The Free Press.

Steinmetz, S. K. (1999). Adolescents in contemporary families. In M. B. Sussman, S. K. Steinmetz, S. K. & G. W. Peterson (Eds.). *Handbook of marriage and the family* (pp. 371-423). New York: Plenum Press.

Stryker, S. (2001). Traditional symbolic interactionism, role theory, and structural symbolic interactionism: The road to identity theory. In J. H. Turner (Ed.). *Handbook of sociological theory* (pp. 211-231). New York: Kluwer Academic/Plenum Publishers.

Super, C. H. (1981). Behavioral development in infancy. R. H. Munroe, R. L. Munroe, & B. B. Whiting (Eds.). *Handbook of cross-cultural human development*. New York: Garland.

Trevathan, W. R., & McKenna, J. J. (1994). Evolutionary environments of human birth and infancy: Insights to apply to contemporary life. *Children's Environments, 11*, 88-104.

Trommsdorff, G., & Kornat, H. (2003). parent-youth relations in cross-cultural perspective. In L. Kuczynski (Ed.). *Handbook of dynamics in parent-youth relations* (pp. 271-306). Thousand Oaks, CA: Sage Publications.

Tylor, E. B. (1871). *Primitive culture* (vol. 2). London: Murray.

White, J. M., & Klein, D. M. (2002). *Family theories* (2nd Ed.). Thousand Oaks, CA: Sage Publications.

Wilson, S. M., Ngige, L. W., & Trollinger, L. (in press). Connecting generations: Kamba and Maasai paths to marriage in Kenya. In R. R. Hamon & B. B. Ingoldsby (Eds.). *Couples formation across cultures*. Thousand Oaks, CA: Sage.

Wilson, S. M., & Peterson, G. W. (2000). The experience of growing up in Appalachia: Cultural and economic influences on adolescent development. In R. Montemayor, G. R. Adams, & T. P. Gullotta (Eds.). *Advances in adolescent development, Vol. 9. Adolescent experiences: Cultural and economic diversity in adolescent development* (pp. 75-109). Newbury Park, CA: Sage.

Yang, K. S. (2000). Monocultural and cross-cultural indigenous perspectives. *Asian Journal of Social Psychology, 3*, 241-263.

Parenting Style and Child Outcomes in Chinese and Immigrant Chinese Families– Current Findings and Cross-Cultural Considerations in Conceptualization and Research

Soh-Leong Lim
Ben K. Lim

ABSTRACT. Parenting style is an important familial variable in the study of child development. Unlike research on white populations, results on how parenting style affects child outcomes are less conclusive in Chinese and Chinese immigrant families. This is largely due to problems associated with applying western typologies, such as Baumrind's prototypes, in research on Chinese families. Studies that use an orthogonal approach, in which different parenting dimensions are examined, yield more interpretable data. This article examines current research on the associations between the two key parenting dimensions of warmth and control on child outcomes in Chinese and Chinese immigrant families. Warmth is associated with positive child outcomes. However, the effect of parental control on child psychosocial outcomes is unclear. Qualitative differences in Chinese parenting call for more research that focuses on conceptualizing and operationalizing di-

Soh-Leong Lim is currently a volunteer with a refugee population in San Diego, CA, and will be Visiting Professor in the Department of Counseling and School Psychology at San Diego State University, San Diego, in fall 2003 (E-mail: sohleong@cox.net). Ben K. Lim is Associate Professor in Marriage and Family Therapy, Bethel Seminary, San Diego, CA (E-mail: blim@bethel.edu).

http://www.haworthpress.com/store/product.asp?sku=J002
© 2003 by The Haworth Press, Inc. All rights reserved.
10.1300/J002v35n03_03

mensions of Chinese parenting that are both culturally specific and culturally sensitive. *[Article copies available for a fee from The Haworth Document Delivery Service: 1-800-HAWORTH. E-mail address: <docdelivery@haworthpress. com> Website: <http://www.HaworthPress.com> © 2003 by The Haworth Press, Inc. All rights reserved.]*

KEYWORDS. Adolescent, child, parenting style, Chinese families, immigrant Chinese families, parental control, parental warmth

INTRODUCTION

Parenting affects family and child outcomes (Maccoby, 1980) and the influences of parenting styles have been studied in both white and non-white populations with differing results. While studies on white populations have consistently showed that authoritative parenting is associated with positive developmental outcomes in children (Baumrind, 1971; Dornbusch, Ritter, Leiderman, Roberts, & Fraleigh, 1987; Maccoby & Martin, 1983; Steinberg, Mounts, Lamborn, & Dornbusch, 1991), research on parenting style as it affects child outcomes in non-white populations demonstrates conflicting results. This paper examines the current research on parenting style and family outcomes and highlights some research considerations, especially that of conceptualization and cross-cultural validity, in the study of parenting style in Chinese populations as well as immigrant Chinese populations in a western cultural context.

CONCEPTUALIZATION OF PARENTING STYLES

Research on parenting has differed in its conceptualization of parenting styles, depending on whether a configurational or orthogonal approach is taken. A configurational approach measures and classifies parenting style according to a set of attributes, such as values, behaviors, and attitudes. In contrast, an orthogonal approach measures parenting style along separate key dimensions. Besides the differences in conceptualization, there are variations in the way constructs are operationalized. This has added to the complexity in understanding parenting as it relates to child outcomes. There is a need for clarity in the way constructs are conceptualized and operationalized for meaningful comparisons between studies.

Baumrind's (1971) widely used typology of parenting styles is configurational: it classifies three types of parenting–permissive, authoritarian, and authoritative. Authoritative parenting, according to Baumrind's typology, is characterized by high parental standards, appropriate autonomy granting, and emotional support consisting of verbal give and take, reason, warmth, and flexibility. Authoritative parents value both autonomous self-will and disciplined conformity: they use both reason and power to achieve their objectives. Authoritarian parents, in contrast, have a set of standards by which they attempt to shape, control, and evaluate the attitudes and behavior of their children. They tend to be highly directive with their children and value unquestioning obedience. Permissive parents are likely to make fewer demands on their children, allowing them to regulate their own activities as much as possible.

Other studies on parenting styles use an orthogonal approach, in which parenting styles are conceptualized according to a two-dimensional framework (Maccoby & Martin, 1983). Maccoby and Martin's (1983) two-dimensional framework attempts to merge Baumrind's (1971) configurational approach with earlier orthogonal approaches. What emerges are four parenting styles based on the dimensions of demandingness and responsiveness. These are (a) authoritative parenting, which is high in both demandingness and responsiveness, (b) authoritarian parenting, which is high in demandingness but low in responsiveness, (c) indulgent parenting, which is high in responsiveness and low in demandingness, and (d) neglectful parenting, which is low in both responsiveness and demandingness.

Research on parenting styles uses the terms authoritarian, authoritative, and permissive either from Baumrind's (1971) conceptualization or Maccoby and Martin's (1983) framework. The two approaches do not directly correspond to each other, but closely approximate each other (Darling & Steinberg, 1993). This clarification is important because results must be understood according to the way these parenting constructs are defined and operationalized. For example, in Maccoby and Martin's orthogonal framework, control is largely measured by the degree of demandingness in the parenting relationship. In contrast, Baumrind incorporates other distinguishing features, such as restrictiveness, autonomy granting, and coerciveness. These conceptual differences must be kept in mind for the data to be understood and compared meaningfully.

As in Maccoby and Martin's (1983) orthogonal approach, most studies on parenting style suggest that parents differ from one another on two important dimensions. Corresponding to Maccoby and Martin's dimension of responsiveness is the dimension of warmth. This dimension has been conceptualized in different ways including (a) affection, in contrast to coldness and rejection (Roe & Siegelman, 1963); (b) acceptance, which included positive evaluation, sharing, expression of affection, emotional support, and equalitarian treatment, in contrast to ignoring, neglect, and rejection (Schaefer, 1965); and (c) care, defined by affection, emotional warmth, empathy, and closeness, in contrast to emotional coldness, indifference, and neglect (Parker, Tupling, & Brown, 1979). The warmth dimension has been identified theoretically and supported empirically as the major dimension in parenting. It is also not a controversial dimension because most would agree that children do well with parental affection (Maccoby, 1980).

The second is the dimension of control, which corresponds to Maccoby and Martin's (1983) dimension of demandingness. This dimension has been variously conceptualized as psychological autonomy versus psychological control (Schaefer, 1965), overprotection versus allowance of autonomy and independence (Parker et al., 1979), and permissiveness versus restrictiveness (Maccoby, 1980). The control dimension further varies in the way it is operationalized in different studies. Some of the ways this dimension has been operationalized include: (a) restriction, characterized by high demand without democratic exchange or negotiation (Stewart et al., 1998); (b) overprotection, characterized by excessive intrusion, infantalization, and interference in the child's plans and relationships (McFarlane, Bellissimo, & Norman, 1995; Shucksmith, Hendry, & Glendinning, 1995); (c) harsh discipline (Wagner, Cohen, & Brook, 1996); (d) psychological autonomy, characterized by non-coercive, democratic discipline and the encouragement of adolescent individuality within the family (Steinberg et al., 1991). The dimension of control is more controversial because there is little consensus on what constitutes optimal levels of control in parenting.

Research on Western Populations

Parenting style and its influence on developmental outcomes have been extensively studied in western societies. There is empirical evidence on links between parenting style and school performance (Dornbusch et al., 1987; Steinberg et al., 1991), family functioning (McFarlane et al., 1995; Mupinga, Garrison, & Pierce, 2002), well-being (McFarlane et al., 1995; Shucksmith et al., 1995), depression (Mackinnon, Henderson, & Andrews, 1993; Parker, 1983), and self-esteem and self-concept (Coopersmith, 1967). Parker's (1983) study, for example, report that a parenting style characterized by low care and high protection was associated with depression. Shucksmith et al. (1995) found that parenting characterized by care and empathy, and not by excessive intrusion and infantilization, correlates with the best family functioning and adolescent well-being.

In terms of authoritative and authoritarian parenting, research on parenting styles has shown with consistency the kind of parenting that is conducive to the successful socialization of children to the mainline culture in the U.S. (Maccoby & Martin, 1983). Studies among white populations have yielded consistent results that show authoritative parenting associated with positive outcomes, including better academic performance (Dornbusch et al., 1987; Steinberg et al., 1991), social maturity and responsibility (Baumrind, 1971), and with a wide variety of measures of competence, self-esteem, and mental health (Buri, 1989; Maccoby & Martin, 1983). However, the evidence on the effect of parenting styles on non-western populations is not as clear.

Cross-Cultural Studies

Research shows that the authoritarian parenting style is endorsed more by Chinese or Asian-Americans than by Euro-American parents (Chao, 1994, 2000; Dornbusch et al., 1987; Steinberg, Dornbusch, & Brown, 1992). Although current research suggest transcontextual validity (Weisz, 1978) between authoritative parenting and child and adolescent psychosocial outcomes (Chen, Dong, & Zhou, 1997), the cross-cultural validity in the associations between authoritarian parenting and child and adolescent outcomes remains unclear. Some studies suggest cross-cultural applicability (Chen et al., 1997; Leung, Lau, & Lam, 1998), while others are not conclusive, or show results that are contrary to findings for western populations (Steinberg et al., 1991; Quoss & Zhao, 1995). The cross-cultural study by Leung et al. (1998), for example, showed that academic achievement was negatively related to academic authoritarianism for all the three samples studied: Australian, American, and Chinese, suggesting cross-cultural applicability. However, Quoss and Zhao (1995) showed results contrary to that for western populations. In their study, the authors report that in their Chinese sample, democratic parenting did not predict any item on the satisfaction scale, whereas authoritarian parenting predicted satisfaction with the overall parent-child relationship. The results, while being contradictory to western norms, were also not conclusive because the children also expressed dissatisfaction with their family rules and ways of making decisions. In noting the non-conclusive results, the authors call for more empirical investigations into contemporary Chinese parent-child relationships.

In the study by Steinberg et al. (1991), it was shown that the relation between authoritativeness and psychosocial and psychological health was consistent across the four ethnic groups: White, Hispanic-American, African-American, and Asian-American. Authoritative parents in this study were characterized as accepting, firm, and democratic. Adolescents who reported such parenting earned higher grades in school, were more self-reliant, reported less anxiety and depression, and were less likely to engage in delinquent behavior. In a later follow-up study, Steinberg and his colleagues showed that the results observed in the initial cross-sectional analyses were either maintained or increased over time (Steinberg, Lamborn, Darling, Mounts, & Dornbusch, 1994).

However, the relation between authoritativeness and school performance was greater among White and Hispanic adolescents compared to African-American and Asian-American adolescents. This effect was also seen in an earlier study by Dornbusch et al. (1987), in which authoritative parenting was not predictive of academic achievement among African-Americans and Asian-Americans. In their study, Asian-Americans were found to score the highest on the authoritarian style while also scoring highest on academic achievement. The authors concluded that the success of "Asian children in our public schools cannot be adequately explained in terms of the parenting styles we have studied" (p. 1256). In a subsequent study by Steinberg et al. (1992), the authors found that Asian students performed better academically than other students. The better performance was not associated with parenting style, but with the students' belief about education and life success. The authors also found that the Asian group reported the highest level of peer support for academic achievement. It appears that the emphasis and high expectations for education amongst the Chinese at the level of peers, family, the community, and culture are prime factors in the academic success of the Chinese (Chao, 1994; Yao, 1985). These findings underscore the importance of exercising caution in studying how child and adolescent outcomes are predicted by parenting style in Chinese families, particularly in the domain of academic success. Instead, educational achievement appears to have its own meaning and unique position for Chinese families, culture, and history.

Baumrind's Prototypes

Some scholars have questioned the validity of categorizing parenting in the Asian context according to Baumrind's prototypes (Chao, 1994, 2000; Chao & Sue, 1996; Gorman, 1998; McBride-Chang & Chang, 1998). In attempting to explain the paradoxical results for the Chinese population, Chao and Sue (1996) suggest that the Chinese have "parenting patterns that are distinct from other groups" (p. 98). Chao (1994) suggests that the western understanding of authoritarian and authoritative parenting can be misleading when applied to Chinese parenting: it does not seem to capture the essence of Chinese parenting, which incorporates the indigenous elements of "chiao shun" and "guan." "Chiao shun" is a Chinese term that refers to training, which incorporates educating or inculcating children in culturally appropriate behaviors (Chao, 1994, p. 1112). "Guan" speaks of caring for, loving, and governing; it suggests that "parental care, concern, and involvement are synonymous with firm control and governance of the child" (Chao, 1994, p. 1112). The function of governing, which is exercised by teachers and parents, is regarded positively in Chinese culture. The reverse is to be uncaring or negligent in one's role (Chao, 2000). In particular, parental control for the Chinese is largely organized around their desire for their children to be successful, particularly in school. This kind of control is often accompanied by sacrifices on the parents' part, so that their children can be successful. Success is often defined as getting good grades, going to a good university, and being assured of getting a good job and a good income in future (Chao & Sue, 1996).

Chao and Sue (1996) assert that this kind of parenting is different from that which is labeled "authoritarian" as applied to western parenting. What captures the Chinese style of parenting is the training concept, which involves elements of authoritarian parenting in Baumrind's typology as well as elements unique to Chinese parenting. In Chao's (1994) study, Chinese mothers who endorsed obedience, respect for work and traditional order, as well as a set of conduct affirming parental authority (Baumrind's authoritarian), were also reported to be highly involved, sacrificial, and supportive of their children, especially in the area of their schooling. This was also supported in Gorman's (1998) study, in which despite high expectations, the mothers in the study were not "overtly overbearing, but exercised influence in more subtle ways" (p. 79). Further evidence from the study by Quoss and Zhao (1995) confirms that Chinese "authoritarian" parenting may be conceptually different from the western understanding. These authors found that the more authoritarian Chinese parents were, the better the overall relationship was perceived by their children. Thus, it would be an error to assume that these parents are authoritarian in the western sense and raises serious questions about the validity of authoritarianism for cross-cultural populations (Chao & Sue, 1996).

This is further supported in a study by McBride-Chang and Chang (1998) on a sample of Hong Kong Chinese adolescents and their parents. The parents in the sample were largely unclassifiable in the categories of authoritative, authoritarian, and permissive parenting. Moreover, contrary to results obtained in the West (Dornbusch et al., 1987; Steinberg et al., 1991), no association was evident between any of the three parenting prototypes and school achievement. In view of these contradictory results, McBride-Chang and Chang (1998) recommend that multiple dimensions of parenting should be considered in the study of Chinese children and adolescents. They assert that, while there may be utility in conceptualizing parenting in these prototypical ways, these categorizations may be less relevant for Chinese families as compared to western families. A later study by Chao (2000) demonstrated a similar effect: The immigrant Chinese parents endorsed more than one typology when presented with separate measures for each of Baumrind's (1971) parenting style typologies. According to Chao, the Chinese parents may be endorsing more than one typology because they capture different aspects of parenting style that cannot be captured by a single typology. Similar results were obtained by Kim and Rohner (2002) in a study on a Korean American sample in which the authors found that 74% in the sample were unclassifiable based on Baumrind's typology, thus raising questions about its cross-cultural applicability.

PARENTING STYLE AND CHILD OUTCOMES IN CHINESE FAMILIES

Current research shows that parenting variables are associated with adolescent psychosocial outcomes in Chinese populations. For example, parenting style and the quality of the parent-child relationship were found to be related to the personality of children (Chan, 1978), school and social performance (Chen et al., 1997), ethnic pride (Rosenthal & Feldman, 1992), self-concept (Leung & Leung, 1992), well-being (Shek, 1999; Stewart et al., 1998), life satisfaction (Leung & Leung, 1992), and parent-adolescent conflict (Yau & Smetana, 1996). Rosenthal and Feldman (1992) found that ethnic pride in Chinese-American and Chinese-Australian adolescents was associated with family environments that are characterized as warm, yet controlled and regulated, in which rules are provided and enforced.

The impact of immigration on parenting style and child outcomes has not been adequately studied. Research on the effect of acculturation on parenting style is scarce and results from the limited research are inconclusive. Chiu, Feldman, and Rosenthal (1992) examined directly questions of how immigration influences the relationship between parenting behavior and adolescent distress, with particular focus on the domains of warmth, control, and involvement. Results indicated that differences did not exist in the associations between parenting behaviors and child outcomes among immigrant and non-immigrant groups. The authors also found that the experience of immigration affected adolescent perceptions of parental control and involvement, but not warmth.

No significant differences also were found between immigrant and non-immigrant families for the composite dimension of warmth or for the specific components of cohesion and acceptance. Chiu et al.'s (1992) study suggests trans-contextual validity in the research on the dimension of warmth and control on child outcomes. In their words, "Our results suggest that existing theories linking cold, uninvolved, and excessively controlling parental behaviors to high adolescent distress apply to families from different cultures and of differing migrant status" (p. 234).

Research on parenting in immigrant families suggests that immigrant families increasingly adopt the childrearing practices and attitudes of the dominant culture as they become more acculturated (Kelley & Tseng, 1992; Lin & Fu, 1990). The comparative cross-cultural study of Asian-American students by Lui (1990) demonstrated association between acculturation and parenting style. Higher levels of acculturation are associated with less controlling and more nurturing styles of parenting as in white families.

Some authors have suggested that while authoritarian or affectionless-control styles of parenting may be contextually appropriate in a collectivistic context, such styles become problematic in a western cultural milieu (Herz & Gullone, 1999). Seen from a western mindset, extreme parental control over adolescent decision-making may be perceived as infantalization, but, from an Asian cultural perspective, it can be interpreted as filial piety. Within a collectivistic context, low levels of expressed warmth may not be equated with a lack of love and care, but this can become discordant for immigrant children in a western context. For example, Sung (1985) reports that Chinese-American children struggle with knowing that their Chinese parents love them because their experience of their parents as distant and formal stands in sharp contrast to the warmth and affection overtly expressed in the mainstream culture. With shifts in values and meanings in an immigrant context, it is likely that the adoption of western norms in parenting, especially in more nurturing styles of parenting, becomes adaptive for immigrant families.

Parental Control

In Baumrind's (1971) prototypes, both authoritarian and authoritative parenting are high on parental control. While both kinds of parenting sets limits on the child, the nature of control varies. In authoritarian parenting, the control is exercised unilaterally, with children being expected to obey unquestioningly. In contrast, authoritative parenting encourages verbal give and take, and the child is directed in an issue-oriented and rational manner. Children are likely to perceive the exercise of control as unwanted domination in authoritarian families, but as helpful maintenance of order and limit setting in authoritative homes.

There is evidence that Chinese parenting is high in control and restrictiveness (Chao, 1994; Chiu, 1987; Ho, 1986; Kelly & Tseng, 1992; Lin & Fu, 1990; Yao, 1985), but the effect of parental control on child psychosocial outcomes is not clear. Lau and Cheung (1987) suggest that one reason for ambiguous results is the undifferentiated nature of the parental control used in this research. They suggest that there is a need to differentiate between positive kinds of control that are functional and negative kinds of control that are dysfunctional in families. In a study on a sample of Chinese adolescents in Hong Kong, Lau and Cheung tested the effects of two kinds of parental control—one that was dominating and interfering, and the other, labeled organization, was functional in maintaining coordination and order in the family. They found that greater parental control was associated with less cohesion and more conflict, while greater organization was associated with more cohesion and less conflict. Moreover, Chinese parents, in the same study, scored high in organizational control, which was found to correlate with parental warmth.

Chiu (1987) demonstrated that Taiwanese parents and immigrant Chinese parents were found to be more restrictive than the Caucasian-American mothers, but that the restriction and strictness appear more to protect than to inhibit. In Yao's (1985) study, family life in the Asian-American homes were found to be more structured, especially around formal educational experiences for the children, compared to Caucasian-American homes. The study by Lin and Fu (1990) showed that parental control was highest among the Chinese mothers and lowest among the Caucasian-American mothers, with immigrant Chinese mothers in the middle. The authors attribute this to the gradual adoption of western values and practices by immigrant mothers. However, contrary to literature, both Chinese and immigrant Chinese mothers rated higher on encouragement of independence. Evidence suggests a positive relation between parental encouragement of independence and parental emphasis on achievement among parents of Chinese origin.

In a cross-national study of Australian, U.S. and Hong Kong adolescents, Rosenthal and Feldman (1990) showed that Hong Kong adolescents perceived their families to be less reinforcing of autonomous behavior than those from Anglo-Australian and Euro-American families. The authors also reported that the family environment of the immigrant Chinese adolescents showed some shifts towards promoting the norms of their host cultures, particularly those emphasizing autonomy. However, one interesting finding was that adolescents from immigrant families in both the U.S. and Australian samples perceived their families as more structured and controlling, as well as emphasizing achievement more than their non-immigrant counterparts, western or Chinese. The authors suggest that it is possible that immigrant parents become more controlling of their children in an effort to maintain traditional values and to monitor their children's acculturation to western values.

In a separate analysis, Chiu et al. (1992) reported that the immigration experience impacted parental control in families. First generation adolescent immigrants reported more rule setting and decision making in their families, compared to their counterparts in Hong Kong. The authors suggest the possibility that parents may actually be setting more rules and making more decisions to try to maintain control over their children's changing behaviors.

There is evidence showing that Chinese children are not unlike western children in resenting strict and authoritarian parenting (Lau & Cheung, 1987; Stewart et al., 1998). In the study by Lau and Cheung (1987) on a sample of Chinese adolescents in Hong Kong, the authors report that greater independence allowed by the parents was associated with more cohesion and less conflict. Further, the self-esteem of the adolescents was correlated positively with independence and negatively with parental control. Research also shows that Chinese adolescents endorse personal values, such as freedom and personal achievement, though as a culture, they are generally seen as collectivistic (Lau, 1988; 1992). Yau and Smetana (1996) reported similar findings, in which their sample of Chinese adolescents in Hong Kong expressed their desire for more autonomy in decision-making. In Stewart et al.'s (1998) study, Chinese late adolescents showed evidence of negative reactions to excessive parental control.

Chao (1994) notes that Chinese parenting, through "chiao shun" and "guan" (Chao, 1994, p. 1112), incorporates elements of authoritarian parenting (high control and set standard of conduct) with high involvement and concern for the child. "Guan" has been shown to correlate highly with the dimension of warmth in a study by Stewart et al. (1998) on a sample of Hong Kong Chinese late adolescent girls. In Chao's (1994) study, Chinese mothers, in comparison with European-American mothers, endorsed a high level of maternal involvement for promoting success in the child. Together with high involvement is the belief that they are the central caretakers of the child. Whether such beliefs about training, governance, high involvement, and concern are perceived by the immigrant adolescent as intrusive or overprotective is an interesting area to explore.

Parental Warmth

The affective dimension of parenting has been found to be a moderator of stressful life events during adolescence (Wagner et al., 1996). In their study, Wagner and his colleagues found that adolescents who perceived higher levels of warmth in their relationships with their fathers or mothers had fewer symptoms of depression and fewer conduct problems. Similar results were found in the study by Mackinnon et al. (1993), in which the care dimension emerged as the principal dimension in predicting depression. In their study, it was found that the lack of care, rather than overprotection, is the primary risk factor for depression. The warmth dimension has also been found to be associated with higher self- worth and competence in children and adolescents (Coopersmith, 1967; McFarlane et al., 1995).

There is evidence that the association of the warmth dimension with positive child and adolescent outcomes is transculturally valid. In one of the few studies on relationships and the adaptation of immigrant families, Scott and Scott (1989) reported that high warmth was associated with enhanced emotional well-being and self-esteem. This is supported in Chiu et al.'s (1992) study in which warmth was observed to have the strongest negative association with measures of adolescent distress. Parental warmth was found to correlate with a decrease in depression in a sample of immigrant Chinese adolescents (Skinner & Crane, 1999). An analysis of maternal and paternal warmth showed that maternal warmth was the strongest contributor to reduced adolescent depression.

While most parents feel affection for their children, they differ in how openly and how freely they express their affection. They also vary in how much their affection is mixed with feelings of coldness, rejection, and hostility. Current research among Asian populations shows contradictory findings on the warmth factor. Various studies have observed that Asian parents score lower on the warmth-accepting dimension in parenting compared to their western counterparts (Chiu, 1987; Dinh, Sarason, & Sarason, 1994; Hertz & Gullone, 1999). Chiu (1987), for example, reported that compared to Caucasian-American mothers, Chinese-American mothers were more likely to approve of the expression of hostility or rejection. In the study by Dinh et al. (1994), the authors reported that Vietnamese-born students perceived lower levels of acceptance and caring from their parents than American-born adolescents. The authors assert that it is unlikely that the two parental groups differed in how much they cared for their children. They chose to attribute this difference to the "reserved behavior between generations that is typical of the traditional Vietnamese family," which differs from "the typical American style of openly expressing positive emotions" (p. 485). The lower level of acceptance was also a finding in Herz and Gullone's (1999) study, in which Vietnamese-Australian adolescents reported lower levels of parental acceptance compared to Anglo-Australian adolescents. The lower acceptance coupled with higher overprotection was found to relate negatively to self-esteem.

However, Chiu et al.'s (1992) study showed no significant differences between immigrant and non-immigrant families for the composite of warmth or for the specific component of acceptance. This finding on an adolescent population was also consistent with the study by Lin and Fu (1990), in which parents reported on their child-rearing practices on their children from kindergarten to second grade. No difference between Chinese, immigrant Chinese, and Caucasian-American mothers on open expression of affection was reported in this study. The authors suggest that the lack of difference on the warmth factor could be due to ethnic differences in the perception and evaluation of affective expression. Another possibility is that Chinese parents are changing their child-rearing practices, though immigrant Chinese mothers, in the study by Kelley and Tseng (1992), reported less nurturance and responsiveness than Caucasian-American mothers. Children in this study were 3-8 years old, and it appears that different results for the warmth factor in these Asian populations were not dependent on the age of the youngsters involved.

Stewart et al. (1998) found that "guan," the indigenous parenting dimension in Chinese families, overlaps significantly with warmth. Although many of the items do not appear to suggest warmth as understood in the West, they speak of commitment and involvement. The authors suggest, "the warmth/*guan* linkage could reflect the relationship between the etic (warmth) and the emic (*guan*)" (p. 354). They propose that it is then likely that the non-inclusion of *guan* items in western scales underestimates the level of warmth in Chinese families. Chao (2000) underscores this by suggesting that there may be important qualitative distinctions in the warmth dimension. A western understanding of warmth and care incorporates physical and emotional demonstrativeness, whereas an eastern understanding may be based on support through involvement and investment. Whether this is so remains to be ascertained through more research.

Immigrant families may be at different stages of the acculturation process, which could be a primary factor determining the degree of warmth parents are comfortable expressing, as is particularly evidenced by the differing results in immigrant Chinese families. Studies on Chinese families show that Chinese parents tend to be very lax and affectionate toward infants and very young children, but restrictive, with little overt affection, once children become older (Chiu, 1987; Ho, 1986; Suzuki, 1980). Although the relative non-expressiveness of warmth in traditional Chinese families may be contextually appropriate for Chinese families located in Asian societies, it may be a problem within immigrant families located in a western setting. Children, in these contexts, are exposed to western norms in which love is more likely to be expressed overtly and warmly. How adolescents perceive parental warmth is likely to affect the parent-child relationship as well as adolescent psychological well-being.

CONFUCIANISM AND ITS IMPACT ON THE CHINESE FAMILY

The empirically based picture of Chinese-American families, as in other Asian-American families is "fragmented and incomplete" (Uba, 1994, p. 27).

Traditional Chinese families are strongly shaped by Confucian ideology, but evidence indicates that the values of Chinese parents and their children are not only changing in immigrant settings, but in their country of origin as well (Lin & Fu, 1990). Studies have shown that there are gradual changes occurring in the traditional Chinese practices within families in Hong Kong and Taiwan (Dawson & Ng, 1972; Ho & Kang, 1984). Evidence exists, in these societies, that adolescents are increasingly endorsing values such as personal competence and autonomy, values associated with an individualistic framework. Chinese families in the East, and Chinese-American families, in particular, are changing and departing from strictly defined roles (Lin & Fu, 1990). In his analysis of continuity and variation in Chinese patterns of socialization, however, Ho (1989) observes that, despite undeniable changes and departures from traditional norms, even among acculturated Chinese-Americans, features of a traditional pattern are still highly discernable.

In traditional Chinese families, family interactions and structure are largely shaped by the teachings of Confucius, which emphasize filial piety and hierarchical relationships (Chan & Leong, 1994). The strongest value by far is filial piety, which includes children's obligation to respect their parents and the responsibility of the adult children for their elderly parents. Parent-child relationships are hierarchical and characterized as formal, with clearly prescribed role relationships and lines of authority. Ancestors and elders are accorded high respect. The father is the undisputed head, and parents often expect unquestioning obedience from their children. Such obedience is encouraged at an early age and is maintained throughout the child's relationship with the parents, even after adulthood and after the adult has started a family of his or her own. Conformity and family solidarity are emphasized.

In the traditional Chinese family, parents discourage their children from displays of anger and aggression. Children are expected to be unobtrusive and to stay out of trouble. Above all things, children are not to do anything that brings shame and dishonor to the family. Behaviors that bring shame and dishonor to the family include aggression, antisocial behavior, and disobedience. Those that bring honor to the family include achievement, obedience, and obligation to the parents. There is little overt affection in the traditional Chinese family. In one sense, Chinese families are child-centered because more emphasis is placed on the parent-child bond than on the marital bond. In the Confucian social order, the relationship between father and son is considered paramount. The mother is primarily responsible for the care of the children and the family. Parents are concerned that their children do well in school (Chiu, 1987; Ho, 1989; Kelley & Tseng, 1992).

In terms of research on Chinese families, two points are noteworthy: (a) the dynamic nature of culture and (b) the need for a balanced perspective and approach. Foner (1997) reminds us that a truly timeless tradition does not exist, while Lau and Yeung (1996) caution researchers against overgeneralizing cultures by calling for greater awareness of culture's dynamic nature. The latter authors pose the following important questions to readers: "What exactly is (Chinese culture)? Is Chinese culture totally different from western culture?" (p. 34). In so doing, Lau and Yeung challenge researchers and theorists alike on the uniqueness as well as the inter-relatedness of all cultures.

In her study on immigrant Chinese mothers of adolescents, Gorman (1998) reported that most of the immigrant Chinese mothers in her study had difficulties responding to queries regarding cultural values. Most mothers did not seem to be consciously raising their children to "be Chinese." One mother, for example, summed up her thoughts as "The world is changing too quickly; it is difficult to say what is east and what is west" (p. 77). In their study of filial piety among New Zealand-Chinese, Liu, Ng, Weatherall, and Loong (2000) report that this social structure is giving way to modernity and that, in different cultural settings, the traditional ideal of filial piety may be endorsed somewhat differently. The authors suggest that "it is possible that different psychological processes are involved in maintaining support of filial piety across the generations" (p. 221). Those who are western-identified, for example, perceive filial piety more as facilitating regular positive communication between generations, whereas those who are Chinese-identified relate filial piety more in terms of material obligations, such as providing financial assistance. Other studies on immigrant Chinese adolescents in Australia and the U.S., such as that by Rosenthal and Feldman (1990), show value shifts from east to west.

In terms of the need for a balanced perspective and approach, Lau and Yeung (1996) note that one shortcoming of research on the impact of Confucianism on Chinese culture and on Chinese rearing practices is the emphasis on positive effects, especially the academic success of the Chinese (Sue & Okazaki, 1990). Scholars have attributed this to the Asian tradition emphasizing academic excellence and the high parental expectations for academic achievement (Chao, 1994; Chao & Sue, 1996; Steinberg et al., 1992; Yao, 1985). Steinberg et al. (1992) note that Asian-American students were more likely to report that their parents had high expectations for school performance. However, they also report that these students were motivated more by their fear of negative consequences than by their belief that educational success pays off. Lau and Yeung caution researchers to be more balanced in their approach. They note:

> Chinese culture is not as glorious as Westerners perceive it to be. It has
> its dark side, problems, and difficulties . . . researchers should try to take
> note of the diversity of Confucianism how it has exerted positive influ-

ence, and on the other hand, how it may also elicit many controversial matters in the Chinese population as well. (p. 36)

Ho (1986) echoes this concern in noting the psychological costs that may be incurred from aspects of the Confucian heritage. Chinese worldview and orientation toward children is more pragmatic and moralistic than psychological (Suzuki, 1980). Although the Chinese value system has fostered academic excellence, this may have occurred at the expense of quality in the parent-child relationship as well as such positive developmental outcomes as psychological health. This observation is supported by research reporting higher levels of anxiety associated with test taking among Chinese students in Canada compared to their Anglo- and European-Canadian counterparts (Dion & Toner, 1988). Other research found that lower levels of psychological well-being were associated with the stress of living up to the model minority stereotype of being Asian (Ahn Toupin & Son, 1991). Hence, it is important to include other critical variables in the study of the Chinese population.

Academic success is only one aspect of measured success and may or may not be related to psychosocial adjustment as indicated by Rumbaut (2000) in a study from the Children of Immigrants Longitudinal Study (CILS). Specifically, results indicated that foreign-born students, who were more recently arrived in the U.S., earned higher grades than their native-born, co-ethnic peers but scored lower on self-esteem and higher on depressive symptoms. This effect was also observed in a study on immigrant Vietnamese families by Dinh et al. (1994), in which the authors observed that the Vietnamese-born students had significantly higher college grade point averages compared to American-born students. However, these students reported a lower quality of parental relationship and less social integration than their American-born counterparts. Such non-concurrence of academic achievement and other family and developmental variables needs to be noted.

CONCLUSION

According to Darling and Steinberg (1993), "viewing parenting style as a context that facilitates or undermines parents' efforts to socialize their children may hold the greatest promise for future research on familial influences on child and adolescent development" (p. 495). While this may be true, given that parental characteristics and child rearing behaviors influence the personality characteristics of and the social outcomes for children (Peterson & Rollins, 1987), parenting style as a construct remains problematic, especially in cross-cultural research. This is particularly so when parenting style is construed in configurational terms. Research on Chinese and immigrant Chinese populations has shown that most Chinese parenting does not fit into Baumrind's prototypes, and attempts at interpreting research data using such prototypes are confusing. The paradoxical results obtained in associations between authoritarian parenting and child outcomes for Chinese families, for example, suggest that there are important differences between cultures in the area of parenting style, especially in the understanding of authoritarian parenting (Chao, 1994, 2000; Chao & Sue, 1996; McBride-Chang & Chang, 1998).

Orthogonal approaches in which parenting style dimensions are investigated separately are likely to yield more meaningful and interpretable data in cross-cultural studies. This is because parenting style in configurational typologies is too complex and prone to being conceptually loaded with associated attitudes, behaviors, and values that are culturally biased. In view of this, parenting dimensions under investigation may best be examined separately rather than seen as an aspect of a style. Even so, these parenting dimensions can in themselves be complex and multidimensional as well as subject to cultural biases.

This article focuses on two key parenting dimensions–warmth and control. Parenting warmth and control have been defined and operationalized in different ways in different studies, making comparisons between and across studies challenging. When studying parent-child relations across cultures, such as in Chinese populations, the researcher has to be mindful of the need to be highly culturally specific when defining the constructs. For example, a western understanding of warmth incorporates physical demonstrativeness, whereas an eastern understanding may focus more on parental involvement and parental investment in the child (Stewart et al., 1998; Chao, 2000). Further, warmth has been conceptualized and operationalized as parental care in some instruments such as the Parental Bonding Instrument (Parker et al., 1979), which has been used as a measure of parenting style. In scoring lower on this dimension (Hertz & Gullone, 1999), does it mean that the Asian parents care less for their children compared to their higher-scoring western counterparts? Researchers need to be aware of cultural biases inherent in measurement instruments that are developed in a western context.

In spite of the qualitative differences that may exist between cultures in the parenting dimensions, the literature review on the key dimensions of parental warmth and control and its association with child outcomes in Chinese and Chinese immigrant families shows evidence of trans-contextual validity for parental warmth. Parenting warmth is associated with positive child outcomes across different cultures and differing migrant status (Chiu et al., 1992; Skinner & Crane, 1999; Rosenthal & Feldman, 1992). However, the dimension of parental control on child psychosocial outcomes is not clear for Chinese and Chinese immigrant families. Some scholars suggest that the multidimensional and undifferentiated nature of parental control have led to confusing results in associations between control and child outcomes in Chinese families. They suggest the need to differentiate between dysfunctional forms of control and functional forms of control that bring necessary order and organization to the family (Lau & Cheung, 1987).

Considering the unique challenges in conceptualizing parenting style in cross-cultural studies on Chinese populations, more research, both quantitative and qualitative, is needed so that with more valid ways of measurement, data can be interpreted more meaningfully. Research methodologies could include self-report questionnaires, interviews and behavior observations. Chao's (1994, 2000) attempts at defining parenting style in culturally relevant ways for the Chinese population are a start in the right direction. The key dimensions of parental warmth and control as applied to research on Chinese populations need to be more precisely defined to allow for a more accurate understanding of the qualitative differences between cultures and what the associated child outcomes are. Research that takes into consideration these cross-cultural issues in an attempt to yield more meaningful data in the study of parenting style and child outcomes in Chinese and immigrant Chinese populations will greatly add to the literature in this understudied, yet important area.

REFERENCES

Ahn Toupin, E., & Son, L. (1991). Preliminary findings on Asian Americans: "The model minority" in a small private East Coast college. *Journal of Cross-Cultural Psychology, 22,* 404-417.

Baumrind, D. (1971). Current patterns of parental authority. *Developmental Psychology Monographs, 4* (Part 2), 1-103.

Buri, J. R. (1989). Self-esteem and appraisals of parental behavior. *Journal of Adolescent Research, 4,* 33-49.

Chan, J. (1978). Parent-child interaction and personality. *New Horizons, 19,* 44-52.

Chan, S., & Leong, C. (1994). Chinese families in transition: Cultural conflicts and adjustment problems. *Journal of Social Distress and the Homeless, 3*(3), 263-281.

Chao, R. K. (1994). Beyond parental control and authoritarian parenting style: Understanding Chinese parenting through the cultural notion of training. *Child Development, 65,* 1111-1120.

Chao, R. K. (2000). Cultural explanations for the role of parenting in the school success of Asian-American children. In R. D. Taylor & M. C. Wang (Eds.), *Resilience across contexts: Family, work, culture, and community* (pp. 333-363). Mahwah, NJ: Lawrence Erlbaum.

Chao, R. K., & Sue, S. (1996). Chinese parental influence and their children's school success. In S. Lau (Ed.), *Growing up the Chinese way: Chinese child and adolescent development.* Shatin, Hong Kong: The Chinese University Press.

Chen, X., Dong, Q., & Zhou, H. (1997). Authoritative and Authoritarian practices and social and school performance in Chinese children. *International Journal of Behavioral Development, 21,* 855-873.

Chiu, L. H. (1987). Child-rearing attitudes of Chinese, Chinese-American, and Anglo-American mothers. *International Journal of Psychology, 22,* 409-419.

Chiu, M. L., Feldman, S. S., & Rosenthal, D. A. (1992). The influence of immigration on parental behavior and adolescent distress in Chinese families residing in two Western nations. *Journal of Research on Adolescence, 2,* 205-239.

Coopersmith, S. (1967). *The antecedents of self-esteem.* San Francisco: Freeman.

Darling, N., & Steinberg, L. (1993). Parenting style as context: An integrative model. *Psychological Bulletin, 113,* 487-496.

Dawson, J. L., & Ng, W. (1972). Effects of parental attitudes and modern exposure on Chinese traditional-modern attitude formation. *Journal of Cross-Cultural Psychology, 3,* 210-217.

Dinh, K. T., Sarason, B. R., & Sarason, I. G. (1994). Parent-child relationships in Vietnamese immigrant families. *Journal of Family Psychology, 8,* 471-488.

Dion, K. L., & Toner, B. B. (1988). Ethnic differences in test anxiety. *Journal of Social Psychology, 128,* 165-172.

Dornbusch, S. M., Ritter, P. L., Leiderman, P. H., Roberts, D., & Fraleigh, M. (1987). The relation of parenting style to school performance. *Child Development, 58,* 1244-1257.

Foner, N. (1997). The immigrant family: Cultural legacies and cultural changes. *International Migration Review, 31,* 961-974.

Gorman, J. C. (1998). Parenting attitudes and practices of immigrant Chinese mothers of adolescents. *Family Relations, 47,* 73-80.

Hertz, L., & Gullone, E. (1999). The relationship between self-esteem and parenting style: A cross-cultural comparison of Australian and Vietnamese adolescents. *Journal of Cross-Cultural Psychology, 30,* 742-761.

Ho, D. (1989). Continuity and variation in Chinese patterns of socialization. *Journal of Marriage and the Family, 51,* 149-163.

Ho, D. Y. F. (1986). Chinese patterns of socialization: A critical review. In M. H. Bond (Ed.), *The psychology of the Chinese people. (pp. 1-37). New York: Oxford University Press.*

Ho, D. Y. F., & Kang, T. K. (1984). Intergenerational comparisons of child-rearing attitudes and practices in Hong Kong. *Developmental Psychology, 20,* 1004-1006.

Kelley, M., & Tseng, H. (1992). Cultural differences in child rearing: A comparison of immigrant Chinese and Caucasian American mothers. *Journal of Cross-Cultural Psychology, 23,* 444-455.

Kim, K., & Rohner, R. P. (2002). Parental warmth, control, and involvement in schooling: Predicting academic achievement among Korean American adolescents. *Journal of Cross-Cultural Psychology, 33,* 127-140.

Lau, S. (1988). The value orientations of Chinese University students in Hong Kong. *International Journal of Psychology, 23,* 583-596.

Lau, S. (1992). Collectivism's individualism: Value preference, personal control, and the desire for freedom among Chinese in mainland China, Hong Kong, and Singapore. *Personality and Individual Difference, 13,* 361-366.

Lau, S., & Cheung, P. C. (1987). Relations between Chinese adolescent's perception of parental control and organization and their perception of parental warmth. *Developmental Psychology, 23*, 726-729.

Lau, S., & Yeung, P. (1996). Understanding Chinese child development, *Growing up the Chinese way: Chinese child and adolescent development*. Hong Kong: The Chinese University Press.

Leung, J., & Leung, K. (1992). Life satisfaction, self-concept, and relationship with parents in adolescence. *Journal of Youth and Adolescence, 21*, 653-665.

Leung, K., Lau, S., & Lam, W. (1998). Parenting styles and academic achievement: A cross-cultural study. *Merrill-Palmer Quarterly, 44*, 157-172.

Lin, C., & Fu, V. R. (1990). A comparison of child-rearing practices among Chinese, Immigrant-Chinese and Caucasian-American parents. *Child Development, 61*, 429-433.

Liu, J. H., Ng, S., Weatherall, A., & Loong, C. (2000). Filial piety, acculturation, and intergenerational communication among New Zealand Chinese. *Basic and Applied Social Psychology, 22*, 213-223.

Lui, B. (1990). Asian-American child-rearing practices and acculturation: A cross-cultural examination. *Dissertation Abstracts International, 51* (12-B), 6112.

Maccoby, E., & Martin, J. (1983). Socialization in the context of the family: Parent-child interaction. In E. M. Hetherington (Ed.), *Handbook of child psychology: Socialization, personality, and social development* (Vol. 4, pp. 1-101). New York: Wiley.

Maccoby, E. E. (1980). *Social development: Psychological growth and the parent-child relationship*. New York: Harcourt Brace Jovanovich.

Mackinnon, A., Henderson, A. S., & Andrews, G. (1993). Parental 'affectionless control' as an antecedent to adult depression: A risk factor refined. *Psychological Medicine, 23*, 135-141.

McBride-Chang, C., & Chang, L. (1998). Adolescent-parent relations in Hong Kong: Parenting styles, emotional autonomy, and school achievement. *The Journal of Genetic Psychology, 159*, 421-436.

McFarlane, A. H., Bellissimo, A., & Norman, G. R. (1995). Family structure, family functioning and adolescent well-being: The transcendent influence of parental style. *Journal of Child Psychology and Psychiatry, 36*, 847-864.

Mupinga, E. E., Garrison, M. E. B., & Pierce, S. H. (2002). An exploratory study of the relationships between family functioning and parenting styles: The perceptions of mothers of young grade school children. *Family & Consumer Sciences Research Journal, 31*, 112-129.

Parker, G. (1983). Parental "affectionless control" as an antecedent to adult depression. *Archives of General Psychiatry, 40*, 56-60.

Parker, G., Tupling, H., & Brown, L. B. (1979). A parental bonding instrument. *British Journal of Medical Psychology, 52*, 1-10.

Peterson, G. W., & Rollins, B. C. (1987). Parent-child socialization. In M.B. Sussman & S.K. Steinmetz (Eds.), *Handbook of marriage and the family* (pp. 471-507). New York: Plenum Press.

Quoss, B., & Zhao, W. (1995). Parenting styles and children's satisfaction with parenting in China and the United States. *Journal of Comparative Family Studies, 26*, 265-80.

Roe, A., & Siegelman, M. (1963). A parent-child questionnaire. *Child Development, 34*, 355-369.

Rosenthal, D. A., & Feldman, S. S. (1990). The acculturation of Chinese immigrants: Perceived effects on family functioning of length of residence in two cultural contexts. *Journal of Genetic Psychology, 151*, 495-514.

Rosenthal, D. A., & Feldman, S. S. (1992). The relationship between parenting behavior and ethnic identity in Chinese-American and Chinese-Australian adolescents. *International Journal of Psychology, 27*, 19-31.

Rumbaut, R. G. (2000). Profiles in resilience: Educational achievement and ambition among children of immigrants in Southern California. In R. D. Taylor & M. C. Wang (Eds.), *Resilience across contexts: Family, work, culture, and community* (pp. 258-294). Mahwah, NJ: Lawrence Erlbaum Associates.

Schaefer, E. S. (1965). A configural analysis of children's reports of parent behavior. *Journal of Consulting Psychology, 29*, 552-557.

Scott, W. A., & Scott, R. (1989). *Adaptation of immigrants: Individual differences and determinants.* Oxford: Pergamon.

Shek, D. T. L. (1999). Paternal and maternal influences on the psychological well-being of Chinese adolescents. *Genetic, Social, and General Psychology Monographs, 125*, 269-296.

Shucksmith, J., Hendry, L. B., & Glendinning, A. (1995). Models of parenting: Implications for adolescent well-being within different types of family contexts. *Journal of Adolescence, 18*, 253-270.

Skinner, K. B., & Crane, D. R. (1999). *Associations between parenting, acculturation, and adolescent functioning among Chinese in North America.* Poster session presented at the annual conference of the National Council on Family Relations, Irvine, CA.

Steinberg, L., Dornbusch, S. M., & Brown, B. B. (1992). Ethnic differences in adolescent achievement: An ecological perspective. *American Psychologist, 47*, 723-729.

Steinberg, L., Lamborn, S. D., Darling, N., Mounts, N. S., & Dornbusch, S. M. (1994). Over-time changes in adjustment and competence among adolescents from authoritative, authoritarian, indulgent, and neglectful families. *Child Development, 65*, 754-770.

Steinberg, L., Mounts, N., Lamborn, S., & Dornbusch, S. (1991). Authoritative parenting and adolescent adjustment across various ecological niches. *Journal of Research on Adolescence, 1*, 19-36.

Stewart, S., Rao, N., Bond, M., McBride-Chang, C., Fielding, R., & Kennard, B. (1998). Chinese dimensions of parenting: Broadening western predictors and outcomes. *International Journal of Psychology, 33*, 345-358.

Sue, S., & Okazaki, S. (1990). Asian-American educational achievements: A phenomenon in search of an explanation. *American Psychologist, 45*, 913-920.

Sung, B. L. (1985). Bicultural conflicts in Chinese immigrant children. *Journal of Comparative Family Studies, 26*, 255-269.

Suzuki, B. H. (1980). The Asian-American family. In M. O. Fantini & R. Cardenas (Eds.), *Parenting in a multicultural society* (pp. 74-102). New York: Longman.

Uba, L. (1994). *Asian Americans: Personality patterns, identity, and mental health.* New York: The Guilford Press.

Wagner, B. M., Cohen, P., & Brook, J. S. (1996). Parent/adolescent relationships: Moderators of the effects of stressful life events. *Journal of Adolescent Research, 11,* 347-374.

Weisz, J. (1978). Transcontextual validity in developmental research. *Child Development, 49,* 1-12

Yao, E. (1985). A comparison of family characteristics of Asian-American and Anglo-American high achievers. *International Journal of Comparative Sociology, 26,* 198-208.

Yau, J., & Smetana, J. (1996). Adolescent-parent conflict among Chinese adolescents in Hong Kong. *Child Development, 67,* 1262-1275.

Parenting Style in Problem-Solving Situations: A Cultural Exploration Based on Structured Observational Methods in Hong Kong

Vicky C. W. Tam
Rebecca S. Y. Lam

ABSTRACT. This study contributes to the debate on applying parenting style typologies to the Chinese population by using structured observational methods in examining parenting behaviors and styles in parent-child interactions in problem-solving situations. Participants were 81 parent-child dyads in Hong Kong. The four parenting groups identified through cluster analysis were authoritative, authoritarian, disengaged, and task-oriented. This clustering was compared internally on parenting attributes and child's school-related outcomes, as well as externally with the Parent Behavior Report typology assessed through the child-report method. Discussion was based on the conceptual and theoretical implications of this new clustering using observational methods. *[Article copies available for a fee from The Haworth Document Delivery Service: 1-800-HAWORTH. E-mail address: <docdelivery@haworthpress.com> Website: <http://www.HaworthPress.com> © 2003 by The Haworth Press, Inc. All rights reserved.]*

KEYWORDS. Chinese parents, observational methods, parenting style, problem-solving situations

Vicky C. W. Tam and Rebecca S. Y. Lam are Assistant Professors, Department of Education Studies, Hong Kong Baptist University, Kowloon Tong, Hong Kong. Correspondence regarding this manuscript should be sent to the first author (E-mail: vtam@hkbu.edu.hk).

An earlier draft of this paper was presented in the 2001 Society for Research on Child Development Biennial Meeting, April 19-22, 2001, Minneapolis, MN.

http://www.haworthpress.com/store/product.asp?sku=J002
© 2003 by The Haworth Press, Inc. All rights reserved.
10.1300/J002v35n03_04

43

Parenting style is a popular construct used in many studies of parenting performance and its impact on children's outcomes. The most widely known parenting style typology, proposed by Diana Baumrind, builds upon the two dimensions of demandingness and responsiveness postulated by Maccoby and Martin (1983) and describes how parents reconcile the joint needs of children for nurturance and limit-setting (Baumrind, 1991). The typology comprises authoritarian, authoritative, permissive, and neglecting parenting, among which the first two types have received much attention. While both denote child-rearing styles that are characterized by high demandingness, authoritative parents are high in responsiveness whereas authoritarian ones are low in this attribute.

Findings often show that authoritative parenting results in favorable developmental outcome in children and adolescents, including better academic performance (e.g., Dornbusch, Ritter, Leiderman, Roberts, & Fraleigh, 1987) and more adaptive psychosocial adjustment (e.g., Baumrind, 1991; Lamborn, Mounts, Steinberg, & Dornbusch, 1991; Maccoby & Martin, 1983) than children of other parenting style groups. Yet the normativity of the authoritative style across cultures has been contested, especially with the Chinese population upon which research yields inconsistent results. On one hand, studies conducted in Hong Kong and mainland China (e.g., Boys' & Girls' Clubs Association of Hong Kong, 1994; Chen, Dong, & Zhou, 1997; Leung, Lau, & Lam, 1998) replicate the results produced in western culture and support the adaptive performance of children from authoritative families. On the other hand, some studies conducted in the United States conclude that Chinese children, whose parents are more likely to be authoritarian than those of European American and other ethnic groups, have better academic achievement (Steinberg, Lamborn, Darling, Mounts, & Dornbusch, 1994). To a certain extent, the difficulty in arriving at consistent and conclusive results may be attributed to the diversity of outcome domains involved (Lam, 2003), the variations in cultural practices among Chinese populations in different communities, and the wide age range of the child samples. The paradox also draws researchers to probe more deeply into the intricate relationship between parenting style and children's outcome in Chinese families, and the adequacy of the Baumrind typology as a predictor of child outcomes (Chao, 1994).

Increasingly, research attention has focused on the significance of cultural factors in understanding parental functioning and child development. It has been suggested that cultural beliefs and norms held by parents form a developmental niche for the growing child (Harkness & Super, 1995). The increasing attention to the significance of the sociocultural context leads researchers to reexamine theories and constructs of child development in western cultures for applicability to non-western societies (Dasen & Mishra, 2000). Rubin

(1998) pointed out that cultural values and beliefs provide interpretation of the acceptability of individual characteristics as well as the types and ranges of interactions and relationships that are likely or permissible. Parents and adults within different cultural contexts have expectations on the development of children that may be related to culturally specific beliefs and perception (Harwood, Miller, & Irizarry, 1995).

In traditional Chinese culture, emphasis often is put on strict discipline of children so as to ensure that they have the proper training to become a moral person (Ho, 1989). This may explain why Chinese parents are sometimes considered authoritarian. Chao (1994) pointed out the limitation of the authoritarian-authoritative conception of parenting in describing Chinese families. The concept of training was proposed to explain Chinese school success, which outlines the emphasis on filial piety in socialization goals and parental practices that comprise structural involvement (Chao, 2000). Such postulation leads to the consideration of parenting patterns beyond the four basic types of authoritative, authoritarian, permissive, and neglectful.

Further challenge to the authoritarian-authoritative typology is presented by Darling and Steinberg (1993) who queried the adequacy of parenting style in capturing the variety and richness of parenting behaviors. Parenting style, as conceptually defined, involves the general emotional climate expressed by parental behavior but is presumed to be independent of the domain or content of socialization. Darling and Steinberg (1993) thus proposed that, in order to understand the processes through which parenting style influences child development, the model also must include practices used by parents to help children reach socialization goals. Parenting practices comprise specific content and socialization goals, operating in circumscribed socialization domains, and involve behavior such as spanking, showing interest in children's activities, or requiring children to do their homework. This discussion leads researchers to consider the significance of domain- or context-specific parenting behaviors and attributes. Along a similar line, the inclusion of alternative conceptualizations of parenting performance, in addition to parenting style, may be helpful in predicting child outcome. For example, Chao (2001) demonstrated the mediating role of parent-child relationship qualities in studying the effect of parenting style on adolescents. In such regard, parenting style still remains a core construct in explaining parenting behavior and child outcome, but other parenting attributes need to be considered in the full understanding of parental impact on children.

It is the goal of this study to contribute to the understanding of parenting in a Chinese context by identifying culture- and domain-specific patterns of parenting behaviors and examining their impact on children's school-related performance. This endeavor focuses on Chinese families with school-age children in Hong Kong and draws upon observational methods. While most studies on parenting are conducted using a paper-and-pencil method of collecting data from either children or parents, it is certainly an issue whether the findings fully represent the range and depth of parenting behaviors and practices. Self-report methods may not be applicable to younger children who have yet to develop competence in observation and introspection necessary for completing assessment inventories. Self-reports can also be influenced by the social desirability effect of testing, which may be particularly prominent among Chinese respondents (Yang, 1996). Observational methods offer a unique source of data by including a systematic and objective assessment by a third party. When used with rating scales, the methods are well-suited for identifying interactional and relationship properties and are able to incorporate into the rating process the interdependence of behaviors among different parties in interaction (Grotevant & Carlson, 1989). The focus of observation in this study is on the interaction between parents and children engaging in problem-solving situations that resemble homework supervision, a common activity in families with school-age children in Hong Kong. This specific domain of parenting performance is considered to be relevant to the school-related outcome of children. The study analyzed ratings on parent behaviors as observed in the interactions in conjunction with self-report data collected through questionnaires. The analysis focuses on identifying profiles of parenting behaviors in problem-solving contexts and examining the relationships with children's school-related outcomes. Findings of this study thus provide a unique contribution to the debate on Chinese parenting.

METHOD

Data used in this analysis were collected through structured observation and a questionnaire survey. The main component, structured observation, was set up for assessing parenting behaviors and parenting styles. It involved 81 parent-child dyads who volunteered to participate. The mean age of the children was 9.77 years ($SD = 0.94$), with 40 boys and 41 girls. They were studying at Primary Three to Five levels in six local schools, which is equivalent to Third Grade to Fifth Grade in the U.S. school system. These schools were selected by the research team to cover a range of geographic locations and funding sources and operating bodies. There are three types of funding sources for schools in Hong Kong: (a) government schools, funded and run by the government; (b) subsidized schools, government-funded and run by non-profit-making organizations; and (c) private schools, privately funded and run by non-profit-making organizations. The present sample was acquired from one government school, two subsidized schools, and three private schools.

Accompanying the children were 59 mothers and 22 fathers who participated in the observation sessions. Their mean age was 40.91 years ($SD = 4.68$), with a majority (80.2%) that had attained secondary school education or higher. A substantial proportion of the parents (39.5%), mostly mothers, were full-time homemakers, whereas 17.3% were professionals.

A series of structured observation sessions of parent-child dyads in problem-solving situations were conducted. The whole process of interaction, lasting 20 minutes, was videotaped. There were four problem-solving activities involved in the interaction: (a) Discuss the best way to spend a monetary gift of $1,000 from a relative for the child's birthday; (b) show a picture only to the child, who then instructs his/her parent to reproduce the picture according to his/her descriptions; (c) show another picture only to the parent, who also instructs his/her child to reproduce the picture according to his/her descriptions; and (d) list as many ways as possible to make use of empty soda cans. These four activities allowed the parent-child dyad to engage in discussion, collaboration, and joint decision-making that simulated everyday communication at home. The sessions were administered by the research team using standardized procedures in the child's school or on university premises, depending on the arrangement preferred by the school and/or the parents. Roughly the same number of sessions was conducted in the two types of settings.

Coding of parental behavior was based on a manual adapted from the Family Interaction Global Coding System (FIGCS) (Hetherington, Stanley-Hagan, & Eisenberg, 1992). The system consists of twelve general scales describing different dimensions of family interaction and eight parenting scales describing attributes of parenting behaviors. This study made use of 11 general scales (anger/rejection, warmth/support, coercion, assertiveness, involvement, transactional conflict, communication skills, authority/control, depressed mood, positive mood, and problem-solving outcome) and one parenting scale (attempted parental influence) from the system, with the target of observation specified to be the parent. These scales were chosen because of relevance to the tasks and the interactions involved in the observation. Ratings ranged from 1 to 5 and were based on the frequency and intensity of the parent's behaviors. Detailed descriptors were provided in the manual for every rating point on each scale. For example, a rating of 1 on the anger/rejection scale was described as "The parent displays *no* negative, angry, rejecting, or hostile behaviors," whereas a rating of 5 indicated that "The most extreme negative, angry, rejecting, or hostile behavior is of *high intensity*." The FIGCS previously has been used in the study of parenting style and adolescent outcome (Gunnoe, Hetherington, & Reiss, 1999). This study marked the first attempt to use the rating system with Chinese families. As the descriptors for the rating points were generic enough to allow for culture-specific interpretation of behaviors and emotions, the use of the system was deemed appropriate.

Coding was performed on the taped sessions by a research team of five members, with every session coded independently by two coders. The mean scores between the two sets of observation were computed and used for subsequent analyses. Reliability of the coding measures was assessed using intraclass correlations (Rowley, 1976). Regarding inter-rater reliabilities, intraclass correlation coefficients were found to be all significant, with values ranging from .33 ($p < .01$) for anger/rejection to .59 ($p < .001$) for assertiveness. Test-retest reliabilities also were computed for the same coder with a 4-week time span on a random selection of 20 cases. All intraclass correlation coefficients were found to be significant, with values ranging from .38 ($p < .05$) for positive mood to .82 ($p < .001$) for warmth/support.

In the second component of this study, data were drawn from a questionnaire survey in which the 81 parent-child dyads also participated to collect information on child performance and parental behavioral variables as well as demographic characteristics of the family. The survey was conducted on a total of 1,011 Primary Three to Primary Five Chinese students recruited from the same six primary schools (Tam & Lam, in press), with 477 fathers and 512 mothers participating in the survey (or a response rate of 47.1% and 50.6%, respectively). Data on five child outcome variables and five parental attributes drawn from the questionnaires were included in this analysis.

For child outcome, the variables of child's academic achievement, aspiration for education, perceived efficacy for self-regulated learning, peer relationship, and self-esteem were measured using the self-report method. Academic performance was appraised using Hong Kong Attainment Tests (Primary) (Hong Kong Education Department, 2000). These are a battery of standardized tests on the subjects of Chinese, English, and Mathematics designed by the Education Department and annually administered by the schools to students for assessing and monitoring academic attainment. The advantages of this instrument are that it is an objective measurement of academic performance, and it allows comparisons across children in different schools. Self-esteem was assessed using the 10-item Self-Esteem Scale (Rosenberg, 1989) (alpha = .74). Other school-related performance indicators were assessed through self-constructed measures. They include peer relationship (three items, 4-point response format, alpha = .85) (e.g., "Do you think that other students prefer to play with you?"); perceived efficacy in self-regulated learning (seven items, 5-point response format, alpha = .76) (e.g., "How well can you plan and organize your academic activities?"); and aspiration for education (six items,

5-point response format, alpha = .66) (e.g., "I expect to improve my academic performance every term"). The reliabilities of these measures, with Cronbach's alphas ranging from .66 to .85, on the whole were deemed acceptable (Robinson, Shaver, & Wrightsman, 1991).

For parental attributes, the five variables of nurturance, psychological pressure, aspiration for the child's education, involvement in the child's education, and parental academic efficacy were assessed. Nurturance and psychological pressure were measured using the Parent Behavior Report (PBR) (Schludermann & Schludermann, 1988) with data provided by the child. The former dimension of nurturance reflects parental expression of affection to the child, whereas the latter dimension refers to the parental use of psychological pressure techniques. The PBR is an adaptation of the Child's Reports of Parental Behavior Inventory (CRPBI) (Schaefer, 1965). With a total of 23 items, this adaptation is simple and short for use with children and has been used in cross-cultural studies (Schludermann & Schludermann, 1983). A 3-point Likert-type response format was used (1 = "Not like my parent"; 2 = "Somewhat like my parent"; and 3 = "A lot like my parent"). Sample items include "My mother/father is a person who showed interest and support" (nurturance) and "My mother/father is a person who often complained about what I did" (psychological pressure). The PBR dimensions were found to be correlated with the acceptance dimension and the psychological control dimension with the CRPBI. Cronbach's alphas reported in previous studies for the two dimensions ranged from .68 to .73 (Schludermann & Schludermann, 1988). For use in this study, the Parent Behavior Report was translated from English into Chinese by the research team. Effort was made to ensure that the original meaning was kept. Cronbach's alphas on the two dimensions reported separately on fathers and mothers in this study ranged from .75 to .90.

Four parenting styles, indulgent (low in psychological pressure but high in nurturance), inductive (high in both), indifferent (low in both dimensions), and dictatorial (high in psychological pressure but low in nurturance), were classified using median-split procedures. Each child reported their perception of the father's and the mother's behavior separately, while both sets of scores were included in the median-split procedures for classifying parenting styles.

Finally, three other parental attributes were assessed with the self-report method scales developed for this project based on a 5-point response format. Parental aspiration for the child's education (e.g., "I expect my child to improve his/her academic performance every term") had 7 items, with Cronbach's alphas being .69 for the fathers' sample and .72 for the mothers' sample. Six items measured the variable involvement in the child's education (e.g., "I often supervise my child to do his/her homework") as well as parental academic efficacy (e.g., "How much can you do to motivate your children for academic pursuit?"). Cronbach's alphas for these two variables were computed separately for the samples of fathers and mothers, with the values ranging from .68 to .89.

RESULTS

The means of parenting behavior ratings found in the structured observation are listed in Table 1. As a group, the parents scored high in the dimensions of warmth/support, involvement, communication skills, positive mood, and problem-solving outcome, and low in anger/rejection, transactional conflict and depressed mood. These findings show that, on the whole, they were positive in behaviors toward children as observed in the session. Pairwise correlations among parenting behavior dimensions ranged from $-.44$ (warmth/support and anger/rejection) to .72 (assertiveness and involvement). A total of 51 out of the 66 pairs were significantly correlated ($p < .05$), among which 20 pairs showed negative significant correlations. These findings imply that a consistent structure exists among the parenting behaviors. Fathers and mothers, on the whole, did not show differences in behavior, except for a significant difference in communication skills. Specifically, fathers ($M = 3.73$) were found to demonstrate better communications skills than mothers ($M = 3.34$), F (1, 79) = 4.01, $p < .05$.

Parental behaviors toward boys and girls were found to differ in the dimensions of coercion, transactional conflict, and communication skills. Parents were observed to use more coercion with boys ($M = 2.45$) than with girls ($M = 2.02$), F (1, 79) = 4.21, $p < .05$; to show higher levels of transactional conflict with boys ($M = 1.75$) than with girls ($M = 1.44$), F (1, 79) = 4.60, $p < .05$; and to exhibit better communication skills with girls ($M = 3.63$) than with boys ($M = 3.25$), F (1, 79) = 5.02, $p < .05$. However, no difference was observed among different gender combinations of parent-child dyads, except for communications skills, F (3, 77) = 3.25, $p < .05$. Fathers were observed to use better communication skills with daughters than in the case of the other parent-child combinations (father-son and mother-daughter or -son). Finally, differences in parental behaviors were found with grade level of the child in the dimensions of warmth/support, F (2, 78) = 3.98, $p < .05$; positive mood, F (2, 78) = 4.06, $p < .05$; and attempted parental influence, F (2, 78) = 5.44, $p < .01$. Parents of Primary 4 students in general showed a higher level of warmth ($M = 3.77$) and positive mood ($M = 3.73$) than those of Primary 3 and Primary 5 children. Parents of Primary 5 students demonstrated a lower level of attempted influence on their children ($M = 3.00$) than the other two groups of parents with younger children.

TABLE 1. Mean Scores on the Parenting Behavior Scales

Parenting behavior	Entire sample (N = 81)	Child's gender		Parent's gender		Grade level of the child		
		Boys (n = 40)	Girls (n = 41)	Fathers (n = 22)	Mothers (n = 59)	Primary Three (n = 32)	Primary Four (n = 26)	Primary Five (n = 23)
Anger/Rejection	1.73	1.78	1.68	1.77	1.71	1.94	1.62	1.57
Warmth/Support	3.47	3.40	3.54	3.55	3.44	*3.25*	*3.77*	*3.43*
Coercion	2.23	*2.45*	*2.02*	2.00	2.32	2.28	2.15	2.26
Assertiveness	3.35	3.28	3.41	3.55	3.27	3.43	3.62	3.04
Involvement	3.69	3.68	3.71	3.95	3.59	3.78	3.77	3.48
Transactional conflict	1.59	*1.75*	*1.44*	1.59	1.59	1.69	1.69	1.35
Communication skills	3.44	*3.25*	*3.63*	*3.73*	*3.34*	3.41	3.58	3.35
Authority/Control	3.10	3.03	3.17	3.32	3.02	3.19	3.12	2.96
Depressed mood	1.68	1.78	1.59	1.77	1.64	1.81	1.62	1.57
Positive mood	3.41	3.38	3.44	3.41	3.41	*3.22*	*3.73*	*3.30*
Problem-solving outcome	3.35	3.30	3.39	3.64	3.24	2.25	3.50	3.30
Attempted parental influence	3.38	3.40	3.37	3.55	3.32	*3.50*	*3.58*	*3.00*

Note. Figures in italics denote significant ANOVA difference ($p < .05$).

To generate typologies that are based on performance in these 12 behavioral dimensions, cluster analysis was performed on the 12 parenting behaviors using the quick cluster (K-means cluster) method with iterations. The optimal solution chosen consisted of four clusters, with a substantial number of cases included in each cluster and the behavioral profile of each cluster appearing meaningful for interpretation (see Table 2). Cluster One, the authoritarian type, was characterized by the smallest number of parents. These parents had higher scores in the dimensions of Anger/Rejection, Coercion, Transactional Conflict, Depressed Mood, and Attempted Parental Influence, and lower scores in Warmth/Support, Assertiveness, Communication Skills, Authority/Control, Positive Mood, and Problem-Solving Outcome than the other clusters. Cluster Two, the disengaged type, consisted of parents with low scores in Transactional Conflict, Communication Skills, Authority/Control, and Attempted Parental Influence. The third cluster, which was the largest one with 35 members, comprised the authoritative parents. Their scores were higher in Warmth/Support, Assertiveness, Involvement, Communication Skills, Positive Mood, Problem-Solving Outcome, and Attempted Parental Influence, and low in Anger/Rejection, Coercion, Transactional Conflict, and Depressed Mood. The final cluster was the task-oriented group. They had high scores in Involvement, Problem-Solving Outcome, and Attempted Parental Influence. The typology was found to have no association with the child's grade level or the gender of the child and the parent.

The four parenting cluster groups generated from the observation data were compared with one another with regard to child performance and parental attributes assessed through the survey. Five areas of children's performance include academic achievement, aspiration for education, perceived efficacy for self-regulated learning, self-esteem, and peer relationships. Significant group differences were reported in perceived efficacy for self-regulated learning and peer relationship, $F(3, 77) = 3.11$ and 3.90, respectively, $p < .05$ (see Table 3). Based on results of post-hoc Scheffé tests, findings show significant group differences ($p < .05$) between the task-oriented group and the authoritarian group on peer relationships (mean difference = 1.16, $p < .05$) and between the task-oriented and disengaged groups on perceived efficacy for self-regulated learning (mean difference = $.68$, $p < .05$). With regard to parental attributes, the four groups differed significantly in their aspiration for the child's education, $F(3, 75) = 2.86$, $p < .05$, with the authoritative group having the highest score ($M = 4.30$) and the authoritarian group the lowest ($M = 3.83$). There was no significant difference found among the cluster groups on the other four parenting attributes, including nurturance, psychological pressure, parental involvement in the child's education, and parental academic efficacy.

For comparison purposes, the 81 of the parents participating in the observation sessions were classified into four parenting style types using the Parent Behavior Report typology assessed in the questionnaire survey. Results show that the indulgent style, which was marked by high nurturance and low psychological pressure, was the most prevalent ($n = 31$), whereas the smallest group comprised indifferent parents who were characterized as low in both nurturance and psychological pressure ($n = 13$) (see Table 4). The PBR typology was juxtaposed against the parenting cluster groups generated from the observations. Chi square analysis showed that there was no significant association between the two groupings ($\chi^2 = .87$, $p > .05$). However, it was observed from the frequency distribution that authoritative parents tended to be indulgent, whereas task-oriented parents were least likely to be indifferent. Further comparison between the two systems of parenting classification was made by repeating the analysis on group differences on the five child performance variables with the PBR typology. Results of One-way Analysis of Variance show significant group differences in two areas, namely, perceived efficacy for self-regulated learning, $F(3,77) = 5.91$, $p < .01$; and aspiration for

TABLE 2. Mean Scores on Parenting Behavior Ratings Among the Cluster Groups

Parenting behavior	Cluster 1 (Authoritarian) (n = 9)	Cluster 2 (Disengaged) (n = 21)	Cluster 3 (Authoritative) (n = 35)	Cluster 4 (Task-oriented) (n = 16)
Anger/Rejection	2.9	1.7	1.4	2.2
Warmth/Support	2.3	3.2	3.9	3.1
Coercion	3.6	2.1	1.7	2.6
Assertiveness	2.2	2.7	3.9	3.3
Involvement	3.3	3.0	4.1	3.6
Transactional conflict	2.4	1.5	1.3	2.0
Communication skills	2.6	2.8	3.9	3.4
Authority/Control	2.8	2.6	3.4	3.0
Depressed mood	2.8	1.7	1.4	2.0
Positive mood	2.4	3.2	3.8	3.2
Problem-solving outcome	2.4	2.8	3.8	3.6
Attempted parental influence	3.6	2.8	3.5	3.7

Note. $N = 81$

TABLE 3. One-way ANOVA Comparison on Children of Parenting Groups

Variable	Parenting group	Mean	df	F	p
Perceived efficacy for self-regulated learning	Authoritarian (n = 9)	2.44	3, 77	3.11	p < .05
	Disengaged (n = 21)	2.38			
	Authoritative (n = 35)	2.72			
	Task-oriented (n = 16)	3.05			
Peer relationships	Authoritarian (n = 9)	1.30	3, 77	3.90	p < .05
	Disengaged (n = 21)	2.00			
	Authoritative (n = 35)	1.93			
	Task-oriented (n = 16)	2.46			

Note. $N = 81$

education, $F(3,77) = 3.28$, $p < .05$. Based on results of post-hoc Scheffé tests, findings indicated significant group differences ($p < .05$) on perceived efficacy for self-regulated learning between the indulgent type and the indifferent type (mean difference = .77, $p < .05$) and between the indulgent type and the dictatorial type (mean difference = .60, $p < .05$).

DISCUSSION

Results of this study provide a glimpse into the profiles of parenting behaviors among Chinese parents in Hong Kong. The study used a combination of observational and questionnaire data. The results revealed intricate relationships among parenting behaviors and school-related outcomes of children that are worthy of further research.

Cluster analysis in this study shows that Chinese parents in Hong Kong behaved in patterns identified as authoritarian, authoritative, disengaged, and task-oriented. This new typology on the whole resembled Baumrind's parenting styles; it shows that the Baumrind typology still has its applicability in the Chinese community of Hong Kong. However, there were at least two points of deviation observed. Researchers need to consider domain- and culture-specific contexts. First, the largest type of parenting group identified in this study was authoritative, whereas the authoritarian type was the smallest group. This observation deviates from the literature in which Chinese parents have often been identified as authoritarian in style.

Second, permissive parenting did not emerge as a prominent type in the analysis. Instead, a new style, the task-oriented, was identified as task-oriented in which parents can be described as higher in involvement in children's schoolwork. Both in terms of attempted parental influence and the outcome of dyadic problem-solving was observed to be better when compared to the other groups. Although this observation relates to the nature of problem-solving activities involved in the interaction, it also is linked to the Chinese cultural emphasis on educational achievement and the significant role of parents in the promotion of children's learning (Chen, Lee, & Stevenson, 1996; Ho, 1981). This situation is amplified in contemporary Chinese societies such as Hong Kong, where education is considered a major channel of upward social mobility. A similar push for children's academic success has also been noted in Shanghai (Xiao & Chang, 2003) where many Chinese parents are heavily involved in their children's schoolwork through close homework supervision as a means of pushing their children to excel in school. A task-oriented style vividly portrays the profile of such parents, an approach to parenting that was not found to be associated with parent and child demographic characteristics. Instead, task-oriented parents were reported to have children performing better in school than those from the other three groups, with measurements being in terms of perceived efficacy for self-regulated learning and peer relationships.

These findings add to the paradox of parenting influence on children's academic success by moving the discussion beyond the authoritarian-authoritative debate toward recognizing that other parenting patterns exist which have influence on children's school performance. Task-oriented parenting bears concep-

TABLE 4. Cross-Tabulation on Frequencies of the PBR Typology and Parenting Cluster Grouping

PBR Typology	Parenting cluster group generated from observation				Total
	Authoritarian	Disengaged	Authoritative	Task-oriented	
Dictatorial	3	5	7	5	20
Indifferent	2	5	5	1	13
Inductive	1	5	7	4	17
Indulgent	3	6	16	6	31
Total	9	21	35	16	81

tual resemblance to the training concept of Chinese parenting proposed by Chao (1994). In Chinese families, parents put emphasis on training and governing children in the appropriate expected behavior, including performing well in school. The findings thus provide impetus for continuous search for and refinement of indigenous parenting profiles beyond the Baumrind typology with particular consideration given to cultural contexts and parenting domains. Parenting in the domain of children's school performance, a focal point of child-rearing pursuits in Chinese families, should receive further research attention.

The parenting types generated through cluster analysis in this study did not show much correspondence with those assessed through the questionnaires. Specifically, results of cross-tabulation analysis show that the four parenting cluster groups in general did not match the classification made by the Parent Behavior Report with child-report data. The two sets of parenting classification also resulted in somewhat varied patterns of group differences in child performance. Significant group differences were observed in children's efficacy for regulated learning with both sets of parenting classification. Furthermore, differences were reported in peer relationships only with the parenting cluster groups and in the child's aspiration for education only with the PBR typology.

There are two possible explanations for the incongruence. First, the activities in structured observation are problem-solving in nature, which facilitated the identification of the task-oriented parenting type. The activities do not evoke the overall, global climate of parenting style as measured by the Parent Behavior Report, but reflect parent-child interaction in a specific domain such as homework supervision. This indicates that parenting performance is likely to vary across specific domains of child behavior and parent-child interaction. Second, the two sets of data were collected through different sources–as observed by an outsider versus as reported by the child or the parent. Results of this study show that each of these perspectives provides diverse and yet significant information that may not be equivalent to each other. Compared to self-report measures, observation methods offer different and significant ways to capture the essence of parenting behaviors.

It is interesting to note the better performance of fathers on parental behaviors assessed in this study, particularly in the area of communication. Fathers were observed to have better communication with children than mothers and the most optimal communication observed was between fathers and daughters. The results contradict the traditional conception of Chinese fatherhood in which male parents were perceived to be strict disciplinarians in contrast to the nurturant mothers (Ho, 1986). However, with recent changing social circumstances, fathers' child-rearing style may have undergone transformation (Ho & Kang, 1984). Chinese fathers in Hong Kong were found to exhibit more varied parenting patterns than mothers (Tam & Lam, in press). The fathers who participated in the observation were all volunteers. As such, they were a self-selected group who might be particularly supportive of their children's development. It also should be noted that communication is the only construct with significant group differences identified among the 12 behavioral dimensions assessed in this study.

Limitations of the Study. While this study provides a unique contribution to the understanding of Chinese parenting by introducing observation data, conclusions drawn in this study are limited in two ways. First, only one observational context, problem-solving, was used in this study; hence, conclusions have to be interpreted with this caveat in mind. Further research attention in other parenting contexts is recommended. Second, the clustering of parenting types was based on an internal comparison mechanism. Specifically, the performance of individual parents was compared to that of others participating in the same study. The method did not go beyond the constraints of other parenting style classification methods that make use of the median split procedures with child-report or parent-report data. This methodological difference makes comparison of results across studies difficult because the assignment of parental types and styles depends on the comparison group that differs in each research setting. Future research on parenting behavior and styles needs to address this methodological issue in order that results across studies are readily comparable. In such ways it becomes possible to conduct meta-analyses on Chinese parenting across studies.

REFERENCES

Baumrind, D. (1991). The influence of parenting style on adolescent competence and substance use. *Journal of Early Adolescence, 11,* 56-95.

Boys' & Girls' Clubs Association of Hong Kong. (1994). *The relationship between parenting styles and adolescents' behavior.* Hong Kong: Author.

Chao, R. K. (1994). Beyond parental control and authoritarian parenting style: Understanding Chinese parenting through the cultural notion of training. *Child Development, 65,* 1111-1119.

Chao, R. K. (2000). Cultural explanations for the role of parenting in the school success of Asian-American children. In R. D. Taylor & M. C. Wong (Eds.), *Resilience across contexts: Family, work, culture, and community* (pp. 333-363). Mahwah, NJ: Erlbaum.

Chao, R. K. (2001). Extending the consequences of parenting style for Chinese Americans and European Americans. *Child Development, 72,* 1832-1843.

Chen, C. S., Lee, S. Y., & Stevenson, H. W. (1996). Academic achievement and motivation of Chinese students: A cross-national perspective. In S. Lau (Ed.), *Growing up the Chinese way: Chinese child and adolescent development* (pp. 69-92). Hong Kong: Chinese University Press.

Chen, X., Dong, Q., & Zhou, H. (1997). Authoritative and authoritarian parenting practices and social and school performance in Chinese children. *International Journal of Behavioral Development, 21,* 855-873.

Darling, N., & Steinberg, L. (1993). Parenting style as context: An integrative model. *Psychological Bulletin, 113,* 487-496.

Dasen, P. R., & Mishra, R. C. (2000). Cross-cultural views on human development in the third millennium. *International Journal of Behavioral Development, 24,* 428-434.

Dornbusch, S. M., Ritter, P. L., Leiderman, P. H., Roberts, D. F., & Fraleigh, M. J. (1987). The relation of parenting style to adolescent school performance. *Child Development, 58,* 1244-1257.

Grotevant, H. D., & Carlson, C. I. (1989). *Family assessment: A guide to methods and measures.* New York: Guilford.

Gunnoe, M. L., Hetherington, E. M., & Reiss, D. (1999). Parental religiosity, parenting style, and adolescent social responsibility. *Journal of Early Adolescence, 19,* 199-225.

Harkness, S., & Super, C. M. (1995). Culture and parenting. In M. Bornstein (Ed.), *Handbook of parenting: Vol. 2* (pp. 211-234). Hillsdale, NJ: Erlbaum.

Harwood, R. L., Miller, J. G., & Irizarry, N. L. (1995). *Culture and attachment: Perceptions of the child in context.* New York: Guilford.

Hetherington, E. M., Stanley-Hagan, M., & Eisenberg, M. M. (1992). *Family interaction global coding system.* Unpublished manual.

Ho, D. Y. (1981). Traditional patterns of socialization in Chinese society. *Acta Psychologica Taiwanica, 23,* 81-95.

Ho, D. Y. (1986). Chinese patterns of socialization: A critical review. In M. H. Bond (Ed.), *The psychology of the Chinese people* (pp. 1-37). Hong Kong: Oxford University Press.

Ho, D. Y. (1989). Continuity and variation in Chinese patterns of socialization. *Journal of Marriage and the Family, 51,* 149-163.

Ho, D. Y., & Kang, T. K. (1984). Intergenerational comparisons of child-rearing attitudes and practices in Hong Kong. *Developmental psychology, 20,* 1004-1016.

Hong Kong Education Department. (2000). *Hong Kong Attainment Tests (Primary).* Hong Kong: Education Research Section, Hong Kong Education Department.

Lam, S. F. (2003). Chinese parenting and adolescents' susceptibility to peer pressure: A multi-dimensional approach. *Journal of Psychology in Chinese Societies, 3,* 183-205.

Lamborn, S. D., Mounts, N. S., Steinberg, L., & Dornbusch, S. M. (1991). Patterns of competence and adjustment among adolescents from authoritative, authoritarian, indulgent, and neglectful families. *Child Development, 62,* 1049-1065.

Leung, K., Lau, S., & Lam, W. L. (1998). Parenting styles and academic achievement: A cross-cultural study. *Merrill Palmer Quarterly, 44,* 157-172.

Maccoby, E. E., & Martin, J. A. (1983). Socialization in the context of the family: Parent-child interaction. In E. M. Hetherington (Ed.), *Handbook of child psychology: Socialization, personality and social development, Vol. 4* (pp. 1-102). New York: Wiley.

Robinson, J. P., Shaver, P. R., & Wrightsman, L. S. (1991). Criteria for scale selection and evaluation. In J. P. Robinson, P. R. Shaver, & L. S. Wrightsman (Eds.), *Measures of personality and social psychological attributes* (pp. 1-16). San Diego, CA: Academic Press.

Rosenberg, M. (1989). *Society and the adolescent self-image.* Middletown, CT: Wesleyan University Press.

Rowley, G. L. (1976). The reliability of observational measures. *American Educational Research Journal, 13,* 51-59.

Rubin, K. H. (1998). Social and emotional development from a cultural perspective. *Developmental Psychology, 34,* 611-615.

Schaefer, E. (1965). Child's reports of parental behavior: An inventory. *Child Development, 36,* 413-424.

Schludermann, E. H., & Schludermann, S. M. (1988). *Parent behavior report (PBR) for younger children* (Tech. Rep.). Winnipeg, Canada: University of Manitoba, Department of Psychology.

Schludermann, S. M., & Schludermann, E. H. (1983). Sociocultural change and adolescents' perceptions of parent behavior. *Developmental Psychology, 19,* 74-85.

Steinberg, L., Lamborn, S. D., Darling, N., Mounts, N. S., & Dornbusch, S. M. (1994). Overtime changes in adjustment and competence among adolescents from authoritative, authoritarian, indulgent, and neglectful families. *Child Development, 65,* 754-770.

Tam, V. C., & Lam, R. S. (in press). Parenting style of Chinese fathers in Hong Kong: Correlates with children's school-related performance. *International Journal of Adolescent Medicine and Health.*

Xiao, Y., & Chang, W. C. (2003). Stress and coping among school-aged children in China. *Journal of Psychology in Chinese Societies, 3,* 205-231.

Yang, C. F. (1996). *Ru he yan jiu Zhongguo ren* (How to study Chinese people). Taipei: Guiguan. (In Chinese)

Ethnicity and Parenting Styles Among Singapore Families

Stella R. Quah

ABSTRACT. Despite the hopes for an enlightened 21st century expressed by some scholars and observers, and despite the undeniable technological progress of humankind, culture or ethnic divide will not go away in the foreseeable future. Although each generation of parents tends to differ from the preceding generation in its approach to parenting, the pace and nature of change across generations is restrained or mediated by culture or ethnicity and by level of formal education and other factors. More specifically, within the context of continued social change and change within the family as a group of interactive individuals, it is expected that parents with (a) different ethnic backgrounds, and (b) different levels of formal education, differ significantly in their parenting styles. *[Article copies available for a fee from The Haworth Document Delivery Service: 1-800-HAWORTH. E-mail address: <docdelivery@ haworthpress.com> Website: <http://www.HaworthPress.com> © 2003 by The Haworth Press, Inc. All rights reserved.]*

KEYWORDS. Parenting, ethnicity, culture, disciplining, character formation, mother's role, father's role, Singapore

---

Stella R. Quah is affiliated with the Department of Sociology, National University of Singapore, AS1-#03-20 Arts Link, Singapore 117570 (E-mail: socquahs@nus. edu.sg).

This paper is part of a larger study on family relations funded by the Ministry of Community Development, Singapore, and supported by the National University of Singapore. The author acknowledges with thanks the invitation to present the findings at the session on "The Social World of the 21st Century: The future of family and kinship culture," RC07, of the ISA World Congress of Sociology 2002, 11 July 2002, Brisbane, Australia.

http://www.haworthpress.com/store/product.asp?sku=J002
© 2003 by The Haworth Press, Inc. All rights reserved.
10.1300/J002v35n03_05

CONCEPTUAL ARGUMENTS

A combination of conceptual premises from the systemic-ecological per-spective, symbolic interaction, and developmental theories guide this discus-sion. The systemic-ecological perspective asserts the pervasive influence of macro-level phenomena over micro-level processes and proposes that "the parent-child relationship is not an isolated dyadic relationship." Instead, the social environment of the young involves father, mother, and siblings, the ex-tended family, the neighborhood, social networks, the community and the larger social structure (Peterson & Hann, 1999:350). Peterson and Hann identify four main perspectives in the family science literature (parent effects; child effects; reciprocal socialization; and systemic-ecological perspective). They argue that of the four, the systemic-ecological perspective "is best suited to under-stand how social phenomena beyond the dyad redefine both the processes and the outcomes that emerge between parents and children" (Peterson & Hann, 1999:350; Bodman & Peterson, 1995).

Ethnicity is a significant component of the social phenomena influencing parenting styles. Peterson and Hann (1999) follow Broderick (1993) and Bodman and Peterson (1995) in referring to this aspect as the "ethnic-minority context." Their understanding of the dynamics of ethnic influences is basically accurate:

> Children who are members of ethnic groups are exposed to the particular group's shared identity, common ancestry, and common life style that shape different conceptions of competent parenting and social compe-tence in children. (Peterson & Hann, 1999:357)

However, their perspective is limited in two respects. First, by giving prom-inence to the "ethnic minorities" transmission to their children of their shared identity, they unwittingly underplay the same process among the ethnic major-ity. In comparative family research we need to address ethnicity comprehensi-bly, that is, as a constant attribute of every community irrespective of their size relative to the other communities within the same nation-state (Quah, 2002). Secondly, their perspective addresses only the socially constructed dichotomy of a White majority versus non-White or "ethnic minorities" in the United States. This is understandable as they deal with the American situation where the White versus non-White dichotomy is commonly used. However, the posi-tion on ethnic identity adopted in this discussion and inspired by symbolic in-teraction is this: ethnic identity is a pervasive individual characteristic or attribute that shapes a person's self-identity as member of a community or group and his/her subjective perception of the world, just as gender identity or religious affiliation do. This position leaves open the possibility of individuals (and families) changing or modifying their ethnic identities across time.

Ethnicity and Culture

Ethnicity is the focus in this analysis but a word about culture is necessary as the two concepts are closely linked. Culture is one of the most discussed and scrutinized concepts in the social sciences and yet, consensus on its meaning and measurement is still elusive. As Khademian (2002: 88-91) suggests, the lack of agreement results from the three-level nature of the concept: (1) culture as material artifacts, symbols and communication patterns; (2) culture as values, beliefs, attitudes and ideology; and (3) culture as the core of "basic assumptions" about oneself and others. Khademian argues that researchers may not agree on this classification or on which of the three levels is the most important. This problem is resolved in the current discussion by following King's (1962:79) comprehensive definition of ethnic group that encompasses the three levels of culture: What constitutes an ethnic group is the combination of "common backgrounds in language, customs, beliefs, habits, and traditions, frequently of racial stock or country of origin" and more importantly, "a consciousness of kind." King was inspired by Weber's (1978: 387-390) emphasis on "a consciousness of kind" and "ethnic honor" as fundamental features of an ethnic group. While Khademian's (2002) first two levels of culture are important, it is the transmission of a "consciousness of kind" that directly or indirectly permeates parents' approaches to child socialization. Consequently, the first research question tested in this study is "Do parenting styles differ across ethnic groups?" If religion is taken as an additional manifestation of cultural identity, then parenting styles would be expected to vary with religious affiliation.

Social Class

Social class is yet another widely acknowledged influence on parenting styles. The influence of social class as a unitary concept notwithstanding, not all the three main components of social class (income, occupational prestige and level of education) are equally influential to parenting styles. Education is the key factor as it shapes values, beliefs, and attitudes. More importantly, education is intertwined with ethnicity in a variety of fashions, including the fact that both factors are crucial in child socialization. And, as Glazer (2000) emphasized, this link requires further and careful investigation. The second research question explored in this study is: "Do parenting styles differ among parents of different educational backgrounds?"

Occupation

Occupation is included in this analysis in terms of the job obligations of parents. The third research question in this study is: "Does the intensity of job obligations influence parents' approaches to parenting?" The role of parental employment has been extensively investigated over the past decades. The classic studies by Melvin Kohn (Kohn, 1969; Kohn & Schooler, 1983; Kohn & Slomczynski, 1990) brought attention to the significant influence of the lifestyle, conditions and opportunities afforded by different social classes upon family relations and socialization values and patterns. In their review of socialization research, Peterson and Hann (1999:356) confirm Kohn's findings and the more recent influence of dual-earner families and employed mothers on parenting, egalitarian role modeling for children, and increasing participation of fathers in child care (1999). Furthermore, Klute and her colleagues (Klute, Crouter, Sayer, & McHale, 2001) found that occupational attitudes marked by self-direction in dual-earner marriages are associated with a more egalitarian division of household labor, including child care. However, other studies have detected no major departure from the traditional gender-based division of domestic labor among dual-earner couples (Windebank, 2001). The latter finding coincides with the resilience of traditional role definitions proposed by symbolic interaction (Klein & White, 1996).

The Family Life Cycle

Any conceptual analysis of family and parental behavior needs to consider the dynamic nature of these phenomena and the corresponding importance of the time factor. The family developmental framework offers the most explicit and methodical analysis of this characteristic through the concept of family life cycle stages, but most family theories, including the systemic-ecological perspective, recognize the influence of the time factor on family structure and behavior (Klein & White, 1996). The family life cycle has been applied extensively for many years. Two of the most recent studies using this approach are the identification of "cultural and structural segmentation" of families in the Netherlands (Cuyvers, 2000) and the process of youth autonomy from parents in Europe (Fernandez Gordon, 2000). Thus, the fourth research question in this study is "Do parenting styles vary across time in the different stages of the family life cycle?" A comparison of age-cohorts of parents might provide a glimpse of future trends in parenting styles. A glimpse of longitudinal trends partially through retrospection is also attempted by the comparison of the respondents' own childhood experience with their own parenting styles. Thus, the fifth research question in this study is: "Did the discipline method experienced by the respondents as children influence their own parenting styles?"

Two additional explanatory variables in this analysis are the gender of the parent and the number of children. These two variables are included based on previous studies' findings documenting a pervasive gender difference in parental roles and the variation in family duties according to family size (McDaniel & Tepperman, 2000; Quah, 1998; 1999).

METHODS AND MEASUREMENTS

The data discussed in this paper is part of a larger study of family structure and family life in Singapore, conducted from 1997 to 1999 and supported by the Ministry of Community Development. The target population was defined as ever-married citizens and the sampling unit was the individual ever-married citizen, and a disproportioned stratified random sampling procedure was used. Ethnicity was used as the criterion for stratification due to the importance of cultural values and beliefs in family life.

Four ethnic group categories are used in the demographic classification of the Singapore population: Chinese, Malay, Indian, and "Other." This latter category comprises a very small number of people from highly diverse ethnic backgrounds, including Eurasians, Arabs, Japanese, and Caucasians, to name just a few. Such diversity precludes a meaningful analysis of those small groups individually. Thus, I have followed the population census in combining these small groups into the category "Others." According to the 2000 Census of Population (Leow, 2001:viii), 76.8 percent of Singapore residents are Chinese; 13.9 percent are Malay; 7.9 percent are Indian; and 1.4 percent fall into the category "Others." The changes in ethnic distribution from the previous population census in 1990 are negligible. Given this ethnic distribution, proportioned stratified sampling would have resulted in a large Chinese stratum, and the obtained samples of Malays, Indian and Other would be too small for detailed analysis.

Consequently, the sampling frame of all ever-married citizens was divided into four sub-populations (i.e., Chinese, Malay, Indian and "Other") and four independent samples were drawn using simple random sampling (computer-generated random numbers). With the exception of the stratum "Other" (N = 268), the final response rate for each ethnic group, Chinese (N = 452), Malay (N = 484) and Indian (N = 448), matched the targeted sample size rather well. The number of Malay respondents actually exceeded it. The response rate for the group "Other" is lower and the findings on this group should be interpreted with caution. This paper deals only with the findings from the 1,489 respondents who are parents. Relevant details of the sample are presented in Table 1.

Data were collected through personal interviews using a structured questionnaire designed especially for this project. The ethnicity and gender of the interviewers were matched with that of the sampled persons. The respondents were assured that the information they provided would remain confidential. By giving these details to each person before beginning the interview, potential respondents were able to decide freely whether or not they would like to participate in the study. The assurance of confidentiality increases the probability of obtaining frank responses, but deviating cases cannot be discounted in personal interviews.

The paper analyzes eight parenting styles: (1) the parents' emphasis on character formation in their children; (2) the parents' perceived best discipline method; (3) their expectation of child's behavior reflected in the traditional norm "children should be seen, not heard"; (4) their inclination toward open, physical demonstration of affection to their children (as opposed to the felt parental affection that some people believe requires no external signs); (5) the performance of parenting roles by the mother; (6) the performance of parenting roles by the father; (7) the performance of parenting roles by both parents jointly, and; (8) the parents' attitudes toward family-school cooperation in child upbringing. The details of the measurements used for each of these eight dependent variables are presented in Table 2.

The data analysis consisted of factor analysis of the attitudinal scales and logistic regression to explore the likelihood of occurrence of the eight parenting styles as dependent variables. Logistic regression was selected as the best tool for the exploratory analysis of the probability of the dependent variable occurring over the probability of it not occurring (Sanders & Brynin, 1998). To meet the requirements of logistic regression, each of the dependent variables was dichotomized (see Table 2). The parents' emphasis on character formation was classified into two categories based on the sample mean score: "low emphasis" (scores below the mean 2.48) and "high emphasis" (scores above the mean 2.48). The parents' perceived best discipline method was classified into two categories "Reasoning/rules" and "Physical punishment." The parental expectations of child behavior, as expressed in the responses to the statement "I believe that a child should be seen and not heard" were classified as "never" versus "sometimes" or "always." The parents' inclination to demonstrate affection was classified as "never" versus "always/sometimes." The mother's role, father role, and shared parenting were dichotomized as "in charge most of the time" versus "not in charge most of the time." Family-school cooperation scores were recoded into two categories based on the

TABLE 1. Sample Characteristics

Characteristics		Number	%	Mean	Standard deviation
Total sample of parents		**1,489**	**100.0**	--	--
Independent variables					
Gender	Male	703	47.2	--	--
	Female	786	52.8	--	--
Age				46.6	13.7
Ethnicity	Chinese	399	26.8	--	--
	Malay	452	30.4	--	--
	Indian	396	26.6	--	--
	Other	242	16.3	--	--
Years of formal education				8.23	4.23
Religion	Muslim	703	47.2	--	--
	Buddhist/Taoist	260	17.5	--	--
	Hindu/Sikh	228	15.2	--	--
	Christian	252	17.0	--	--
	Other	2	0.1	--	--
	No religion	44	3.0	--	--
Number of children				2.67	1.08
Family cycle stage[1]	Stage 2-Infants/Pre-school children	488	32.8	--	--
	Stage 3-School-age children	531	35.7	--	--
	Stage 4-Young adult children	192	12.9	--	--
	Stage 5-Adult children	278	18.7	--	--
Parents' job obligations	No parent works more than 7 hours daily	344	23.1	--	--
	One parent works 8 hrs/day or longer	786	52.8	--	--
	Both parents work 8 hrs/day or longer	359	24.1	--	--
Most frequent discipline method as a child	No discipline	45	3.0	--	--
	Reasoning/rules	808	54.3	--	--
	Physical punishment	636	42.7	--	--
Dependent variables					
Character formation	Low emphasis (below mean score 2.48)	562	39.0	--	--
	High emphasis (above mean score 2.48)	886	61.0		
Best discipline method	Reasoning/rules	1,328	89.2	--	--
	Physical punishment	161	10.8		
Expected child behavior	Always/Sometimes	1,064	72.1	--	--
	Never	411	27.9		
Open demonstration of affection	Never	203	13.8	--	--
	Always/Sometimes	1,273	86.2		
Mother's role	Performs none of 5 parenting roles	556	37.3	--	--
	Performs 1 or more of 5 parenting roles	933	62.7		
Father's role	Performs none of 5 parenting roles	1,051	70.6	--	--
	Performs 1 or more of 5 parenting roles	438	29.4		
Shared parenting	Mother & father perform none of 5 roles	1,149	77.2	--	--
	Mother & father perform 1 or more of 5 roles	340	22.8		
Family-School cooperation	Low (below mean score 16.7)	707	49.5	--	--
	High (above mean score 16.7)	722	50.5		

1. The first stage of the family life cycle, the pre-parental stage, is excluded because the sample analyzed in this paper is only the sample of parents.

TABLE 2. Measurement of Parenting Styles and Summary Statistics

Measurements	Summary statistics
(1) Character formation ☐ I respect my child's opinions and encourage him/her to express them. ☐ I let my child make many decisions for him/herself. ☐ I talk it over and reason with my child when he/she does something wrong. ☐ I give my child(ren) a good many duties and family responsibilities. ☐ I have strict, well-established rules for my children. ☐ I encourage my child(ren) to be curious, to explore and question things. ☐ I encourage my child(ren) to talk about his/her/their problems. ☐ I encourage my child(ren) to be independent of me Original response categories and scores: Always (3), Only sometimes (2), Never (1). Variable dichotomized as (1) Scores below 2.484 "Low emphasis on character formation"; (2) Scores above 2.484 "High emphasis on character formation" Source: Childrearing Practices Report (CRPR) [Block, J. and Block, J. H. (1980) *California Child Q-set.* Palo Alto, CA: Consulting Psychologists Press.] Selected items	Higher scores indicate parental empha-sis on child's character formation. Range: 1.88 Mean: 2.484 Standard deviation: .338 Sample size: 1489 Reliability coefficient Cronbach's Alpha = .6546
(2) Perceived best discipline method "From your experience, which of the following is the best method of disciplining your child[ren], that is, the method that gives the best results?" (1) Reasoning/rules; (2) Physical punishment.	Mean: 1.111 Standard deviation: .3149 Sample size: 1489
(3) Expected child's behaviour ☐ I believe that a child should be seen and not heard. Response categories and scores: Always/Sometimes (1); Never (2). Source: Childrearing Practices Report (CRPR) [Block, J. and Block, J. H. (1980) *California Child Q-set.* Palo Alto, CA: Consulting Psychologists Press.]	Mean: 1.2786 Standard deviation: .4484 Sample size: 1489
(4) Open demonstration of affection ☐ I express affection by hugging, kissing, and hold-ing my child(ren). Response categories and scores: Always/Sometimes (2), Never (1). Source: Childrearing Practices Report (CRPR) [Block, J. and Block, J. H. (1980) *California Child Q-set.* Palo Alto, CA: Consulting Psychologists Press.]	Mean: 1.8625 Standard deviation: .3445 Sample size: 1489
Parenting Roles From a scale of family division of responsibilities constructed for the larger study. Only the items on parenting roles (mother's role, father's role, and shared parenting) are discussed in this paper.	
(5) Mother's role ☐ Physical care of child(ren) ☐ Disciplining child(ren) ☐ Help child(ren) with schoolwork ☐ Talking to teacher/principal ☐ Taking child(ren) to the doctor Response categories and scores: Mother is in charge most of the time (1); Mother is not in charge most of the time (0)	Mean: 2.024 Standard deviation: 1.917 Sample size: 1489 Range: 5.0 Scores dichotomized as (0) None of the 5 roles; (1) 1 to 5 roles

Measurements	Summary statistics
(6) Father's role ☐ Physical care of child(ren) ☐ Disciplining child(ren) ☐ Help child(ren) with schoolwork ☐ Talking to teacher/principal ☐ Taking child(ren) to the doctor Response categories and scores: Father is in charge most of the time (1); Mother is not in charge most of the time (0)	Mean: .4936 Standard deviation: .9246 Sample size: 1489 Range: 5.0 Scores dichotomized as (0) None of the 5 roles; (1) 1 to 5 roles
(7) Shared parenting ☐ Physical care of child(ren) ☐ Disciplining child(ren) ☐ Help child(ren) with schoolwork ☐ Talking to teacher/principal ☐ Taking child(ren) to the doctor Response categories and scores: Mother and father, jointly, are in charge most of the time (1); Other arrangement most of the time (0)	Mean: .4822 Standard deviation: 1.048 Sample size: 1489 Range: 5.0 Scores dichotomized as (0) None of the 5 roles; (1) 1 to 5 roles
(8) Family-School Cooperation in children's upbringing [Scale designed specifically for this study]	

Talking about your children today, which of these as-
pects of child upbringing should be left entirely to the
family, entirely to the school, to both family and school
together, or should be left to the children to learn by
themselves:
☐ Filial responsibility (being a good son/daughter)
☐ Self-discipline
☐ Personal grooming
☐ Hard work
☐ Courtesy
☐ Thriftiness
☐ Sex education
☐ Mutual respect
☐ Civic responsibility (caring for the needy; being a
   good member of the community)
Response categories and scores:
To be left to the children to learn by themselves (0);
to be taught by the family only (1); the school only (2);
both family and school jointly (3).
	Higher scores indicate higher inclina-
	tion towards family-school cooperation
	in child upbringing.
	
	Range: 27.0
	
	Mean: 16.74
	Standard deviation: 6.09
	Sample size: 1429
	
	Reliability coefficient
	Cronbach's Alpha = .8300
	
	Scores dichotomized as
	(1) Low cooperation [scores below
	   mean 16.74]
	(2) High cooperation [scores above
	   mean 16.74]

mean score (16.74): "low cooperation" (scores below 16.74) and "high cooperation" (scores above 16.74).

Several independent variables were tested, and those that were not significant were dropped from the model. Four sets of significant explanatory variables are included in this analysis: sociocontextual factors; family structure;
parent's job obligations; and the developmental (or time) dimension. The
sociocontextual factors comprise the respondents' ethnicity, religious affiliation, level of formal education, and gender. The categorical variable, ethnicity,
covered the four main ethnic groups: Chinese, Malays, Indians, and "Others,"
and the reference group was Chinese. Religious affiliation was set as two
dummy variables: Muslim/non-Muslim and Buddhist-Taoist/non-Bud-

dhist-Taoist. Muslims and Buddhist-Taoists were the two religious groups with the most significant differences in parenting styles. Education was ascertained as total years of formal education. The indicator of family structure was number of children, whereas parental job obligations were measured by the daily hours parents spend on the job, from none to 8 hours or more. The developmental dimension comprises three variables: age, the stage of the family life cycle, and past socialization. For the logistic regression analysis the respondents' age was simply measured in years (ratio scale). The indicator of past socialization influence was the most frequent discipline method used by the respondent's parents when the respondent was 10 to 12 years old as recalled and perceived by the respondent. These variables are described in Table 1.

RESULTS

This paper explores five research questions. The first three are derived mainly from the systemic-ecological and symbolic interaction perspectives: (1) Do parenting styles differ across ethnic groups? (2) Do parenting styles differ among parents of different educational backgrounds? and (3) Does the intensity of job obligations influence parents' approaches to parenting? The other two research questions refer to premises from the developmental perspective: (4) Do parenting styles vary across time in particular among different stages of the family life cycle and different age-cohorts? and (5) Does the discipline method experienced by the respondents as children influence their own parenting styles? Eight parenting styles are analyzed: parents' emphasis on character formation; their perceived best discipline method; their attitudes towards open demonstration of affection; the performance of mother's role; father's role; shared parenting; and parents' attitudes towards family-school cooperation on child upbringing.

The main findings from the logistic regression analysis are summarized in Table 3. The impact of the four sets of independent variables on each of the eight parenting styles is indicated by the exponentiated coefficients (ExpB) or odds ratios. Odds of 1 signify no change in the dependent variables, and each coefficient represents the increase or reduction in the log odds of the particular parenting dimension occurring. The scores of the eight dependent variables were dichotomized for the linear regression analysis as follows: high versus low emphasis on child's character formation; use of reasoning rather than physical punishment; traditional as opposed to non-traditional expectations of child behavior; open demonstration of affection as opposed to none; performance of mother's, father's, and shared parenting roles most of the time as opposed to some of the time or no performance; and high versus low inclination towards family-school cooperation in child upbringing (see Table 2). Only ExpB coefficients with a level of significance equal to or smaller than .05 are considered statistically significant.

Parents' Emphasis on Character Formation

In contrast to a parent who does not emphasize character formation, a parent who uses this approach in his/her childrearing approach communicates respect for the child's opinions and encourages the child to express them; lets the child make many decisions by him/herself; talks it over and reasons with the child when the child does something wrong; gives the child duties and family

TABLE 3. Logistic Regression Model Predicting Eight Parenting Styles

Variables in the Model		Estimated Odds Ratio [Exp(B)]			
		(a) Character formation	(b) Best discipline method	(c) Expected child behavior	(d) Open demonstration of affection
Sociocontextual factors					
Ethnicity	[Chinese]	.664	.781	1.212	****.241
	[Malay]	.700	.893	****.290	***.360
	[Indian]	1.363	**.465	**.626	.620
Religion	Muslim	.877	**.496	.721	1.541
	Buddhist/Taoist	**.567	*1.992	.963	**.512
Gender [female]		*1.280	***.520	.780	****.435
Years of formal education		****1.070	.995	*****1.086	***1.073
Family structure					
Number of children		1.045	***1.272	1.002	.893
Parents' job obligations					
Parents' hours at work		1.084	.757	.815	1.140
The developmental (time) dimension					
Age		.997	1.022	.995	.980
Stage of family cycle		***1.350	.747	.951	.898
Past socialization		.954	****2.410	**1.330	1.103
Nagelkerke R Square		**.101**	**.136**	**.148**	**.236**
Variance predicted correct		**63.6%**	**89.1%**	**73.1%**	**87.0%**

TABLE 3 (continued)

Variables in the Model		Estimated Odds Ratio [Exp(B)]			
		(e) Mother's role	(f) Father's role	(g) Shared parenting	(h) Family-school cooperation
Sociocontextual factors					
Ethnicity	[Chinese]	1.134	.631	1.196	***1.943
	[Malay]	**1.847	1.121	.723	***.585
	[Indian]	***1.870	**1.647	****.445	1.213
Religion	Muslim	1.258	1.316	.804	.996
	Buddhist/Taoist	**1.978	*1.819	.712	.942
Gender [female]		.879	****2.122	*1.361	1.217
Years of formal education		.999	1.013	***1.062	****1.109
Family structure					
Number of children		.909	1.039	.953	1.093
Parents' job obligations					
Parents' hours at work		.985	****1.460	1.240	1.153
The developmental (time) dimension					
Age		***.967	1.002	.983	1.005
Stage of family cycle		****.292	****.585	****.525	.878
Past socialization		1.074	1.139	.876	1.115
Nagelkerke R Square		**.513**	**.180**	**.222**	**.132**
Variance predicted correct		**84.5%**	**71.5%**	**77.8%**	**63.2%**

Notes
Sample size = 1489 parents
  *   Statistically significant at p = .04 to .05
  **   Statistically significant at p = .01 to .03
  *** Statistically significant at p = .001 to .009
  **** Statistically significant at p = .0001 or less

responsibilities; has strict and well-established rules for the children; encourages the child to be curious, explore and question things, talk about his/her problems, and be independent (see scale items and scoring in Table 2). The more that these characteristics are exhibited by a parent, the higher is his/her emphasis on character formation.

The Nagelkerke R Square of .101 (Table 3, column a) suggests that 10 percent of the overall variation in the emphasis on character formation is predicted by the variables in the model. The model predicted correctly the emphasis on character formation among parents 63.6 percent of the time. Of the four sets of independent variables, the sociocontextual, and developmental factors were influential. Religion, gender, and education were important sociocontextual factors.

Religion. The logistic regression coefficients in Table 3 (column a) indicate that the odds of parents emphasizing character formation as outlined above decreased by 56 percent if the parent is Buddhist or Taoist. Parents most likely to emphasize character formation in their approach to parenting are non-Buddhist/Taoist. No significant differences were found among ethnic groups, but the impact of culture is nevertheless revealed in the contrast between Buddhist/Taoist parents and parents categorized as having "no" or "other" religious affiliation. Buddhist/ Taoist parents are more inclined to discount and discourage child's opinions; to emphasize obedience and respect for authority over reasoning; and to avoid giving children family responsibilities. These parents are less likely to encourage children to ask questions and to explore things; or to talk about their problems. As will be shown later, they are not inclined to demonstrate their affection openly by hugging, kissing, and holding their children. In general, Buddhist/Taoist parents use a style of parenting that is in clear contrast with the features of character formation outlined above.

Gender. There were differences between mothers and fathers in the emphasis on character formation. The Exp(B) coefficient in Table 3 (column a) suggests that fathers are 28 percent more likely to emphasize character formation compared to mothers. This difference between mothers and fathers is explained in part by certain informal and almost habitual "division" of child rearing duties as will be discussed in the section below. Concerning education, one unit increase in formal education above the mean is associated with a seven percent increase in the probability of parents focusing on character formation. Put differently, the higher the parent's level of education, the more likely he/she is to be concerned with character formation.

Stage in the Family Life Cycle. The developmental or time dimension, as indicated by the stage in the family life cycle, was also significant. In contrast to parents of infants or preschoolers, being a parent at later stages of the family life cycle corresponds to a 35 percent increase in the probability of emphasizing character formation. It appears that parents are more permissive in the preschool stage while attention to rules, responsibilities, respect for the child's opinions, and the other features of character formation (among parents who exhibit them) tend to begin after their children enter school.

Perceived Best Discipline Method

Parents were asked to indicate, based on their experience, which of a list of child disciplining methods is the best method "that is, the method that gives you the best results." The meaning of "best" results was left to the parent to define. The methods listed varied from reasoning to using rules such as setting curfew and cutting allowances, to spanking, smacking and caning. For the logistic regression analysis, the responses were dichotomized into (1) reasoning/rules and (2) physical punishment.

The variables in the model contribute about 13.6 percent of the variance in parents' perception of best discipline method and the variance was predicted correctly by the model 89 percent of the time (Table 3 column b). Of the sociocontextual variables, ethnicity, religion, and gender showed significant influence. Parents more likely to consider reasoning and rules (in contrast to physical punishment) as the best method of discipline are found among the Indian and Malay communities and among Muslims. On the other hand, the odds of preferring physical punishment as the best method of discipline increase significantly if the parent is Buddhist or Taoist.

Congruent with the findings on character formation, fathers are more likely than mothers to prefer reasoning and rules to physical punishment. The number of children is also important: the odds of using physical punishment increase by 27 percent among large families (i.e., those with three or more children).

Of the three developmental dimension variables, past socialization was significantly associated with the perception that the most effective discipline method is physical punishment. Parents who underwent physical punishment as children were significantly more inclined to see physical punishment as the best discipline method for their own children.

Expectations of Child Behavior

Parents' expectations on child behavior were tapped by their opinions on how to bring up children: "I believe that a child should be seen, not heard." The variables in the model (Table 3, column c) explain 14.8 percent of the variation in the expectations of child behavior (Nagelkerke R Square = .148) and variance in this dependent variable was explained correctly 73 percent of the time. Of the sociocontextual variables, ethnicity and education were found to be significantly associated with this expectation. The coefficients in Table 3 indicate that Malay and, to a lesser extent Indian parents, are significantly more inclined to agree with this expectation than Chinese parents or parents of other ethnic groups. Expecting children to be seen, not heard, is also predominantly associated with the level of education of the parents. The higher the level of a parent's education, the more inclined the parent is to reject this expectation.

Interestingly, the expected influence of past experiences is confirmed by the findings. Parents who experienced strict discipline in their own childhood are significantly more likely than those who did not, to prefer that children should be seen, not heard. This trend is compatible with the influence of past socialization on parental preferences for best discipline method discussed earlier.

Open Demonstration of Affection

One of the issues covered on child upbringing practices was parents' open demonstration of affection to their children. Parents were asked whether they "always," "only sometimes," or "never" expressed affection to their children by hugging, kissing, and holding them. The manner in which one expresses emotions and affection is shaped not only by one's personality and other individual characteristics, but also by the values and norms of one's culture in terms of the sense of propriety and social expectations of role performance. As indicated in Table 3 (column d), the probability of parents demonstrating affection to their children by hugging, kissing, and holding them, varies as expected, with the sociocontextual variables ethnicity, religion, gender, and education.

In contrast to Malay parents, Indian parents, or parents from other ethnic groups, Chinese parents are the least likely to demonstrate their affection by hugging, kissing, and holding their children. It is characteristic of traditional norms of propriety among the Chinese to be parsimonious in the open manifestation of emotions. This trend is particularly evident among Chinese parents who are Buddhist/Taoist compared to non-Buddhist/Taoist Chinese parents. Being a Buddhist or Taoist parent is associated with a 51 percent decrease in the odds of demonstrating affection to the children by hugging, kissing, and holding them. It is important to note that the absence of open demonstration of affection does not necessarily mean absence of affection. Like all world religions, Buddhism and Taoism stress the importance of love and harmony in the family and the duty of parents. Mothers are expected to love and care for their children to the point of being prepared to sacrifice their own lives to protect them. However, at the same time, Buddhism advocates strict self-discipline and equanimity in one's behavior (Morgan, 1996), virtues that lead to the perception of hugging, kissing, and holding loved ones as effusive behavior.

Significant variations in the probability of open demonstration of affection are also influenced by the parent's gender and education level. The inclination to openly demonstrate their affection to children is stronger among mothers than fathers. The influence of education also follows the expected direction. The higher the level of education of parents, the more likely they are to be openly affectionate with their children. Altogether, the variables in the model explained 23.6 percent of the variation in open demonstration of affection (Nagelkerke R Square = .236), with the variance in this dependent variable being predicted correctly 87 percent of the time.

Parenting Roles

Three parenting roles were included among the eight parenting styles (dependent variables) in this study: the mother's role, the father's role, and shared parenting. In the larger study, the respondents were shown a list of 14 duties and asked, "Most people have to deal with the many duties of running a home. Here is a list of some of those duties. Please tell me who is in charge of each duty in your home *most of the time,* that is, whether it is usually the wife, the husband, the children, grandparents, or someone else." Only the five duties that deal directly with parenting were incorporated in this analysis and are described in Table 2. These duties are: physical care of the children, disciplining the children, helping the children with schoolwork; talking to the teacher or school principal; and taking the children to the doctor. The two categories of these three dummy variables are: (0) none of the five duties, and (1) the performance of any or all of the five duties.

Mother's Role. Of the three roles, the model was most successful in predicting the mother's duties (or mother's role) that are performed by the wife/mother most of the time. The Nagelkerke R Square of .513 (Table 3, column e) suggests that 51.3 percent of the overall variation in the mother's role is predicted by the variables in the model. The model correctly predicted the mother's role 84.5 percent of the time. As expected, ethnicity and religion play a significant part in shaping the mother's role. In contrast to Chinese mothers and mothers from other ethnic groups, Malay and Indian mothers are the most likely to practice one or more of the five roles. This finding may be tentatively explained by anecdotal evidence indicating that the financial ability to hire child care assistance or domestic help appears to be higher among Singaporean Chinese mothers. Yet, religious affiliation introduces an important qualification. Not all Chinese mothers depend on hired child care. When religious affiliations of Chinese mothers is taken into account, Buddhist and Taoist mothers (all of whom are Chinese) are more likely to be busy with one or more of the mother's roles, compared to Chinese mothers who have other or no religious affiliation.

The developmental variables age and stage of the family life cycle are influential on mother's engagement in roles. Younger mothers (below the sample mean age of 46.6 years) are significantly more engaged in the five mother's roles compared to older mothers. This impact of age corresponds to the first two life cycle parental stages (Table 1) when the children (infants/preschoolers and school-age children) demand most attention.

Father's Roles. The model does not fare as well in the prediction of the father's role (Table 3, column f). As indicated by the Nagelkerke R Square, about 18 percent of the variation in father's role is explained by the variables in the model (variance was correctly predicted 71.5 percent of the time). The probability of fathers engaging in one or more of the five roles is higher among Indian fathers and non-Buddhist/Taoist fathers. Mothers differed from fathers in their report of fathers' role performance. In contrast to mothers, fathers are more inclined to perceive themselves as performing one of more of the five child upbringing roles.

It is noteworthy that of the eight dependent variables in the study, the variable "parents' job obligations" only contributes significantly to variation in father's role. Being part of a dual-earner couple, who works eight or more hours daily, is associated with a 46 percent increase in the probability of the father contributing to one of more of the five child upbringing roles. Adding the developmental dimension, the probability of the father's involvement in those roles is highest during the first two stages of the family life cycle (infants/preschoolers and school-age children).

Shared Parenting Roles. Shared parenting refers to the performance of the five roles by both parents jointly most of the time (see Table 2). As shown in Table 3, column g, shared parenting is least likely among Indian families, compared to families in other ethnic groups, and most likely among couples with high level of education. As in the case of the father's role, fathers tend to differ from mothers in their perception of their contribution to the five roles. The stage of the family life cycle is significant: shared parenting is least likely to occur at the two late stages, characterized by the presence of young or mature adult children. The variables in the model help to predict 22 percent of the variation in shared parenting (variance predicted correctly 77.8 percent of the time).

Family-School Cooperation

A substantial aspect of child upbringing has to do with the school given that, among other things, the school is where children spend the largest proportion of their time from age six (or earlier, if play, school, and kindergarten are included) to age 18 or 19. American studies have shown that parent-teacher cooperation constitutes a positive factor in the child's academic achievement and/or behavior (Izzo, Weissberg, Kasprow, & Fendrich, 1999; McNeal, 2001) despite cultural differences in targeted school outcomes and approaches between parents and teachers (Diamond, 1999; Greenfield, Quiroz, & Raeff, 2000). A list of nine aspects of child upbringing was shown to the parents, and they were asked to indicate which of those aspects should be left entirely to the family, entirely to the school, to both family and school together, or should be left to the children to learn by themselves (see Table 2).

The variables in the model predict 13.2 percent of the variation in family-school cooperation (variance was correctly predicted 63.2 percent of the time) as indicated in Table 3, column h. Two sociocontextual variables are significant in the prediction of family-school cooperation: ethnicity and level of formal education. The main contrast in attitudes toward family-school cooperation was found between Chinese and Malay parents. In contrast to Malay parents, Chinese parents are significantly more inclined to favor family-school cooperation. The impact of education is in the predicted direction: the higher the level of education of the parents, the more likely they are to favor family-school cooperation.

CONCLUSION

The model appears to work best for the prediction of parenting roles, especially the mother's role, and the open demonstration of affection, in that order. In general, the influence of culture, operationalized as ethnicity and religious affiliation, has been found as predicted. The values, beliefs, and customs associated with of parents' ethnic group identity and religious affiliation significantly influence seven of the eight parenting styles discussed in this paper.

Thus, the impact of culture is modified, but not eliminated by other variables in the model, especially gender and level of education. In their study of families in Canada, McDaniel and Tepperman (2000:194) found that "people within cultural and class groups are becoming more different, while groups as a whole become more similar." The Singapore data suggest that education diminishes somewhat the cultural differences in parenting styles among Chinese, Malay, and Indian Singaporeans, but the cultural differences (as a combination of ethnic identity and religious affiliation) prevail.

Finally, the analysis is useful, not only for the variables found significant, but also for the expected influences that did not occur. Parental job obligations were not as influential as expected, with the only effect on a parental approach being on the father's role. One may speculate that this was due to the strong tendency to follow traditional role obligations in Singapore (Quah, 1998) in which women tend to perform most if not all household and child care duties (Quah, 1999). Consequently, employed mothers appear to handle job obligations in a manner that fails to interrupt their parental obligations in a serious way. The number of children was another variable that, against expectations, did not influence any of the parenting styles except the perception of the best discipline method. This might be due to the narrow variation (mean = 2.67; SD = 1.08) of the number of children within families in Singapore.

REFERENCES

Bodman, D., & Peterson, G. W. (1995). Parenting processes. In R. D. Day, K. Gilbert, B. Settles & W. R. Burr (Eds.), *Research and theory in family science* (pp. 205-225). Pacific Grove, CA: Brooks & Cole.

Broderick, C. (1993). *Understanding family process: Basics of family systems theory.* Newbury Park, CA: Sage.

Cuyvers, P. (2000). You can't have it all–at least at the same time: Segmentation in the modern life course as a threat to intergenerational communication and solidarity. In S. Trnka (Ed.), *Family issues between generations* (pp. 30-43). Luxembourg: European Commission.

Diamond, J. B. (1999). Beyond social class: Cultural resources and educational participation among low-income Black parents. *Berkeley Journal of Sociology, 1999-2000, 44,* 15-54.

Fernandez-Gordon, J. A. (2000). Youth as a transition to full autonomy. *Family Observer, 3,* 4-11.

Glazer, N. (2000). Disaggregating culture. In L. E. Harrison, & S. P. Huntington (Eds.), *Culture matters: How values shape human progress* (pp. 219-230). New York: Basic Books.

Greenfield, P. M., Quiroz, B., & Raeff, C. (2000). Cross-cultural conflict and harmony in the social construction of the child. *New Directions for Child and Adolescent Development, 87,* 93-108.

Izzo, C. V., Weissberg, R. P., Kasprow, W. J., & Fendrich, M. (1999). A longitudinal assessment of teacher perceptions of parental involvement in children's education and school performance. *American Journal of Community Psychology, 27,* 817-839.

Khademian, A. M. (2002). *Working with culture: The way the job gets done in public programs.* Washington, DC: CQ Press.

King, S. H. (1962). *Perceptions of illness and medical practice.* New York: Russell Sage Foundation.

Klute, M. M., Crouter, A. C., Sayer, A. G., & McHale, S. M. (2001). Occupational self-direction, values, and egalitarian relationships: A study of dual-earner couples. *Journal of Marriage and the Family, 64,* 139-151.

Kohn, M. L. (1969). *Class and conformity. A study in values.* Homewood, IL: Dorsey Press.

Kohn, M. L., & Schooler, C. (1983). *Work and personality. An inquiry into the impact of social stratification.* Norwood, NJ: Ablex.

Kohn, M. L., & Slomczynski, K. M. (1990). *Social structure and self-direction: A comparative analysis of the United States and Poland.* Oxford, UK: Basil Blackwell.

Leow, B. G. (2001). *Census of population 2000: Demographic characteristics.* Singapore: Singapore Department of Statistics.

McDaniel, S. A., & Tepperman, L. (2000). *Close relations. An introduction to the sociology of families.* Scarborough, Canada: Prentice-Hall.

McNeal, R. B. (2001). Differential effects of parental involvement on cognitive and behavioral outcomes by socioeconomic status. *Journal of Socio-Economics, 30,* 171-179.

Morgan, P. (1996). Buddhism. In P. Morgan & C. Lawton (Eds.), *Ethical issues in six religious traditions* (pp. 55-98). Edinburgh: Edinburgh University Press.

Peterson, G. W., & Hann, D. (1999). Socializing children and parents in families. In M. B. Sussman, S. K. Steinmetz, & Peterson, G. W. (Eds.), *Handbook of marriage and the family* (2nd Ed.) (pp. 327-370). New York: Plenum Press.

Quah, S. R. (1998). *Family in Singapore. Sociological perspectives.* Singapore: Times Academic Press.

Quah, S. R. (1999). *Study on the Singapore family.* Singapore: MCDS.

Quah, S. R. (2002). Conceptualizing ethnicity: In search of cognitive innovations. In N. Genov (Ed.), *Advances in sociological knowledge* (pp. 284-311). Paris: International Social Science Council.

Sanders, D., & Brynin, M. (1998). Ordinary least squares and logistic regression analysis. In E. Scarbrough & E. Tanenbaum (Eds.), *Research strategies in the social sciences. A guide to new approaches* (pp. 29-52). Oxford, UK: Oxford University Press.

Weber, M. (1978). *Economy and society.* Berkeley, CA: University of California Press.

Windebank, J. (2001). Dual-earner couples in Britain and France: Gender divisions of domestic labor and parenting work in different welfare states. *Work, Employment and Society, 15,* 269-290.

Cross-National Perspectives on Parental Acceptance-Rejection Theory

Ronald P. Rohner
Abdul Khaleque
David E. Cournoyer

ABSTRACT. Parental acceptance-rejection theory (PARTheory) is a theory of socialization that seeks to predict and explain major causes, consequences, and other correlates of parental acceptance-rejection worldwide. In effect, the theory searches for verifiable universals in parent-child relations insofar as these universals relate to issues surrounding perceived parental acceptance-rejection. In this article, we focus on four major issues within the theory. First, we review the common meaning-structure used by children cross-nationally to assess the extent to which they are accepted or rejected by their parents. Second, we describe the apparently universal psychological outcome of experiencing specific degrees of parental acceptance or rejection. Third, we review sociocultural factors that tend to be associated cross-nationally with variations in parental acceptance-rejection. Finally, we review other sociocultural factors, especially expressive correlates such as a people's institutionalized religious beliefs, that are known to be associated cross-nationally (universally) with perceived acceptance-rejection. *[Article copies available for a fee from The Haworth Document Delivery Service: 1-800-HAWORTH. E-mail address: <docdelivery@haworthpress.com> Website:*

Ronald P. Rohner and Abdul Khaleque are affiliated with the Ronald and Nancy Rohner Center for the Study of Parental Acceptance and Rejection, University of Connecticut. David E. Cournoyer is affiliated with the School of Social Work and the Ronald and Nancy Rohner Center for the Study of Parental Acceptance and Rejection, University of Connecticut.

Address correspondence to: Ronald P. Rohner, Ronald and Nancy Rohner Center for the Study of Parental Acceptance and Rejection, University of Connecticut, U-2058 School of Family Studies, Storrs, CT 06269-2058 (E-mail: Rohner@uconn.edu).

http://www.haworthpress.com/store/product.asp?sku=J002
© 2003 by The Haworth Press, Inc. All rights reserved.

10.1300/J002v35n03_06

<http://www.HaworthPress.com> © 2003 by The Haworth Press, Inc. All rights reserved.]

KEYWORDS. Cross cultural, parental acceptance-rejection, psychological adjustment, socialization

Parental acceptance-rejection theory (PARTheory) is a theory of socialization that attempts to predict and explain major causes, consequences, and other correlates of parental acceptance and rejection within the United States and worldwide (Rohner, 1975, 1986, 2003; Rohner & Rohner, 1980). Perhaps the most notable feature of the theory is its search for verifiable universals in parent-child relations as they relate to perceived parental acceptance-rejection, as well as its search for universal effects of the acceptance-rejection process (Cournoyer, 2000). In effect, this is a quest for identifying empirically derived generalization about human behavior–generalizations that can be shown to hold true across all races, languages, genders, cultures, ethnicities, and other such defining conditions of humankind. In order to achieve this objective, PARTheory researchers have spent more than four decades investigating the details of parent-child relations within a great many communities cross-nationally as well as parent-child relationships and developmental issues revealed in more than 200 ethnographies based on long-term participant observation research of anthropologists (Rohner, 1975; Rohner & Rohner, 1981).

This program of research has revealed a common meaning-structure used by children and adults everywhere to assess the extent to which they are loved (accepted) or not (rejected) by their parents and other attachment figures. This universal meaning-structure, described below, underlies the rich diversity of individualistic parenting styles found in communities throughout the world. This meaning-structure also tends to be associated with a specific set of psychological outcomes for children and adults. That is, individuals everywhere tend to respond in the same way psychologically to the experience of parental acceptance-rejection. These two issues of perceived parental acceptance-rejection and its psychological effects form a core portion of PARTheory, and constitute a major thrust of this article. Additionally, we review here cross-national evidence bearing on the question of why parents in some societies tend to be warmer and more loving than parents in other societies. And we review very briefly a few of the other sociocultural correlates–especially expressive correlates–known to be associated cross-nationally with perceived parental acceptance-rejection. First, however, it is important to describe the acceptance-rejection process, or what we call the warmth dimension of parenting.

THE WARMTH DIMENSION OF PARENTING

Parental acceptance and rejection are the basis for the "warmth" dimension of parenting. This is a dimension or continuum on which all humans can be placed because everyone during their childhood has experienced more or less love at the hands of major caregivers. Thus, the warmth dimension has to do with the quality of the affectional bond between parents and their children, and with the physical and verbal behaviors parents use to express these feelings. One end of the continuum is marked by parental acceptance, which refers to the warmth, affection, care, comfort, concern, nurturance, support, or simply love that parents can feel and express toward their children. The other end of the continuum is marked by parental rejection, which refers to the absence or significant withdrawal of these feelings and behaviors and by the presence of a variety of physically and psychologically hurtful behaviors and affects. The studies cited by Rohner and colleagues, above, reveals that parental rejection can be shown by any combination of four principal expressions: (1) cold and unaffectionate, the opposite of being warm and affectionate, (2) hostile and aggressive, (3) indifferent and neglecting, and (4) undifferentiated rejecting. Undifferentiated rejection refers to children's beliefs that their parents do not really care about them or love them, even though there might not be clear behavioral indicators that the parents are neglecting, unaffectionate, or aggressive toward them.

These behaviors are shown graphically in Figure 1. Elements to the left of the slash marks (warmth, hostility, and indifference) in the figure refer to internal, psychological feelings of the parents. That is, parents may feel warm (or cold and unloving) toward their children, or they may feel hostile, angry, bitter, resentful, irritable, impatient, or antagonistic toward them. Alternatively, parents may feel indifferent toward their children, feel unconcerned and uncaring about them, or have a restricted interest in their overall well-being. Elements to the right of the slash marks in the figure (affection, aggression, and neglect) refer to observable behaviors that result when parents act on these emotions. Thus, when parents act on their feelings of love, they are likely to be affectionate. As noted in the figure, parental affection can be shown either physically (e.g., hugging, kissing, caressing, and comforting) or verbally (e.g., praising, complimenting, and saying nice things to or about the child). These and many other caring, nurturing, supportive, and loving behaviors help define the behavioral expressions of parental acceptance.

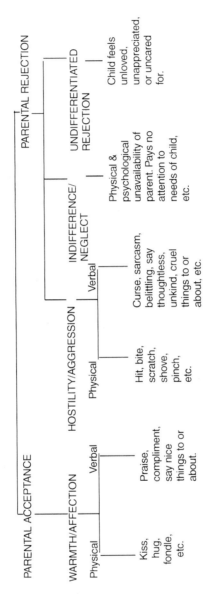

FIGURE 1. The Warmth Dimension of Parenting

When parents act on feelings of hostility, anger, resentment, or enmity, the resulting behavior is generally called aggression. As construed in PARTheory, aggression is any behavior where there is the intention of hurting someone, something, or oneself. Figure 1 shows that parents may be physically aggressive (e.g., hitting, pushing, throwing things, and pinching) and verbally aggressive (e.g., sarcastic, cursing, mocking, shouting, saying thoughtless, humiliating, or disparaging things to or about the child). Additionally, parents may use hurtful, nonverbal symbolic gestures toward their children.

The connection between indifference as an internal motivator and neglect as a behavioral response is not as direct as the connection between hostility and aggression. This is true because parents may neglect their children for many reasons that have nothing to do with indifference. For example, parents may neglect their children as a way of trying to cope with their anger toward them. Neglect is not simply a matter of failing to provide for the material and physical needs of children, however. It also pertains to parents' failure to attend appropriately to children's social and emotional needs. Often, for example, neglecting parents pay little attention to children's needs for comfort, solace, help, or attention. They may also remain physically as well as psychologically unresponsive or even unavailable or inaccessible. All these behaviors–individually and collectively–are likely to induce children to feel unloved or rejected.

Even in warm and loving families, however, children are likely to experience, at least occasionally, a few of these hurtful emotions and behaviors. Thus, it is important to be aware that parental acceptance- rejection can be viewed and studied from either of two perspectives. That is, acceptance-rejection can be studied as perceived or subjectively experienced by the child (the phenomenological perspective), or it can be studied as reported by a second person (the behavioral perspective). Usually, but not always, the two perspectives lead to similar conclusions. Results of PARTheory research suggest, however, that if the conclusions are very discrepant, one should generally trust information derived from the phenomenological perspective. This is true because a child may feel unloved (as in undifferentiated rejection), but outside observers may fail to detect any observable indicators of parental rejection.

Alternatively, observers may report a significant amount of parental aggression or neglect, but the child may not feel rejected. This occurs with some regularity in reports of child abuse and neglect. Thus, there is a problematic relation between official reports of abuse, rejection, and neglect on the one hand and children's perceptions of parental acceptance-rejection on the other. As Kagan (1978: 57) put it, "parental rejection is not a specific set of actions by parents but a belief held by the child."

In effect, much of parental acceptance-rejection is symbolic. Therefore, to understand why rejection has consistent effects cross-nationally, one must understand its symbolic nature. Certainly in the context of ethnic and cross-national studies, one must be sensitive to people's symbolic, culturally based interpretations of parents' love-related behaviors. That is, even though parents everywhere may express, to some degree, acceptance (warmth, affection, care, concern) and rejection (coldness, lack of affection, hostility, aggression, indifference, neglect), the way they do it is highly variable and saturated with cultural or sometimes idiosyncratic meaning. For example, parents anywhere might praise or compliment their children, but the way in which they do it in one sociocultural setting might have no meaning (or might have a totally different meaning) in a second setting. This is illustrated in the following incident:

> A few years ago, the senior author, Rohner, interviewed a high caste Hindu woman about family matters in India. Another woman seated nearby distracted my attention. The second woman quietly and carefully peeled an orange and then removed the seeds from each segment. Her 9-year-old daughter became increasingly animated as her mother progressed. Later, my Bengali interpreter asked me if I had noticed what the woman was doing. I answered that I had, but that I had not paid much attention to it. "Should I have?" "Well," she answered, "you want to know about parental love and affection in West Bengal, so you should know. . . ." She went on to explain that when a Bengali mother wants to praise her child–to show approval and affection for her child–she might give the child a peeled and seeded orange. Bengali children understand completely that their mothers have done something special for them, even though mothers may not use words of praise, for to do so would be unseemly, much like praising themselves. (Rohner, 1994:113; see also Rohner & Chaki-Sircar, 1988)

In everyday American English, the word rejection implies bad parenting and sometimes even bad people. In cross-national and multiethnic research, however, one must attempt to view the word as being descriptive of parents' behavior, not judgmental or evaluative. This is so because parents in about 25% of the world's societies behave in ways that are consistent with the definition of rejection given here (Rohner, 1975; Rohner & Rohner, 1981). However, in the great majority of cases, including the United States, these parents behave toward their children the way they believe good, responsible parents should behave, as defined by cultural norms. Therefore, in the context of cross-national research on parental acceptance-rejection, a major goal is to determine whether children everywhere respond the same way when they experience themselves to be accepted or rejected.

PARTHEORY'S PERSONALITY SUBTHEORY

PARTheory's personality subtheory attempts to predict and explain major personality, and psychological or mental health-related consequences of perceived parental acceptance and rejection. The subtheory begins with the probably untestable assumption that over the course of evolution humans have developed the enduring, biologically based emotional need for positive response from the people most important to them. The need for positive response includes an emotional wish, desire, or yearning (whether consciously recognized or not) for comfort, support, care, concern, nurturance, and the like. In adulthood, the need becomes more complex and differentiated to include the wish (recognized or unrecognized) for positive regard from people with whom one has an affectional bond of attachment. People who can best satisfy this need are typically parents for infants and children, but include significant others and non-parental attachment figures for adolescents and adults. From the global perspective emphasized in PARTheory, a parent is any person who has more-or-less long-term, primary caregiving responsibility for a child. This person may be a mother, father, grandparent, other relative, or even a non-kinsperson such as a foster parent or parent surrogate in an institutional setting.

As construed in PARTheory, a "significant other" is any person with whom a child has a relatively long-lasting emotional tie, who is uniquely important to the child, and who is interchangeable with no one else. In this sense, parents are generally significant others, but parents also tend to have one additional quality not shared by most significant others. That is, children's sense of emotional security and comfort tends to be dependent on the quality of their relationship with their parents. Because of that, parents are usually the kind of significant other called attachment figures in both PARTheory and attachment theory (Ainsworth, 1989; Bowlby, 1982; Colin, 1996). Thus, parents are uniquely important to children because the security and other emotional and psychological states of offspring are dependent on the quality of relationship with their parent(s). It is for this reason that parental acceptance and rejection is postulated in PARTheory to have unparalleled influence in shaping children's personality development over time. Indeed, PARTheory argues that children's experiences of parental acceptance-rejection are likely to have greater developmental consequences than any other single parental influence.

Personality, as defined in personality subtheory, is an individual's more or less stable set of predispositions to respond (i.e., affective, cognitive, perceptual, and motivational dispositions) and actual modes of responding (i.e., observable behaviors) in various life situations or contexts. This definition recognizes that behavior is motivated or influenced by external factors (e.g., environmental) as well as internal factors (e.g., emotional, biological, and learning) and usually has regularity or orderliness about it across time and space. PARTheory's personality subtheory postulates that the emotional need for positive response from significant others and attachment figures is a powerful motivator, and when children do not get this need satisfied adequately by their parents, they are predisposed to respond emotionally and behaviorally in specific ways. According to the subtheory, rejected children are likely to feel anxious and insecure. In an attempt to allay these feelings and to satisfy their needs, rejected children often increase their bids for positive response, but only up to a point. That is, they tend to become more dependent, as shown in Figure 2.

The term "dependence" in the theory refers to the internal, psychologically felt wish or yearning for emotional (as opposed to instrumental or task-oriented) support, care, comfort, attention, nurturance, and similar behaviors from attachment figures. The term also refers to the actual behavioral bids children make for such responsiveness. For young children, these bids may include clinging to parents, whining or crying when parents unexpectedly depart, and seeking physical proximity with them when they return. In times of distress, older children and adolescents may express their need for positive response more symbolically by seeking reassurance, approval, or support, as well as comfort, affection, or solace from people who are most important to them. Dependence is construed in PARTheory as a continuum, with independence defining one end of the continuum and dependence the other. Independent children, are those who have their need for positive response met sufficiently so that they are free from frequent or intense yearning or behavioral bids for succor from significant others. Very dependent children on the other hand are those who have a frequent and intense desire for positive response, and are likely to make many bids for response. As with all the personality dispositions continuum studied in PARTheory, humans can be placed somewhere along the of being more or less dependent or independent. According to the theory, much of the variation in dependence among children is contingent on the extent to which they perceive themselves to be accepted or rejected. Many rejected children feel the need for constant reassurance and emotional support.

FIGURE 2. Dependence/Independence in Relation to Parental Acceptance-Rejection

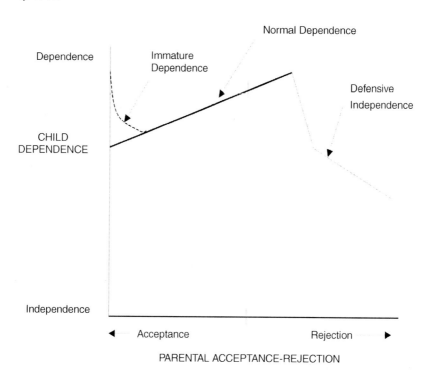

According to personality subtheory, parental rejection also leads to other personality outcomes, in addition to dependence. These include: hostility, aggression, passive aggression, or psychological problems with the management of hostility and aggression; emotional unresponsiveness; immature dependence or defensive independence depending on the form, frequency, duration, and intensity of perceived rejection and parental control; impaired self-esteem; impaired self-adequacy; emotional instability; and negative worldview. Theoretically, these dispositions are expected to emerge because of the intense psychological pain produced by rejection. More specifically, beyond a certain point that varies from individual to individual, children who experience significant rejection are likely to feel ever-increasing anger, resentment, and other destructive emotions that may become intensely painful. As a result, many rejected children emotionally close down in an effort to protect themselves from the hurt of further rejection, and they become less emotionally responsive. In so doing, they often have problems being able or willing to express love and in knowing how to or even being capable of accepting it from others.

Because of all this psychological hurt, some rejected children, especially during adolescence, become defensively independent. Defensive independence is like healthy independence in that youths make relatively few behavioral bids for positive response. It is unlike healthy indepen- dence, however, in that defensively independent youths continue to crave warmth and support–positive responses–though they sometimes do not recognize or admit it. Indeed, because of the overlay of anger, distrust, and other negative emotions generated by chronic rejection, they often positively deny this need, saying in effect, "To hell with you! I don't need you. I don't need anybody!" Defensive independence with its associated emotions and behaviors sometimes leads to a process of counter rejection, where rejected youths reject the person(s) who reject them. Not surprisingly, this process sometimes escalates into a cycle of violence.

In addition to dependence or defensive independence, rejected children are predicted in PARTheory's personality subtheory to develop feelings of impaired self-esteem and impaired self-adequacy. This comes about because, as noted in symbolic interaction theory (Cooley, 1902; Mead, 1934), individuals tend to view themselves as they think their parents or significant others view them. Thus, children and adults who feel that their attachment figures do not love them are likely to feel they are unlovable, perhaps even unworthy of being loved.

Whereas self-esteem pertains to children's feelings of self-worth or value, self-adequacy pertains to their feelings of competence or mastery to perform daily tasks adequately and to satisfy their own instrumental (task-oriented) needs. When children feel they are not very good people, they are also apt to feel they are not very good at satisfying their personal needs and tend to think less well of themselves more globally.

Anger, negative self-feelings, and the other consequences of perceived rejection tend to diminish rejected children's capacity to deal effectively with stress. Because of this, rejected children often tend to be less emotionally stable than those who feel accepted. They often become emotionally upset, even tearful or angry when confronted with stressful situations that accepted youths are able to handle with greater emotional equanimity. All these acutely painful feelings associated with perceived rejection tend to induce children to develop a negative worldview. PARTheory suggest that rejected children are likely to develop a view of the world as being hostile, unfriendly, emotionally unsafe, threatening, or dangerous. These thoughts and feelings often extend to youths' beliefs about the nature of the supernatural world (Rohner, 1975, 1986).

Negative worldview, negative self-esteem, negative self-adequacy, and some of the other personality dispositions described above are important elements in the social-cognition or mental representations of rejected children. In PARTheory, the concept of mental representation refers to an individual's more-or-less coherent but usually implicit conception of reality. The conception consists largely of generalizations about self, others, and the experiential world constructed from emotionally significant past and current experiences. Along with one's emotional state, which both influences and is influenced by one's conception of reality, mental representations tend to shape the way in which children perceive, construe, and react to new experiences, including interpersonal relationships. Mental representations also influence what and how children store and remember experiences (Baldwin, 1992; Clausen, 1972; Crick & Dodge, 1994; Epstein, 1994).

Once created, children's mental representations of self, of significant others, and of the world around them tend to induce them to seek or to avoid certain situations and kinds of people. In effect, the way children think about themselves and their world shapes the way they live their lives. This is most notably true of rejected children. For example, many rejected children have a tendency to perceive hostility where there is none, or to devalue their sense of personal worth in the face of strong counter-information. Moreover, rejected youths are likely to seek, create, interpret, or perceive experiences, situations, and relationships in ways that are consistent with their distorted mental representations. And they often tend to avoid or mentally reinterpret situations that are inconsistent with these representations. Additionally, rejected children often construct mental images of personal relationships as being unpredictable, untrustworthy, and perhaps hurtful. This mental representation may be carried forward into new relationships where rejected youths find it difficult to trust others emotionally, or where they may become hyper vigilant and hypersensitive to any slights or signs of emotional undependability. Because of all this selective attention, selective perception, faulty styles of causal attribution, and distorted cognitive information processing, rejected children everywhere are expected in PARTheory to self-propel along qualitatively different developmental pathways from accepted or loved children.

A meta-analysis of 43 studies containing a total of 7,563 respondents cross-nationally (Khaleque & Rohner, 2002)[1] supports the major postulates of PARTheory's personality subtheory. In fact, every study in the sample reached the same conclusion: The experience of parental acceptance (or rejection) tended to be associated with the form of psychological adjustment (or maladjustment) just described in personality subtheory.[2] Additionally, results showed no significant heterogeneity in effect sizes in different samples cross-nationally or within U.S. ethnic groups.

At a more general level, results of cross-national research with over 14,000 respondents in more than 100 studies (Rohner, 2003; Rohner & Britner, 2002), including the 43 studies mentioned in the meta-analysis, lend substantial support to PARTheory's expectations shown graphically in Figure 3. That is, PARTheory expects that within a band of individual variation, children's mental health status is likely to become impaired in direct proportion to the frequency, severity, and duration of rejection experienced.

Some individuals who come from loving families, however, also display the constellation of psychological problems typically shown by rejected youths. These people, termed "troubled" in PARTheory's personality subtheory, generally appear to have less than satisfying interpersonal relationships with non-parental attachment figures (Rohner & Khaleque, 2003). Finally, PARTheory expects that a small minority of children and adolescents will be able to thrive emotionally despite having experienced significant rejection by parents. As shown in Figure 3, these youths are called copers. They are the focus of PARTheory's coping subtheory, discussed in Rohner (1986).

PARTHEORY'S SOCIOCULTURAL SYSTEMS MODEL AND SUBTHEORY

Parental acceptance-rejection occurs in a complex ecological (familial, community, and sociocultural) context. PARTheory's sociocultural systems model shown in Figure 4 provides a way of thinking about the antecedents, consequence, and other correlates of parental acceptance-rejection within individuals and total societies. The model shows, for example, that the likelihood of parents (element 3 in the model) displaying any given form of behavior (e.g., acceptance-rejection) is shaped in important ways by the maintenance systems of that society. This maintenance system includes family structure, household organization, economic organization, political organization, system of defense, and other institutions that bear directly on the survival of a culturally organized population within its natural environment (element 1 in the model). The model also shows that parents accepting-rejecting and other behaviors impact directly on children's personality development and behavior (as postulated in personality subtheory).

FIGURE 3. Copers and Troubled Individuals in Relation to PARTheory's Personality Subtheory

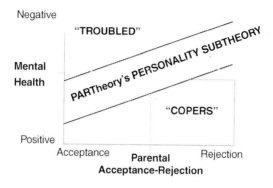

The double-headed arrow in the model, indicating interaction, shows that personal characteristics of children such as their temperament and behavioral dispositions shape, to a significant extent, the form and quality of parents' behavior toward them. In addition to family experiences, the arrows in the model also reveal that youths have a wide variety of often-influential experiences (element 5, intervening developmental experiences) in the context of the natural environment in which they live, the maintenance systems of their society, peers, and adults in the community (element 6), and the institutionalized expressive systems of their society (element 7).

Institutionalized expressive systems and behaviors refer to the religious traditions and behaviors of a people, to their artistic traditions and preferences, to their musical and folkloric traditions and preferences, and to other such symbolic, mostly non-utilitarian, and nonsurvival-related beliefs and behaviors. They are called "expressive" in PARTheory because they are believed to express or reflect people's internal, psychological states, at least initially when the expressive systems were first created. Thus, expressive systems are believed in PARTheory to be symbolic creations, created over time by multiple individuals within a society. As the people change, the expressive systems and behaviors also tend to change, especially if the systems have been codified in writing. It is important to note that according to sociocultural systems subtheory, expressive systems are ultimately human creations, that once created and incorporated into the sociocultural system, tend to loop back on individuals, shaping their future beliefs and behaviors.

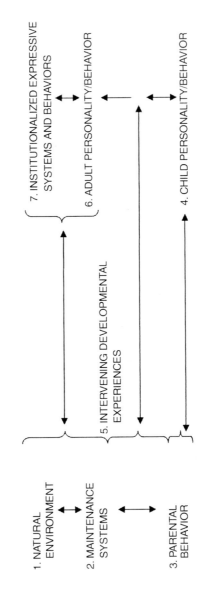

FIGURE 4. PARtheory's Sociocultural Systems Model

Guided by the sociocultural systems model, PARTheory's sociocultural systems subtheory attempts to predict and explain worldwide causes of parental acceptance and rejection. Among other questions, the subtheory asks why parents in the great majority of societies described by anthropologists in cross-cultural surveys using two large samples of the world's known and adequately described sociocultural systems[3] (Rohner, 1975, 1986; Rohner & Rohner, 1981), tend to be warm and loving, but in about 25% of the world's societies, they tend to be mildly to severely rejecting. To illustrate, Arab Sudanese parents living in the community of Buurri Al Lamaab (Barclay, 1964) are described by anthropologists as being typically warm and loving, as are Serbs living in the community of Orasac (Halpern, 1958), Taiwanese in the community of Hsin Hsing (Gallin, 1966), and rural Australians living in Mallee Town (Oester & Emery, 1954). Contrasting sharply with these loving styles of parenting, as described by anthropologists, is the rejecting style characteristic of Colombian Mestizo living in the community of Aritama (Reichel-Dolmatoff & Reichel-Dolmatoff, 1961), Palauans living on the South Pacific island of Babeldaob (Barnett, 1960), and the Alorese living in the Indonesian community of Atimelang (Dubois, 1944).

What factors account for these cross-national differences and for individual variations in parenting within different societies cross-nationally? The more complex the sociocultural system, the more likely children are to be rejected (Rohner, 1975, 1986). Every industrialized nation of the world for which adequate information is available appears to have significant problems with parental rejection and other forms of child maltreatment. On the other hand, virtually all the most technologically simple people, those for whom hunting provides the primary mode of subsistence, such as the traditional Greenland Eskimo (Mirskly, 1937), tend to be warm and loving toward their children (Levinson, 1989; Rohner, 1975).

True hunters such as the Eskimo or the Plains Indians in the United States during aboriginal times–the Cheyenne Indians, for example–not only did not reject their children, but could not reject them if that kind of society was to survive, because rejection produces characteristics that are probably maladaptive for successful hunting. It seems plausible, for example, that personality dispositions such as emotional stability, positive feelings of self-adequacy and self-esteem, a sense of self-determination, and a positive worldview–all of which are associated with parental acceptance–are more adaptive in a hunting context than are their contraries. Persons who have these dispositions can, psychologically, more easily leave the security of the campsite to go on a food quest in an often hazardous, demanding, and uncertain environment. Insofar as they are successful, their families are likely to survive, their children are more likely to reach reproductive age, to marry, and to bear children of their own–and to raise their children in the way they had been raised, with warmth and affection.

Hunters who have been seriously rejected do not have this constellation of adaptive personality traits. As a result, one might expect the families of these people to fare less well over time than families of accepted hunters who have a selective advantage, in a Darwinian sense (Konner, 1982). Fewer offspring of the rejecting hunters reach childbearing age. Those who do and who treat their own children as they have been treated (that is, rejected) place their offspring at risk. As the generations pass, fewer and fewer of these people survive to perpetuate the rejection cycle. The net effect is–if rejecting hunters ever existed in the course of human evolution over the past several million years–they have now vanished in favor of the adaptive "accepting" style of parenting.

At a more personal level, conditions that promote the breakdown of primary emotional relationships and social supports are also among the significant factors associated cross-nationally with the incidence of parental rejection. Thus, young, economically deprived single parents, most often mothers, living in social isolation without social and emotional supports, appear to be at greatest risk for withdrawing love and affection from their children (Rohner, 1986). It is useful to note that from a global perspective, poverty, by itself, is not necessarily associated with increased rejection. Rather, it is poverty in association with these other social and emotional conditions that place children at greatest risk.

In addition to predicting and explaining worldwide causes of parental acceptance-rejection, PARTheory's sociocultural systems subtheory also attempts to predict and explain expressive correlates of parental acceptance and rejection. As the subtheory predicts, there is substantial cross-national evidence to suggest that in societies where children tend to be rejected, cultural beliefs about the supernatural world usually portray supernaturals as being malevolent, i.e., hostile, treacherous, unpredictable, capricious, destructive, or negative in some other way (Levinson & Malone, 1980; Rohner, 1975, 1986; see also Dickie, Eshleman, Merasco, Shepard, Venderwilt, & Johnson, 1997).

However, the supernatural world is usually thought to be benevolent (warm, supportive, generous, protective, or kindly in some other way) in societies where most children are raised with loving acceptance. No doubt these cultural differences are the result of aggregated individual differences in the mental representations of accepted versus rejected people within these two different kinds of societies. Parental acceptance and rejection are also known to be associated cross-nationally with many other expressive sociocultural correlates such as the artistic traditions characteristic of individual societies, as well as the artistic preferences of individuals within these societies (Rohner & Frampton, 1982). Additionally, evidence suggests that the recreational and occupational choices adults make may be associated with childhood experiences of acceptance and rejection

(Aronoff, 1967; Mantell, 1974; Rohner, 1986). All these and other expressive behaviors and beliefs appear to be byproducts of the emotional and social-cognitive effects of parental acceptance-rejection discussed earlier.

CONCLUSION

The quest in PARTheory for cross-nationally valid principles of behavior is based on the assumption that with a scientific understanding of the worldwide antecedents, consequences, and other correlates of parental acceptance-rejection comes the possibility of formulating culture-fair and practicable programs, policies, and interventions affecting families and children everywhere. Social policies and programs of prevention, intervention, and treatment based on idiosyncratic beliefs at a particular point in history are likely to prove unworkable for some and probably even prejudicial for many populations. Policies and programs based on demonstrable principles of human behavior, however, stand a good chance of working as nations and people change.

It is thoughts such as these that motivated a great part of PARTheory research. Now, after more than four decades of research with more than 14,000 children, adolescents, and adults in many nations internationally and with members of every major American ethnic group, we feel confident in drawing at least two overarching conclusions. First, the same classes of behaviors appear universally to convey the symbolic message that "my parent (or other attachment figure) loves me" (or does not love me, care about me, want me, i.e., rejects me). These classes of behavior include the perception of warmth/affection, hostility/aggression, indifference/neglect, and undifferentiated rejection, as defined at the beginning of this article. Second, differences in nationality, ethnicity, social class, race, gender, and other such factors do not exert enough influence to override the apparently universal tendency for youths everywhere to respond in essentially the same way when they perceive themselves to be accepted or rejected by their parents. Having said this, however, we must also stress that the association between perceived acceptance-rejection and psychological outcomes for youths is far from perfect. Part of the unexplained variability in these relations no doubt results from sociocultural and other such influences. Nonetheless, results of almost all research completed so far are so robust and stable cross-nationally that we believe professionals everywhere should feel confident in developing policies and practice-applications based on the central tenets of PARTheory, especially PARTheory's personality subtheory.

NOTES

1. The sample consisted of 848 African Americans, 357 Asian Americans, 3,660 European Americans and 100 Hispanic Americans. The remainder of the sample came from Africa (Egypt and Nigeria; $N = 593$), Asia (Bahrain, Pakistan, India, China, Japan, and Korea; $N = 508$), Europe (Czechoslovakia, England, Greece, and Italy; $N = 739$), and South America and the Caribbean (Mexico, Peru, and St. Kitts, West Indies; $N = 748$). All studies in the sample used one or more versions of the Parental Acceptance-Rejection Questionnaire and the Personality Assessment Questionnaire (Rohner, 2003).

2. An analysis of fail-safe N (Cooper, 1979; Rosenthal, 1979) in the meta-analysis showed that 3,433 additional studies, all with nonsignificant results, would be required to disconfirm the conclusion that perceived acceptance-rejection is panculturally associated with children's psychological adjustment.

3. One sample consisted of the ethnographies of 101 societies and formed the basis of *They Love Me, They Love Me Not* (Rohner, 1975). A description of the methodology used in this holocultural research is described in the book. The second sample, consisting of 186 societies, is the widely-used "standard cross-cultural sample" developed by G. P. Murdock and D. White (Murdock's) *Outline of Cultural Materials*. Details about the sample and coding process are reported in the Rohner and Rohner (1981). Results from both samples are reported in *The Warmth Dimension* (Rohner, 1986). In both samples the actual ethnographies, not HRAF materials are used.

REFERENCES

Ainsworth, M. D. S. (1989). Attachment beyond infancy. *American Psychologist, 44*, 709-716.

Aronoff, J. (1967). *Psychological needs and cultural systems: A case study*. Princeton, NJ: D. Van Nostrand.

Baldwin, M. W. (1992). Relational schemas and the processing of societal information. *Psychological Bulletin, 112*, 461-484.

Barclay, H. B. (1964). *Buurri Al Lamaab: A suburban village in the Sudan*. Ithaca: Cornell University Press.

Barnett, H. (1960). *Being a Palauan*. New York: Holt, Rinehart and Winston.

Bowlby, J. (1982). *Attachment and Loss, Vol. 1: Attachment*, 2nd edition. New York: Basic Books.

Clausen, J. A. (1972). The life course of individuals. In M. W. Riley, M. Johnson, & A. Foner (Eds.), *Aging in society, 3*. New York: Russell Sage Foundation.

Colin, V. L. (1996). *Human attachment*. New York: McGraw-Hill.

Cooley, C. H. (1902). *Human nature and the social order*. New York: Scribner's.

Cooper, H. M. (1979). Statistically combining independent studies: A meta-analysis of sex differences in conformity research. *Journal of Personality and Social Psychology, 37*, 131-146.

Cournoyer, D. E. (2000). Universalist research: Examples drawing from the methods and findings of parental acceptance-rejection theory. In A. L. Comunian & U. Gielen (Eds.), *International Perspective on Human Development* (pp. 213-232). Berlin, Germany: Pabst Science Publishers.

Crick, N. R., & Dodge, K. A. (1994). A review and reformulation of social informa-tion-processing mechanisms in children's social adjustment. *Psychological Bulle-tin, 115*, 74-101.

Dickie, J. R., Eshleman, A. K., Merasco, D. M., Shepard, A., Venderwilt, M., & John-son, M. (1997). Parent-child relationships and children's images of God. *Journal for the Scientific Study of Religion, 36*, 25-43.

DuBois, C. (1944). *The people of Alor: A social-psychological study of an East Indian island.* Minneapolis: University of Minnesota Press.

Epstein, S. (1994). Integration of the cognitive and the psychodynamic unconscious. *American Psychologist, 49*, 709-724.

Gallin, B. (1966). *Hsin Hsing, Taiwan: A Chinese village in change.* Berkeley: Univer-sity of California Press.

Halpern, J. M. (1958). *A Serbian village.* New York: Columbia University Press.

Kagan, J. (1978). *The growth of the child: Reflections on human development.* New York: W.W. Norton.

Khaleque, A., & Rohner, R. P. (2002). Perceived parental acceptance-rejection and psychological adjustment: A meta-analysis of cross-cultural and intracultural stud-ies. *Journal of Marriage and the Family, 64*, 54-64.

Konner, M. (1982). *The tangled wing.* New York: Harper & Row.

Levinson, D. (1989). *Family violence in cross-cultural perspective.* Newbury Park, CA: Sage Publications.

Levinson, D., & Malone, M. J. (1980). *Toward explaining human culture: A critical re-view of the findings of worldwide cross-cultural research.* New Haven, CT: HRAF Press.

Mantell, D. (1974). *True Americanism: Green Berets and war resisters: A study of commitment.* New York: Teachers College Press.

Mead, G. H. (1934). *Mind, self, and society.* Chicago: University of Chicago Press.

Mirsky, J. (1937). *The Eskimo of Greenland.* In M. Mead (Ed.), *Cooperation and com-petition among primitive peoples* (pp. 51-81). New York, McGraw-Hill.

Oeser, O. A., & Emery, F. E. (1954). *Social structure and personality in a rural com-munity.* London: Routledge and Kegan Paul.

Reichel-Dolmatoff, G., & Reichel-Dolmatoff, A. (1961). *The people of Aritama: The cultural personality of a Colombian Mestizo village.* Chicago: University of Chi-cago Press.

Rohner, R. P. (1975). *They love me, they love me not: A worldwide study of the effects of parental acceptance and rejection.* New Haven, CT: HRAF Press (Available from Rohner Research Publications).

Rohner, R. P. (1986). *The warmth dimension: Foundations of parental acceptance-re-jection theory.* Beverly Hills, CA: Sage Publications, Inc. (Available from Rohner Research Publications).

Rohner, R. P. (1994). Patterns of parenting: The warmth dimension in cross-cultural perspective. In W. J. Lonner and R. S. Malpass (Eds.), *Readings in psychology and culture* (pp. 113-120). Needham Heights, MA: Allyn and Bacon.

Rohner, R. P. (2003). Parental acceptance-rejection bibliography. Retrieved February 5, 2003, from *http://vm.uconn.edu/~rohner/*

Rohner, R. P., & Britner, P. A. (2002). Worldwide mental health correlates of parental acceptance-rejection: Review of cross-cultural and intracultural evidence. *Cross-Cultural Research, 36,* 16-47.

Rohner, R. P., & Chaki-Sircar, M. (1988). *Women and children in a Bengali village.* Hanover, NH: University Press of New England.

Rohner, R. P., & Frampton, S. (1982). Perceived parental acceptance-rejection and artistic preference: An unexplained contradiction. *Journal of Cross-Cultural Psychology, 13,* 250-259.

Rohner, R. P., & Khaleque, A. (2003). Relations between partner acceptance and parental acceptance, behavioral control, and psychosocial adjustment among heterosexual adult women. Manuscript submitted for publication.

Rohner, R. P., & Rohner, E. C. (1980). Worldwide tests of parental acceptance-rejection theory. *Behavior Science Research, 15,* 1-88.

Rohner, R. P., & Rohner, E. C. (1981). Parental acceptance-rejection and parental control: Cross-cultural codes. *Ethnology, 20,* 245-260.

Rosenthal, R. (1979). The 'file drawer' problem and tolerance for null results. *Psychological Bulletin, 86,* 638-641.

A Multi-National Study of Interparental Conflict, Parenting, and Adolescent Functioning: South Africa, Bangladesh, China, India, Bosnia, Germany, Palestine, Colombia, and the United States

Kay Bradford
Brian K. Barber
Joseph A. Olsen
Suzanne L. Maughan
Lance D. Erickson
Deborah Ward
Heidi E. Stolz

ABSTRACT. This study assessed the associations between interparental conflict (IPC), parenting, and individual functioning among data gathered from school-going adolescents in *Bangladesh, China, India,*

Kay Bradford is affiliated with the University of Kentucky. Brian K. Barber is affiliated with the University of Tennessee. Joseph A. Olsen is affiliated with Brigham Young University. Suzanne L. Maughan is affiliated with the University of Nebraska at Kearney. Lance D. Erickson is affiliated with the University of North Carolina at Chapel Hill. Deborah Ward is affiliated with Aspen Systems. Heidi E. Stolz is affiliated with California State University, San Bernardino.

Address correspondence to: Kay Bradford, University of Kentucky, 319A Funkhouser, Lexington, KY 40506 (E-mail: kbrad@uky.edu).

This study was supported in part by a FIRST Award from the National Institute of Mental Health (R29-MH47067-03) to Brian K. Barber, with additional funding from the College of Family Home and Social Sciences, the Family Studies Center, and the Kennedy Center for International Studies, all at Brigham Young University.

http://www.haworthpress.com/store/product.asp?sku=J002
© 2003 by The Haworth Press, Inc. All rights reserved.

10.1300/J002v35n03_07

Bosnia, Germany, Palestine, Colombia, United States and three ethnic groups within South Africa. Specifically, we tested the validity of the spillover dynamic found in much research in the U.S., whereby marital conflict spills over into parenting and into the psychological and social functioning of children and adolescents. Previous analyses of these same data showed complete invariance in the linkages between parenting and adolescent functioning. This study thus provided a meaningful extension to the substantive literature on family processes. We followed recommendations within cross-cultural psychology to "transport and test" models validated in one culture to other cultures as an initial step in systematic comparative research. The findings revealed substantial invariance across the samples in documenting significant direct and indirect associations. Similar to prior research in the U.S., IPC was associated with youth outcomes directly, and more often indirectly, via parenting. *[Article copies available for a fee from The Haworth Document Delivery Service: 1-800-HAWORTH. E-mail address: <docdelivery@haworthpress.com> Website: <http://www.HaworthPress.com> © 2003 by The Haworth Press, Inc. All rights reserved.]*

KEYWORDS. Cross-cultural research, marital conflict, parenting, youth adjustment

INTRODUCTION

Parents' marital functioning is widely recognized as having significant impact on children's adjustment (Fincham, 1998). Research over the past decade has documented the "spillover," or carryover of marital interactions into parent-child relationships and child outcomes (Buehler, Anthony, Krishnakumar, Stone, Gerard, & Pemberton, 1997; Erel & Burman, 1995; Krishnakumar & Buehler, 2000). Marital conflict, often referred to as interparental conflict (IPC), has been associated with problems in child development both directly (e.g., Cummings, 1987; Emery, Fincham, & Cummings, 1992), and indirectly, through its effects on parenting (e.g., Buehler, Krishnakumar, Anthony, Tittsworth, & Stone, 1994; Fauber, Forehand, Thomas, & Wierson, 1990; Harold, Fincham, Osborne, & Conger, 1997; Stone, Buehler, & Barber, 2002). Scholars have noted, however, that these findings are based mostly on studies of European American families (Buehler et al., 1997; Krishnakumar & Buehler, 2000). There is a need to study diverse samples to better understand the extent to which these findings represent family functioning generally.

This study is one in a series of articles presenting data from a new multinational/ethnic group study of adolescents (Cross-National Adolescence Project [C-NAP]; Barber, Stolz, Olsen, & Maughan, 2003, under review). The purpose of this present study is to test the validity of the spillover dynamic found in many U.S. samples. Data from eleven cross-national samples, *drawn from Bangladesh, China, India, Bosnia, Germany, Palestine, Colombia, the United States, and three distinct ethnic groups within South Africa*, are tested to discern (1) the direct relationships between interparental conflict (IPC) and youth outcomes, and (2) the direct and indirect relationships between IPC, parenting, and youth outcomes. Specifically, we examine the links between IPC and youth adjustment via three central dimensions of parenting: support, psychological control, and behavioral control. Interparental conflict (IPC) is examined, rather than marital satisfaction, because conflict between parents has been found to have a stronger impact on youth outcomes than does global marital satisfaction (Cummings, Davies, & Simpson, 1994; Katz & Gottman, 1993). In operationalizing IPC, we distinguish between overt and covert conflict styles. Furthermore, most studies have examined either global conflict between parents, or have focused on overt conflict (see Buehler et al., 1997). This study responds to calls in the literature to differentiate styles of conflict. We also distinguish between externalizing and internalizing problem behaviors. Overall, IPC has been linked to both types of problem behaviors; however, the link may be somewhat stronger for externalizing problem behaviors (Buehler et al., 1997). In addition, there is evidence that the mediating role of parenting between IPC and youth problem behaviors varies widely. In one study, psychological control strongly mediated the relationship between IPC and internalizing behaviors, whereas lax control was only a weak mediator of IPC and externalizing behaviors (Fauber et al., 1990).

Styles of Interparental Conflict

Interparental conflict (IPC) has been defined as disagreement between parents about various issues in family life, and is differentiated from mundane discord by the mode of expression, frequency, intensity, chronicity, content, and degree of resolution (Buehler et al., 1997; Buehler et al., 1994; Cummings & Davies, 1994; Fincham & Osborne, 1993; Krishnakumar & Buehler, 2000). While disagreements and problem solving are common to daily family life (Cummings & Davies, 1994; Davies & Cummings, 1994), interparental conflict, as described and measured in the literature, is typically intense and harmful. Buehler and colleagues distinguish five modes of conflict: overt, which includes verbal and physical conflict, covert, cooperative, avoidant, and withdrawn (Buehler et al., 1994; Buehler et al., 1997). Most studies have focused on hostile overt conflict, while a few have also measured covert conflict (Buehler et al., 1994). Overt styles of conflict include open disagreement between partners, with actions such as threatening, yelling, insults and disrespect, and name-calling (Buehler et al., 1997). Covert conflict is characterized by passive-aggressive tactics, such as triangulating children into conflict or denigrating the other parent in the presence of the child, as well as global covert behaviors such as resentment or unverbalized tension between parents manifest in indirect behaviors not directly involving the children. Few studies focus on the other modes of expressing conflict expression (i.e., cooperative, avoidant, and withdrawn).

In their meta-analysis, Buehler and colleagues (1997) reported an average effect size for the association between overt conflict style and youth problem behaviors of .35 (126 effect sizes), and an average effect size for the association between covert conflict style and youth problem behaviors of .28 (24 effect sizes). Findings from another study suggest that overt styles of conflict may be specifically associated with externalizing behaviors, and covert styles of conflict associated with internalizing behaviors (Buehler et al., 1998). Based on these findings, we focus on overt and covert conflict.

INTERPARENTAL CONFLICT: DIRECT AND INDIRECT EFFECTS

Research in the last decade indicates that the effects of interparental conflict are often both direct and indirect (e.g., Stone et al., 2002), but there is some consensus that more of the effects of interparental conflict tend to be indirect, often via parenting (Buehler et al., 1994). We now briefly review past research on the associations between (1) IPC and youth problem behaviors, (2) IPC and parenting, (3) parenting and youth problem behaviors, and finally, (4) parenting as an intervening variable between IPC and youth problem behaviors.

Interparental Conflict and Adolescent Problem Behaviors

Two meta-analytic reviews reported mild to moderate associations between IPC and youth problem behaviors (Buehler et al., 1997; Reid & Crisafulli, 1990). Another study found a moderate direct link between overt IPC and externalizing youth problem behaviors in a sample of intact families despite the inclusion of three parenting variables as mediators (Fauber et al., 1990). In addition, the work of Cummings and Davies provides experimental evidence that interadult anger causes arousal in children, which may translate into aggression and anger in children (see Cummings, Pellegrini, Notarius, & Cummings, 1989; Davies & Cummings, 1994).

Interparental Conflict and Parenting

A recent meta-analysis showed that interparental conflict is moderately associated with diminished warmth and support in parents, poor parental monitoring and behavioral control, and increased verbal criticism and physical punishment in parents (Krishnakumar & Buehler, 2000). The strongest associations were those between marital hostility and higher levels of parental harsh discipline, and lower levels of parental love, support, and sensitivity. Effect sizes calculated from longitudinal data were almost as high as those calculated from cross-sectional data. Another meta-analysis also found a positive relationship between marital conflict and the quality of parent-child relationships (Erel & Burman, 1995). In a recent study, IPC was linked with maternal psychological control and decreased parental monitoring for both European and African American families (Stone et al., 2002).

Parenting and Adolescent Problem Behaviors

The association between parenting and youth functioning has long been the topic of much investigation, and accordingly, the literature is voluminous. Two common approaches have been used to classify parenting behaviors: (1) the dimensional approach, which focuses on discrete parenting behaviors, and (2) the typological approach, which includes patterns of parenting behaviors (cf. Darling & Steinberg, 1993). Barber (1997; Barber et al., 2003) has noted that at least three central elements of parenting are common to both approaches, namely: parental support, psychological control, and behavioral control. These are the basic dimensions of parenting identified in the earliest work on parent-child relations (e.g., Becker, 1964; Schaefer, 1965). They are also the components of many recent attempts to replicate in self-reported data the authoritative parenting typology (e.g., Steinberg, Elmen, & Mounts, 1989; Steinberg, Lamborn, Dornbusch, & Darling, 1992; Steinberg, Mounts, Lamborn, & Dornbusch, 1991). Although Baumrind did not explicitly use these labels in her typological configurations, her conceptualizations clearly include the essence of these same parenting behaviors (e.g., Baumrind, 1971).

Recently, Barber (Barber et al., 2003) found unique effects on key aspects of adolescent social and psychological functioning in sequential cross-sectional analyses and longitudinal analyses in a U.S. sample. Parental support was found to be consistently related to higher adolescent social competence and lower depression; parental psychological control was related to higher levels of depression and antisocial behavior; and parental behavioral control was found to be uniquely related to lower levels of antisocial behavior. Further, these same linkages were found when the model was tested on the 11 samples studied in this present investigation. This present study builds on this work by expanding the model to incorporate the marital relationship.

Parenting as an Intervening Variable Between IPC and Adolescent Problem Behaviors

There is a small but growing body of literature that examines the relationship between IPC and youth adjustment as mediated by various parenting variables (Fauber et al., 1990; Gonzales, Pitts, Hill, & Roosa, 2000; Harold et al., 1997; Osborne & Fincham, 1996; Stone, Buehler, & Barber, 2002). Krishnakumar, Buehler, and Barber (2003) discovered that 11 such investigations supported a partial or fully mediated relationship, while four investigations did not support the mediated relationship. In addition, Krishnakumar and colleagues tested a mediational model similar to our present model and found that African American and European American families showed no difference on three of five spillover pathways. The authors concluded that the key elements of individual development and family process function similarly across the two ethnic groups. However, in a meta-analytic study of the associations between IPC and parenting behaviors (138 effect sizes), the association was approximately two-thirds of a standard deviation stronger for samples consisting solely of European American families than it was for mixed samples (Krishnakumar & Buehler, 2000). Such findings underscore the need to understand possible differences based on culture and other contextual factors.

TESTING ACROSS CULTURE

In justifying this study, we have followed the recommendation that cross-cultural research should occur in stages. Stage one consists of transporting and testing in other cultures models that have been validated in one culture (Berry, Poortinga, Segall, & Dasen, 1992). Stage two includes *emic* analyses within cultures to understand or extend these findings. Stage three consists of another cross-cultural analysis that is informed by what has been learned by the prior two steps. This study is part of stage one. The C-NAP project will also include these latter two stages once analyses like the present one and others have been completed.

The justification for testing the parenting and youth outcome portions of the model comes most directly from the work of Barber et al. (2003), in which the same variables were found to have significant and invariant linkages in data from the same sites used here. A detailed review of the supporting theory and research for the common relevance of basic parenting dimensions can be found in Barber et al. (2003). Briefly, it includes notions of the common role of parents across cultures to the development of children (e.g., Bornstein, 1991; Chen & Rubin, 1994; Heath, 1995; Whiting & Edwards, 1988); the specific positive association between parental supportive behavior and adolescent psychological functioning across cultures (e.g., Cheng, 1998; Offer, Ostrov, Howard, & Atkinson, 1988; Scott & Scott, 1998); and the specific negative association of parental psychological control to child and adolescent psychosocial functioning across ethnic groups (e.g., Eccles, Early, Frasier, Belansky, & McCarthy, 1997) and cultures (e.g., Olsen, Yang, Hart, Robinson, Wu, Nelson, Nelson, Jin, & Wo, 2002).

The consistent evidence in U.S. data for the relevance of the direct and indirect effects of interparental conflict styles on youth functioning from the extensive work by Buehler and colleagues reviewed above qualifies these constructs and processes for "transporting and testing" in other cultures. This justification is enhanced by the cross-ethnic validations of some of the parameters of the model in U.S. data reviewed above. Further, although there is not yet substantial evidence from other cultures of the relevance of interparental conflict styles to child functioning, the evidence that does exist suggests the same types of effects. Of particular note is a large-scale study of college students from 39 nations on six continents, comprising a range of collectivist and individualist countries. Marital conflict among the parents of students was consistently found to have long-term, negative consequences for the students' well-being (Gohm, Oishi, Darlington, & Diener, 1998). Notably, the negative association between marital conflict and both life satisfaction and affective experience of adult offspring was consistent regardless of the culture's classification as individualist or collectivist, and regardless of gender. The negative linkage between marital conflict and life satisfaction held in countries with both high and low rates of divorce, and was also consistent in remarried families (Gohm et al., 1998). In another study, marital harmony was associated with parental acceptance in a Chinese sample (Chen & Rubin, 1994), a finding that supports the notion that a lack of conflict may allow parents to behave in an affectionate and accepting manner, regardless of cultural context.

Hypotheses

To our knowledge, no study has yet attempted a cross-national test of the spillover of interparental conflict to youth problem behaviors through parenting. Based on prior findings in the North American literature, we hypothesized a positive, direct relationship between IPC and depression, and between IPC and antisocial behavior. Because it was a basic criterion variable in the parenting model upon which we are building here (Barber et al., 2003), we also included social initiative as an outcome variable in this study. To our knowledge, no work has tested the association between marital conflict and youth social initiative, but we see no reason to expect other than a negative, direct relationship between IPC and social initiative as well.

For the indirect effects of IPC, we hypothesized that IPC would be negatively related to parental support, positively related to psychological control, and negatively related to parental behavioral control. The parenting effects were predicted to be the same as for the Barber et al. (2003) findings; specifically, that parental support would positively predict social initiative, and negatively predict depression; psychological control would positively predict depression and antisocial behavior; and, parental behavioral control would negatively predict antisocial behavior. Based on prior work, we further hypothesized that adding the three central elements of parenting to the IPC/problem behavior model would help explain the relationship between IPC and youth functioning with at least some degree of clarity and consistency. We saw no reason to expect that this dynamic would vary systematically by nation or ethnic group.

METHOD

Sample

Data for this study consist of self-reported survey data from 9,050 school-going adolescents from 11 national or within-nation ethnic groups whose ages ranged between 14 and 17 years. The groups include: South Africa-Black (N = 635), South Africa-Colored ("colored" is the self-referent term employed in South Africa for mixed-race individuals) (N = 520), South Africa-White (N = 579); Bangladesh (N = 1084); China (N = 1027); India (N = 976); Bosnia (N = 584); Germany (N = 970); Palestine (N = 978); United States (N = 749); and Colombia (N = 948). The data were collected between 1997 and 2000, with oversight and consultation from an on-site, native colleague for every sample. Surveys were administered in classroom groups in schools in metropolitan school districts. Schools were selected to maximize the socioeconomic and ethnic diversity that exists in those districts. Surveys were written originally in English and were back-translated into all languages of instruction for the samples: Afrikaans, Arabic, Bangla, Bosnian, German, Mandarin, Spanish, and Xhosa. English was the language of instruction for the Indian sample. See Barber et al. (2003) for a full report of the C-NAP methodology.

Measures

Table 1 presents the reliability coefficients for the constructs of IPC, parenting, and youth outcomes respective to each of the 11 samples.

IPC. Interparental conflict was measured using seven of eight items from Buehler and colleagues' measures of IPC (Buehler et al., 1998). For overt conflict, there were three items on which youth rated how often they see and hear conflict between their parents, such as "threaten each other" and "insult each other." There were four items assessing youth involvement in interparental covert conflict, including "How often does one of your parents try to get you to side with one of them?" and "How often do you feel caught in the middle when your parents fight?" The responses ranged from *never* (1) to *very often* (4). Cronbach's alpha levels in the original two-sample study (Buehler et al., 1998) were .87 and .87 for overt conflict style, four items, and .82 and .78 for covert conflict style, four items. In the present study, Cronbach's alpha levels for overt conflict were acceptable and ranged between .66 (Colombia) and .84 (United States). Bangledesh fell short of the criteria with an alpha of .58. For covert conflict, Cronbach's alpha levels ranged from .60 (China) to .84 (United States). The covert conflict alpha level for Bangladesh was .39, again markedly low. Prior work supports the validity of the use of youth ratings of parental conflict (Cummings, Davies, & Simpson, 1994; Grych & Fincham, 1990).

Parenting. Parental support was assessed using the 10-item acceptance subscale from the Child Report of Parent Behavior Inventory (CRPBI) (Schaefer, 1965). Reporting separately for mothers and fathers, youth responded to items such as "My mother or father is a person who . . . makes me feel better after talking over my worries with her/him . . . is able to make me feel better when I am upset . . . cheers me up when I am sad." The response format ranged from *not like her/him* (1) to *a lot like her/him* (3). Mother and father scores were averaged to create a parent support score. Cronbach's alpha for parental support ranged from .86 (South Africa Black) to .93 (United States).

Psychological control was measured using the eight-item Psychological Control Scale Youth Self-Report (Barber, 1996). Reporting separately for

TABLE 1. Reliability Coefficients for IPC, Parenting, and Youth Outcomes

	Africa			Asia			Europe		Middle East	North America	South America
	S. A. Black	S. A. Coloured	S. A. White	Bangladesh	China	India	Bosnia	Germany	Palestine	Utah	Colombia
Conflict											
Overt IPC	.82	.81	.81	.58	.81	.70	.76	.76	.76	.84	.66
Covert IPC	.61	.84	.78	.39	.60	.73	.79	.75	.64	.84	.72
Parenting											
Support	.86	.90	.92	.88	.91	.87	.90	.91	.90	.93	.88
Psy. Control	.74	.80	.83	.76	.82	.78	.84	.83	.72	.89	.78
Beh. Control	.78	.83	.85	.79	.87	.78	.88	.86	.75	.88	.85
Youth Outcomes											
Depression	.79	.66	.77	.55	.77	.70	.75	.78	.64	.82	.76
Antisoc. Beh.	.75	.72	.70	.65	.70	.74	.72	.68	.64	.80	.65
Soc. Initiative	.83	.81	.83	.73	.88	.84	.83	.77	.83	.87	.83

mothers and fathers, youth rated their perceptions of their parents, including items such as "My mother or father is a person who . . . is always trying to change how I feel or think about things . . . often interrupts me . . . brings up past mistakes when s/he criticizes me." The response format ranged from *not like her/him* (1) to *a lot like her/him* (3). Mother and father scores were averaged to create a parent score. Cronbach's alpha for parental psychological control in these samples ranged from .72 (Palestine) to .89 (United States).

Behavioral control was assessed using a five-item scale originally referred to as parental monitoring of adolescent behaviors (Brown et al., 1993), but we now refer to as parental knowledge of adolescent behaviors and activities based on recent conceptual clarifications (Crouter & Head, in press; Kerr & Stattin, 2000; Stattin & Kerr, 2000). Youth rated how much their parents "really know" about their activities such as "who your friends are . . . how you spend your money . . . where you are most afternoons after school." The response scale was *doesn't know* (1) to *knows a lot* (3). Cronbach's alpha levels for parental behavioral control in these samples ranged from .75 (Palestine) to .88 (Bosnia and the United States).

Adolescent Outcomes. Social initiative was assessed using 13 items from Bachman and colleagues (1993; Barber & Erikson, 2001). Sample items include "I enjoy doing things and talking with peers," "I share feelings and ideas with peers," and "I talk to teachers and staff about things other than class." The response format ranged from *never/almost never* (1) to *very often/always* (5). Cronbach's alphas for social initiative in these samples ranged from .73 (Bangladesh) to .88 (China). Depression was measured with the 10-item Child Depression Inventory (Kovacs, 1992). Youth rated themselves on items such as "I am sad . . . once in a while/many times/all the time" and "I feel like crying every day/many days/once in a while." Responses were coded 1-3, and the appropriate scores were reversed such that a higher score indicates a higher level of depression. Cronbach's alpha levels for depression in these samples ranged from .55 (Bangladesh) to .82 (United States). Antisocial behavior was assessed using six items from the Child Behavior Checklist (Achenbach & Edelbrock, 1987). Sample items include "I hang around kids who get in trouble," "I lie or cheat," and "I steal things from places other than home." The response format ranged from *not true* (1) to *very true or often true* (3). Cronbach's alphas for antisocial behavior in these samples ranged from .64 (Palestine) to .80 (United States).

RESULTS

Bivariate Correlations

Preliminary bivariate intercorrelations revealed mostly significant relationships in the expected directions. Overt IPC was positively correlated with depression and antisocial behavior in all 11 samples, and covert IPC was correlated positively with depression and antisocial behavior in samples, excepting Bangladesh. The correlations between IPC and social initiative were somewhat weak and inconsistent. Significant correlations ranged from .06 (covert IPC and antisocial behavior) to .34 (covert IPC and psychological control). These results justified a multivariate test of the direct effects of IPC on youth outcomes. Full bivariate results can be obtained from the first author.

Structural equation modeling (SEM) was used to test two models for each of the 11 samples. Scale scores were used to indicate latent constructs. The first model–the direct effects model–assessed the direct relationships between IPC and youth outcomes. The second–the full effects model–tested the spillover model, with the three parenting measures inserted as intervening variables between the IPC and outcome variables. Because the analyses are performed simultaneously for each culture, a single chi-square and set of goodness of fit indices are calculated. Unstandardized coefficients are reported such that each sample can be compared to the others along any particular parameter.

Direct Effects Model

Before testing the full effects model, it was first necessary to test whether a direct relationship existed between the predictor variables and the criterion variables (Holmbeck, 1997). Hence, we first tested a direct model of the relationships between the two interparental conflict variables and the three youth outcomes.

Table 2 presents the direct associations between overt and covert conflict and youth outcomes for each nation/ethnic group. The multivariate coefficients for the constrained model–that is, constraining parameters to be equal across all 11 samples–are reported in the far right column of the table. Parameters from the various unconstrained models for each nation/ethnic group were then compared via modification indices to determine any significant differences in parameters among samples from the constrained model. Although a total of six were found to be significantly different, freeing these parameters did not markedly improve the model's fit. The chi-square for the unconstrained model reached 0, with 0 degrees of freedom, and a comparative fit index of 1. The fit of the constrained model was acceptable ($\Pi 2 = 273.48$, $df = 60$. $p = .000$).

Overt conflict was associated with increased depression (nine samples, 82%) and with increased antisocial behavior (10 samples, 91%). Overt conflict was associated with decreased social initiative in four of eleven samples (36%). Covert conflict was associated with higher depression in eight samples (73%), and with higher antisocial behavior in six samples (55%). Covert conflict was positively associated with youth social initiative for South Africa-Black and Bangladesh, but was non-significant for all other samples. Thus, both forms of conflict were directly related to depression in 17 of 22 tests (77%), directly related to antisocial behavior in 16 of 22 parameter tests (73%), and directly related to social initiative in six of 22 (27%) tests. Looking at the entire direct effects model, IPC was significantly related to measures of youth functioning in 39 of 66 tests (59%).

Full Effects Model

Having established direct links between IPC and youth outcomes, the next step involved adding the parenting variables to the model in order to test for possible indirect effects. This model tested both direct associations of overt and covert conflict with youth outcomes and indirect effects of both forms of conflict through the three intervening parenting variables.

Tables 3a through 3c present the results of the full effects model. These tables contain three categories of parameters for each nation/ethnic group: (1) Table 3a presents the direct associations between IPC and youth outcomes, controlling now for the presence of the parenting variables; (2) Table 3b presents the direct associations between IPC and parenting; and, (3) Table 3c presents the direct associations between the parenting variables and youth outcomes. Again, the coefficients for the constrained model are reported in the far right column of the tables. As with the reduced form model, the unconstrained parameters for each nation/ethnic group were compared to the constrained parameters using modification indices to determine any significant differences. In this full effects model, none of the primary parameters' coefficients of interest differed significantly from the constrained model, although eleven correlated error terms had coefficients with significance levels in excess of 10.00. The unconstrained model had a good fit ($II2 = 445.71$, $df = 209$, $p = .000$), as did the constrained model ($II2 = 1410.78$, $df = 371$, $p = .000$). See Table 3b for other goodness of fit measures.

Interparental Conflict and Youth Outcomes. Once the three parenting variables were added to create the full effects model, overt IPC was no longer directly associated with depression in any of the 11 samples. Overt IPC was associated significantly with antisocial behavior in six samples (55%), as compared to ten samples in the direct effects model. Overt conflict was positively related with youth social initiative in three samples. Coefficients for covert conflict showed less change from the direct to the full effects model. Covert conflict was directly related to increased depression, but only in three samples (27%), compared to eight samples in the direct effects model. Covert conflict was significantly related directly to increased antisocial behavior in

TABLE 2. Direct Effects Model: Direct Effects of Interparental Conflict on Youth Outcomes

| | Unconstrained Model by Sample† | | | | | | | | | | | Constrained† |
| | Africa | | | Asia | | | Europe | | Middle East | North America | South America | |
	S. A. Black	S. A. Coloured	S. A. White	Bangladesh	China	India	Bosnia	Germany	Palestine	Utah	Colombia	
Overt Conflict												
Depression	.03	.06*	.05**	.06***	.07***	.03	.10***	.11***	.09***	.05*	.04*	.06***
Antisocial Behavior	.13***	.01	.13***	.10***	.08***	.15***	.06*	.10***	.06***	.13***	.05*	.08***
Social Initiative	-.16**	.03	-.10	-.11***	-.13***	-.10*	-.07	-.02	.03	-.11	-.04	-.07***
Covert Conflict												
Depression	.03	.08***	.11***	-.01	.07***	.04*	.02	.05*	.06**	.13***	.11***	.06***
Antisocial Behavior	.06	.07*	.00	.01	.05**	.10***	.08***	.02	.07***	.10**	.02	.04***
Social Initiative	.19**	-.08	.04	.14***	.01	.08	.08	.01	.06	-.04	-.03	.05***

*$p < .05$ **$p < .01$ ***$p < .001$
† Unstandardized coefficients

Goodness of Fit Indicators—Reduced Form Model		
	Unconstrained Model	Constrained Model
χ^2	0	273.48
df	0	60
p		.000
Comparative Fit Index (CFI)	1	.998
Tucker-Lewis Index (TLI)		.994
RMSEA		.021

112

but two (18%) samples, compared to eight samples in the direct effects model. In the full effects model, covert conflict was positively associated directly with youth social initiative in three samples (27%). Thus, both types of IPC were directly related to depression, antisocial behavior, and social initiative in the full effects model, but much less frequently than in the direct effects model.

Interparental Conflict and Parenting. Overt IPC was found to have consistent, significant relationships to the three dimensions of parenting. Universally consistent with the hypotheses, overt conflict was associated with significantly less parental support (11 samples, 100%), with increased levels of psychological control (nine samples, 82%), and lower levels of parental behavioral control (10 samples, 91%). Covert conflict was also significantly related to parenting in the expected directions, but to a lesser extent. Covert IPC was significantly associated with decreased levels of parental support (six samples, 55%), and associated with increased parental support in one sample (Bangladesh). Covert conflict was consistently associated with increased parental psychological control (11 samples, 100%), and with decreased parental behavioral control (five samples, 45%).

Parenting and Youth Outcomes. The associations between the three dimensions of parenting and youth outcomes were mainly consistent with hypothesized expectations. Parental support was consistently associated with higher youth social initiative (11 samples, 100%), and consistently related to lower youth depression (11 samples, 100%). Ratings of parental psychological control were significantly associated with higher youth depression (10 of 11 samples, 91%), and with higher antisocial behavior (five samples, 45%). Parental behavioral control was significantly related to lower youth antisocial behavior (10 samples, 91%). Essentially, therefore, the associations among the parenting and youth variables did not change from the Barber et al. (2003) findings once tested in conjunction with the IPC variables in this analysis, except for the less consistent association between psychological control and antisocial behavior. This finding is actually consistent with the initial theorizing about the more purely internalized, versus externalized, problem behavior consequences of psychological control (Barber, 1992, 2002).

The Intervening Role of Parenting for the Links Between IPC and Youth Outcomes

Tables 4a through 4c present a summary overview of (1) the direct associations between IPC and youth outcomes, (2) the direct associations between

TABLE 3a. Full Effects Model: Effects of Interparental Conflict on Youth Outcomes

| | Unconstrained Model by Sample† | | | | | | | | | | | Constrained† |
| | Africa | | | Asia | | | Europe | | Middle East | North America | South America | |
	S. A. Black	S. A. Coloured	S. A. White	Bangladesh	China	India	Bosnia	Germany	Palestine	Utah	Colombia	
Overt Conflict												
Depression	.01	−.02	−.03	.00	−.01	−.01	.02	.02	.04	−.02	.00	.00
Antisocial Behavior	.12***	−.04	.06*	.05**	.03	.11***	.00	.01	.04*	.07*	.01	.05***
Social Initiative	−.09	.14*	.06	−.03	.00	.00	.04	.10*	.14*	.08	.03	.02
Covert Conflict												
Depression	.00	.03	.06**	.00	.03	.00	.01	−.03	.02	.07**	.08***	.03***
Antisocial Behavior	.04	.05	−.04	.01	.01	.09***	.04	−.04	.05*	.00	.03	.03***
Social Initiative	.16*	−.05	.06	.11**	.05	.15**	.10	.05	.12	.05	.03	.08***

*p < .05   **p < .01   ***p < .001
† Unstandardized coefficients

TABLE 3b. Full Effects Model: Effects of Interparental Conflict on Parenting

| | Unconstrained Model by Sample† | | | | | | | | | | | Constrained† |
| | Africa | | | Asia | | | Europe | | Middle East | North America | South America | |
Overt Conflict	S.A. Black	S.A. Coloured	S.A. White	Bangladesh	China	India	Bosnia	Germany	Palestine	Utah	Colombia	
Support	−.09***	−.16***	−.17***	−.16***	−.21***	−.11***	−.25***	−.19***	−.19***	−.14***	−.11***	−.15***
Psy. Control	.02	.12***	.11***	.13***	.15***	.10***	.19***	.13***	.04	.13***	.09***	.11***
Beh. Control	−.01	−.08*	−.11***	−.20***	−.14***	−.13***	−.13***	−.07***	−.11***	−.08**	−.10***	−.10***
Covert Conflict												
Support	.03	−.04	−.02	.06**	−.06*	−.09*	−.04	−.06*	−.09**	−.08*	−.08**	−.04***
Psy. Control	.08*	.13***	.14***	.05*	.18***	.10***	.10***	.14***	.13***	.23***	.16***	.13***
Beh. Control	−.05	−.01	−.04	.02	−.01	−.05*	−.11**	−.03*	−.04	−.12***	−.06*	−.03***

*$p < .05$ **$p < .01$ ***$p < .001$
†Unstandardized coefficients

TABLE 3c. Full Effects Model: Effects of Parenting on Youth Outcomes

Parenting:	Africa			Asia			Europe		Middle East	North America	South America	Constrained†
	S.A. Black	S.A. Coloured	S.A. White	Bangladesh	China	India	Bosnia	Germany	Palestine	Utah	Colombia	
Support												
Soc. Initiat.	.76**	.71***	.87***	.47***	.61***	.83***	.47***	.61***	.58***	1.14***	.65***	.65***
Depression	-.32**	-.29***	-.30***	-.31***	-.28***	-.26***	-.23***	-.42***	-.26**	-.34***	-.35***	-.30**
Psych.Control												
Depression	.54***	.28**	.32***	.06*	.08*	.17***	.09*	.36***	.13**	.16**	.04	.13***
Antisoc. Beh.	.11	.15	.16	.04	.18***	.08	.14***	.22***	.15***	.13	.14***	.11***
Beh. Control												
Antisoc. Beh	-.12	-.34***	-.46***	-.26***	-.18***	-.20***	-.26***	-1.09***	-.15**	-.60***	-.35***	-.22***

*p < .05   **p < .01   ***p < .001
†Unstandardized coefficients

Goodness of Fit Indicators–Mediational Model

	Unconstrained Model	Constrained Model
x^2	445.71	1410.78
df	209	371
p	.000	.000
Comparative Fit Index (CFI)	.989	.954
Tucker-Lewis Index (TLI)	.970	.925
RMSEA	.012	.016

IPC and parenting, and (3) parenting as an intervening variable between IPC and youth outcomes.

As stated earlier, we found in the initial direct effects model that IPC was significantly related to youth functioning in 39 of 66 total parameters (59%). However, when parenting was added to the model, only 11 of the original 39 direct effects remained. Taking the results together, we found that the impact of IPC on youth outcomes became fully indirect for 25 of the 39 parameters (64%). Both significant direct and indirect pathways were observed for 10 of the 39 originally significant parameters (26%). See Table 4c for a full report of direct and indirect effects.

The Intervening Role of Parenting for Overt Conflict. Table 4c presents a summary of direct and indirect effects. Of the nine direct associations originally between overt IPC and youth depression, all nine became fully indirect via parental support and psychological control, except for Palestine, where the intervening variable was parental support only. In other words, for these associations, parenting fully mediated the effect of IPC on depression. Thus, the risk to youth of heightened depression as a consequence of overt IPC was explained by the decreased parenting quality (lower support and higher psychological control) associated with IPC.

The link between overt IPC and youth antisocial behavior became fully indirect in four samples (out of 10 originally direct relationships; 40%) via parents' psychological control and behavioral control. Overt IPC had both direct and indirect effects in five of the ten samples where the direct effect was initially observed (50%). Parental psychological control was an intervening variable only for China, Bosnia, Germany, Palestine, and Colombia. Parental behavioral control, on the other hand, was a significant intervening variable in nine of ten samples where indirect effects existed. Thus, the risk to antisocial behavior from overt IPC is partly explained by the decreased parenting quality associated with overt IPC.

Finally, parental support intervened completely between overt IPC and social initiative in all four samples where overt IPC was directly related to social initiative. Thus, the risk to youth for decreased social initiative posed by overt IPC is explained by the decrease in parenting support that accompanied overt IPC. In sum, there was substantial evidence that risk to adolescent functioning associated with the presence of overt IPC can be explained by way of decreased parenting quality that accompanies overt IPC.

The Intervening Role of Parenting for Covert Conflict. Of the eight initial direct links between covert IPC and youth depression, five (63%) became fully indirect, and three had significant direct and indirect links (37%). Four of the links between covert IPC and depression became fully indirect via both parental support and psychological control: China, India, Germany, and Pales-

TABLE 4a. Summary of Direct Effects Model (See Table 2 for Coefficients)

	Is Interparental Conflict Associated with *Youth Functioning* Across C-NAP Countries?*										
	Africa			Asia			Europe		Middle East	North America	South America
	S. A. Black	S. A. Coloured	S. A. White	Bangladesh	China	India	Bosnia	Germany	Palestine	Utah	Colombia
Overt Conflict											
Depression		+X	+X	+X	+X	+X	+X	+X	+X	+X	+X
Antisocial Behavior	+X	+X	+X	+X	+X	+X	+X	+X	+X	+X	+X
Social Initiative	−X			−X	−X	−X					
Covert Conflict											
Depression		+X	+X		+X	+X		+X	+X	+X	+X
Antisocial Behavior		+X			+X	+X	+X		+X		+X
Social Initiative	+X			+X							

*An X indicates a significant effect.
Positive and negative associations are noted.

118

TABLE 4b. Summary of the Effects of IPC on Parenting (See Table 3b for Coefficients)

	Is Interparental Conflict Associated with *Parenting* Across C-NAP Countries?*										
	Africa			Asia			Europe		Middle East	North America	South America
	S. A. Black	S. A. Coloured	S. A. White	Bangladesh	China	India	Bosnia	Germany	Palestine	Utah	Colombia
Overt Conflict											
Parental Support	−X	−X	−X	−X	−X	−X	−X	−X	−X	−X	−X
Psychological Control		+X	+X	+X	+X	+X	+X	+X		+X	+X
Behavioral Control	−X	−X	−X	−X	−X	−X	−X	−X	−X	−X	−X
Covert Conflict											
Parental Support	+X				−X	−X		−X	−X	−X	−X
Psychological Control	+X	+X	+X	+X	+X	+X	+X	+X	+X	+X	+X
Behavioral Control						−X	−X	−X		−X	−X

*An X indicates a significant effect.
Positive and negative associations are noted.

TABLE 4c. Summary of the Full Effects Model (See Tables 3a-c for Coefficients)

	Africa			Asia			Europe		Middle East	North America	South America
Do the Three Central Parenting Variables *Intervene* in the Associations Between Interparental Conflict and Youth Functioning?*	S. A. Black	S. A. Coloured	S. A. White	Bangladesh	China	India	Bosnia	Germany	Palestine	Utah	Colombia
Overt Conflict											
Depression		Indirect *φ	Indirect*φ	Indirect*φ	Indirect*φ		Indirect*φ	Indirect*φ	Indirect*	Indirect*φ	Indirect*φ
Antisocial Behavior	Direct		Both†	Both†	Indirectφ†	Both†	Indirect††	Indirect†	Both††	Both†	Indirect††
Social Initiative	Indirect*			Indirect*	Indirect*	Indirect*					
Covert Conflict											
Depression		Indirectφ	Bothφ		Indirect *φ	Indirect *φ		Indirect *φ	Indirect *φ	Both *φ	Both *
Antisocial Behavior		Direct			Indirectφ	Both†	Indirectφ†		Bothφ		Indirectφ†
Social Initiative	Direct			Direct							

Intervening Variables:
*Parental Support
φParental Psychological Control
† Parental Behavioral Control

tine. Both the direct and indirect paths remained significant for the U.S. and Colombia; the effect was indirect via only psychological control for South Africa-Black. Both direct and indirect paths via psychological control, but not via behavioral control, were significant for the South Africa-White sample. In the link between covert IPC and antisocial behavior, both psychological control and behavioral control were significant intervening variables for Bosnia and Colombia; psychological control fully mediated the same link for China. Covert IPC had both direct and indirect effects in the Palestine sample (indirect effect via psychological control) and in the India sample (indirect effect via behavioral control). There were no indirect links for the South Africa-Colored sample. Refer to Table 4c for an overview of these results. In sum, as was the case for overt IPC, the negative associations between covert IPC and youth functioning were largely explained by the decreased parenting quality that was associated with covert IPC.

Controlling for Age and Sex

In order to assess how generalizable these findings were across key subgroups of the sample, we next included both adolescent age and sex in the models.

Age. The inclusion of age in both the direct and full effects models for the combined samples revealed very few differences in model parameters. There was neither strength nor patterns to these few significant differences, and thus we concluded that the found effects were not contingent on the age of the youth.

Sex. Sex of youth in the direct model revealed no significant changes in model parameters for the combined sample. However, a significant change in fit for the full effects model for males and females was found (chi-squared difference: 39.21, $df = 17$, $p = .002$). Due to the complexity of the analyses conducted here, we did not pinpoint the specific locations of these sex differences. This will be pursued in future analyses.

DISCUSSION

This study assessed the associations between interparental conflict (IPC), parenting, and individual functioning in data gathered from samples of school-going adolescents in 11 national/ethnic groups. Specifically, the model tested the validity of the spillover dynamic found in much research in the U.S., whereby marital conflict spills over into parenting and, directly and/or indirectly, into the psychological and social functioning of children and adolescents. This study built on previous analyses of these same data that showed consistent linkages between parenting and adolescent functioning, and thereby provided a meaningful extension to the substantive literature on family processes. We followed recommendations within cross-cultural psychology to "transport and test" models validated in one culture to other cultures as an initial step in systematic comparative research. The findings of this study will be used to design future within- and across-culture extensions to more precisely understand these processes and if, when, and how they vary by population group.

As complex as the analyses were in terms of assessing multiple multivariate models in 11 samples, the findings are relatively straightforward. Most basically, the findings provide meaningful support to the distinction between overt and covert interparental conflict as substantively different forms of conflict. In most samples, these constructs were reliably measured, even when translated into numerous different languages, and they were significantly associated with measures of internalized and externalized problem behaviors as forecasted by theory and prior research in the very large majority of samples (see Table 4a). The relative lack of prediction to social initiative will be discussed below. There was no evidence either from the occasional instance of no association or any other aspect of the associations—strength or direction, for example—that suggested that these forms of conflict had anything but common salience to youth across these samples.

Children's modeling of their parents' conflict is one of the most immediate and well-documented direct effects of interparental conflict on child problem behaviors (Buehler, Krishnakumar, Anthony, Tittsworth, & Stone, 1994; Grych & Fincham, 1990). As children learn that conflict is overtly or tacitly acceptable, they may become aggressive with their peers or younger siblings (Cummings & Davies, 1994). Others have described conflict between parents as triggering a phenomenon of developmental overload, which overwhelms children's ability to cope with the stress, or to self-soothe (Fincham, Grych, & Osborne, 1994).

The value of these aspects of interparental conflict was strengthened by their consistent association across sites in these data with the three parenting variables (see Table 4b). Not only was their overall prediction from the conflict to the parenting variables (i.e., both forms of conflict were predictive of parenting variables in the majority, and, in some cases, all of the samples), but the patterns of prediction were common and in accord with past research and theory (e.g., the particularly specialized and consistent association between covert conflict and parental psychological control). The relatively less consistent prediction from covert conflict (e.g., inconsistently related to support and behavioral control), as compared to overt conflict, which was widely predictive of all three forms of parenting, reinforces the unique compatibility and co-incidence of insidious and passive family processes represented by overt conflict and psychological control (see Stone et al., 2002 for an elaboration). It is not immediately clear why covert conflict was less consistent in predicting parenting across samples, especially given that these particular samples vary by region, level of economic development, minority versus majority status, and so forth. The notable exception is psychological control, which was related to parents' covert conflict in all 11 samples.

Despite the complexity of the analyses–three intervening variables between two independent and two dependent variables across 11 sites–these findings are also quite consistent, both with substantive expectations and across sites (see Table 4c). Overall, the findings provide consistent support for the relevance of parenting in explaining the risk to youth development from IPC. In a large majority of tests, IPC was related to youth problem behaviors indirectly through parenting; direct effects were less common but still present in some cases even when parenting was added to the model. The relevance of parenting was particularly consistent for the theorized linkages; that is, consistent for the association between overt conflict and antisocial behavior through parental behavioral control, and for the association between covert conflict and depression through parental psychological control. These findings are quite consistent with previous work in various multi-ethnic U.S. samples and further solidify the distinction between overt behavioral dynamics and covert process within families.

The inclusion of the social initiative construct was not guided by theory or research on marital conflict and youth difficulty. Rather, it was included because it was part of the parenting model that was validated using these same data (Barber et al., 2003). It is perhaps not surprising, therefore, that it proved to be a relatively unimportant variable in these analyses. Not only was it relatively rarely predicted by the conflict variables, but it was also inconsistent in terms of direction. This (non)finding helps circumscribe the relevance of marital conflict by showing that, at least in the case of this measure, conflict poses risk for problem behaviors, but does not necessarily compromise adaptive functioning.

Limitation

The most accurate way to summarize the findings of this study is to say that they have offered multiple replications of a model of family dynamics; that is, the essential parameters of the hypothesized model were supported in multiple, highly varying samples. Thus, one can have greater confidence that the model is not limited in its relevance to the western populations in which it was developed and tested. We state this conclusion without specific reference to culture not just because of the relatively invariant findings across samples, but because very few of the C-NAP samples, only South Africa and Germany, were drawn with national or cultural representation as a goal. It would, therefore, be inaccurate to interpret a variant finding as a cultural difference.

This, therefore, can be considered one of the limitations of the C-NAP data set, and of this study specifically, if cultural insights are expected. Significant as the findings are, we can say no more than that the model works across multiple samples. Clearly, we expect that the ways in which the samples vary (e.g., demographically, politically, economically, religiously) do in part reflect important cultural differences, but conclusions that directly implicate culture await replication on samples that are adequately representative of the cultures in question.

We wish also to make clear that, despite the reliability and validity of the constructs investigated here, we in no way conclude that the measures used in this study are the best ways to represent the family processes under study. What the findings of this study have done is to demonstrate that these constructs are similarly understood by youth of very different backgrounds and experiences, and that, therefore, the constructs have common meaning. It is entirely likely, however, that more ethnically, nationally, and culturally sensitive measures of these family constructs could be discerned. Such progress can only be made through more cultural-intensive, or *emic* investigations where information is sought directly and thoroughly from members of the various groups under study. In other words, there may be "better" ways to conceive of and measure family conflict, parenting, and youth problem behaviors. Such a direction is precisely where an initial "transport and test" study is designed to lead.

It is also important to recognize that the C-NAP samples only include school-going youth. In most societies, school attendance, or continuing attendance, represents advantage of some kind. Therefore, it would not be justified to conclude that the common family patterns revealed in these findings would be the same in families whose children were not attending school.

Naturally, causal assertions among these variables are not justified before more evidence of temporal ordering is obtained. Also, the single-informant design of this study is, of course, subject to criticism. Similar findings achieved through multiple methods and sources of information are often more credible. Given the limitations listed above, however, we are relatively comfortable in the credibility of these findings for a number of reasons. First, using many of the same variables, it has been shown that these patterns are durable once controlling for the response bias of single-informant studies (e.g., correlating manifest variable error terms across exogenous and endogenous variables; Buehler et al., 1998). Second, as noted previously, many of the variables assessed in this study are arguably more, or only reliable, when reported by youth, given their subjective nature. Most important, perhaps, is the invariance in findings across such diverse samples. It would seem that something "real" is happening when the same patterns are discernable in the lives of youth from such widely varying languages, heritages, religions, social classes, and so forth.

In sum, notwithstanding numerous limitations, this study has provided evidence for the commonality of patterns among negative processes in human families. It appears more certain than previously that marital conflict can, in part, be understood in terms of overt and covert manifestations, and that these relate reliably and consistently with diminished parenting, which in large part transmits the conflict to maladaptive behavior in adolescents in many parts of the world.

REFERENCES

Achenbach, T. M., & Edelbrock, C. (1987). *Manual for the youth self-report and profile.* Burlington, VT: University of Vermont, Department of Psychiatry.

Barber, B. K. (2002). Introduction. In B. K. Barber (Ed). *Intrusive parenting: How psychological control affects children and adolescents.* Washington, DC: American Psychological Association Press.

Barber, B. K. (1997). Introduction: Adolescent socialization in context: The role of connection, regulation, and autonomy in the family. *Journal of Adolescent Research, 12,* 5-11.

Barber, B. K. (1996). Parental psychological control: Revisiting a neglected construct. *Child Development, 67,* 3296-3319.

Barber, B. K. (1992). Family, personality, and problem behaviors. *Journal of Marriage and the Family, 54,* 69-79.

Barber, B. K., & Erickson, L. D. (2001). Adolescent social initiative: Antecedents in the ecology of social connections. *Journal of Adolescent Research, 16,* 326-354.

Barber, B. K., Stolz, H. E., Olsen, J. A., & Maughan, S. L. (2003). Parental support, psychological control, and behavioral control: Validations across time, analytic method, and culture. Manuscript under review for publication.

Baumrind, D. (1971). Current patterns of parental authority. *Developmental Psychology Monographs, 4,* 1-102.

Becker, W. C. (1964). Consequences of different kinds of parental discipline. In M. L. Hoffman & W. W. Hoffman (Eds.), *Review of child development research* (Vol. 1, pp. 169-208). New York: Russell Sage Foundation.

Berry, J. W., Poortinga, Y. H., Segall, M. H., & Dasen, P. R. (1992). *Cross-cultural psychology: Research and applications.* Cambridge, UK: Cambridge University Press.

Bornstein, M. H. (1991). Approaches to parenting in culture. In M. H. Bornstein (Ed.), *Cultural approaches to parenting*. Hillsdale, NJ: Lawrence Erlbaum.

Brown, B. B., Mounts, N., Lamborn, S. D., & Steinberg, L. (1993). Parenting practices and peer group affiliation in adolescence. *Child Development, 63*, 391-400.

Buehler, C., Anthony, C., Krishnakumar, A., Stone, G., Gerard, J., & Pemberton, S. (1997). Interparental conflict and youth problem behaviors: A meta-analysis. *Journal of Child and Family Studies, 6*, 233-247.

Buehler, C., Krishnakumar, A., Anthony, C., Tittsworth, S., & Stone, G. (1994). Hostile interparental conflict and youth maladjustment. *Family Relations, 43*, 409-416.

Buehler, C., Krishnakumar, A., Stone, G., Anthony, C., Pemberton, S., Gerard, J., & Barber, B. K. (1998). Interparental conflict styles and youth problem behaviors: A two sample replication. *Journal of Marriage and the Family, 60*, 119-132.

Chen, X., & Rubin, K. H. (1994). Family conditions, parental acceptance, and social competence and aggression in Chinese children. *Social Development, 3*, 269-290.

Cheng, C. (1998). Getting the right kind of support: Functional differences in the types of social support of depression for Chinese adolescents. *Journal of Clinical Psychology, 54*, 845-849.

Crouter, A. C., & Head, M. R. (in press). Parental monitoring and knowledge of children. In M. Bornstein (Ed.), *The handbook of parenting*. Hillsdale, NJ: Lawrence Erlbaum.

Cummings, E. M. (1987). Coping with background anger in early childhood. *Child Development, 58*, 976-984.

Cummings, E. M., & Davies, P. (1994). Children and marital conflict: The impact of family dispute and resolution. New York: The Guilford Press.

Cummings, E. M., Davies, P. T., & Simpson, K. S. (1994). Marital conflict, gender, and children's appraisals and coping efficacy as mediators of child adjustment. *Journal of Family Psychology, 8*, 141-149.

Cummings, J. S., Pellegrini, D., Notarius, C., & Cummings, E. M. (1989). Children's responses to angry adult behavior as a function of marital distress and history of interparental hostility. *Child Development, 60*, 1035-1043.

Davies, P. T., & Cummings, E. M. (1994). Marital conflict and child adjustment: An emotional security hypothesis. *Psychological Bulletin, 116*, 387-411.

Darling, N., & Steinberg, L. (1993). Parenting style as context: An integrative model. *Psychological Bulletin, 113*, 487-496.

Eccles, J. S., Early, D., Frasier, K., Belansky, E., & McCarthy, K. (1997). The relation of connection, regulation, and support for autonomy to adolescents functioning. *Journal of Adolescent Research, 12*, 263-286.

Emery, R. E., Fincham, F. D., & Cummings, E. M. (1992). Parenting in context: Systemic thinking about parental conflict and its influence on children. *Journal of Consulting and Clinical Psychology, 10*, 11-24.

Erel, O., & Burman, B. (1995). Interrelatedness of marital relations and parent-child relations: A meta-analytic review. *Psychological Bulletin, 118*, 108-132.

Fauber, R., Forehand, R., Thomas, A. M., & Wierson, M. (1990). A mediational model of the impact of marital conflict on adolescent adjustment in intact and divorced families: The role of disrupted parenting. *Child Development, 61*, 1112-1123.

Fincham, F. D. (1998). Child development and marital relations. *Child Development, 69 (2)*, 543-574.

Fincham, F. D., Grych, J. H., & Osborne, L. N. (1994). Does marital conflict cause child maladjustment? Directions and challenges for longitudinal research. *Journal of Family Psychology, 8,* 128-140.

Fincham, F. D., & Osborne, L. N. (1993). Marital conflict and children: Retrospect and prospect. *Clinical Psychology Review, 13,* 75-88.

Gohm, C. L., Oishi, S., Darlington, J., & Diener, E. (1998). Culture, parental conflict, parental marital status, and the subjective well-being of young adults. *Journal of Marriage and the Family, 60,* 319-334.

Gonzales, N. A., Pitts, S. C., Hill, N. E., & Roosa, M. W. (2000). A mediational model of the impact of interparental conflict on child adjustment in a multiethnic, ethnic low-income sample. *Journal of Family Psychology, 14,* 365-379.

Grych, J. H., & Fincham, F. D. (1990). Marital conflict and children's adjustment: A cognitive-contextual framework. *Psychological Bulletin, 108,* 267-290.

Harold, G. T., Fincham, F. D., Osborne, L. N., & Conger, R. D. (1997). Mom and dad are at it again: Adolescent perceptions of marital conflict and adolescent psychological distress. *Developmental Psychology, 33,* 333-350.

Heath, D. T. (1995). Parents' socialization of children. In B. B. Ingoldsby & S. Smith (Eds.), *Families in multicultural perspective* (pp. 161-186). New York: Guilford.

Holmbeck, G. N. (1997). Toward terminological, conceptual, and statistical clarity in the study of mediators and moderators: Examples from the child-clinical and pediatric psychology literatures. *Journal of Consulting and Clinical Psychology, 65,* 599-610.

Katz, L. F., & Gottman, J. M. (1993). Patterns of marital conflict predict children's internalizing and externalizing behaviors. *Developmental Psychology, 29,* 940-950.

Kerr, M., & Sattin, H. (2000). What parents know, how they know it, and several forms of adolescent adjustment: Further support for a reinterpretation of monitoring. *Developmental Psychology, 36,* 1-15.

Kovacs, M. (1992). *Children's depression inventory.* Niagara Falls, NY: Multi-Health Systems.

Krishnakumar, A., & Buehler, C. (2000). Interpersonal conflict and parenting behaviors: A meta-analytic review. *Family Relations, 49,* 25-44.

Krishnakumar, A., Buehler, C., & Barber, B. K. (2003). Youth perceptions of interparental conflict, ineffective parenting, and youth problem behaviors in European-American and African-American families. *Journal of Personality and Social Relationships, 20,* 239-260.

Offer, D., Ostrov, E., Howard, K. I., & Atkinson, R. (1988). *The teenage world: Adolescents' self-image in ten countries.* New York: Plenum.

Olsen, S. F., Yang, C., Hart, C. G., Robinson, C. C., Wu, P., Nelson, D. N., Nelson, L. J., Jin, S., & Wo, J. (2002). Mothers' psychological control and pre-school children's behavioral outcomes in China, Russia, and the United States. In B. K. Barber (Ed.), *Intrusive parenting: How psychological control affects children and adolescents* (pp. 235-262). Washington, DC, US: American Psychological Association.

Osborne, L. N., & Fincham, F. D. (1996). Marital conflict, parent-child relationships, and child adjustment: Does gender matter: *Merrill-Palmer Quarterly, 42,* 48-75.

Reid, W., & Crisafulli, A. (1990). Marital discord and child behavior problems: A meta-analysis. *Journal of Abnormal Child Psychology, 18,* 10-117.

Schaefer, E. S. (1965). Children's report of parental behavior: An inventory. *Child Development, 36,* 413-424.

Scott, R., & Scott, W. A. (1998). Adjustment of adolescents: Cross-cultural similarities and differences. London: Routledge.

Stattin, H., & Kerr, M. (2000). Parental monitoring: A reinterpretation. *Child Development, 71,* 1072-1085.

Steinberg, L., Elmen, J. D., & Mounts, N. S. (1989). Authoritative parenting, psychosocial maturity, and academic success among adolescents. *Child Development, 60,* 1424-1436.

Steinberg, L., Lamborn, S. D., Dornbusch, S. M., & Darling, N. (1992). Impact of parenting practices on adolescent achievement: Authoritative parenting, school involvement, and encouragement to succeed. *Child Development, 63,* 1266-1281.

Steinberg, L., Mounts, N. S., Lamborn, S. D., & Dornbusch, S. M. (1991). Authoritative parenting and adolescent adjustment across varied ecological niches. *Journal of Research on Adolescence, 1,* 19-36.

Stone, G., Buehler, C., & Barber, B. K. (2002). Interparental conflict, parental psychological control, and youth problem behavior. In B. K. Barber (Ed.), *Intrusive parenting: How psychological control affects children and adolescents* (pp. 53-95). Washington, DC: American Psychological Association.

Whiting, B. B., & Edwards, C. P. (1988). Children of different worlds: The formation of social behavior. Harvard University Press, Cambridge, MA.

The Relationship Between Parenting Behaviors and Adolescent Achievement and Self-Efficacy in Chile and Ecuador

Bron Ingoldsby
Paul Schvaneveldt
Andrew Supple
Kevin Bush

ABSTRACT. The purpose of this study was to examine the relationship between the perception of parenting behaviors (positive induction, monitoring, autonomy granting, punitiveness, and permissiveness) on adolescent achievement orientation and self-efficacy among samples of Chilean and Ecuadorian adolescents. Hierarchical regression analyses indicated that parental positive induction significantly predicted a greater achievement orientation for Ecuadorian youth. Achievement orientation and self-efficacy was positively predicted by the perception of Chilean mothers' and fathers' monitoring of behaviors. By contrast, a perception of greater parental punitiveness by Chilean youth negatively predicted self-efficacy and achievement orientation. Similarly, parental punitiveness and permissiveness negatively predicted self-efficacy among Ecuadorian youth. This study yields important insights into the diversity of Latin American culture and parenting behaviors that foster greater adolescent competency. *[Article copies available for a fee from The Haworth Document Delivery Service: 1-800-HAWORTH. E-mail address: <docdelivery@haworthpress. com> Website: <http://www.HaworthPress.com> © 2003 by The Haworth Press, Inc. All rights reserved.]*

Bron Ingoldsby is affiliated with Brigham Young University. Paul Schvaneveldt is affiliated with Weber State University. Andrew Supple is affiliated with the University of North Carolina-Greensboro. Kevin Bush is affiliated with the University of Georgia.

Address correspondence to: Bron Ingoldsby, School of Family Life, Brigham Young University, Provo, UT 84602-5325 (E-mail: bron_ingoldsby@byu.edu).

http://www.haworthpress.com/store/product.asp?sku=J002
© 2003 by The Haworth Press, Inc. All rights reserved.
10.1300/J002v35n03_08

129

KEYWORDS. Achievement orientation, Chile, Ecuador, parenting, self-efficacy

The purpose of this study is to examine the predictability of key dimensions of parental behaviors on the achievement orientation and self-efficacy of adolescents attending public schools in large urban cities in Chile and Ecuador. Although numerous investigations have examined the relationships between parental influences and adolescent academic achievement, few studies have examined parental influences on the development of adolescent self-efficacy (Hoeltje, Zubrick, Silburn, & Garton, 1996). Moreover, no studies to date have examined these relationships among adolescents living in Chile and Ecuador.

LITERATURE REVIEW

A considerable body of research has investigated the importance of parenting styles and behavior in relation to adolescent development, with Baumrind's (1966) typology being quite useful. Authoritarian parents demand obedience and conformity from their children, and favor punitive methods in gaining compliance. Permissive parents have few standards and avoid control. They tend to indulge rather than force or guide their children into acceptable behaviors. Authoritative parents have firm limits but are warm and nurturing in their approach. They prefer reasoning to coercion. Research tends to confirm that the latter approach is most likely to result in children who manifest social competence and responsibility, achievement, and friendliness (Heath, 1995).

Another way of examining the relationship between parenting influences and adolescent development is to divide parenting styles into its major components. Three broad dimensions of parental behavior have been identified as significant contributors to healthy adolescent development: parental support/connection, parental firm control, and punitive or harsh control (Barber, 1997; Barber & Olsen, 1997; Peterson & Hann, 1999). Adolescents reared by parents using high levels of support and firm control (e.g., monitoring), and low levels of punitiveness have typically been found to experience more positive developmental outcomes such as academic achievement, positive feelings toward the self, and avoidance of risky behavior (Amato & Fowler, 2002; Barber, Chadwick, & Oerter, 1992; Peterson & Hann, 1999).

While studies have consistently identified aspects of parenting behaviors and styles that are optimal in promoting social competence among adolescents in the U.S., controversy exists regarding the applicability of this body of research to adolescents in other cultures. Research findings examining parent-adolescent relationships in diverse samples of adolescents in the U.S., for example, suggest the positive influence of authoritative parenting may not be as positive for African and Asian American adolescents (Dornbusch, Ritter, Leiderman, Roberts, & Fraleigh, 1987; Steinberg, Dornbusch, & Brown, 1992). Differences in the influence of parenting on adolescent development may be related to parental style approaches, but this methodological focus on styles may not fully capture parenting processes for non-European American groups (Chao, 1994; Chao & Sue, 1996). Moreover, few studies have examined parent-adolescent relationships among non-western or collectivist cultural groups outside of US samples, especially in families from South America. Thus, little is known about the potential generalizability of current research findings to the parental socialization of adolescents across countries or ethnic groups within a nation.

Academic Achievement Orientation

Because of the increasingly complex and competitive nature of the modern world, academic achievement has become extremely important to adolescent psychosocial competence. As technological advances are made, fewer jobs will be available for less educated people. Therefore, it is important for researchers to identify the predictors of adolescent academic achievement and develop prevention programs to target those at risk for poor academic achievement.

Little data is available relating to the family and school experiences of young people in Chile and Ecuador. However, considering the high dropout rate and poverty levels in Latin American countries (Maddaleno & Silber, 1993), it is useful to examine factors that influence adolescent academic achievement and self-efficacy. Moreover, it is important to identify influential parenting behaviors that can be targeted by intervention efforts.

Studies done in the U.S. have consistently demonstrated the importance of parents in facilitating academic achievement among children and adolescents (e.g., Dornbusch et al., 1987; Steinberg et al., 1992; Steinberg, Mounts, Lamborn, & Dornbusch, 1991). However, the findings across diverse ethnic groups are not as clear since it appears that the patterns of relationships between parenting styles/behaviors and adolescent academic achievement vary across cultural groups (Asakawa & Csikszentmihalyi, 1998; Chao, 1996; Dornbusch et al., 1987; Steinberg et al., 1992). For example, Dornbusch et al. (1987) did not find the same positive effects of authoritative parenting for ethnic minority adolescents. In addition, authoritarian parenting was more strongly associated with poor school performance in Hispanic females than it was for Hispanic males, even though both sexes were equally likely to experience it. Dornbusch et al. (1987) also concluded that the benefits of authoritative parenting in relation to adolescent school performance were stronger for European Americans and Hispanics than for Asian Americans and African Americans.

In a subsequent study of the same data, Steinberg et al. (1991) examined the benefits of authoritative parenting compared to non-authoritative parenting across 16 ecological niches defined by SES, family structure, and ethnicity. The authors found that across each of the 16 niches, an authoritative parenting style was related to fewer problem behaviors of adolescents and higher academic achievement and self-reliance. In addition, they concluded that the benefits of authoritative parenting were stronger or more apparent among European American adolescents, middle-class adolescents, and adolescents in intact families. Similar to the findings of Dornbusch et al. (1987), authoritative parenting was less beneficial for academic achievement among African Americans and Asian Americans.

Herman, Dornbush, Herron and Herting (1997) disaggregated parenting styles and found that parental support, firm parental control, and punitive parenting predicted academic achievement for Anglo, African, Asian, and Hispanic Americans. Results from this study suggest the importance of examining specific dimensions of parental behavior when investigating parent-adolescent relationships among non-European American samples.

In summary, research has consistently found significant positive relationships between authoritative parenting and adolescent academic achievement. However, these results are less consistent across cultural groups. When specific dimensions of parental behavior are operationalized separately, parental support, firm control, and punitiveness appear to be consistent predictors of adolescent academic achievement across ethnic minority groups in the US. Therefore, parental support, induction, monitoring, and autonomy granting are hypothesized to be significant positive predictors of academic orientation among adolescents in Chile and Ecuador. In contrast, parental punitive behavior and permissiveness is expected to be a negative predictor across both groups.

Adolescent Self-Efficacy

The extent to which adolescents view themselves as competent and able to deal with normal life challenges refers to adolescents' sense of general self-efficacy (Bandura, 1977; Hoeltje et al., 1996). The development of a sense of general self-efficacy is viewed as a central developmental task of adolescence

(Greve, Anderson, & Krampen, 2001). Self-efficacy enhancement is one method of promoting successful adaptation for children and adolescents living in adversity (Rutter, 1990). Self-efficacy has been found to be significantly related to academic performance and various mental health disorders and problem behaviors among adolescents (Bandura, 1986; Hoeltje et al., 1996). Considering the high levels of poverty and school dropout rates in Latin America, understanding how parents help facilitate the development of adolescent self-efficacy could be an important mechanism for improving educational outcomes among youth in these countries. Another useful outcome is increased knowledge about potential ways to reduce mental health disorders and problem behaviors by adolescents through learning how to enhance youthful feelings of self-efficacy.

Although few studies have examined the relationships between parenting influences and adolescent self-efficacy, the work that does exist demonstrates consistent results across diverse cultural groups. Hoeltje et al. (1996) examined the family and adjustment correlates of self-efficacy among Australian adolescents. Results from this study indicated that parental nurturance was a positive predictor of adolescent self-efficacy, while parental rejection was a negative predictor. Similarly, Whitbeck, Simons, Conger, Wickrama, Ackley, and Elder (1997) found that parental induction was a positive predictor while harsh parental behaviors negatively predicted self-efficacy among a US sample of European American adolescents. Moreover, in a study examining the longitudinal impact of supportive parenting, Juang and Silbereisen (1999) reported that adolescents in East and West Germany who experienced consistent supportive parenting had higher levels of self-efficacy and school achievement over a three-year period.

In summary, the available research suggests that parental support, induction, and punitive parenting are predictive of adolescent self-efficacy development. Although previous research has not been conducted among Hispanic or Latin American samples, the following general predictions are made regarding adolescents living in Chile and Ecuadore: (1) It is expected that parental support, induction, monitoring, and autonomy granting will be positive predictors of adolescent self-efficacy; (2) Parental punitiveness and permissiveness will be negative predictors of adolescent self-efficacy.

This study contributes to the literature by exploring the hypothesized relationships within and across two countries for which little empirical research currently exists. Because of the exploratory nature of this study, differences between the Chile and Ecuador samples were not hypothesized. The present investigation improves upon previous studies by examining the relationship between specific parental behaviors and adolescent outcomes versus the reliance on parental styles that may not generalize across cultures. Additionally, the current study improves upon previous research by including adolescent perceptions of fathers' parenting. Previous research suggests that differences may exist in the patterns of influence between mothers and fathers on developmental outcomes of boys and girls (Block, 1983; Demo, Small, & Savin-Williams, 1987). Therefore, we examine models separately by gender of the parent to examine potential differences in adolescent perceptions of paternal versus maternal influence on adolescent outcomes for youth in Ecuador and Chile.

METHODS

Sample

The sample consisted of 185 adolescents from Ecuador and 245 adolescents from Chile. The ages ranged from 11 to 18 years (mean age = 15.15; sd = 1.08) and were nearly even in distribution of gender (50.4% female, 49.6% male). Self-administered questionnaires were distributed in the classroom setting by teachers trained in research protocols and the principal investigator. Schools of mostly middle class students in Cuenca allowed the investigators to take class periods for data collection for the Ecuador sample. Two public schools in Santiago Chile allowed teachers (trained in the standardized protocol) to recruit potential students and administer surveys to student volunteers during normal class periods.

Given that these samples were generated using a convenience strategy, they may not be representative of Ecuador or Chile as a whole. Moreover, we do not claim that these two countries are representative of Latin America as a whole, or that there are reasons to consider them to be especially similar or distinctive in reference to other Latin American countries.

Survey Instrument

The questionnaire consisted of scales and items that measure a variety of social psychological variables that are relevant to the characteristics of parents, social outcomes of adolescents, and the parent-adolescent relationship. All of the items and scales measuring maternal and paternal parenting behaviors and family dynamics are from the perspective of the adolescent. Likert-type responses were used for all the scale items, in the form of 4-point responses (0 indicating never to 4 indicating always, or 1 corresponding to strongly disagree and 4 corresponding to strongly agree). Items were recoded so that higher scores on scales indicate greater frequency of behaviors or more agreement on the part of the adolescent on each statement. Back translation procedures were applied to the survey instrument in the translation of the questionnaire from English to Spanish.

The survey consists of scales and items which measure sociodemographic variables, self-efficacy, autonomy granting, educational aspirations, parenting behaviors, grade point average, and academic orientations.

Measures

It was hypothesized that the various indicators of parenting would predict the adolescent's achievement orientation and self-efficacy. Parental monitoring, positive induction, punitiveness, permissiveness, and autonomy granting were measured by items from the Parent Behavior Measure (PBM), a shortened version of the Rollins and Thomas Parent Inventory resulting from previous factor analytic studies (Henry, Wilson, & Peterson, 1989; Peterson, Bush, & Supple, 1999). Six items measured parental monitoring and captured the extent to which the parents know how the adolescent spends free time, money, and who his or her friends are. Results of factor analyses, using a maximum likelihood analysis with a direct oblimin rotation, indicated that all six items reflecting parental monitoring for both mothers and fathers in Chile and Ecuador loaded well onto this construct and were retained for subsequent analyses (Cronbach alpha ranged from $\alpha = .83$ to $\alpha = .89$).

Parental positive induction was assessed by eleven items that were intended to measure the extent to which mothers and fathers are perceived as explaining to adolescents how their behavior affects other people, and being accepting, warm, approving, and nurturant. Factor analyses, with a maximum likelihood analysis and a direct oblimin rotation, indicated that three items reflecting positive induction should be dropped due to poor factor loadings for perception of Ecuadorian mothers' positive induction (e.g., parent shares activities; parent does things with me; parent approves of me and things I do). This resulted in eight items reflecting positive induction ($\alpha = .92$). Four items were dropped due to poor factor loadings for perception of Chilean mothers' positive induction (parent made me feel she would be there if needed; parent approves of me and things I do; parent enjoys doing things with me; parent shares activity with me). Seven items reflected maternal positive induction for the Chilean youth ($\alpha = .85$). Perceptions of paternal positive induction for Ecuadorian youth were best represented by seven items with four items dropped due to poor factor loadings (parent made me feel she would be there if needed; parent approves of me and things I do; parent enjoys doing things with me; parent shares activity with me; $\alpha = .90$). Paternal positive induction for the Chilean youth was best represented by six items with five items dropped due to poor factor loading (parent made me feel she would be there if needed; parent approves of me and things I do; parent enjoys doing things with me; parent shares activity with me; parent explained I should feel good when I share with other family members; $\alpha = .87$).

Parental punitiveness was measured by 14 items that tap into the adolescents' perceptions that mothers and fathers use of verbal and physical threats and behaviors. Factor analyses, using a maximum likelihood analysis and direct oblimin rotation, indicated that four items should be dropped due to poor factor loadings for perception of Ecuadorian mother's punitiveness (parent will not talk when displeased; parent avoids looking at me when disappointed; parent tells me about things he/she has done for me; parent tells me all things she has done for me; $\alpha = .91$). Maternal punitiveness as perceived in Chile was best represented by 12 items and two items were dropped (parent will not talk when displeased; parent tells me about things he/she has done for me; $\alpha = .92$). Paternal punitiveness in Ecuador is best represented by 12 items, and two items were dropped from this construct due to poor factor loadings (parent punished me by not letting me do what I enjoy; parent tells me about things he/she has done for me; $\alpha = .93$). Paternal punitiveness in the Chilean data was best reflected by 11 items, and three were dropped due to poor factor loadings (parent will not talk when displeased; parent avoids looking at me when disappointed; parent tells me about things he/she has done for me; $\alpha = .93$).

Parental permissiveness was reflected by three items intending to show how much the parent permits the adolescent to do things on his/her own. Factor analyses with a maximum likelihood analysis and direct oblimin rotation indicated all items load well in representing this construct for both mothers and fathers in the Chilean and Ecuadorian data. Reliability (measured by Cronbach's alpha) ranged from .73 to .74 for the permissiveness measure. A full list of the measurement items are listed in Table 1.

Adolescent reports of behavioral autonomy granted by the parents were measured by a scale of 10 items based on previous studies of youthful development of autonomy (see Peterson et al., 1999). These items measure the extent to which the young person make decisions and engages in activities without excessive parental intrusion or control regarding choices about friendships, dating, clothing selection, educational goals, and career plans.

Factor analyses, using a maximum likelihood analysis and direct oblimin rotation of the Ecuadorian data, show that five items best represent this construct for mothers. The retained items are: parent allows me to make decisions about career; parent allows me to make decisions about education; parent allows me to be my own person; parent has confidence in my ability to make decisions; parent encourages me to help make family decisions. The resulting reliability as measured by the Cronbach Alpha was .73. Five items also represented this construct for perception of mothers in Chile (parent allows me to make decisions about career; parent allows me to make decisions about education; parent gives me enough freedom; parent has confidence in my ability to make decisions; parent encourages me to help make family decisions; α = .78).

Six items best represented paternal autonomy granting for youth in Ecuador (parent gives me enough freedom, parent allows me to choose own friends, parent allows me to choose right from wrong, parent has confidence in my ability to make own decisions, parent encourages me to make decisions about family matters, parent lets me be my own person; α = .71). Four items best represented paternal autonomy granting for the Chilean youth (parent allows me to choose own dating partners, parent allows me to decide what clothes to wear, parent allows me to decide right from wrong, parent allows me to choose own friends; α = .70).

Self-reported academic orientations of the teenaged respondents also were measured. Academic orientation was assessed by a five-item scale that taps into effort exerted at school, the importance of education, whether assignments are completed on time, and whether the adolescent likes school. A sample item for this scale is: I try hard in school. Factor analyses, using a maximum likelihood analysis and direct oblimin rotation, indicated all five items loaded well together for both the Ecuadorian (α = .81) and Chilean (α = .85) youth. Self-efficacy was measured by 15 items (with several items reversed coded), to reflect the adolescent's perception of perceptions of competency and initiative. Factor analyses showed that nine items best reflected this item, and six items were dropped due to poor factor loadings for both the Ecuadorian (α = .87) and Chilean (α = .88) youth (I cannot get down to work when I should, If I can't do the job the first time, I keep trying, When I have something unpleasant, I stick to it until finished, When decide to do something, I go right to work, Failure makes me try harder, I am a self-reliant person).

Analyses

Hierarchical multiple regression analyses were used to test the hypotheses that parenting behaviors would predict greater self-efficacy and achievement orientation among adolescents. Separate statistical models were tested for mothers' and fathers' parental behaviors as predictors of adolescent self-efficacy and achievement orientation to help prevent multi-collinearity among

TABLE 1. Hypothesized Factor Structure of Parenting Items

Positive Induction (11 items)	
Explains how good I should feel when I do something that he/she liked	Parent would be there for me
Explains how good I should feel when I share things	Parent approves of me
Explains how good I should feel when I do what is right	Parent tells me how much she/he loves me
Explains that when I share with other family members, that I am liked by other family	Parent says nice things about me
Tells me how good others feel when I do what is right	Parent enjoys doing things with me
Parent shares many activities with me	
Punitiveness (14 items)	
Hits me when he/she thinks I am doing something wrong	Is always finding fault with me
Does not give me any peace until I do what he/she says	Punishes me by sending me out of the room
Punishes me by not letting me do things that I really enjoy	Punishes me by hitting me
Yells at me a lot without a good reason	Tells me if I loved him/her, I would do what he/she wants me to do
Punishes me by not letting me do things with other teenagers	Tells me about all the things he/she has done for me
Tells me that I will be sorry I wasn't better behaved	This parent will not talk to me when I displeased him/her
Tells me someday I will be punished for my behavior	This parent avoids looking at me when I have disappointed him/her
Monitoring (6 items)	
Knows where I am after school	Knows the parents of my friends
I tell this parent who I am going to be with when I go out	Knows who my friends are
When I go out, this parent knows where I am	Knows how I spend my money
Autonomy Granting (10 items)	
Gives me enough freedom	Has confidence in my ability to make my own decisions
Allows me to choose my own friends	Encourages me to help in making decisions about family matters
Allows me to decide what is right and wrong without interfering	Allows me to make my own decisions about career goals without interfering
Allows me to decide what clothes to wear without interfering	Allows me to make my own decisions about educational goals without interfering
Allows me to choose my own dating partner	Lets me be my own person in enough situations
Permissiveness (3 items)	
Allows me to do anything I want to do	Allows me to have any friends I want without questioning me
Allows me to be out on my own as often as it pleases me	

Achievement Orientation (5 items)	
I try hard in school	Education is so important that it's worth it to put up with things about school I don't like
Grades are very important to me	In general, I like school
I usually finish my homework on time	
Self-Efficacy (15 items)	
I cannot get down to work when I should	When unexpected problems occur, I don't handle them well
If I can't do a job the first time, I keep trying until I can	I avoid trying to learn new things when they look too difficult
When I set important goals for myself, I rarely achieve them	Failure just makes me try harder
I give up on things before completing them	I feel insecure about my ability to do things
I avoid facing difficulties	I am a self-reliant person
If something looks complicated, I will not bother to try	I give up easily
When I have something unpleasant to do, I stick to it until I finish it	When I decide to do something, I go right to work on it
When trying something new, I soon give up if not initially successful	

adolescent perceptions of the same parental behaviors for each parent. Also, separate statistical models were tested among the Chilean and Ecuadorian data. An initial inclination to merge the data files was rejected because many differences were identified between the two countries in the item composition of the parental measures. Furthermore, the smaller sample sizes from each country prohibited the use of structural equation modeling procedures, which led to the choice of hierarchical multiple regression analyses.

RESULTS

The demographic variables of age of adolescent, gender of adolescent, and father's educational attainment were included as a control variable block in the hierarchical regression models. Results are presented separately for adolescents' perceptions of mothers and fathers, and by country of origin.

Achievement Orientation

Ecuador, Maternal Model. Standardized regression coefficients indicated that age and father's education failed to attain statistical significance (see Table 2). Standardized regression coefficients indicated that gender significantly predicted achievement orientation ($\beta = .248$; $p < .05$), indicating that female adolescents scored higher on achievement orientation. Parenting variables significantly predicting an achievement orientation were maternal autonomy granting (ß = −.208; p < .10) and positive induction (ß = .487; p < .001). Thus, it appears that Ecuadorian adolescents who perceive their mothers as granting a high degree of autonomy reported a lowered achievement orientation, whereas, maternal positive induction was a positive predictor of achievement orientation.

Ecuador, Paternal Model. As with the perception of Ecuadorian mothers, standardized regression coefficients for fathers showed gender to significantly predict achievement orientation (ß = .226; p < .05), indicating female adolescents scored higher on achievement orientation, while age and father's education were not significantly related to achievement orientation (see Table 2). Paternal monitoring of behaviors demonstrated a positive association with achievement orientation (ß = .263; p < .05) as did positive induction (ß = .418; p < .001). This indicates that greater paternal monitoring and positive induction had a positive effect on the achievement orientation of adolescents from Ecuador.

Chile, Maternal Model. Gender significantly predicted achievement orientation (ß = .124; p < .10; see Table 2) meaning that Chilean female adolescents score higher than males on this measure. Maternal monitoring of behaviors had a significant and positive effect on achievement orientation (ß = .343; p < .001), whereas, punitiveness had a negative effect (ß = −.145; p < .10). This indicates that Chilean adolescents who perceived their mothers as monitoring their behaviors were more likely to have a positive achievement orientation. Furthermore, those who perceived their mothers as being punitive were less likely to have a positive achievement orientation.

Chile, Paternal Model. The gender of the adolescent was related to achievement orientation (ß = .175; p < .05). This indicates that Chilean females, on average, have a higher achievement orientation than males. Paternal monitoring demonstrated a positive association with achievement orientation (ß = .313; p < .01) while paternal punitiveness was a negative predictor (ß = −.216; p < .01; see Table 2). This indicates that greater monitoring by Chilean fathers predicts a higher achievement orientation among Chilean adolescents, whereas greater punitiveness predicts a lower achievement orientation. These results are similar to those that were found in the Chilean maternal model.

Self-Efficacy

Ecuador, Maternal Model. The demographic variables failed to predict self-efficacy. Ecuadorian youth perceived that maternal punitiveness had a negative impact on self-efficacy (ß = −.469; p < .01) as did permissiveness (ß = −.172; p < .10), while induction was positively related (β = .245; p < .05; see

TABLE 2

Ecuadorian Model: Multiple Regression Analysis for Ecuadorian Mothers' and Fathers'
Parenting Behaviors as Predictors of Achievement Orientation

Predictor Variables	b (father in parentheses)	SE ß (father in parentheses)	ß (father in parentheses)
Demographic Variables			
Age of Adolescent	−.268 (−.161)	.220 (.270)	−.116 (−.069)
Gender of Adolescent	1.129 (1.181)	.506 (.609)	.248** (.226**)
Father's Education	−.003 (−.009)	.086 (.096)	−.038 (.012)
Paternal Behaviors			
Monitoring	.036 (.149)	.064 (.069)	.064 (.263**)
Autonomy Granting	−.153 (.052)	.091 (.130)	−.208* (.060)
Punitiveness	−.032 (.009)	.033 (.033)	−.098 (.032)
Positive Induction	.297 (.259)	.070 (.078)	.487*** (.418***)
Permissiveness	−.095 (−.124)	.140 (.158)	.077 (−.110)

Multiple Correlation R .558 (.604)   R-Square .311 (.365)
F-Value 4.635 (4.665)   Significance F .000*** (.000***)
n = 185 (185)

Chilean Model: Multiple Regression Analysis for Chilean Mothers' and Fathers'
Parenting Behaviors as Predictors of Achievement Orientation

Predictor Variables	b (father in parentheses)	SE ß (father in parentheses)	ß (father in parentheses)
Demographic Variables			
Age of Adolescent	.363 (.322)	.289 (.292)	.096 (.088)
Gender of Adolescent	.799 (1.117)	.514 (.531)	.124* (.175**)
Father's Education	.062 (.057)	.122 (.121)	.038 (.037)
Paternal Behaviors			
Monitoring	.346 (.258)	.089 (.076)	.343*** (.313***)
Autonomy Granting	−.038 (−.118)	.105 (.123)	−.032 (−.089)
Punitiveness	−.060 (−.083)	.034 (.032)	−.145* (−.216***)
Positive Induction	.061 (.004)	.080 (.087)	.071 (.005)
Permissiveness	−.021 (.187)	.147 (.145)	−.013 (.124)

Multiple Correlation R .475 (.239)   R-Square .226 (.193)
F-Value 5.096 (5.186)   Significance F .000*** (.000***)
n = 245 (245)
b = unstandardized betas;   ß = standardized betas;   SE ß = standard error of standardized beta
*p < .10;   **p < .05;   ***p < .01

Table 3). This indicates that adolescents who perceived their mothers as being punitive and permissive reported lower levels of self-efficacy, and that experiencing their relationship as rational and supportive resulted in higher levels of self-efficacy.

Ecuador, Paternal Model. Fathers educational attainment had a significant and positive impact on the self-efficacy of the adolescent ($\beta = .237$; $p < .05$), whereas age and gender did not impact self-efficacy. Greater paternal punitiveness negatively predicted self-efficacy ($\beta = -.459$; $p < .01$) as did greater paternal permissiveness ($\beta = -.303$; $p < .05$; see Table 3). This indicates that adolescents who perceived their fathers (as they did with their mothers) as being punitive and permissive reported lower levels of self-efficacy.

Chile, Maternal Model. The father's level of education significantly predicted self-efficacy ($\beta = .165$; $p < .05$). This indicates that a higher level of father's education predicted greater self-efficacy. Greater maternal monitoring of behaviors also predicted self-efficacy ($\beta = .177$; $p < .05$). Maternal punitiveness negatively predicted self-efficacy ($\beta = -.545$; $p < .01$; see Table 3). This indicates that greater monitoring of behaviors had a positive effect on self-efficacy and punitiveness had a negative impact on the adolescent's self-efficacy.

Chile, Paternal Model. Father's level of education significantly predicted self-efficacy ($\beta = .173$; $p < .05$). Paternal monitoring of behaviors also had a significant and positive impact on self-efficacy ($\beta = .267$; $p < .05$) and punitiveness had a negative impact on self-efficacy ($\beta = -.493$; $p < .01$; see Table 3). These results are similar to those found for Chilean mothers, where greater monitoring had a positive impact on self-efficacy and greater punitiveness had a negative impact.

DISCUSSION

Based on the review of the literature, we hypothesized that adolescents in Chile and Ecuador, as in the U.S., would have a higher achievement orientation (educational effort) and experience greater self- efficacy (sense of competence and initiative) when their parents interact with them using strategies of positive induction (reasoning and support), monitoring (keeping track of the child's activities), and autonomy (freedom granting). Parental punitiveness (punishing behaviors) and permissiveness (lack of control) were expected to result in lower levels of achievement orientation and self-efficacy.

A total of 430 students from urban areas in Ecuador and Chile responded to a self-report survey designed to assess their perceptions of a wide-range of parenting behaviors and their own academic orientation and feelings of self-efficacy. The sample consisted of nearly equal numbers of males and females, whose average age was fifteen. Analyses were run separately for mothers and fathers and by country, as factor analyses revealed a number of apparent gender and cultural differences in how the measures were conceptualized by the respondents. This was expected to some degree, as differences in attitudes and understandings are an important part of being a separate and identifiable culture or society.

Achievement Orientation. Overall, examination of the findings suggests differences in the development of achievement orientation across gender of adolescent and across cultural group. Female adolescents tended to manifest a higher level of achievement orientation than did males. These findings are consistent with similar research among US samples of European American adolescents. For example, Pomerantz, Altermatt, and Saxon (2002) reported that early adolescent girls performed higher than boys in their school grades (i.e., language arts, social studies, science, and math). Moreover, within an ethnically diverse US sample of adolescents, Miller and Byrnes (2001) found that girls in the 11th grade reported higher levels of achievement orientation than boys in the 11th grade.

Interesting differences across Chilean and Ecuadorian samples were also found. Consistent with research among European American samples (e.g., Herman et al., 1997), parental positive induction, as well as monitoring (by fathers) predicted achievement orientation in Ecuador. Autonomy granting, on the other hand, was associated with lowered achievement orientation, which is contrary to previous empirical and theoretical work among US samples (e.g., Herman et al., 1997; Peterson & Hann, 1999). This finding also contrasts with recent empirical work, suggesting that Mexican American adolescents expect behavioral autonomy at similar levels to European American adolescents (Fuligni, 1998). Therefore, it seems autonomy granting, at least as conceptualized and measured in this particular study, is not as important to the development of academic orientation (or self-efficacy) among these Chilean and Ecuadorian adolescents.

In Chile, similar to studies of European American adolescents (e.g., Herman et al., 1997), monitoring from both parents had a positive effect while punitiveness had a negative effect. In general, the most consistent predictors of a high achievement orientation for Chilean and Ecuadorian adolescents was being female and having parents who are rational or supportive (in Ecuador) and monitor their behaviors without being punitive.

Self-Efficacy. Overall, the development of self-efficacy among Chilean and Ecuadorian adolescents were similar across age and gender of adolescent, with a few differences found across gender of parent, SES, and cultural group. Father's education served as our measure of family SES, and the findings sug-

TABLE 3

Ecuadorian Model: Multiple Regression Analysis for Ecuadorian Mothers' and Fathers' Parenting Behaviors as Predictors of Self-Efficacy

Predictor Variables	b (father in parentheses)	SE ß (father in parentheses)	ß (father in parentheses)
Demographic Variables			
Age of Adolescent	.032 (−.226)	.503 (.584)	.006 (−.040)
Gender of Adolescent	.079 (.371)	1.229 (1.134)	.002 (.028)
Father's Education	.273 (.489)	.204 (.222)	.140 (.237**)
Paternal Behaviors			
Monitoring	−.002 (−.158)	.182 (.197)	−.002 (−.101)
Autonomy Granting	−.330 (063)	.223 (.346)	−.181 (.029)
Punitiveness	−.385 (−.342)	.084 (.084)	−.469*** (−.459***)
Positive Induction	.355 (.241)	.178 (.214)	.245** (.151)
Permissiveness	−.528 (−.844)	.336 (.406)	−.172* (−.303**)

Multiple Correlation R .581 (.644)   R-Square .338 (.415)
F-Value 4.843 (5.229)   Significance F .000*** (.000***)
n = 185 (185)

Chilean Model: Multiple Regression Analysis for Chilean Mothers' and Fathers' Parenting Behaviors as Predictors of Self-Efficacy

Predictor Variables	b (father in parentheses)	SE ß (father in parentheses)	ß (father in parentheses)
Demographic Variables			
Age of Adolescent	.292 (.193)	.428 (.458)	.047 (.031)
Gender of Adolescent	−1.143 (−.659)	.766 (.840)	−.108 (−.061)
Father's Education	.434 (.452)	.180 (.187)	.165** (.173**)
Paternal Behaviors			
Monitoring	.291 (.365)	.130 (.118)	.177** (.267**)
Autonomy Granting	−.192 (.194)	.154 (.189)	−.098 (−.088)
Punitiveness	−.364 (−.312)	.049 (.048)	−.545*** (−.493***)
Positive Induction	.125 (−.096)	.119 (.139)	.089 (−.065)
Permissiveness	−.089 (−.092)	.218 (.229)	−.035 (−.004)

Multiple Correlation R .620 (.599)   R-Square .384 (.358)
F-Value 10.601 (8.938)   Significance F .000*** (.000***)
n = 245 (245)

b = unstandardized betas; ß = standardized betas; SE ß = standard error of standardized beta
*p < .10; **p < .05; ***p < .01

gest that higher levels of paternal education predict greater feelings of self-efficacy among boys and girls in Chile and Ecuador.

In Ecuador, punitiveness and permissiveness resulted in lower self-efficacy, while positive induction from mothers was connected to greater self-efficacy. In Chile, monitoring resulted in greater self-efficacy, and punitiveness had the opposite effect. These significant findings are in the expected directions and consistent with previous studies among US (Whitbeck et al., 1997) and Australian (Hoeltje et al., 1996) samples. However, similar to the findings for academic orientation, there were some differences across the two cultural groups.

CONCLUSIONS

In general, our results are similar to those found in the US. Parental induction and monitoring contribute to positive outcomes for adolescents, while being overly permissive or punishing have the opposite effect. Being female and from higher SES families are also helpful in attaining higher levels of academic orientation and self-efficacy.

It is intriguing that autonomy granting only appears as significant one time (with Ecuadorian mothers and achievement orientation) and that it is a negative predictor. It seems that for the most part it is simply not important either way. There is some evidence that Hispanic parents do not grant their children as much freedom as do parents in the US, and that, therefore, it loses its predictive value.

The most powerful parental behavior seems to be monitoring. Knowing where their children are and what they are doing has a positive impact on achievement motivation in both countries and on self-efficacy in Chile. The biggest surprise was that positive parental induction was not as powerful as it has tended to be in other studies. The research reviewed from Chile points to significant behavioral, health, and educational problems in that country (Urzua, 1993). It may be, therefore, that their situation calls for a firm (though not punitive) hand in guiding youth so that they will have a successful educational experience.

Overall, these findings underscore the diversity of adolescent socialization experiences and development in Latin America. Many culture differences (i.e., across gender of parent, gender of adolescent, age of adolescent, and SES) were found within both the Chilean and Ecuadorian samples, highlighting intriguing differences within, and well as between Ecuadorian and Chilean families. For example, parental induction and permissiveness show up in Ecuador more often as significant variables, and monitoring less often. In Chile, it is clear that it is important for parents to monitor their children's activities and avoid punitive responses. Ecuadorian adolescents seem to have a special relationship with their mothers not found with other samples. While our samples were neither huge nor truly random (a practical impossibility in most cross-cultural research), they were sufficient for our statistical analyses. It seems likely that a more sensitive, perhaps qualitative approach is needed in future research in order to tease out these likely societal and gender differences in parenting approaches and their impact on adolescent outcomes.

REFERENCES

Amato, P. R., & Fowler, F. (2002). Parenting practices, child adjustment, and family diversity. *Journal of Marriage and Family, 64*, 703-716.

Asakawa, K., & Csikszentmihalyi, M. (1998). The quality of experience of Asian American adolescents in activities related to future goals. *Journal of Youth and Adolescence, 27*, 141-163.

Bandura, A. (1977). Self-efficacy: Toward a unifying theory of behavioral change. *Psychological Review, 84*, 191-215.

Bandura, A. (1986). Self-efficacy. In A. Bandura (Ed.), *Social foundations of thought and action: A social cognitive theory* (pp. 390-453). Englewood Cliffs, NJ: Prentice-Hall.

Barber, B. K. (1997). Introduction: Adolescent socialization in context–The role of connection, regulation, and autonomy in the family. *Journal of Adolescent Research, 12*, 5-11.

Barber, B., Chadwick, B., & Oerter, R. (1992). Parental behaviors and adolescent self-esteem in the United States and Germany. *Journal of Marriage and the Family, 54*, 128-141.

Barber, B. K., & Olsen, J. A. (1997). Socialization in context: Connection, regulation, and autonomy in the family, school, and neighborhood, and with peers. *Journal of Adolescent Research, 12*, 287-315.

Baumrind, D. (1966). Effects of authoritative parental control on child behavior. *Child Development, 37*, 887-906.

Block, J. H. (1983). Differential premises arising from differential socialization of the sexes: Some conjectures. *Child Development, 54*, 1335-1354.

Chao, R. K. (1994). Beyond parental control and authoritarian parenting style: Understanding Chinese parenting through the cultural notion of training. *Child Development, 65*, 1111-1119.

Chao, R. K., & Sue, S. (1996). Chinese parental influence and their children's school success: A paradox in the literature on parenting styles. In S. Lau and N. T. Sha Tin (Eds.), *Growing up the Chinese way: Chinese child and adolescent development* (pp. 93-120). Hong Kong: The Chinese University Press.

Demo, D. H., Small, S. A., & Savin-Williams, R. C. (1987). Family relations and the self-esteem of adolescents and their parents. *Journal of Marriage and the Family, 49*, 705-715.

Dornbusch, S., Ritter, P., Leiderman, P., Roberts, D., & Fraleigh, M. (1987). The relation of parenting style to adolescent school performance. *Child Development, 65,* 754-770.

Fuligni, A. J. (1998). Authority, autonomy, and parent-adolescent conflict and cohesion: A study of adolescents from Mexican, Chinese, Filipino, and European backgrounds. *Developmental Psychology, 34,* 782-792.

Greve, W., Anderson, A., & Krampen, G. (2001). Self-efficacy and externality in adolescence: Theoretical conceptions and measurement in New Zealand and German secondary school students. *Identity: An International Journal of Theory and Research, 1,* 321-344.

Heath, T. (1995). Parents' socialization of children. In B. Ingoldsby & S. Smith (Eds.), *Families in multicultural perspective* (pp. 161-186). New York: Guilford Press.

Henry, S., Wilson, S. M., & Peterson, G. W. (1989). Parental power bases and processes as predictors of adolescent conformity. *Journal of Adolescent Research, 4,* 15-32.

Herman, M., Dornbusch, S., Herron, M., & Herting. (1997). The influence of family behavioral control, connection, and psychological autonomy on six measures of adolescent functioning. *Journal of Adolescent Research, 12,* 34-67.

Hoeltje, C. O., Zubrick, S. R., Silburn, S. R. & Garton, A. F. (1996). Generalized self-efficacy: Family and adjustment correlates. *Journal of Clinical Child Psychology, 24,* 446-453.

Juang, L. P., & Silbereisen, R. K. (1999). Supportive parenting and adolescent adjustment across time in former East and West Germany. *Journal of Adolescence, 22,* 719-736.

Maddaleno, M., & Silber, T. (1993). An epidemiological view of adolescent health in Latin America. *Journal of Adolescent Health, 14,* 595-604.

Miller, D. C., & Byrnes, J. P. (2001). To achieve or not to achieve: A self-regulation perspective on adolescents' academic decision making. *Journal of Educational Psychology, 93,* 677-685.

Peterson, G. W., Bush, K. R., & Supple, A. J. (1999). Predicting adolescent autonomy from parents: Relationship connectedness and restrictiveness. *Sociological Inquiry, 69,* 431-457.

Peterson, G. W., & Hann, D. (1999). Socializing parents and families. In M. Sussman, S. K. Steinmetz, & Peterson, G. W. (Eds.), *Handbook of marriage and the family* (pp. 471-506). New York: Plenum Press.

Pomerantz, E. M., Altermatt, E. R., & Saxon, J. L. (2002). Making the grade but feeling distressed: Gender differences in academic performance and internal distress. *Journal of Educational Psychology, 94,* 396-404.

Rutter, M. (1990). Psychological resilience and protective mechanisms. In J. Rolf, A. S. Masten, D. Cicchetti, K. H. Neuchterlein, & S. Weintraub (Eds.), *Risk and protective factors in the development of psychopathology* (pp. 181-214), Cambridge, England: Cambridge University Press.

Steinberg, L., Dornbusch, S. M., & Brown, B. B. (1992). Ethnic differences in adolescent achievement: An ecological perspective. *American Psychologist, 47,* 723-729.

Steinberg, L., Mounts, N. S., Lamborn, S. D., & Dornbusch, S. M. (1991). Authoritative parenting and adolescent adjustment across varied ecological niches. *Journal of Research on Adolescence, 1*, 19-36.

Urzua, R. (1993). Risk factors and youth: The role of family and community. *Journal of Adolescent Health, 14*, 619-625.

Whitbeck, L. B., Simons, R. L., Conger, R. D., Wickrama, K. A. S., Ackley, K. A., & Elder, G. H. (1997). The effects of parents' working conditions and family economic hardship on parenting behaviors and children's self-efficacy. *Social Psychology Quarterly, 60*, 291-303.

Parent-Adolescent Relations and Problem Behaviors: Hungary, the Netherlands, Switzerland, and the United States

Alexander T. Vazsonyi

ABSTRACT. The current investigation examined the predictive strength of mother/father-adolescent relations (closeness, support, and monitoring) and of low self-control for a variety of adolescent problem behaviors in samples from Hungary, the Netherlands, Switzerland, and the United States. Based on data from over $N = 6,900$ middle and late adolescents, findings indicated the following: (1) each family process dimension was predictive of adolescent problem behaviors in all national contexts. And, despite some overlap between maternal and paternal measures of parent-adolescent relations, each measure had unique and additive explanatory power in adolescent problem behaviors; (2) family processes were predictive of all types of problem behaviors ranging from trivial school misconduct to more serious behaviors such as assault; (3) pairwise comparisons of partial regression coefficients of individual family process dimensions predicting problem behaviors in-

Alexander T. Vazsonyi is affiliated with the Department of Human Development and Family Studies, Auburn University, 284 Spidle Hall, Auburn, AL 36849 USA (E-mail: vazsonyi@auburn.edu).

This research was supported in part by a grant from the Auburn University Competitive Research Grant-in-Aid Program. The author would like to thank Marianne Junger and Dick Hessing for coordinating and supporting the Dutch data collection as well as Lara Belliston and Lloyd Pickering for their assistance with data entry and coding. The author also thanks all administrators, teachers, and students for making this study possible.

http://www.haworthpress.com/store/product.asp?sku=J002
© 2003 by The Haworth Press, Inc. All rights reserved.
10.1300/J002v35n03_09

dicated that they were largely identical cross-nationally; (4) final prediction models accounted for between 30% (Swiss youth) and 37% (American and Dutch youth) of the variance in problem behaviors. These findings provide further support for the idea of universal developmental processes. *[Article copies available for a fee from The Haworth Document Delivery Service: 1-800-HAWORTH. E-mail address: <docdelivery@ haworthpress.com> Website: <http://www.HaworthPress.com> © 2003 by The Haworth Press, Inc. All rights reserved.]*

KEYWORDS. Family process, closeness, support, monitoring, deviance, cross-cultural

INTRODUCTION

Over the past decade, there has been a renewed interest in cross-national comparative research on the *etiology* of adolescent problem behaviors, deviance, and more generally, adjustment (Barber & Harmon, 2001; Barber, Chadwick, & Oerter, 1992; Bush, 2000; Chen, Greenberger, Lester, Don, & Guo, 1998; Chirkov & Ryan, 2001; Crystal, Chen, Fuligni, & Stevenson, 1994; Dekovic, Engels, Shirai, De Kort, & Anker, 2002; Feldman, Rosenthal, Mont-Reynaud, Leung, & Lau, 1991; Feldman & Rosenthal, 1994; Greenberger, Chen, Beam, Whang, & Dong, 2000; Vazsonyi, Hibbert, & Snider, 2003). In part, this is due to the availability of representative samples in diverse developmental contexts and due to more sophisticated psychometric methods and analytic techniques (Chen & Farruggia, 2002). In turn, this has contributed to more rigorous inquiries–inquiries that have been interested in answering whether developmental processes, namely the patterns of association between predictors and outcomes of interest, were similar or different in diverse countries. This is in contrast to most previous cross-cultural comparative investigations (e.g., Weigert & Thomas, 1979) in the tradition of cultural anthropology, cultural psychology, or relativist theories. These latter studies primarily focused on cultural or national differences in mean levels of both parenting practices and outcomes. A number of such studies found substantial evidence of differences in mean levels of parenting, and in some cases have speculated without substantial empirical evidence about the implications of observed cross-national differences in parenting for the observed differences in outcomes (e.g., Devereux, Bronfenbrenner, & Suci, 1962; Devereux, Bronfenbrenner, & Rodgers, 1969).

Cross-national comparative inquiry is an important methodological tool in the study of human development. In fact, van de Vijver and Leung (1997) argue that cross-cultural studies are quasi-experiments, where cultural or national groups are compared in order to "unpack" the effects of culture or country (the independent variable). Cross-national comparative inquiry is also important because diverse national contexts provide a larger natural range and diversity in human development and behavior (Vazsonyi, 2003). In turn, this greater variability lends itself to confirm or disconfirm hypotheses (van de Vijver and Leung call this verifying or falsifying the effects of culture) on human development and on the etiology of human behaviors. These tests would be aimed, in turn, at issues defined by previous empirical work in other national contexts or based on theoretical propositions.

One such key hypothesis is whether human beings have similar socialization goals and mechanisms to achieve them across societies (Chirkov & Ryan, 2001). In other words, do socialization mechanisms function in a similar or different fashion across developmental contexts. Based on the assumption that human beings everywhere seem to be interested in successfully socializing their children into "confirming citizens" in society, it is plausible to suggest that socialization efforts or parenting efforts may be a generalizable human quality. This would mean that a socialization mechanism would be observed in different cultures and societies as well as have similar effects across cultural groups. Recent evidence in a review by Rohner and Britner (2002), for example, supports this idea of universality in reference to the dimension of parental acceptance-rejection and measures of adjustment. These proposals about universality were based on a large number of investigations in different national contexts. Consequently, the current investigation sought to address this issue, namely whether the relationships between perceived parenting behaviors (both maternal and paternal) and measures of problem behaviors were similar or different cross-nationally.

Previous Empirical Investigations

This is by no means a new idea, yet surprisingly few studies have examined this question employing the cross-national comparative framework (e.g., Barber & Harmon, 2001; Feldman et al., 1991; Chen et al., 1998; Vazsonyi et al., 2003), in part due to the complexity of such work. Feldman and colleagues (1991) completed an important cross-national study that focused on the etiological importance of "the family" in adolescent misconduct. Based on samples from Australia, Hong Kong, and the United States, the authors found strong evidence that family processes, especially parental monitoring, accounted for misconduct in a largely invariant fashion across the three groups. In addition, the authors also concluded that the predictor variables tested in their model, that included family processes, reduced cultural variability in misconduct by 70% to about 3% of the total variance explained. In a similar study by Chen and colleagues (1998), the authors also were interested in the effects of family and peer correlates on measures of adolescent misconduct. Based on samples from China, Taiwan, and the United States (Caucasian and Chinese youth), they found consistent evidence that a higher order parent-adolescent relationship construct (measured by conflict, warmth, and monitoring) was related to adolescent misconduct in a highly similar fashion cross-nationally. It is important to note that the authors did not employ a direct statistical test to examine whether these relationships differed by country, while Feldman and Rosenthal used an ANCOVA procedure to assess whether the regression planes were parallel. Finally, in a recent chapter by Barber and Harmon (2001), the authors presented preliminary evidence of cross-national similarity in relationships between psychological control and antisocial behavior based on samples from six different countries, nine cultural groups. More specifically, they found that parental psychological control was consistently associated with a measure of antisocial behavior, namely between $r = .21$ and $r = .29$ (average $r = .24$). In addition to such cross-national comparative efforts, a number of analogous cross-cultural comparisons between different racial groups have been completed in the United States over the past decade that have provided strong evidence of similarity or generalizability–both on measurement of parenting constructs and outcomes (e.g., Knight, Tein, Shell, & Roosa, 1992; Knight, Virdin, & Roosa, 1994) as well as the relationships between predictors and outcomes (e.g., Rowe, Vazsonyi, & Flannery, 1994).

Parent-Adolescent Relations: Harmony, Autonomy, and Conflict

Steinberg and Silk (2002) succinctly summarized three core developmental changes that take place during adolescence in the parent-adolescent relationship, and thereby also provided an overview of the key parenting constructs and their importance in adolescent adjustment.

Harmony. Harmony includes the affective tie between parents and adolescents that is key in understanding adolescent adjustment. Despite some evidence of a decreased frequency of interaction during the adolescent years, research has documented that children and youth who enjoy warm, close, and intimate relations with their parents are better adjusted in comparison to adolescents who do not enjoy such ties. Better adjustment refers to being more self-reliant, having a higher sense of self-worth, scoring higher on indicators of psychological well-being, and being lower on measures of problem behaviors or deviance.

Autonomy. Autonomy is the relational quality in the parent-adolescent dyad that undergoes the greatest changes. Gradually, adolescents may (parents permitting) be allowed to individuate and learn how to function independently, autonomously. These youth continue to enjoy their parents and family life, and generally speaking, are most self-reliant and socially competent. On the other hand, parents who are intrusive or overprotective (psychologically or behaviorally) have the opposite effect on adolescent development; youth in these families do not individuate and learn how to function independently. Studies have shown that adolescents from overprotective (psychologically) homes often face internalizing problems (anxiety and depression) or externalizing problems (problem behaviors, substance use and deviance).

Conflict. Finally, Steinberg and Silk (2002) discuss the developmental changes and importance of *conflict* and note that conflict per se may be part of most parent-adolescent relations; however, the frequency (rate) and the affective intensity (affect) of conflict that gradually decrease and increase, respectively, may be able to account for variability in adolescent adjustment. Interestingly, research does not document a simple association with positive or negative developmental outcomes. In fact, Steinberg and Silk (2002) conclude that it depends–in a supportive family, one that let's their children individuate and one that maintains close affective ties, conflict may have little or no effect on adolescent adjustment. On the other hand, the same intensity of conflict in a family that can be characterized as overprotective and as lacking warmth may be associated with adverse effects on adolescent adjustment. The authors conclude that one of the most promising areas of research on parent-adolescent relations has been the dimensional conceptualization of parenting (in comparison to a typological one); this approach allows the simultaneous measurement of multiple, interdependent parenting processes that, in turn, individually or interactively are predictive of adolescent adjustment.

Based on this broad conceptualization, Vazsonyi and colleagues (2003), found strong empirical evidence of the cross-national validity of a six dimensional parenting or family process measure, the Adolescent Family Process (AFP) measure. More specifically, based on samples from four countries (Hungary, the Netherlands, Switzerland, and the United States), a series of confirmatory factor analyses provided consistent evidence for the cross-national validity of the measure that independently assessed both *maternal* and *paternal* closeness, support, monitoring, communication, conflict, and peer approval. In addition, the same evidence was found in comparisons across countries for males, females, middle adolescents, and late adolescents. Finally, based on a model-free LISREL analytic technique, great similarity in developmental processes was also found across the four countries for maternal and paternal measures of family processes–namely the patterns of relationships between six family process subscales and measures of both internalizing and externalizing behaviors.

The Current Investigation

The current study extends this previous work on the measurement of family processes in different countries and on the relationships between family processes and adolescent developmental outcomes in four important ways. First, it examined the combined predictive strength of the three most salient maternal and paternal family processes (closeness, support, and monitoring) in adolescent problem behaviors across samples of adolescents from four countries. Previous work has established each of these parenting dimensions as important in understanding adolescent socialization, in particular with regards to the etiology of problem behaviors in youth, both in the United States as well as cross- nationally (Barber, 1992; Chen et al., 1998; Feldman et al., 1991; Steinberg & Silk, 2002; Vazsonyi et al., 2003). Second, the study examined the potentially overlapping or additive predictive effects of maternal and paternal family processes in adolescent problem behaviors. Most investigations to date have exclusively focused on parenting efforts by the mother or have simply averaged perceived maternal and paternal parenting efforts (e.g., Lamborn, Mounts, Steinberg, & Dornbusch, 1991). Third, based on conceptual and theoretical rationale (e.g., Gottfredson & Hirschi, 1994; Jessor & Jessor, 1977), the study examined the importance of family processes for a wide variety of adolescent problem behaviors, ranging from more "trivial" school misconduct to assault (Gottfredson & Hirschi's concept of versatility or generality of problem behaviors). And finally, based on prediction by Gottfredson and Hirschi's (1994) General Theory of Adolescent Problem Behaviors, the study also tested the importance of low self-control in problem behaviors after accounting for family process effects. Barber (1992) has argued that one of the greatest criticisms of socialization research has been the omission of individual difference variables in etiological studies.

Gottfredson and Hirschi (1994) suggest that low self-control, the tendency to act in ways to maximize immediate gratification with no regard for consequences or the future, is the common element found across all problem behaviors, ranging from sexual promiscuity to auto theft. They also suggest "in families in which parents care about their children, monitor their actions, recognize deviant behavior, and sanction it negatively, self-control will become a stable characteristic of the child" (p. 44). In other words, early rearing experiences in the family context socialize an individual to be able to delay gratification or to develop a sense of self-control; families that do not develop a strong affective bond with their children and that do not monitor the behavior of their children do not instill the ability to delay gratification or to develop a sense of self-control. In a sense, children from such families simply have an inability to control impulses–a low level of self-control. These youth are at greatest risk for engaging in problem behaviors according to Gottfredson and Hirschi (1994). Since parenting and family processes are causally antecedent to self-control or a lack thereof, the current study attempted to examine the additional explanatory power of low self-control above and beyond the effects by family processes.

METHODS

Procedures

The data were collected as part of the International Study of Adolescent Development (ISAD), a multinational, multisite investigation consisting of about 8,500 subjects from four different countries (Hungary, the Netherlands, Switzerland, and the United States). The purpose of ISAD is to examine the etiology of adolescent problem behaviors and deviance utilizing large representative samples from different countries (Vazsonyi, Pickering, Junger, & Hessing, 2001; Vazsonyi, Pickering, Belliston, Hessing, & Junger, 2002). A standard data collection protocol was used for all study locations and approval was acquired from the university Institutional Review Board. A self-report instrument was used for data collection that included instructions on how to complete the survey, a description of the ISAD project, and assurances of anonymity. Questionnaires were administered to participants during a 1 to 2 hour period.

Substantial attention was devoted to developing the ISAD survey instrument, particularly by creating new or employing existing measures that could be used cross-culturally without losing nuances or changing meanings. This included an evaluation of survey items to whether they assessed a readily observable and "ratable" behavior in each of the countries included in the current study. The survey was translated from English into each of the target languages (Dutch, German, and Hungarian) and then back-translated by bilingual translators. Additional bilingual translators examined the surveys, and, when translation was difficult or ambiguous, consensus was used to produce the final translation.

Sample

Data were collected from $N = 8,417$ adolescents in four countries: Hungary ($n = 871$), Netherlands ($n = 1,315$), Switzerland ($n = 4,018$), and the United

States (n = 2,213). In all locations, medium-sized cities of similar size were selected for participation. For each country, different schools were invited for
participation to obtain locally representative samples of the adolescent population. For European samples, this included schools for university-bound students (Gymnasium) as well as schools specializing in vocational/technical
training for students in apprenticeships. In the United States, the samples included high school students, community college students, and university students (for a more detailed description of the samples, see Vazsonyi et al.,
2001).

In the current study, a common "age band" including 15- to 19-year- olds
across all country samples reduced the sample to n = 6,914 (82% of the total
sample). The numbers for each country in final study sample were: 1,516
Americans, 1,040 Dutch, 797 Hungarians, and 3,561 Swiss. In the total sample,
there were 3,913 males (mean age = 17.5, sd = 1.3) and 2,939 females (mean
age = 17.5, sd = 1.4) in this sample. Sixty-two participants did not identify
their gender. In the Hungarian sample, there were 544 males and 242 female
(11 Hungarian subjects did not identify their gender). The Dutch adolescents
sample has 495 males and 540 females (5 Dutch subjects did not identify their
gender). There were 2,235 males and 1,291 females in the Swiss sample (35
Swiss subjects did not identify their gender). Finally, the American sample included 639 males and 866 females (11 American subjects did not identify their
gender).

Measures

Participants from all countries were asked to fill out the same questionnaire
that included demographic and background variables (age, gender, family
structure, and socioeconomic status), maternal and paternal family process
measures, low self-control, and measures of problem behaviors and deviance.

Age. Participants were asked to indicate the month and year in which they
were born. The 15th day of each respective month was used to calculate subjects' specific ages.

Gender. Participants were asked to indicate their gender on a single item:
"What is your gender?" Responses were given as 1 = male and 2 = female.

Family structure. An adolescent's home situation was assessed by a single
item: "Which of the following home situations best applies to you?" Responses in the survey included: 1 = biological parents, 2 = biological mother
only, 3 = biological father only, 4 = biological mother and stepfather, 5 = biological father and stepmother, 6 = biological parent and significant other, and
7 = other. Due to the small number of participants who selected categories 5
and above, responses were recoded for subsequent analyses into: 1 = biologi-

cal parents, 2 = biological mother only or father only, 3 = biological mother/father and step-parent, and 4 = other.

Socioeconomic status (SES). SES was measure by two items. First, participants were asked to indicate the type of work performed by the primary wage earner in the family. Six categories collapsed from Hollingshead's (1975) original nine categories and modified to be applicable in each of the four countries were specified that would readily map on professions found in each of the four study countries. Each category contained descriptions of sample jobs which would fit into each of them. Responses were given by indicating the number of the category which contained the closest or most accurate description of the family's primary wage earner's job. The categories, listed here with condensed descriptions, were as follows: 1 = owner of a large business, executive; 2 = owner of a small business, professional; 3 = semi-professional, skilled laborer; 4 = clerical staff; 5 = semiskilled laborer; and 6 = laborer or service worker. The second item simply asked participants to rate the approximate annual family income: "Please pick one of the following choices describing your family's approximate total annual income": 1 = $20,000 or less, 2 = $20,000 to $35,000, 3 = $35,000 to $60,000, 4 = $60,000 to $100,000, and 5 = $100,000 or more. Equivalent response options (not simple conversions) were provided in each country in local currency (Dutch Guilder, Hungarian Forint, or Swiss Franc). Based on a commonly used procedure, SES was assessed by standardizing each item and then forming an average based on the two items (e.g., Capaldi, Stoolmiller, Clark, & Owen, 2002).

Country. Participants were each identified in the data according to their national membership (American, Swiss, Hungarian, or Dutch). In some analyses, this variable (national membership) was used as a dummy coded predictor with three (n-1) dichotomous variables. Table 1 includes frequencies of demographic information for males and females by country.

Family processes. Family processes were measured by the *Adolescent Family Process* (AFP) measure (Vazsonyi et al., 2003), an instrument that assessed six dimensions of parenting. The AFP included items that measured parenting by mothers or mother figures/caretakers and items that measured parenting by fathers or father figures/caretakers. The current study focused on three maternal and paternal family process subscales, namely maternal and paternal closeness (6 items each), support (4 items each), and monitoring (5 items each). All items were rated by participants on a 5-point Likert-type scale: 1 = strongly disagree, 2 = disagree, 3 = neither disagree nor agree, 4 = agree, 5 = strongly agree. The scales were internally consistent across all four countries, for both males and females. Table 2 includes scale descriptions and reliability estimates of all scalar measures by country and by sex.

Low self-control. A revised version of Grasmick, Tittle, Bursik, and Arneklev's (1993) low self-control scale was used to measure low self-control (Vazsonyi et al., 2001). This scale included 22 items, and ratings were completed on a 5-point Likert type scale (1 = strongly disagree, 2 = disagree, 3 = neither disagree nor agree, 4 = agree, 5 = strongly agree). A high score indicated low self-control. The measure was also reliable across all samples (see Table 2).

Problem behaviors. Problem behaviors and deviance (these two terms are used interchangeably) was measured by the 55-item *Normative Deviance Scale* (NDS; for more detail on the measure, see Vazsonyi et al., 2001). The scale was developed to measure problem behaviors and deviance in general adolescent populations cross-nationally and to provide epidemiological data, and, therefore, examined a broad range of deviant activities.

The current investigation examined all seven subscales of the NDS, namely vandalism (8 items), alcohol (7 items), drugs (9 items), school misconduct (7 items), general deviance (11 items), theft (7 items), and assault (6 items). A total deviance score was also computed by averaging all 55 items. Responses for all items in the NDS were given on a 5-point Likert type scale and identified lifetime frequency of specific behaviors (1 = never, 2 = one time, 3 = 2-3 times, 4 = 4-6 times, and 5 = more than 6 times). Reliability coefficients indicated that the subscales were internally consistent (see Table 2).

RESULTS

Initial analyses examined the associations between maternal and paternal family processes, low self-control, and measures of problem behaviors. Table 3 includes partial correlations by country, where age, sex, family structure, and SES were entered as control variables. Consistent with expectations, measures of maternal and paternal family processes were negatively associated with all eight (seven subscales and total deviance) measures of problem behaviors. There was a striking amount of similarity in how individual dimensions of family processes were correlated with different measures of problem behaviors within each country; in addition, there was also great similarity in these relationships across countries. For example, maternal closeness and the total deviance measure were correlated $r = -.24$, $r = -.19$, $r = -.22$, $r = -.23$ for adolescents from Hungary, the Netherlands, Switzerland, and the United States, respectively. Similar findings were made for low self-control. Very consistent patterns of positive associations between low self-control and measures of problem behaviors were found both within each country as well as between countries (see Table 3).

TABLE 1. Background Variables by Country and by Sex

		Hungary		Netherlands		Switzerland		United States	
		Males	Females	Males	Females	Males	Females	Males	Females
Age (years)		16.8	16.3	16.5	16.4	17.9	17.9	17.7	18.0
Family Structure	Two biological parents	78.7	81.0	85.5	87.7	82.2	84.4	71.0	70.4
	One biological parent only	2.0	1.2	1.4	1.3	1.3	1.0	1.9	1.2
	Biological and step parent	6.6	7.4	3.8	4.2	3.1	3.4	10.6	10.7
	Other	3.9	4.5	4.2	1.8	5.2	4.4	4.9	4.2
Primary Wage Earner	Laborer, service worker	1.8	0.8	1.0	0.5	2.1	0.7	1.1	0.5
	Semi-skilled worker	8.6	9.9	3.0	2.2	3.5	2.6	2.8	5.2
	Clerical staff, sales	35.3	26.9	10.5	9.8	11.7	13.2	5.9	6.6
	Semi-professional	18.2	15.3	24.8	24.3	34.1	25.9	12.7	11.8
	Professional	21.9	23.1	30.9	35.2	32.3	37.4	34.0	38.6
	Executive, business owner	13.1	21.9	16.4	17.2	14.1	18.1	31.9	29.3
Annual Family Income[1]	$20,000 or less	8.6	4.1	6.9	5.4	4.3	4.6	4.9	4.5
	$20,000 to $35,000	24.3	22.3	19.6	13.2	21.9	21.3	9.1	9.9
	$35,000 to $60,000	29.2	32.2	24.4	20.9	32.6	31.3	26.4	22.2
	$60,000 to $100,000	23.9	26.4	17.2	12.3	19.9	19.7	30.4	32.3
	$100,000 or more	10.8	8.3	8.3	6.2	15.5	11.1	24.7	25.1

Note. [1]Youth responded to a question with local currency (see methods). Frequencies do not add to 100%; balance is missing data in each group.

TABLE 2. Descriptive Statistics and Reliabilities of Scales

Males		Hungary			Netherlands			Switzerland			United States		
		M	SD	α	M	SD	α	M	SD	α	M	SD	α
Maternal Family Processes	Closeness	3.87	.72	.79	3.65	.63	.71	3.84	.70	.73	4.05	.81	.84
	Support	3.62	.80	.66	3.70	.86	.71	4.04	.84	.74	3.85	1.03	.83
	Monitoring	3.55	.84	.73	3.34	.85	.71	3.40	.96	.77	3.49	.93	.77
Paternal Family Processes	Closeness	3.48	.88	.84	3.46	.69	.72	3.56	.82	.78	3.76	.98	.89
	Support	3.57	.86	.73	3.77	.88	.75	3.97	.87	.84	3.81	.98	.79
	Monitoring	3.13	.98	.84	2.67	.96	.82	2.82	1.06	.81	3.00	1.02	.87
Low Self-Control		2.82	.49	.83	2.91	.48	.82	2.50	.42	.81	2.83	.62	.89
Deviance	Vandalism	1.77	.80	.85	1.82	.82	.82	1.85	.80	.84	1.87	.89	.87
	Alcohol Use	2.43	.98	.83	2.48	.86	.76	2.33	.95	.81	2.73	1.35	.91
	Drug Use	1.61	.75	.83	1.82	1.04	.89	2.28	1.14	.90	2.11	1.17	.91
	School Misc.	2.15	.79	.76	2.37	.83	.76	2.17	.80	.77	2.28	1.02	.84
	General	1.91	.76	.85	2.26	.77	.79	2.20	.83	.83	2.12	.86	.85
	Theft	1.41	.63	.82	1.54	.66	.72	1.69	.83	.86	1.62	.81	.84
	Assault	1.72	.71	.74	1.75	.72	.73	1.80	.77	.76	1.76	.79	.80
Total Deviance		1.85	.63	.96	2.02	.67	.95	2.07	.72	.96	2.08	.82	.97

Females		M	SD	α	M	SD	α	M	SD	α	M	SD	α
Maternal Family Processes	Closeness	3.99	.63	.77	3.76	.66	.76	3.98	.69	.75	4.25	.78	.85
	Support	3.75	.82	.76	3.72	.89	.75	4.10	.85	.77	3.99	1.01	.83
	Monitoring	3.88	.75	.76	3.75	.77	.71	3.91	.86	.78	3.94	.84	.76
Paternal Family Processes	Closeness	3.62	.78	.84	3.50	.74	.78	3.61	.84	.81	3.94	.98	.83
	Support	3.73	.81	.76	3.74	.90	.77	4.05	.87	.79	4.00	.99	.90
	Monitoring	3.29	.92	.84	2.87	.96	.83	3.03	1.10	.87	3.26	1.11	.79
Low Self-Control		2.78	.45	.83	2.78	.49	.85	2.41	.36	.79	2.64	.56	.87
Deviance	Vandalism	1.31	.46	.80	1.28	.44	.79	1.32	.43	.72	1.30	.49	.81
	Alcohol Use	1.85	.75	.80	2.19	.78	.75	1.88	.80	.79	2.66	1.22	.89
	Drug Use	1.22	.43	.80	1.48	.69	.82	1.81	.95	.89	1.84	.98	.88
	School Misc.	1.84	.65	.74	2.13	.71	.71	2.11	.71	.75	1.90	.79	.79
	General	1.46	.48	.82	1.81	.56	.73	1.78	.57	.74	1.68	.60	.78
	Theft	1.16	.35	.80	1.25	.45	.74	1.32	.48	.73	1.24	.47	.78
	Assault	1.30	.46	.73	1.40	.53	.68	1.32	.46	.63	1.27	.49	.73
Total Deviance		1.44	.41	.87	1.65	.46	.93	1.67	.50	.93	1.70	.57	.95

In a next step, the importance of family processes in adolescent problem behaviors was examined using a multiple regression framework. For this purpose, a series of hierarchical regression analyses by country were completed, where the following strategy was used. First, four background variables were entered separately to examine their importance in predicting total deviance (age, sex, family structure, and SES). Next, because maternal and paternal measures (e.g., maternal closeness and paternal closeness) were only moderately correlated (partial correlations with four controls between $r = .43$ for monitoring and $r = .48$ for closeness), three maternal family process subscales were entered in a set, followed by a set of paternal family processes. In order to examine the unique and additive effects of maternal and paternal family processes, the order of entry of the two family process blocks was also subsequently reversed, where paternal family processes preceded maternal ones. Finally, low self-control was entered in a final model step. Table 4 presents the findings of the regressions for total deviance by country. Values in parentheses in Table 4 are based on the second order of entry of the family process variables, where paternal measures were entered first followed by maternal measures.

With the exception of participant sex, background variables explained very little variance in total deviance across the four countries. On average across the four groups, age accounted for less than 2% of the variance, family structure for less than 1.5%, and SES for less than 1%. In contrast, gender accounted for about 8% of the variance in total deviance across all four countries. Family processes, namely both maternal and paternal subscales, accounted for 13% in American, 7% in Dutch, 12% in Hungarian, and 10% in Swiss youth. Based on the reverse analytic procedure, findings indicated that both maternal family processes and paternal family processes each uniquely accounted for about 5% of the variance in total deviance. For American youth, for example, of the 13% of total variance explained by family processes in total deviance, 5% were explained by maternal family process, 5% by paternal family process, and 3% were accounted for by a "shared" component between maternal and paternal family processes. This finding was largely the same across all four countries (see Table 4), though paternal family processes only uniquely accounted for 3% in Dutch youth, while they explained 6% in Hungarian adolescents. Finally, low self-control explained between 8% of the variance in total deviance for Hungarians and 9% for Swiss adolescents to 14% for Americans and 15% for Dutch youth. The final model accounted for between 30% (Swiss) to 37% (American and Dutch) of the variance in total deviance.

In order to further examine the relationship of both sets of family process measures and low self-control on diverse measures of problem behaviors, the

TABLE 3. Partial Correlations Between Family Processes, Low Self-Control, and Problem Behavior Measures by Country

Country	Problem Behavior	Maternal			Paternal			Low Self-Control
		Closeness	Support	Monitoring	Closeness	Support	Monitoring	
Hungary	Vandalism	-.24	-.21	-.22	-.18	-.25	-.16	.36
	Alcohol Use	-.16	-.13	-.19	-.16	-.19	-.16	.32
	Drug Use	-.25	-.13	-.24	-.20	-.20	-.18	.24
	School Misconduct	-.15	-.18	-.15	-.13	-.22	-.15	.37
	General Deviance	-.15	-.13	-.18	-.09	-.23	-.15	.33
	Theft	-.23	-.15	-.19	-.19	-.21	-.16	.21
	Assault	-.19	-.14	-.20	-.15	-.21	-.18	.26
	Total Deviance	-.24	-.19	-.24	-.19	-.27	-.21	.38
Netherlands	Vandalism	-.17	-.17	-.12	-.17	-.15	-.07*	.39
	Alcohol Use	-.09	-.13	-.09	-.10	-.14	-.08*	.34
	Drug Use	-.14	-.17	-.15	-.18	-.18	-.11	.34
	School Misconduct	-.19	-.18	-.18	-.16	-.14	-.10	.36
	General Deviance	-.15	-.15	-.13	-.15	-.10	-.09	.42
	Theft	-.18	-.19	-.16	-.15	-.10	-.08*	.33
	Assault	-.14	-.16	-.13	-.10	-.13	-.07*	.36
	Total Deviance	-.19	-.21	-.17	-.18	-.17	-.11	.46

TABLE 3 (continued)

Country	Problem Behavior	Maternal			Paternal			Low Self-Control
		Closeness	Support	Monitoring	Closeness	Support	Monitoring	
Switzerland	Vandalism	−.20	−.21	−.21	−.16	−.21	−.12	.35
	Alcohol Use	−.15	−.12	−.20	−.12	−.12	−.14	.30
	Drug Use	−.16	−.13	−.22	−.15	−.14	−.15	.29
	School Misconduct	−.16	−.15	−.18	−.15	−.14	−.16	.27
	General Deviance	−.18	−.16	−.23	−.15	−.14	−.16	.34
	Theft	−.19	−.19	−.20	−.19	−.20	−.15	.29
	Assault	−.18	−.21	−.14	−.14	−.20	−.06	.25
	Total Deviance	−.22	−.20	−.25	−.19	−.20	−.17	.38
United States	Vandalism	−.25	−.22	−.25	−.22	−.24	−.15	.39
	Alcohol Use	−.10	−.08	−.22	−.08	−.12	−.11	.39
	Drug Use	−.17	−.14	−.26	−.16	−.20	−.13	.38
	School Misconduct	−.19	−.17	−.21	−.17	−.20	−.14	.43
	General Deviance	−.21	−.20	−.27	−.16	−.20	−.18	.41
	Theft	−.27	−.23	−.24	−.22	−.22	−.14	.33
	Assault	−.25	−.20	−.18	−.19	−.17	−.09	.35
	Total Deviance	−.23	−.21	−.29	−.20	−.23	−.17	.48

Note: Controls included age, family structure, and SES. All correlations statistically significant at $p < .01$ unless noted: *($p < .05$).

same analytic approach was used for each deviance subscale. To simplify presentation, background variables were collapsed in Table 5 into a single step. Findings from these analyses indicated that background variables were associated with deviance subscales in a similar manner as with total deviance. The majority of variability explained in the different deviance measures by background variables was due to gender. The model performed in a very similar fashion as described for the total deviance measure, although family processes accounted for smaller amounts of variance in individual problem behavior subscales in comparison to the total deviance measure.

Finally, the importance of family processes in each national context was more closely examined. Although partial correlations and regression analyses provide some evidence of similarity in developmental process by country, a more conservative test was used to confirm similarity. For this purpose, a pairwise comparison of unstandardized regression coefficients (b) of individual AFP subscales was used as suggested by Cohen and Cohen (1983; b to z transformations). Despite evidence of very limited effects of background variables, partial regression coefficients were used (controls: age, sex, family structure, and SES). In addition, in the pairwise comparisons of paternal family process dimensions, the effects of the three maternal family processes were also partialled out. Six comparisons were completed for each variable or dimension—that is, for maternal closeness, for example, six pairwise comparisons were completed across the four countries—for a total of 36 comparisons. Results of these computations are included in Table 6.

TABLE 4. Hierarchical Regression Analyses Predicting Total Deviance by Country

	Hungary ΔR^2	Netherlands ΔR^2	Switzerland ΔR^2	United States ΔR^2
Age	.04	.02	.00	.01
Sex	.07	.10	.08	.08
Family Structure	*.01*	.02	.03	.01*
SES	.01	.03	.00	*.00*
Maternal (Paternal) FP	.08 (.10)	.06 (.04)	.09 (.06)	.11 (.07)
Paternal (Maternal) FP	.04 (.03)	.01* (.03)	.01 (.04)	.02 (.06)
Low Self-Control	.08	.15	.09	.14
Total R^2	.33	.37	.30	.37

Note. FP = Family Processes. All ΔR^2 statistically significant at $p < .01$ unless noted: *$p < .05$. Non-significant ΔR^2 italicized. Total R^2 is actual value from analyses and may be slightly different from the sum of individual predictors due to rounding.

For maternal family processes, only 2 of 18 pairwise comparisons reached statistical significance. The unstandardized partial regression coefficient on the monitoring measures from the American sample was significantly different (larger) from the Dutch and Hungarian ones. For paternal family processes, 6 of 18 tests indicated significantly different partial coefficients. Again, three were found on the monitoring measure, where the Hungarian coefficient was significantly different (larger) from the American, Dutch, and Swiss one. Similarly, for paternal support, the Dutch coefficient was significantly different (smaller and not significant) from the American and Hungarian ones; in addition, the Hungarian coefficient differed (larger) significantly from the Swiss one.

DISCUSSION

The current investigation adds to the literature on parent-adolescent relationships in a number of important ways. First, the study examined the predictive strength of the three most commonly tested parenting dimensions, namely closeness, support, and monitoring, for adolescent problem behaviors in samples of adolescents from four countries. For this purpose, both maternal and paternal family processes were included as well as a measure of problem behaviors that ranged in severity from trivial norm-violating conduct (school misbehavior) to more serious law-breaking behaviors (theft and assault). Findings indicated that each of the family process dimensions was negatively associated with each measure of problem behaviors. The combined effect of both maternal and paternal family processes on total deviance ranged from 7% for Dutch youth to 13% for American youth. Family processes explained the least amount of variance in alcohol use, namely 2% for Dutch youth and 6% for adolescents from each of the other three countries.

Perhaps the most striking thing about the findings is the way that individual family process dimensions were related to measures of problem behaviors in a largely invariant manner across the four samples. This was especially true for maternal family processes, where with the exception of two significant differences between American and both Dutch and Hungarian youth, partial regression coefficients did not differ by country. It is also worth noting that the two differences that were found simply indicate that maternal monitoring of adolescents seems to have a stronger deterrent effect in the United States in comparison to Hungary and the Netherlands–or that a lack of monitoring seems to explain more of adolescent problem behaviors. It does not mean that maternal monitoring works in a fundamentally different manner across national con-

TABLE 5. Hierarchical Regression Analyses Predicting Seven Deviance Subscales by Country

		Hungary ΔR^2	Netherlands ΔR^2	Switzerland ΔR^2	United States ΔR^2
Vandalism	Background Variables	.09	.18	.14	.16
	Maternal (Paternal) FP	.08 (.08)	.04 (.03)	.07 (.05)	.09 (.05)
	Paternal (Maternal) FP	.03 (.03)	.01 (.02)	.01 (.04)	.02 (.08)
	Low Self-Control	.07	.10	.07	.08
	Total R^2	.27	.33	.29	.35
Alcohol Use	Background Variables	.15	.10	.08	.13
	Maternal (Paternal) FP	.04 (.05)	.02 (.02)	.05 (.03)	.05 (.02)
	Paternal (Maternal) FP	.02 (.01)	.01 (.00)	.01 (.02)	.01 (.03)
	Low Self-Control	.06	.09	.07	.10
	Total R^2	.28	.22	.26	.28
Drug Use	Background Variables	.13	.11	.09	.06
	Maternal (Paternal) FP	.07 (.02)	.04 (.04)	.05 (.04)	.08 (.05)
	Paternal (Maternal) FP	.02 (.06)	.02 (.02)	.01 (.03)	.02 (.05)
	Low Self-Control	.03	.08	.06	.09
	Total R^2	.25	.25	.21	.24
School Misconduct	Background Variables	.09	.09	.04	.06
	Maternal (Paternal) FP	.05 (.06)	.06 (.03)	.05 (.04)	.07 (.05)
	Paternal (Maternal) FP	.03 (.01)	.00 (.03)	.01 (.02)	.02 (.03)
	Low Self-Control	.09	.09	.05	.12
	Total R^2	.26	.24	.15	.26
General Deviance	Background Variables	.10	.15	.09	.11
	Maternal (Paternal) FP	.04 (.08)	.03 (.02)	.07 (.04)	.10 (.06)
	Paternal (Maternal) FP	.06 (.01)	.00 (.02)	.01 (.03)	.02 (.05)
	Low Self-Control	.07	.13	.08	.10
	Total R^2	.26	.32	.24	.32

TABLE 5 (continued)

		Hungary ΔR^2	Netherlands ΔR^2	Switzerland ΔR^2	United States ΔR^2
Theft	Background Variables	.06	.10	.08	.10
	Maternal (Paternal) FP	.06 (.07)	.05 (.02)	.07 (.06)	.10 (.06)
	Paternal (Maternal) FP	.03 (.02)	*.00* (.03)	.02 (.03)	.02 (.05)
	Low Self-Control	.02	.08	.05	.06
	Total R^2	.17	.23	.22	.27
Assault	Background Variables	.08	.09	.12	.17
	Maternal (Paternal) FP	.05 (.07)	.04 (.02)	.06 (.04)	.07 (.04)
	Paternal (Maternal) FP	.03 (.02)	*.00* (.02)	.01 (.03)	.01 (.04)
	Low Self-Control	.04	.10	.03	.07
	Total R^2	.20	.23	.22	.32

FP = Family processes. All model steps were statistically significant at $p < .05$; non-significant ΔR^2 italicized. Total R^2 is actual value from analyses and may be slightly different from the sum of individual predictors due to rounding.

text. In fact, the evidence suggests that developmental processes are highly similar.

Comparisons of paternal family processes also indicated similarity, although some differences were found. One-third of comparisons by country indicated significant differences of which most involved Hungarian youth. The data suggested that in comparison to Dutch and Swiss adolescents, the perceptions of paternal support and monitoring were more strongly related to problem behaviors in Hungarian youth. However, as found for maternal family processes, data from all countries supported the expectation that paternal closeness, support, and monitoring deterred problem behaviors or that a lack of parenting is predictive of problem behaviors. It is important to note that individual family process dimensions already have modest associations with problem behaviors; therefore, once six measures are combined into a single model, small effects become even smaller, and in some cases, not significant due to redundancy.

Second, findings also suggested that consistent with previous work (Baumrind, 1991), considerable overlap exists in explaining problem behaviors in terms of maternal and paternal family processes. At the same time, the

TABLE 6. Pairwise Comparisons of Unstandardized Partial Regression Coefficients of Family Processes by Country (Total Deviance)

		Hungary		Netherlands		Switzerland		United States		Pairwise Comparisons
		b	SE	b	SE	b	SE	b	SE	
Maternal	Closeness	−.089	.040	−.023	.038	−.052	.020	−.057	.029	
	Support	−.021	.030	−.079	.027	−.074	.016	−.060	.021	
	Monitoring	−.080	.031	−.084	.026	−.129	.014	−.172	.022	3 5
Paternal	Closeness	−.037	.034	−.062	.034	−.017	.018	−.009	.025	
	Support	−.154	.028	−.035	.026	−.083	.015	−.101	.021	1 2 5
	Monitoring	−.091	.027	−.003	.022	−.034	.012	−.027	.019	1 2 3

Note. Unstandardized partial regression coefficients after entry of age, sex, family structure, and SES. Individual subscales entered in sets by parent, maternal and then paternal family processes. Non-significant *B*'s are italicized. Pairwise contrasts include: 1 = Hungarian/Dutch, 2 = Hungarian/Swiss, 3 = Hungarian/American, 4 = Dutch/Swiss, 5 = Dutch/American, and 6 = Swiss/American. Only significantly different unstandardized partial regression coefficients ($z > +/- 1.96$) are noted under pairwise comparisons.

study also provides evidence that both maternal and paternal family processes added uniquely to our understanding of adolescent problem behaviors (see also Fletcher, Steinberg, & Seller, 1999). Therefore, much like the study by Gray and Steinberg (1999) demonstrated about involvement, autonomy granting, and supervision for a sample of American youth, the current study suggests that maternal and paternal closeness, support, and monitoring have independent, additive effects in explaining adolescent problem behaviors across all four national contexts. Third, consistent with predictions and previous conceptualizations of problem behaviors (Jessor & Jessor, 1977; Gottfredson & Hirschi, 1994), the data suggest that the etiology of a variety of problem behaviors is very similar, both within individual countries as well as across countries.

These findings are also consistent with previous work (Vazsonyi et al., 2003) in which a model-free LISREL analytic approach was used to examine similarity versus differences. In the current study, findings did indicate some differences in the amount of variance explained in different measures of problem behavior. For example, family processes accounted for a comparatively small amount of variance in alcohol use in comparison to other measures. However, no direct statistical test was used to conclude these observed differences were statistically significant. Finally, low self-control was predictive of deviance above and beyond measures of family process. For example, it predicted between 8% in Hungarian youth to 15% in Dutch youth of the variance in total deviance. Similar effects of low self-control were also found across all seven subscales of problem behaviors. Although the low self-control-devi-ance relationship has been well established cross-nationally (Vazsonyi et al., 2001), no previous work has examined its effects together with family pro-cesses in samples from different countries.

Whereas the findings provide evidence of similarity in developmental pro-cess, the study also has a number of limitations that require some discussion. First of all, the countries selected for participation were not random, but rather based on established relationships by the investigator. In addition, one could make the argument that Dutch and Swiss youth are fairly similar on a number of indicators and that both groups are geographically proximate, namely in Western Europe. In this sense, one could also argue that Western European youth are probably the most similar to American youth, and therefore, one would expect similarities in developmental processes and behaviors. How-ever, previous work has documented how this perception may in fact be quite inaccurate because even two populations that speak the same language and that share a common cultural heritage, such as American and British adoles-cents, differ substantially in how they experience parental socialization (Devereux et al., 1969). In addition, in the current study, Hungarian youth were very different in terms of cultural context, one where a democracy and free market economy have only recently emerged. It would certainly be im-portant in future work to include adolescents from cultures that are dramati-cally different in a number of respects, such as Japan, Taiwan, or China. Interestingly, previous work that has compared youth from such contexts to adolescents in the United States also found great similarity in the importance of family processes for problem behaviors (Chen et al., 1998; Feldman et al., 1991).

Secondly, the samples in the investigation were convenience samples. Therefore, findings from the current study are not generalizable beyond the sampling framework used. For example, although Switzerland has four dis-tinct language and cultural regions, the current sample only included popula-tion members from one of these regions, namely the German speaking part. Clearly, replication efforts need to include Swiss youth from other parts of Switzerland in order to draw generalizable conclusions about Swiss youth. Related to this, the findings can also not be generalized beyond the samples employed in the sense that adolescents who did not attend school, due to drop out for example, were not included in the current study.

A final limitation is that the current study of family processes is based on youth self-reports. Including other sources of information would have cer-tainly strengthened measurement of family processes. It is also possible that us-ing different assessments of family processes, such as observational measures, could lead to different conclusions about similarities. At the same time, adolescent self-reports of parenting are a very well accepted way of measuring family processes; in fact, most previous cross-national comparative efforts are based on self-reports. In addition, some have suggested that when studying the etiology of adolescent adjustment, adolescent self-reports of parenting may even be more relevant and more appropriate measures (see Gray & Steinberg, 1999 for a discussion). Finally, previous work that has extensively compared different informants on family processes found that adolescent and parent reports of parenting may be assessing very different things because the concordance rates were surprisingly low. Therefore, while adding additional informants is important, it is also not clear that this would change the substantive finding of great similarities in developmental processes across the four countries sampled.

In conclusion, the current study adds to the rather small literature that has examined the importance of family socialization variables in problem behaviors across different national groups (Barber & Harmon, 2001; Chen et al., 1998; Feldman et al., 1991; Feldman & Rosenthal, 1994; Rohner & Britner, 2002). Most previous studies have found evidence of similarity in developmental processes, although none have examined the breadth of family processes included in the current investigation. Furthermore, another unique contribution is that other studies included comparatively few indicators of problem behaviors, mostly less serious forms of misconduct. The current study found evidence for similarity in developmental processes in more serious forms of problem behaviors, such as theft and assault. Finally, with the exception of the work by Feldman and colleagues and by Vazsonyi et al., 2003, previous studies have not employed rigorous disconfirmation analytic techniques to compare similarities versus differences in developmental processes by country. Despite the use of these techniques, the study provides substantial evidence that maternal and paternal family processes are important in a highly similar, generalizable manner for our understanding of a variety of problem behaviors across the four countries sampled.

REFERENCES

Barber, B. K. (1992). Family, personality, and adolescent problem behaviors. *Journal of Marriage and the Family*, *54*, 69-79.

Barber, B. K., Chadwick, B. A., & Oerter, R. (1992). Parental behaviors and adolescent self esteem in the United States and Germany. *Journal of Marriage and the Family*, *54*, 128-141.

Barber, B. K., & Harmon, E. L. (2001). Violating the self: Parental psychological control of children and adolescents. In B. K. Barber (Ed.), *Intrusive parenting: How psychological control affects children and adolescents* (pp. 15-52). Washington, DC: APA.

Baumrind, D. (1991). Parenting styles and adolescent development. In J. Brooks-Gunn, R. Lerner, & A. C. Peterson (Eds.), *The encyclopedia of adolescence.* New York: Garland.

Bush, K. R. (2000). Separatedness and connectedness in the parent-adolescent relationship as predictors of adolescent self-esteem in US and Chinese samples. *Marriage and Family Review, 30,* 153-178.

Capaldi, D. M., Stoolmiller, M., Clark, S., & Owen, L. D. (2002). Heterosexual risk behaviors in at-risk young men from early adolescence to young adulthood: Prevalence, prediction, and association with STD contraction. *Developmental Psychology, 38,* 394-406.

Chen, C., & Farruggia, S. (2002). Culture and adolescent development. In W. J. Lonner, D. L. Dinnel, S. A. Hayes, & D. N. Sattler (Eds.), *Online readings in psychology and culture* (Unit 11, Chapter 2), (http://www.wwu.edu/~culture), Center for Cross-Cultural Research, Western Washington University, Bellingham, WA.

Chen, C., Greenberger, E., Lester, J., Don, Q., & Guo, M. (1998). A cross-cultural study of peer correlates of adolescent misconduct. *Developmental Psychology, 34,* 770-781.

Chirkov, V. I., & Ryan, R. M. (2001). Parent and teacher autonomy-support in Russian and U.S. adolescents: Common effects on well-being and academic motivation. *Journal of Cross-Cultural Psychology, 32,* 618-635.

Cohen, J., & Cohen P. (1983). *Applied multiple regression/correlation analysis for the behavioral sciences.* Hillsdale, NJ: Lawrence Erlbaum Associates.

Crystal, D. S., Chen, C., Fuligni, A. J., & Stevenson, H. W. (1994). Psychological maladjustment and academic achievement: A cross-cultural study of Japanese, Chinese, and American high school students. *Child Development, 65,* 738-753.

Dekovic, M., Engels, R. C. M. E., Shirai, T., De Kort, G., & Anker, A. L. (2002). The role of peer relations in adolescent development in two cultures: The Netherlands and Japan. *Journal of Cross-Cultural Psychology, 33,* 577-595.

Devereux, E. C., Bronfenbrenner, U., & Suci, G. J. (1962). Patterns of present behavior in the United States of America and the Federal Republic of Germany: A cross-national comparison. *International Social Science Journal, 14,* 488-506.

Devereux, E. C., Bronfenbrenner, U., & Rodgers, R. R. (1969). Child-rearing in England and the United States: A cross-national comparison. *Journal of Marriage and Family, 31,* 257-270.

Feldman, S. S., Rosenthal, D. A., Mont-Reynaud, R., Leung, K., & Lau, S. (1991). Ain't misbehavin': Adolescent values and family environments as correlates of misconduct in Australia, Hong Kong, and the United States. *Journal of Research on Adolescence, 1, 109-134.*

Feldman, S. S., & Rosenthal, D. A. (1994). Culture makes a difference . . . or does it? A comparison of adolescents in Hong Kong, Australia, and the United States. In R. K. Silbereisen & E. Todt (Eds.), *Adolescence in context* (pp. 99-124). New York: Springer.

Fletcher, A. C., Steinberg, L., & Seller, E. B. (1999). Adolescents' well-being as a function of perceived interparental consistency. *Journal of Marriage and the Family, 61*, 599-610.

Gottfredson, M. R., & Hirschi, T. (1994). A general theory of adolescent problem behavior: Problems and prospects. In R. D. Ketterlinus & M. E. Lamb (Eds.), *Adolescent problem behaviors: Issues and research* (pp. 41-56). Hillsdale, NJ: Lawrence Erlbaum Associates.

Grasmick, H. G., Tittle, C. R., Bursik, R. J., & Arneklev, B. J. (1993). Testing the core empirical implications of Gottfredson and Hirschi's General Theory of Crime. *Journal of Research in Crime and Delinquency 30*, 5-29.

Gray, M. R., & Steinberg, L. (1999). Unpacking authoritative parenting: Reassessing a multidimenisonal construct. *Journal of Marriage and the Family, 61*, 574-587.

Greenberger, E., Chen, C., Beam, M., Whang, S. M., & Dong, Q. (2000). The perceived social contexts of adolescent misconduct: A comparative study of youths in three cultures. *Journal of Adolescent Research, 13*, 365-388.

Hollingshead, A. B. (1975). *Four-factor index of social status*, Yale University Department of Sociology, New Haven, CT.

Jessor, R., & Jessor, S. (1977). *Problem behavior and psychosocial development: A longitudinal study of youth*. New York: Academic Press.

Knight, G. P., Tein, J. Y., Shell, R., & Roosa, M. (1992). The cross-ethnic equivalence of parenting and family interaction measures among Hispanic and Anglo-American families. *Child Development, 63*, 1392-1403.

Knight, G. P., Virdin, L. M., & Roosa, M. (1994). Socialization and family correlates of mental health outcomes among Hispanic and Anglo American children: Consideration of cross-ethnic scalar equivalence. *Child Development, 65*, 212-224.

Lamborn, S., Mounts, N., Steinberg, L., & Dornbusch, S. (1991). Patterns of competence and adjustment among adolescents from authoritative, authoritarian, indulgent, and neglectful homes. *Child Development, 62*, 1049-1065.

Rohner, R. P., & Britner, P. A. (2002). Worldwide mental health correlates of parental acceptance-rejection: Review of cross-cultural evidence. *Cross-Cultural Research, 36*, 16-47.

Rowe, D. C., Vazsonyi, A. T., & Flannery, D. J. (1994). No more than skin deep: Ethnic and racial similarity in developmental process. *Psychological Review, 101*, 396-417.

Steinberg, L., & Silk, J. S. (2002). Parenting adolescents. In M. H. Bornstein (Ed.), *Handbook of parenting* (Vol. 1, pp. 103-133). Mahwah: Lawrence Erlbaum Associates.

Van de Vijver, F., & Leung, K. (1997). *Methods and data analysis for cross-cultural research*. Thousand Oaks: Sage.

Vazsonyi, A. T., Hibbert, J. R. & Snider, J. B. (2003). Exotic enterprise no more? Adolescent reports of family and parenting process in adolescents from four countries. *Journal of Research on Adolescence, 13*, 129-160.

Vazsonyi, A. T. (2003). Cross-national comparative research in criminology: Content or simply methodology? In C. Britt & M. R. Gottfredson (Eds.), *Control theories of crime and delinquency* (pp. 179-211), Advances in criminological theory (Vol. 12). New Brunswick, NJ: Transaction Publishers.

Vazsonyi, A. T., Pickering, L. E., Belliston, L., Hessing, D., & Junger, M. (2002). Routine activities and deviant behaviors: American, Dutch, Hungarian and Swiss youth. *Journal of Quantitative Criminology, 18,* 397-422.

Vazsonyi, A. T., Pickering, L. E., Junger, M., & Hessing, D. (2001). An empirical test of A General Theory of Crime: A four-nation comparative study of self-control and the prediction of deviance. *Journal of Research in Crime and Delinquency, 38,* 91-131.

Weigert, A. J., & Thomas, D. L. (1979). Family socialization and adolescent conformity and religiosity: An extension to Germany and Spain. *Journal of Comparative Family Studies, 10,* 371-383.

PART II

COMPLEMENTARY APPROACHES IN CROSS-CULTURAL PARENT-YOUTH RESEARCH

Introduction:
Complementary Approaches
in Cross-Cultural Parent-Youth Research

Gary W. Peterson
Suzanne K. Steinmetz
Stephan M. Wilson

The articles in the second part of this collection illustrate the diversity of perspectives and methodologies that can be used to pursue both culture and cross-cultural issues in the study of parent-youth relationships. The articles are particularly notable for the diversity of sampled respondents that are drawn from many cultures located on the continents of North America, South America, Europe, Asia, and Africa. Other features of these papers include how they illustrate the utility of searching for nuances of unique socialization patterns and meanings provided by each culture (i.e., *cultural relativism*) as well as identifying relationship patterns shared across cultures that might approach universality (i.e., *cultural universalism*).

Although leaning in one direction or another, in actuality, all of these papers can be characterized as falling somewhere in-between the extremes of *relativism* versus *universalism*. The article by Stolz, Barber, Olsen, Erickson, Bradford, Maughan, and Ward, for example, is primarily intended to make cross-cultural comparisons of survey data and search for common relationship patterns between parents and their young. Although generalizable patterns are identified across several cultures for the influence of family relationship predictors on adolescent academic achievement, the authors also point to considerable variability in their findings in terms of gender differences and across samples (or cultures). Leaning toward the other end of the universal-relativist continuum is the paper by Kaltenborn, which explores in-depth subjective meanings of a single case example within one culture (i.e., Germany). Also

http://www.haworthpress.com/web/MFR
© 2004 by The Haworth Press, Inc. All rights reserved.
Digital Object Identifier: 10.1300/J002v36n01_01

177

evident in this study, however, are Kaltenborn's efforts to demonstrate how the recommended relativist approach can inform mainstream research (i.e., from survey methodologies and quantitative strategies) conducted within other societies on how parental divorce impacts children.

The predominant approach of the remaining papers in this section falls somewhere in-between the more universalist strategy of the Stolz et al. article and the relativist leanings of the Kaltenborn paper. Specifically, these articles use survey methodologies conducted within one culture and seek to relate their findings to similar research from other cultures, but most particularly from Western scholarship. Such efforts to compare and contrast cultural similarities and differences are clear indicators that relativist and universalist strategies are complementary rather than contradictory approaches. Perhaps it is true, therefore, that one can best establish the generalizability (or commonality) of a socialization pattern when it appears repeatedly in contexts that are dissimilar in other ways. At the same time, we must always be sensitive to different nuances of meaning that each context provides and the variations on a theme that may be prevalent.

What comes to mind here, of course, is the Hegelian philosophical concept of the "dialectic," which originally referred to a discussion or discourse leading to greater understanding. From this perspective, all reality, all understanding, involves ideas in constant evolution toward a more complex stage through a process involving the resolution of opposing ideas or internal contradictions. Using the dialectical method of thesis, antithesis, and synthesis in discourse, an idea is initially posed, confronted, interpreted, and ultimately united with its opposite. Despite initial contradictions, therefore, ideas or seemingly opposite approaches to studying cultural issues (i.e., relativism versus universalism) in the parent-youth relationships can be synthesized into a larger whole involving an integration of competing conceptions. In other words, relativistic and universalistic strategies are truly not opposites in the sense of being contradictory. Instead, these strategies can work hand in hand to provide deeper understanding about the similarities and differences of parent-youth relations across cultures and societies. Ultimately, we may get beyond the identification of sameness and distinctiveness to a deeper understanding at a more general level of meaning and synthesis.

Turning to the specifics of the papers in this section, the article by Stolz and associates examines aspects of both family and school socialization contexts as predictors of adolescent academic achievement. This study is an example of high quality comparative research aimed at identifying common patterns across ten national/ethnic groups. The specific hypothesized predictors within both family and school contexts consisted of connection, regulation, and respect for psychological autonomy. Of particular interest were the goals of determining whether the identified dimensions of family and school socialization can be measured in similar fashion within both contexts (i.e., school and family) and to determine the relative contributions of these potential predictors on adolescent achievement separately by gender of youth. The results of this study indicate, in turn, that maternal knowledge, paternal support, and teacher support are consistent predictors of academic achievement across several national/ethnic groups. At the same time, the unique contributions and relative importance of the predictors examined in this study were found to vary across gender and specific sample.

A careful analysis of the current research on parent-child contact after parental separation and divorce is the focus of Kaltenborn's article. Of particular importance is the case study approach used by Kaltenborn with a female subject from early childhood to early adulthood. Child psychiatric evaluations and a personal narrative report were the sources of information used. An insightful critique of the current literature on parental separation and divorce is provided, and recommendations are provided about how the in-depth perceptions of the children can add substantially to our understanding of the influence of parental divorce on children. Kaltenborn takes the position that our current research is quite limited due to excessive reliance on "structural" strategies, characterized by quantitative survey approaches that capture only summarized perceptions of external patterns. The path he proposes is to increasingly recognize that complicated, long-term processes are involved, most of which are beyond the reach of structural research.

The article by Bush, Supple, and Lash is a well-crafted example of extending parent-adolescent variables used in U.S. research to a sample of Mexican youth. Many of the resulting relationships in this study correspond with previous research conducted in the U.S. What is particularly noteworthy in this study, however, is the exploration of both parental behaviors and rarely explored dimensions of parental authority as predictors of both self-esteem and familistic attitudes by the young. The authors appear to recognize that adolescents from Mexico (and perhaps other cultures) are not influenced simply by their parents' socialization behaviors of the moment, but also by youthful perceptions of their parents' competencies and resources. These influential dimensions of parental "authority" are nonbehavioral in nature and are rooted in the lengthy history of adolescents' relationships with their parents. The authors report interesting findings, analyzed separately for gender of parent and adolescent, involving dimensions of parental behavior and authority as predictors of adolescent self-esteem and their beliefs about familism.

Another article that seeks to extend research conducted within the U.S. to a sample from another country is the study by McClellan, Heaton, Forste, and Barber. The goal of this research is to examine how parental conflict and parental behavior influence aggression and depression by adolescents in Colombia, a country characterized by high societal violence. The investigators use both socialization and parenting perspectives as the basis for distinguishing between overt and covert parental conflict and for exploring how these variables may have direct or indirect influence (i.e., mediated by parental behavior) on adolescent aggression and depression. Rather than a strong direct effect of overt parental conflict on aggression through social learning processes, a more influential association was found for overt conflict as a predictor of parental behavior, which, in turn, was a predictor of aggression. Covert parental conflict and parental support were more directly predictive of depression. Overall, therefore, this study underscores the importance of exploring elaborate statistical models with mediated effects and for making important distinctions in family processes such as overt versus covert conflict. Conceptual distinctions of this kind may result in identifying subtle differences in the meaning and consequences of conflict across cultures.

Xia, Xie, Zhou, DeFrain, Meredith, and Combs explore the relationships among decision-making involvement, parent-adolescent communication, and family relationships within a sample of adolescents from mainland China in their paper. Important contributions of this paper include results that challenge some widely held cultural conceptions of Chinese socialization and parent-adolescent relationships. Structural equation modeling revealed that Chinese parents do not make use of authoritarian behavior as much as commonly held conceptions of Chinese parenting would indicate. Moreover, contrary to collectivistic conceptions of Chinese socialization, Xia and her associates find that Chinese adolescents in their sample progress toward autonomy from parents in a manner similar to that of their American counterparts. Moreover, consistent with Western research is the finding that healthy parent-adolescent communication was a positive predictor of cohesion and a negative predictor of conflict. This study also provides some interesting results that highlight the importance of testing for gender-of-adolescent differences in parent-youth relationships.

The study by Yoon examines predictors of sexual behavior in a sample of Korean adolescents' sexual behavior. Results from regression analyses indicate that such variables as alcohol use, love for partner, and similarity of sexual attitude between partners were significant predictors of adolescents' sexual behavior. The strongest predictor of sexual involvement, however, was "dating mood" or passions of the moment that adolescents experience while dating. Perhaps the most important results of this study are its nonsignificant findings that challenge traditional views about family influences being pervasive in Korea. Contrary to expectations, neither parental factors nor sibling influences were significant predictors of adolescent sexuality. Despite the persistence of strong family values, experiences beyond those of family life appear to be determining why Korean adolescents engage in sexual relationships.

Zhan provides insight into a growing dilemma for parent-adult child relations in the People's Republic of China. An implied consequence is that China's one-child policy may have the unintended consequence of creating a future crisis in the ability of adult children to care for their aged parents, a practiced deeply rooted in Chinese cultural heritage. Intergenerational differences in the perceived expectations for and the willingness of adult children to provide care for aged parents is explored with survey data acquired from one-child generation students and current familial caregivers. Findings suggest that current caregivers have very low expectations that they will receive elder care from their own adult children in the future. Although children from one-child families expressed lower levels of willingness to co-reside with their parents in the future than adult children from multiple-child families, one-child youth have a greater sense of obligation to provide future parental care than their multiple-child contemporaries. Socialization factors, such as close contacts with grandparents, were not found to be sources of the one-child generation's sense of personal commitment to provide future parental care. Instead, structural factors, such as family income and respondents' educational levels, seemed to be the primary sources of this type of filial responsibility. The author's conclusion is that the culture of *xiao* (i.e., commitment to future filial responsibility) is not declining, but that pragmatic structural changes like the one-child policy, growing educational opportunities, and greater geographic mobility are making it more difficult for the one-child generation to provide elder care to their parents.

Overall, these articles add depth to generalizations about parent-youth relationships across cultures, but also identify phenomena that may be either unique or characteristic of only some cultures. A logical pattern is that both common and unique solutions will be found in the complicated socialization processes that occur between parents and youth within diverse cultures.

Family and School Socialization
and Adolescent Academic Achievement:
A Cross-National Dominance Analysis
of Achievement Predictors

Heidi E. Stolz
Brian K. Barber
Joseph A. Olsen
Lance D. Erickson
Kay P. Bradford
Suzanne L. Maughan
Deborah Ward

ABSTRACT. This study investigates the socialization conditions of connection, regulation, and respect for psychological autonomy within the family and school contexts as predictors of adolescent academic achievement across 10 national/ethnic groups. We assess the extent to which these socialization dimensions in the family and school can be

Heidi E. Stolz is affiliated with California State University, San Bernardino. Brian K. Barber is affiliated with the University of Tennessee. Joseph A. Olsen is affiliated with Brigham Young University. Lance D. Erickson is affiliated with the University of North Carolina. Kay P. Bradford is affiliated with the University of Kentucky. Suzanne L. Maughan is affiliated with the University of Nebraska, Kearney. Deborah Ward is affiliated with Aspen Systems.

Address correspondence to: Heidi E. Stolz, Department of Psychology, California State University, San Bernardino, 5500 University Parkway, San Bernardino, CA 92407-2397 (E-mail: hstolz@csusb.edu).

This study was supported in part by a FIRST Award from the National Institute of Mental Health (R29-MH47067-03) to Brian K. Barber, with additional funding from the College of Family Home and Social Sciences, the Family Studies Center, and the Kennedy Center for International Studies, all at Brigham Young University.

http://www.haworthpress.com/web/MFR
© 2004 by The Haworth Press, Inc. All rights reserved.
Digital Object Identifier: 10.1300/J002v36n01_02

similarly measured within these samples. The correlations are evaluated for unique contributions, and the relative importance of these predictors is examined for adolescent achievement in each sample, separately by gender of youth. Results suggest a consistent association of maternal knowledge, paternal support, and teacher support with academic achievement in these national/ethnic groups. However, some variability across gender and sample in regard to the unique contributions and relative importance of these predictors was indicated. *[Article copies available for a fee from The Haworth Document Delivery Service: 1-800-HAWORTH. E-mail address: <docdelivery@haworthpress.com> Website: <http://www.HaworthPress. com> © 2004 by The Haworth Press, Inc. All rights reserved.]*

KEYWORDS. Academic achievement, family influence, school influence, cross-national adolescent development

INTRODUCTION

One broad approach to the study of schools and adolescent development is to explicate the factors and processes within the school and elsewhere that promote success in school. Given the well-documented connection between school success measures (e.g., academic achievement) and decreased delinquency (Maguin & Loeber, 1996), compliance with social norms, and selection of prosocial peer groups (Catalano & Hawkins, 1996), a focus on the facilitators of school success seems justified. In an effort to extend this research, the present study investigated contributions of socialization dimensions in school and family contexts to academic achievement, and assessed the relative importance of these factors in 10 national/ethnic groups.

Building on theory and the substantial evidence for the role of parental support, psychological control, and behavioral control in the development of children and adolescents (e.g., Baumrind, 1971; 1991; Becker, 1964; Ryan, Stiller, & Lynch, 1994; Schaefer, 1965; Steinberg, 1990), Barber (1997) suggested that there are family-level analogues of consequential conditions that occur generally in the social life of children and adolescents (as well as adults). He recommended, therefore, a broader conceptualization of these conditions that could be descriptive of socialization in multiple contexts. The first of these conditions, *connection*, refers to consistent, positive, stable relationships with significant others. Connection provides the foundation for the development of social skills and communicates to the adolescent that the world is safe and predictable. The second of these conditions, *regulation* of behavior by adults, refers to supervision, monitoring, and rule-setting that foster self-regulation in the adolescent and otherwise protects them from associations with deviant peers. Regulation encompasses mechanisms consistently found to be associated with lower levels of antisocial behavior, *respect for the psychological autonomy* of adolescents, and the avoidance of manipulative or intrusive behaviors (i.e., psychological control) that interfere with the adolescent's developing identity. Recent empirical evidence supports the utility of this framework for studying the socialization of adolescents (e.g., Barber & Olsen, 1997; Eccles, Early, Frasier, Belansky, & McCarthy, 1997; Herman, Dornbusch, Herron, & Hertig, 1997).

One objective, therefore, is to conceptualize and assess the individual contributions (via correlations) and unique, additive contributions (via multiple regressions) of measures from the school and family contexts to academic achievement. This study also examined the relative importance of these measures in predicting achievement by assessing the unique contribution of predictive variables through regression-based analytical methods that provide information about the extent to which one variable explains variance above and beyond (i.e., unique) the other independent variables. Consequently, the present study employs a dominance analysis framework, testing for the relative importance of each socialization dimension to academic achievement. Thus, we pit the family context (mothering and fathering) and school context against each other in 10 national/ethnic groups to address the question, "Which of the theorized dimensions (connection, regulation, and respect for psychological autonomy) from which context is the most useful/important predictor of academic achievement?"

ACADEMIC ACHIEVEMENT

Academic achievement, as measured by test scores or grades, is considered an important measure of overall success in middle childhood and adolescence (Roeser, Eccles, & Sameroff, 2000; Masten & Coatsworth, 1998). Studies suggest that individual resources (Bernard, 1993; Ford, 1992; Mickelson, 1990; Sanders, 1998; Stevenson, Chen, & Lee, 1993), characteristics of the community (Bowen & Bowen, 1999; Coleman, 1988), and characteristics of the peer system (Barber & Olsen, 1997) are associated with academic achievement. The predictors of achievement stemming from the family and school contexts, which are the focus of the present investigation, are reviewed below.

The Family Context

A well-established association has been found between factors present in the family context and adolescent academic achievement. For example, much support exists for the link between authoritative parenting (an aggregate of parental support, psychological control, and behavioral control) and academic outcomes (Dornbusch, Ritter, Leiderman, Roberts, & Fraleigh, 1987; Lamborn, Mounts, Steinberg, & Dornbusch, 1991; Steinberg, Mounts, Lamborn, & Dornbusch, 1991) as well as between parental responsiveness/demandingness and academic success (Paulson, 1994). Moreover, the protective effect of authoritative parenting was found for numerous indices of social and psychological functioning, regardless of the ethnicity, social class, and family structure of the adolescents' families (e.g., Avenevoli, Sessa, & Steinberg, 1999; Chao, 2000; Steinberg, Darling, & Fletcher, 1995). Most relevant to the current study, this same literature has found academic achievement to be the only type of measured adolescent functioning not universally predicted by authoritative parenting, specifically not for Black and Hispanic U.S. youth. Apparently for these minority groups, factors outside the family (e.g., peer relations) modified the otherwise ubiquitous effect of authoritative parenting.

Thus, this specific literature on authoritative parenting is useful to the present study for three reasons: first, because it is comprised of the same dimensions of the parenting context used here; second, it suggests the need to more clearly understand for which cultures the parenting environment is salient to school functioning; and, third, because it invokes the role of nonfamily contexts in understanding school functioning. Our method of treating the constituents of authoritative parenting independently may aid in understanding why (i.e., which components of) authoritative parenting are not predictive of academic achievement in some minority groups. The sampling of multiple ethnic groups from one nation (South Africa), for example, permits us to replicate this minority group-based finding.

Family connection. In correlational analyses, connection in the family environment, measured as perceived support from parents, has been predictive of school performance for samples of predominantly white 5th and 8th graders in Utah (Barber & Olsen, 1997), predominantly white and Asian American high school students in California (Herman et al., 1997), and predominantly Black 7th graders from Maryland (Eccles et al., 1997). Additionally, Grolnick and Ryan (1989), Sanders (1998), and Connell and Wellborn (1991) all report a relationship between parental support/involvement and youth school achievement.

Family regulation. School success measures such as academic alienation and grade point average (G.P.A.) have been linked to parental regulation, measured as a composite of locus of decision making, monitoring, and household organization (Herman et al., 1997) and a composite of monitoring and family management (Eccles et al., 1997). Parental knowledge (i.e., the extent to which a parent knows how and with whom the adolescent spends her/his time) and monitoring are components of regulation which have received widespread support as a family context predictor of achievement (Barber & Olsen, 1997; Crouter, MacDermid, McHale, & Perry-Jenkins, 1990; Grolnick & Ryan, 1989).

Family psychological autonomy. Family relationships characterized by respect for psychological autonomy have received less attention as individual predictors of adolescent academic achievement than have measures of connection and regulation. However, correlational evidence suggests that school success is predicted by measures of autonomy or closely related conceptions such as noncoercive, democratic discipline and the encouragement of individuality of expression (Herman et al., 1997), the absence of overcontrolling and overprotective behaviors (Eccles et al., 1997), encouragement of participation in decision making (Grolnick & Ryan, 1989), and the absence of psychologically controlling behaviors (Barber & Olsen, 1997).

Overall, much support exists for the hypothesis that adolescent relationships with parents characterized by (1) consistent, positive, emotional connections, (2) regulation of behavior (e.g., knowledge, supervision, monitoring, and rule-setting), and (3) respect for psychological autonomy (by avoiding psychologically controlling behavior) are likely to provide the developing adolescent with personal resources needed to succeed in the school environment. The fact that these findings appear robust across different measures, ages, ethnic groups, and family structures provides the basis for the hypothesis that across all 10 cultures, these provisions will be individually (i.e., bivariate) related to academic achievement.

The School Context

Several school context factors that predict achievement can be conceptualized as tapping the level of connection, regulation, and respect for autonomy that adolescents experience with adults (cf. Eccles, Midgley, Wigfield, Buchanan, Reuman, Flanagan, & MacIver, 1993).

School connection. Adolescents who report feeling connected or bonded to the school and adults within it tend to obtain better grades than those lacking connection. Many studies point to the critical role of teacher support, particularly with minority students (Alva, 1991; Holliday, 1985). Similarly, Barber and Olsen (1997) and Roeser and Eccles (1998) report a significant relationship between school connection and academic achievement. More recently, Barber and Olsen (in press), using the U.S. sample from the data examined in this study, have demonstrated that, during the transitions to middle school and high school, significant changes in school success were predicted by changes in students' reported connection with teachers.

School regulation. Regulation within the school setting involves the ability of adults to provide a structured, safe environment characterized by clear, consistent rules. Connell and Wellborn (1991) asserted that social contexts offering structure best meet the developing adolescent's need for competence, autonomy, and relatedness, thus resulting in enhanced performance in that setting. Masten and Coatsworth (1995) indicate that a link exists between rule-governed behavior and academic achievement. Regulation, as measured by "kids are expected to do well in their work," "the academic program is very good," and "there is good discipline" (Eccles, Early, Frasier, Belansky, & Mc-Carthy, 1997), was also reported as predicting both academic alienation (negatively) and G.P.A.

School psychological autonomy. Findings regarding the relationship between psychological autonomy in the school context and academic success are mixed. Eccles et al. (1997) report no correlation between school autonomy and achievement, and Barber and Olsen (1997) report a significant correlation for girls, but not boys. Further, Barber and Olsen (in press) found no consistent prediction from classroom autonomy to school achievement across multiple grade and school transitions. Other evidence exists, however, indicating that students tend to excel academically when they are given more autonomous control over their learning environment. Eccles and Midgley (1989) and Connell and Wellborn (1991) suggest that adolescence is a time of increased desire for autonomy and decision making. When youth believe they have an opportunity to participate in their own learning, they are more motivated in the school arena (Ames, 1992; Deci & Ryan, 1985; Eccles et al., 1993; Maehr & Midgley, 1991).

Overall, at the bivariate level, school conditions characterized by high connection, appropriate regulation, and psychological autonomy are expected to facilitate adolescent academic achievement. However, the reviewed research is complicated by the use of different measures and by inconsistent findings. Thus, we approach this study aware of the need to critically evaluate the conceptual framework within the school setting and to assess the strengths and weaknesses of our measures relative to the framework in an effort to add clarity to this issue.

Additive/Unique Effects of Family and School Contexts

Facilitators of achievement from the family and school domains also have been evaluated jointly. Using a multiple regression framework to parse out the unique contributions of individual predictors, Barber and Olsen (1997) found that *family* connection, regulation, and psychological autonomy were *not* significantly associated with grades, but *school* connection and regulation (for both boys and girls) and psychological autonomy (for girls only) were predictive of grades. Applying a similar framework, Eccles et al. (1997) found that of the three dimensions in each of the two contexts, *family* autonomy predicted G.P.A. for both boys and girls, and *school* connection predicted for girls only. The other key dimensions were nonsignificant. Given these prior mixed findings regarding unique contributions of school and family contexts to achievement, the present study aims to advance this research by addressing the question with multisite data. While we approach this as a replication effort, we are also aware of the need to appropriately consider potential cultural mechanisms that might account for different patterns across these sites.

Family and School in Non-U.S. Cultures

Nearly all of the research cited thus far was conducted in the United States. As noted, although there is substantial evidence for the role of family factors in adolescent academic achievement, there is less evidence for the role of school factors. Even less evidence exists for the joint effects of family and school. The justification for extending this research across multiple national and ethnic groups, therefore, is both firm and tentative; it is firm in that the well-established findings for family influence should be tested across cultures (cf. Berry, Poortinga, Segall, & Dasen, 1992; Yau-Fai Ho, 1994), and is tentative in that the school and joint school/family linkages are exploratory. Unlike other studies using the data for this project where cross-national/ethnic group invariance was both expected and found regarding family processes and adolescent functioning (e.g., Barber, Stolz, Olsen, & Maughan, under review; Bradford, Barber, Olsen, Maughan, Erickson, Ward, & Stolz, in press), sound reasons exist to expect differences across samples when focusing on school achievement and its association with family and school socialization.

Comparative studies on the school context and academic achievement which suggests several important cultural mechanisms that could vary has been so far documented as a Western school/family/academic achievement pattern reviewed above. First, it is possible that these patterns might differ for boys and girls, given that academic achievement is often valued more for males than for females in many non-U.S. countries. Interestingly, this difference might be offset by the fact that nearly all cultures reinforce aggressive behavior in boys and passive behavior in girls, a mechanism that might, in turn, facilitate girls' school success (Gibson-Cline, 1996). Additionally, Oerter (1986) cautions that individual outcomes such as school achievement may be viewed as less important in cultures emphasizing community and belonging.

This prior work suggests that our findings might differ more by gender of youth than by national/ethnic group, and that we might be less able to predict achievement with these socialization measures in collectivist cultures such as Palestine, Bangladesh, and India.

Cross-cultural research also points to structural difference in schools as important features on the effects of the school context. For example, in the People's Republic of China, the goal of schools is to replace the community of the home, with students remaining in the same class with the same teacher for several years (Gibson-Cline, 1996). Higher levels of connection with the school/teachers and perhaps stronger relationships between school connection and academic achievement may exist in China. Another school structure issue which might affect the investigated relationships is the type of school(s) included in the sample. Key schools in the People's Republic of China (Dong, Lin, Ollendick, Xia, & Yang, 1995; Gibson-Cline, 1996) and Gymnasiums in Germany (Hurrelmann & Engel, 1992) include only top achievers, thus potential exists for different mechanisms to be working in elite compared to nonelite schools. Findings might be different in China and Germany, for example, where we combined responses from youth in different types of schools. Additionally, cultures with such limited access school systems tend to promote increased emphasis on achievement (Hurrelmann & Engel, 1992).

Summary and Goals

As demonstrated above, evidence exists that relationships with adults in the family context, and to a lesser extent in the school context, characterized by high connection, appropriate regulation, and respect for psychological autonomy meet the psychological needs of adolescents and allow them to excel in academic avenues. Mixed findings exist concerning the unique/additive contributions of these combined contexts. Thus, we attempted to extend the knowledge base regarding the facilitators of school success in three ways by (1) assessing the extent to which these socialization dimensions in the family and school contexts can be similarly measured across a variety of cultures, (2) evaluating the generalizability of the "facilitation hypothesis" by examining both bivariate correlations and the unique effects of connection, regulation, and psychological autonomy with academic achievement within the family and school contexts across a variety of cultures. Thus, we assess the fundamental (as opposed to primarily Western) nature of connection, regulation, and psychological autonomy in the family and the school in reference to school outcomes. Finally, (3) we introduce the notion of relative importance of predictors, and conduct dominance analyses on each national/ethnic sample to assess the universality of dominance patterns. These analyses are conducted separately on boys and girls to address gender-culture interactions.

METHODOLOGY

Sample and Instrument

Data for these analyses stem from the Cross-National Adolescence Project (C-NAP), a survey and interview study designed to test the commonality of key socialization conditions in the lives of adolescents across many parts of the world and their associations with basic elements of adolescent psychosocial functioning (Barber , Stolz, Olsen, & Maughan, nd). Paper-pencil surveys were administered to school-going youth ages 14-17 in classrooms of selected schools within metropolitan school districts. Schools were selected to maximize the existing ethnic and/or socioeconomic diversity present. Data were gathered in Cape Town, South Africa; Dhaka, Bangladesh; Beijing, China; Bangalore, India; Sarajevo, Bosnia; Darnstadt, Germany; Gaza Strip, Palestine; and Ogden, Utah, USA. Three different ethnic groups sampled in Cape Town are referred to as South Africa Black, South Africa Coloured, and South Africa White. The language of the survey for each assessment were as follows: (1) South Africa Black, Xhosa, (2) South Africa Coloured, Afrikaans, (3) South Africa White, English, (4) Bangladesh, Bangla, (5) China, Mandarin, (6) India, Bangalore, (7) Bosnia, Bosnian, (8) Germany, German, (9) Palestine, Arabic, and (10) Utah, USA, English.

The assessments were conducted between 1997 and 2000, with oversight and consultation from an on-site, native colleague for every sample. The survey included basic demographic information and numerous scales and questions tapping adolescent psychosocial well-being and their experiences in the family, peer, school, community, and religious contexts.

Family Context Measures

At this stage in the exploration of these family dynamics, we did not concentrate on item equivalence of measures. Rather, we were concerned with the constructs, all of which have some empirical support in multiple populations. Maternal and paternal scales were constructed with the full set of items in each sample. The 60 distinct reliability coefficients for the maternal and paternal scales ranged from .60 to .90 across the multiple samples, except for the following low reliabilities: (1) maternal knowledge .54, South Africa Black, (2) maternal psychological control .59, Bangladesh, (3) paternal psychological control .57, Bangladesh, (4) maternal psychological control .54, Palestine, and (5) paternal psychological control .54, Palestine. The scale means and standard deviations are reported in Table 1.

Parental support. As a measure of the broad construct of parental connection, maternal and paternal support measures were constructed separately for mothers and fathers using the 10-item Acceptance subscale of the 30-item revision of the Child Report of Parent Behavior Inventory (Schaefer, 1965; Schludermann & Schludermann, 1983). Youth rated each parent on a 3-point scale (1 = not at all like her/him, 2 = somewhat like her/him, 3 = very much like her/him) on a series of 10 items. Sample items include "makes me feel better after talking over my worries with her/him" and "enjoys doing things with me."

Parental knowledge. Parental knowledge of youth activities, one component of parental regulation, was measured by a five-item scale frequently used in family research with adolescents (e.g., Brown, Mounts, Lamborn, & Steinberg, 1993). Youth responded to a 3-point scale from 1 "Doesn't know" to 3 "Knows a lot" concerning how much their parents "really know" (a) "Where you go at night," (b) "Where you are most afternoons after school," (c) "How you spend your money," (d) "What you do with your free time," and (e) "Who your friends are." These items have previously been considered measurements of monitoring, but recent clarifications and reconceptualizations support the label parental knowledge (cf. Crouter & Head, 2002; Kerr & Stattin, 2000; Stattin & Kerr, 2000). Separate scales were constructed for maternal and paternal knowledge.

Parental psychological control. The eight-item Psychological Control Scale-Youth Self Report (PCS-YSR; Barber, 1996) was used to assess mother's and father's psychological control, a violation of psychological autonomy in the family context. Respondents were asked to evaluate on a 3-point scale (1 = not like her/him, 2 = somewhat like her/him, 3 = a lot like her/him) the extent to which their mother/father "is a person who . . ." behaves in a particular way. Sample items include: "changes the subject, whenever I have something to say," "is always trying to change how I feel or think about things," and "brings up my past mistakes when he/she criticizes me."

School Context Measures

Because there is less theoretical and empirical support for the school context measures than the family context measures, exploratory factor analyses were conducted on the 15 hypothesized school context items in each separate national/ethnic group. The 15 items were hypothesized to tap four constructs within the school context: teacher support, school connection (support, more

TABLE 1. Academic Achievement and Predictor Means and Standard Deviations by Culture*

Geographic Area	National/Ethnic Group	Academic Achievement (1-9)	Maternal Support (1-3)	Paternal Support (1-3)	Maternal Knowledge (1-3)	Paternal Knowledge (1-3)	Maternal Psych Control (1-3)	Paternal Psych Control (1-3)	Teacher Connection (1-5)	School Regulation (1-5)
Africa	S.A. - Black	5.87 (2.38)	2.42 (.50)	2.20 (.54)	2.27 (.45)	1.96 (.60)	1.79 (.47)	1.89 (.51)	3.65 (.96)	2.27 (1.17)
	S.A. - Coloured	5.87 (1.88)	2.34 (.52)	2.08 (.55)	2.43 (.45)	2.08 (.58)	1.61 (.44)	1.63 (.47)	3.66 (.86)	2.92 (.93)
	S.A. - White	6.03 (2.01)	2.42 (.512)	2.19 (.56)	2.55 (.45)	2.14 (.60)	1.53 (.43)	1.55 (.47)	3.80 (.82)	2.99 (.99)
Asia	Bangladesh	6.14 (1.47)	2.52 (.38)	2.38 (.41)	2.56 (.39)	2.20 (.51)	1.78 (.36)	1.74 (.36)	3.46 (.78)	2.11 (.98)
	China	5.52 (2.00)	2.20 (.49)	2.07 (.49)	2.33 (.52)	2.00 (.59)	1.65 (.41)	1.57 (.40)	3.37 (.92)	2.30 (1.13)
	India	6.97 (1.79)	2.46 (.43)	2.38 (.44)	2.44 (.44)	2.16 (.51)	1.72 (.41)	1.71 (.42)	3.63 (.90)	3.54 (1.29)
Europe	Bosnia	5.25 (1.91)	2.56 (.44)	2.45 (.45)	2.69 (.41)	2.45 (.54)	1.52 (.40)	1.50 (.41)	3.16 (.88)	3.66 (1.26)
	Germany	5.18 (1.65)	2.39 (.48)	2.17 (.52)	2.36 (.48)	2.00 (.57)	1.40 (.38)	1.43 (.41)	2.72 (.82)	3.10 (1.05)
Middle East	Palestine	6.37 (2.05)	2.32 (.45)	2.24 (.48)	2.44 (.42)	2.18 (.50)	1.72 (.36)	1.71 (.38)	3.60 (.97)	3.41 (1.42)
North America	U.S. - Utah	5.76 (2.42)	2.49 (.49)	2.25 (.58)	2.53 (.49)	2.12 (.65)	1.50 (.46)	1.51 (.49)	3.78 (.93)	3.04 (.95)

* Means in bold; standard deviations in parentheses.

broadly defined), school regulation, and school psychological autonomy. Two of the four hypothesized factors, teacher support and school regulation, appeared interpretable and showed similarity across the 10 national/ethnic groups. These measures are described below. The other two hypothesized factors, school support and school autonomy, were not interpretable in a similar fashion across the 10 groups and were excluded from subsequent analyses. The 20 distinct reliability coefficients for the teacher support and school regulation ranged from .60 to .90 across the multiple samples, except for a coefficient of .49 for the teacher support scale administered in Bangladesh. The means and standard deviations for these scales are reported in Table 1.

Teacher support. All four items hypothesized as relating to support from teachers loaded on this factor across all 10 samples. This measure was intended to tap a property of the teachers, rather than of the schools or the individual students. Thus, a teacher support scale was based on youth reports of "how many of [their] teachers" behave in a variety of supportive ways. Youth reported on a 5-point response scale ranging from 1 "None" to 5 "All."

School regulation. All three items hypothesized as relating to appropriate regulation in the school environment loaded on this factor across all 10 samples. These items were therefore averaged to construct the school regulation scale within each culture. Youth were asked, "How much need is there at your school for more rules to (a) stop stealing?, (b) stop drug use?, and (c) stop violence and fighting?" The 5-point response scale ranged from 1 "No need at all" to 5 "Extreme need." These items were reverse-scored so that higher scores would reflect less need for more rules, evidencing higher levels of current school regulation. This measure was intended to tap a property of the school, rather than of the individual. Limited data from one culture in which school identification codes were collected (India) suggests variability across the 21 sampled schools, with mean school regulation ranging from 1.00 to 3.30. This offers some evidence that our measures indeed tap a school-level, rather than individual-level, property.

Academic Achievement Measure

In the U.S. sample, youth were asked to report their grades on a 9-point scale ranging from 1 = A through 9 = D. In all other national/ethnic groups, youth were asked, "In general, how well did you do in school? Would you say your grades were . . ." Response categories ranged from 1 "Well above average" through 3 "Average" to 5 "Well below average." These items were reverse-scored so higher scores would reflect higher levels of achievement, and the 5-point responses were converted to a 9-point scale for comparison with the U.S. sample. Means and standard deviations of academic achievement by culture are reported in Table 1.

Multiple Regressions and Dominance Analyses

Ordinary Least Squares (OLS) multiple regressions were estimated for academic achievement on all eight theoretically meaningful predictors in each of the 10 cultures, separately for boys and girls. This procedure provides a means to parse out the contributions of each independent variable beyond the explanatory power shared with other predictors.

Dominance analysis (Budescu, 1993) provides a method of assessing the relative importance of predictor variables in situations where theoretically justified hierarchy is not possible. In contrast to multiple regression, which parses out the unique contributions beyond any effect shared with another predictor, this relatively new technique explicitly considers the shared variance by assessing the unique variance and any partial joint variance contributed by each predictor in a multiple regression equation. Thus, dominance analysis provides an assessment of the overall predictive power of each variable. A useful measure of variable importance must (1) be based on the extent to which the predictor variable reduces error in a criterion variable, (2) allow for a direct comparison of the relative importance of a variety of predictors, and (3) include direct effects, total effects, and partial effects. Dominance analysis meets these criteria by performing a pairwise comparison of all predictors, evaluating their contribution to R-squared in all possible subset models.

For example, in a simple multiple regression with two independent variables (mothers' support [MS] and teacher support [TS]) predicting youth adolescent achievement (Ach), if MS has a unique effect on Ach and TS does not (i.e., if the coefficient on MS is significant and the coefficient on TS is not), then MS will also dominate TS in predicting Ach. However, in more complex models that more accurately reflect the situations of youth in multiple contexts (i.e., where youth receive a variety of theoretically meaningful commodities from mothers, fathers, and other socializing contexts), a measure that is shown to contribute uniquely to achievement might not actually be the most important predictor in an overall sense.

Budescu (1993) suggested that variable A can be said to dominate variable B if it is a stronger predictor in all subset regressions. In other words, if the additional contribution of A to R-squared is greater than or equal to the additional contribution of B to R-squared in all the regression models that could be estimated with all possible combinations of the independent variables, then variable A dominates variable B. More recently, Azen and Budescu (2003) have refined Budescu's (1993) definition and have established criteria whereby three levels of dominance can be evaluated. Budescu's original criteria are now considered a test of "complete dominance" (Azen & Budescu, 2003: 11), and two less stringent levels of dominance are also outlined. "Conditional dominance" is calculated by first averaging additional contributions to R-squared across all same size subsets. Then, if variable A makes a greater additional contribution, on average, to models of all sizes than variable B does, it can be said that variable A dominates variable B conditionally. "General dominance," the least stringent, is calculated by averaging the paired R-squared comparisons across subset models of all sizes.

As an example of these three levels of dominance, consider a simplified version of the research question to be addressed in this study, the relative importance of maternal support (MS), paternal support (PS), and teacher support (TS) in predicting adolescent academic achievement in only one culture. If the results of the dominance analysis indicate that the contribution of MS to R-squared is greater than the contributions of PS and TS to R-squared in every subset model (i.e., as bivariate, the three models with two independent variables, and the model with three independent variables) then it can be said that MS completely dominates PS and TS in predicting achievement. If there are some models in which MS does not make a greater additional contribution than one of the other independent variables, but still contributes more on average to the models of each subset size, MS will be said to dominate PS and TS conditionally in predicting achievement. If MS does not dominate PS and TS completely or conditionally (for example, if MS makes a greater bivariate contribution and a greater additional contribution to the two variable models on average, but TS makes a greater additional contribution to the three variable model) it is still possible that paternal MS dominates PS and TS generally if MS makes a greater additional contribution than the other predictors on average when combining all the models together.

Twenty dominance analyses were therefore performed (ten for boys and ten for girls), each addressing the relative importance of the eight predictors of youth academic achievement in a separate national/ethnic group. All observations with missing data on achievement or any predictor variable were excluded from the analyses. After the separate models were evaluated for patterns of dominance, national/ethnic groups could be visually compared. Results were then interpreted based on Azen and Budescu's (2003) three dominance levels.

RESULTS

Scale reliabilities of the constructed scales differ across samples, with the largest cross-national differences found on the constructs of maternal knowledge (ranging .54 to .84), and maternal and paternal psychological control (ranging .54 to .83). Additionally, the Bangladesh teacher support scale (alpha = .49) is considerably lower than all other teacher support alphas which range from .66 to .86. In addition to comparing scale reliabilities across national/ethnic groups, reliability coefficients can also be summarized within culture (across construct). For this purpose, an average alpha within each culture is more descriptive than a range, as an overall measure of the extent to which items tapped the intended construct within that culture. Average alphas of the eight constructed scales (within each sample) are as follows (from highest to lowest): U.S. (.85), S.A. White, China, and Bosnia (.80), Germany (.79), S.A. Coloured (.78), S.A. Black (.73), India (.72), Palestine (.69), and Bangladesh (.66).

Table 1 reports the means and standard deviations of academic achievement and the eight theorized predictors across national/ethnic group. No formal statistical tests were conducted for these means; however, raw differences, variability measures and sample sizes would suggest that significant differences do exist. There is little support for the one hypothesized difference, that Chinese youth might report higher levels of teacher support due to spending longer periods with the same teacher. China ranks 9th out of the 10 samples on the reported level of teacher support.

Table 2 summarizes the bivariate correlations of all eight predictors with academic achievement across the 10 samples. Overall, 24 of 30 maternal measures (80%), 23 of 30 paternal measures (77%), and 14 of 20 school measures (70%) were bivariately related to academic achievement in the expected direction. The most predictive measures at the bivariate level across the national/ethnic groups were maternal knowledge, teacher support, and paternal support, which were significantly associated with achievement in 10, 10, and 9 samples (out of 10), respectively.

Multiple regression results and dominance analysis results are summarized in Table 3, separately for female and male youth. With regard to the OLS regression results (i.e., the unique contributions) of the eight predictors across the samples (indicated by a one), maternal knowledge and teacher support (each contributing uniquely in three cultures) were most often predictive of girls' achievement, while teacher support (contributing uniquely in five samples), school regulation, paternal psychological control, and maternal support (each contributing uniquely in three samples) were most predictive of achievement for boys. There is a wide range of R^2 values for these separate models (.02 to .25), suggesting that the theorized model explains academic achievement much better in some sample/gender-of-child combinations than in others. The average R^2 value for male-only models across all sites is similar to the average R^2 value for female-only models; however, within many samples there is substantial difference between the R^2 values for females and males.

The results of the dominance analysis allow us to assess whether one measure dominates all others in predicting achievement across all cultures. This approach yields additional information beyond the OLS regression results. Here we briefly digress from the focus on cross-national findings to clarify the contribution of dominance analysis in general. Consider the model predicting achievement of male youths in the U.S. (Utah sample). Five predictors are significant ($p < .05$) in the OLS model. Thus, each of the five predictors contributes uniquely (i.e., beyond the others) to youth achievement. Given this situation of five important and correlated predictors, OLS regression does not offer an answer to the question of which predictor matters more. Rather, through standardized coefficients it is only possible to ascertain which predictor makes the largest unique contribution, but not the largest overall contribution. The dominance results, however, indicate that paternal knowledge conditionally dominates all other predictors. In other words, in this particular sample, paternal knowledge is the variable that "covers the most territory" of shared and unique influence on achievement. Assuming, for the moment, that the direction of effect is from the predictors to the outcome, and assuming policymakers (or practitioners) were able to design interventions targeting all five significant predictors, there would be a larger pay-off (in terms of achievement) for improving paternal knowledge in this culture than for improving any of the other significant predictors.

Returning now to the cross-national findings, as Table 3 suggests, there is no "universally dominant" predictor of academic achievement across these 20 national/sex-of-youth groups. In terms of individual measures, maternal and paternal psychological control (each dominant in 0 of 20 samples) and paternal knowledge (dominant in only 1 of 20 samples) are clearly relatively less important than teacher support (dominant in 8 of 20 samples). Comparing contributions of the school context with those of the family context, family measures dominate in 50% of the samples, while school measures dominate in the other 50% of the samples. Comparing dominance patterns across sex-of-youth rather than across national group, it is noteworthy that in only one of ten national/ethnic groups (Germany) did the same measure dominate in predicting achievement for both males and females. Overall, these findings offer moderate support for teacher support as a facilitator of achievement and point to variability in predicting achievement across gender and sample requiring further explanation.

DISCUSSION

The overall goal of this study was to test the robustness of theorized school and family context measures to adolescent school functioning across multiple national or ethnic groups throughout the world. More specifically, the study was designed to provide greater understanding of how two key contexts of socialization (family and school) are associated with a key marker of adolescent

TABLE 2. Correlations of Academic Achievement with Constructed Scales by Culture

Geographic Area	National/Ethnic Group	Maternal Support	Paternal Support	Maternal Knowledge	Paternal Knowledge	Maternal Psych Control	Paternal Psych Control	Teacher Connection	School Regulation	# of Significant Predictors in Culture
Africa	S.A. - Black	–	.10[1]	.08[1]	.12[1]	–	–	.12[2]	–	4
	S.A. - Coloured	.14[2]	–	.17[3]	.11[1]	–.14[2]	–.12[2]	.16[3]	–	6
	S.A. - White	.12[2]	.13[2]	.14[3]	–	–.14[3]	–.10[1]	.16[3]	.14[3]	7
Asia	Bangladesh	.10[3]	.14[3]	.09[2]	.12[3]	–	–	.14[3]	–	5
	China	.19[3]	.18[3]	.14[3]	.08[2]	–	–.09[2]	.19[3]	–	6
	India	–	.11[3]	.14[3]	.12[3]	–.09[2]	–.10[2]	.14[3]	–	6
Europe	Bosnia	.11[2]	.15[3]	.11[2]	–	–	–.14[2]	.11[2]	.22[3]	6
	Germany	.16[3]	.09[2]	.20[3]	.11[3]	–.11[3]	–	.30[3]	.06[1]	7
Middle East	Palestine	.10[2]	.09[2]	.08[1]	–	–.07[1]	–.11[3]	.10[2]	.08[2]	7
North America	U.S. - Utah	.23[3]	.30[3]	.27[3]	.31[3]	–.14[3]	–.17[3]	.32[3]	–	7
	# of Cultures in Which Scale Is Predictive	8	9	10	7	6	7	10	4	

[3] $p < .001$
[2] $p < .01$
[1] $p < .05$
– nonsignificant

positive functioning (academic achievement). A particular contribution of the design was the use of a new analytical method of assessing the relative importance of multiple predictors from the two contexts.

As to measurement, the maternal and paternal support scales, in particular, demonstrate high reliability across these national/ethnic groups, providing further evidence for the "universal" nature of parental support, as well as for

TABLE 3. Results of Regressions and Dominance Analyses

Geographic Area	Africa			Asia			Europe		Mid. East	N.A.
National/Ethnic Group	S.A. - Black	S.A. - Coloured	S.A. - White	Bangladesh	China	India	Bosnia	Germany	Palestine	U.S. - Utah
FEMALE YOUTH										
N =	163	232	245	499	529	434	265	439	519	334
Maternal Support	1,3									
Paternal Support					2			4		1
Maternal Knowledge			1			1,4		1	2	
Paternal Knowledge										
Maternal Psych Control										
Paternal Psych Control										
Teacher Support		1,3			4			1,4		1,2
School Regulation			1,3							
R^2 =	.10	.11	.10	.03	.02	.07	.04	.20	.03	.18
MALE YOUTH										
N =	161	227	268	498	441	432	237	433	371	316
Maternal Support					1,2				1,4	1
Paternal Support	1,4			1						
Maternal Knowledge		1,4								
Paternal Knowledge										1,2
Maternal Psych Control										1
Paternal Psych Control				1					1	1
Teacher Support			1,4	1,4		2	1	1,4		1
School Regulation					1		1,4	1		
R^2 =	.08	.07	.06	.06	.14	.04	.14	.08	.04	.25

4   *Complete Dominance* (Measure makes a greater additional contribution to R^2 than any other measure in every subset regression.)

3   *Conditional Dominance* (Measure makes a greater average additional contribution to R^2 than any other measure to subset regressions of every size.)

2   *General Dominance* (Measure makes a greater average additional contribution to R^2 than any other measure overall.)

1   *Unique Contribution* (Measure contributes uniquely in the within-culture multiple regression.)

the ability of this Western-based scale to tap that dimension of parent-child relationships across a variety of cultures. Additionally, it is noteworthy that despite differences in mothers' and fathers' roles in these cultures, the single measure of parental support used here appears to tap perceived support from mothers and perceived support from fathers equally well within and across these cultures. In other words, there is evidence here that the same types of specific behaviors lead youth in a variety of cultures to feel supported by both fathers and mothers. The two school-related scales also demonstrate moderate reliability across these samples, with the exception of the teacher support scale in Bangladesh. Future item-level and within-culture analyses will allow us to fine-tune these scales and evaluate sample-specific and/or cultural mechanisms; however, there appears to be substantial common ground across these samples concerning the constructs of teacher support and school regulation as well as the specific items that tap these constructs. The items used in this study are somewhat less able to generally tap the remaining three constructs: maternal/paternal psychological control and maternal knowledge, as well as the two additional theorized constructs: school connection and school psychological autonomy (Barber et al., nd).

Concerning the robustness of these school and family context measures at the predictive level, most (76%) of the hypothesized bivariate correlations between context variables and academic achievement were significant. Near invariance occurred across the sites in regard to the salience of paternal support, maternal knowledge, and teacher support. Some nonsignificant bivariate correlations might be due to the aforementioned low scale reliabilities of the scales in those cultures. Excluding scales with reliabilities less than .65, the invariance rate (i.e., ratio of significant bivariate correlations to theorized ones) increases from 76% to 81%.

With that overall pattern in mind, there are several exceptions worth noting and exploring in future research. First, in terms of the number of significant predictors, our framework appears less suited to explaining achievement among South African Blacks and Bengali youth than within other sampled cultural/ethnic groups (with only 4 and 5 predictors, respectively, significantly correlated with achievement out of the 8 hypothesized). Second, there are instances where particular predictors (among the 5 noted above) are not correlated with achievement in certain samples (see Table 2). These anomalies should be examined in future within-culture work. At this stage of the investigation, it would be inappropriate to conclude that these exceptions are culturally based, since the Bangladesh sample was not drawn to be representative of the culture(s) as a whole. (This was the case for most of the C-NAP samples.) Thus, we do not know if this exceptional finding refers to Bangladesh culture or the subsample that was surveyed. Further, although the South African samples were drawn to be representative (at least of the school-going populations in the Cape), it is not immediately clear what would be culturally common among the South African Black and Bangladesh samples to permit a culturally based explanation for these differences. When additional research provides more reliable measures of these constructs in more representative samples of these national/ethnic groups, it will be possible to address the cultural universality of these constructs as fundamental predictors of academic achievement.

In addition to these correlational findings, two different methodologies were employed to evaluate the effects on achievement of family socialization dimensions in combination with socializing factors from the school domain. In evaluating the findings from these approaches, it is first noteworthy that the predictive ability of these school and family factors (taken together) varies across these gender-national/ethnic groups. Overall, the model is best able to predict achievement within the U.S. sample. Thus, while connection, regulation, and respect for psychological autonomy have been shown to facilitate a variety of healthy adolescent outcomes across a range of cultures (e.g., Barber et al., nd; Steinberg et al., 1991), the relationship between these socialization dimensions and achievement, specifically, appears not to be generalizable across the multiple sites investigated in this study. For example, the framework employed here is much less able to predict achievement in Bangladesh, Palestine, and India than in the U.S. sample. Perhaps intra-individual factors (e.g., ability, motivation), school-specific support (e.g., help with homework, parent-teacher communication), and/or broader contextual factors (e.g., neighborhood, family structure, peer value on achievement) that were not included in the present study play a more substantial role in determining achievement outcomes in these cultures. This was the case, for example, in Steinberg's U.S. findings where the otherwise ubiquitous prediction of academic achievement by authoritative parenting (and perhaps authoritative school experiences, had they been measured) did not hold for U.S. Black and Hispanic youth, whose academic achievement was explained more fully when considering other socialization forces.

Also, there appears to be a gender-culture interaction in operation within some national/ethnic groups. For example, the socializing dimensions considered in the present study were stronger predictors of achievement among German females than males, but were stronger predictors among Chinese and Bosnian males than females. This phenomenon remains, at this point, unexplained. Future work with qualitative data from these cultures may address this issue.

In addition to considering the cross-national predictive ability of this set of facilitators of achievement, we also (a) considered whether a smaller number of predictors emerged as "universally" important and (b) compared the roles of school and family factors in facilitating academic achievement. With regard to the first issue, identifying a smaller number of universally important predictors, neither the regression findings (which identify the variables that predict beyond the others in the model) nor the dominance findings (which identify the variables that are most important in an overall sense, taking into account the variance shared with other predictors) suggest that there is any universally important predictor of achievement across these national/ethnic groups. The only pattern that could perhaps be labeled a cross-national "trend" is the tendency for teacher support to dominate other predictors of achievement. This finding is very consistent with that of the Barber and Olsen (in press) study where it was connection to teacher (tested in conjunction with school regulation and respect for psychological autonomy) that significantly explained changes in student academic, personal, and social functioning at grade transitions across adolescence. This finding, now supported with these cross-national findings, argues strongly for the role of the teacher in facilitating student performance. As was the case with assessments regarding the robust nature of these constructs at the predictive level, the study of relative importance of predictors will likewise benefit from more reliable measures as well as from qualitative research to uncover the meanings of differences across cultures, where they exist.

In comparing the facilitating roles of connection, regulation, and respect for psychological autonomy in the family context with the same dimensions in the school context, the present study again suggests that the school and family contexts contribute to academic achievement differently in different gender-culture subgroups. For example, for South African Black and Palestinian boys and girls, as well as for South African Coloured boys and Bengali, Indian, and Bosnian girls, achievement can be optimally predicted from family variables alone. However, for South African White, Indian, Bosnian, and German boys, as well as South African Coloured and Chinese girls, achievement can be optimally predicted with school context variables alone. While explanation of these patterns will need to come from future culture-level work, the present study suggests that the Western notion of the school and family as somewhat interchangeable in facilitating achievement (i.e., that a good teacher can compensate for a poor family context and a strong family can compensate for low quality schools and teachers) might not be the best initial template for understanding academic achievement cross-nationally.

As a final comment on these findings, it is instructive to note how different and more complex they are than are the findings from previous analyses of this same data set. Those analyses found, first, that the three parenting variables employed in this study were invariantly associated across samples with key (nonacademic) dimensions of adolescent social and psychological functioning for males and females alike (Barber et al., 2003). Second, when a multidimensional index of interparental conflict was added to that same model, again, patterns of direct and indirect effects (through the parenting variables) of marital conflict on youth functioning were largely invariant across samples (Bradford et al., in press). The contrast between this invariability in findings with the substantial variability found in the present study helps clarify the source of the variability. At least in this sample, it is the shift to academic achievement as the measure of adolescent functioning, and the move outside the family realm (to include the school realm) that has uncovered some of the complexity and variability of understanding youth socialization. The tentative conclusion here would be that family experiences, and their impact on basic dimensions of psychological health and social competence/conformity, are much more commonly experienced and understood by adolescents in diverse populations around the world. The greater complexity of the school setting, both its social provisions to youth and youth performance in the institution, is likely attributable to the greater extent that this social context is influenced by varying values, beliefs, and opportunity.

The present study is an initial effort to apply a well-tested Western socialization framework to cross-national academic achievement. Strengths include a defined conceptual framework, the large sample sizes, and the diversity of the national/ethnic groups investigated. The study is limited by the cross-sectional nature of the data, which may suggest reverse causation, with high achieving students viewing their school and family contexts more positively than low achieving students. Another limitation was the inability to reliably tap some theoretically salient constructs. Additionally, a limitation of nonculturally representative sampling strategies is that differences between national/ethnic groups might be due to the differential national representativeness of the samples, rather than to actual differences between youth experiences in the larger populations. Lastly, while efforts were made to ensure that all independent variables represented school or family properties, rather than properties of the individual, our findings may be inflated due to shared method variance. That is, the same respondents reported on their grades and their contexts, and may reflect that some quality of the individual affected both of these reports. Future research should assess the theoretically meaningfulness of the constructs that this study was unable to address as well as those constructs for which we found marginal reliabilities. Moreover, within-culture work is needed to shed additional light on the differing roles of family and school facilitators of achievement uncovered by the present work, and their gender variations.

REFERENCES

Alva, S. A. (1991). Academic invulnerability among Mexican-American students: The importance of protective resources and appraisals. *Hispanic Journal of Behavioral Sciences, 13,* 18-34.

Ames, C. (1992). Achievement goals and the classroom motivational climate. In D. H. Schunk & D. L. Meese (Eds.), *Student perceptions in the classroom* (pp. 327-348). Hillsdale, NJ: Erlbaum.

Avenevoli, S., Sessa, F. M., & Steinberg, L. (1999). Family structure, parenting practices, and adolescent adjustment: An ecological examination. In E. M. Hetherington (Ed.), *Coping with divorce, single parenting, and remarriage: A risk and resiliency perspective* (pp. 65-90). Mahwah, NJ: Lawrence Erlbaum Associates.

Azen, R., & Budescu, D. V. (2003). Dominance analysis: A method for comparing predictors in multiple regression. *Psychological Methods, 8,* 129-148.

Barber, B. K. (1996). Parental psychological control: Revisiting a neglected construct. *Child Development, 67,* 3296-3319.

Barber, B. K. (1997). Introduction: Adolescent socialization in context–connection, regulation, and autonomy in multiple contexts. *Journal of Adolescent Research, 12,* 173-177.

Barber, B. K., & Olsen, J. A. (1997). Socialization in context: Connection, regulation, and autonomy in the family, school, and neighborhood, and with peers. *Journal of Adolescent Research, 12,* 287-315.

Barber, B. K., & Olsen, J. A. (in press). Assessing the transition to middle and high school. *Journal of Adolescent Research, 19.*

Barber, B. K., Stolz, H. E., Olsen, J. A., & Maughan, S. L. (nd). *Parental support, psychological control, and behavioral control: Validations across time, analytic method, and culture.* (Manuscript in preparation).

Baumrind, D. (1971). Current patterns of parental authority. *Developmental Psychology Monographs, 4* (1, part 2).

Baumrind, D. (1991). The influence of parenting style on adolescent competence and substance use. *Journal of Early Adolescence, 11,* 56-95.

Becker, W. C. (1964). Consequences on different kinds of parental discipline. In M. L. Hoffman & W. W. Hoffman (Eds.), *Review of child development research* (Vol 1, pp. 169-208). New York: Russell Sage Foundation.

Bernard, B. (1993). Fostering resiliency in kids. *Educational Leadership, 51,* 44-48.

Berry, J. W., Poortinga, Y. H., Segall, M. H., & Dasen, P. R. (1992). *Cross-cultural psychology: Research and applications.* Cambridge, UK: Cambridge University Press.

Bowen, N. K., & Bowen, G. L. (1999). Effects of crime and violence in neighborhoods and schools on the school behavior and performance of adolescents. *Journal of Adolescent Research, 14,* 319-342.

Bradford, K. P., Barber, B. K., Olsen, J. A., Maughan, S. L., Erickson, L. D., Ward, D., & Stolz, H. E. (in press). When parents fight: A multi-national study of interparental conflict, parenting, and adolescent functioning. *Marriage and Family Review.*

Brown, B. B., Mounts, N., Lamborn, S. D., & Steinberg, L. (1993). Parenting practices and peer group affiliation in adolescence. *Child Development, 63,* 391-400.

Budescu, D. V. (1993). Dominance analysis: A new approach to the problem of relative importance of predictors in multiple regression. *Psychological Bulletin, 114,* 542-551.

Catalano, R. F., & Hawkins, J. D. (1996). The social development model: A theory of antisocial behavior. In J. D. Hawkins (Ed.), *Delinquency and crime: Current theories* (pp. 149-197). New York: Cambridge University Press.

Chao, R. K. (2000). Cultural explanations for the role of parenting in the school success of Asian-American children. In R. D. Taylor & M. C. Wang (Eds.), *Resilience across contexts: Family, work, culture, and community* (pp. 333-363). Mahwah, NJ: Erlbaum.

Coleman, J. S. (1988). Social capital in the creation of human capital. *American Journal of Sociology, 94* (Suppl.), S95-S120.

Connell, J. P., & Wellborn, J. G. (1991). Competence, autonomy, and relatedness: A motivational analysis of self-system processes. In M. R. Gunnar & L. A. Sroufe (Eds.), *Self-processes and development: The Minnesota symposium on child psychology* (Vol. 23, pp. 43-77). Hillsdale, NJ: Erlbaum.

Crouter, A. C., & Head, M. R. (2002). Parental monitoring and knowledge of children. In M. Bornstein (Ed.), *The handbook of parenting: Vol. 3. Being and becoming a parent* (2nd ed., pp. 461-483). Mahwah, NJ: Erlbaum.

Crouter, A. C., MacDermid, S. M., McHale, S. M., & Perry-Jenkins, M. (1990). Parental monitoring and perceptions of children's school performance and conduct in dual- and single-earner families. *Developmental Psychology, 26,* 649-657.

Deci, E. L., & Ryan, R. M. (1985). *Intrinsic motivation and self-determination in human behavior.* New York: Plenum.

Dong, Q., Lin, L., Ollendick, T. H., Xia, Y., & Yang, B. (1995). Only children and children with sibling in the People's Republic of China: Levels of fear, anxiety, and depression. *Child Development, 66,* 1301-1311.

Dornbusch, S. M., Ritter, P. L., Leiderman, P. H., Roberts, D. F., & Fraleigh, M. J. (1987). The relation of parenting style to adolescent school performance. *Child Development, 58,* 1244-1257.

Eccles, J. S., Early, D., Frasier, K., Belansky, E., & McCarthy, K. (1997). The relation of connection, regulation, and support for autonomy to adolescents' functioning. *Journal of Adolescent Research, 12,* 263-286.

Eccles, J. S., & Midgley, C. (1989). Stage/environment fit: Developmentally appropriate classrooms for early adolescents. In C. Ames & R. Ames (Eds.), *Research on motivation in education* (Vol. 3, pp. 139-186). New York: Academic Press.

Eccles, J. S., Midgley, C., Wigfield, A., Buchanan, C. M., Reuman, D., Flanagan, C., & MacIver, D. (1993). Development during adolescence: The impact of stage-environment fit on young adolescents' experiences in schools and in families. *American Psychologist, 48,* 90-101.

Ford, M. E. (1992). *Motivating humans: Goals, emotions, and personal agency beliefs.* Newbury Park, CA: Sage.

Gibson-Cline, J. (1996). *Adolescence from crisis to coping: A thirteen nation study.* Oxford: Butterworth-Heinemann.

Grolnick, W. S., & Ryan, R. M. (1989). Parent styles associated with children's self-regulation and competence in school. *Journal of Educational Psychology, 81,* 143-154.

Herman, M. R., Dornbusch, S. M., Herron, M. C., & Hertig, J. R. (1997). The influence of family regulation, connection, and psychological autonomy on six measures of adolescent functioning. *Journal of Adolescent Research, 12,* 34-67.

Holliday, B. G. (1985). Towards a model of teacher-child transactional processes affecting black children's academic achievement. In M. B. Spencer & G. K. Brookins (Eds.), *Beginnings: The social and affective development of black children* (pp. 117-130). Hillsdale, NJ: Erlbaum.

Hurrelmann, K., & Engel, U. (1992). Delinquency as a symptom of adolescents' orientation toward status and success. *Journal of Youth and Adolescence, 21,* 119-138.

Kerr, M., & Stattin, H. (2000). What parents know, how they know it, and several forms of adolescent adjustment: Further support for a reinterpretation of monitoring. *Developmental Psychology, 36,* 1-15.

Lamborn, S. D., Mounts, N. S., Steinberg, L., & Dornbusch, S. M. (1991). Patterns of competence and adjustment among adolescents from authoritative, authoritarian, indulgent, and neglectful families. *Child Development, 62,* 1049-1065.

Maehr, M. L., & Midgley, C. (1991). Enhancing student motivation: A school-wide approach. *Educational Psychologist, 26,* 399-427.

Maguin, E., & Loeber, R. (1996). Academic performance and delinquency. In M. Tonry (Ed.), *Crime and justice: A review of research* (Vol. 20, pp. 145-264). Chicago: University of Chicago Press.

Masten, A. S., & Coatsworth, J. D. (1995). Competence, resilience, and psychopathology: In D. Cicchetti & D. Cohen (Eds.), *Developmental psychopathology: Vol 2. Risk, disorder, and adaptation* (pp. 715-752). New York: Wiley.

Masten, A. S., & Coatsworth, J. D. (1998). The development of competence in favorable and unfavorable environments: Lessons from research on successful children. *American Psychologist, 53,* 205-220.

Mickelson, R. A. (1990). The attitude-achievement paradox among Black adolescents. *Sociology of Education, 63,* 44-61.

Oerter, R. (1986). Developmental tasks through the lifespan: A new approach to an old concept. In P. B. Baltes, D. L. Featherman, & R. M. Lerner (Eds.), *Lifespan development and behavior* (Vol 7, pp. 233-269). Hillsdale, NJ: Erlbaum.

Paulson, S. E. (1994). Relations of parenting style and parental involvement with ninth grade students' achievement. *Journal of Early Adolescence, 14,* 250-267.

Roeser, R. W., & Eccles, J. S. (1998). Adolescents' perceptions of middle school: Relation to longitudinal changes in academic and psychological adjustment. *Journal of Research on Adolescence, 8,* 123-158.

Roeser, R. W., Eccles, J. S., & Sameroff, A. J. (2000). School as a context of early adolescents' academic and social-emotional development: A summary of research findings. *The Elementary School Journal, 100,* 443-471.

Ryan, R. M., Stiller, J. D., & Lynch, J. H. (1994). Representations of relationships to teachers, parents and friends as predictors of academic motivation and self-esteem. *Journal of Early Adolescence, 14,* 226-249.

Sanders, M. G. (1998). The effects of school, family, and community support on the academic achievement of African American adolescents. *Urban Education, 33,* 385-409.

Schaefer, E. S. (1965). Children's reports of parental behavior: An inventory. *Child Development, 36,* 413-424.

Schludermann, S. M., & Schludermann, E. H. (1983). Sociocultural change and adolescents' perceptions of parent behavior. *Developmental Psychology, 19,* 674-685.

Stattin, H., & Kerr, M. (2000). Parental monitoring: A reinterpretation. *Child Development, 71,* 1072-1085.

Steinberg, L. (1990). Autonomy, conflict, and harmony in the family context. In S. S. Feldman & G. R. Elliot (Eds.), *At the threshold: The developing adolescent* (pp. 255-276). Cambridge, MA: Harvard University Press.

Steinberg, L., Darling, N. E., & Fletcher, A. C. (1995). Authoritative parenting and adolescent adjustment: An ecological journey. In P. Moen & G. H. Elder Jr. (Eds.), *Examining lives in context: Perspectives on the ecology of human development* (pp. 423-466). Washington, DC: American Psychological Association.

Steinberg, L., Mounts, N. S., Lamborn, S. D., & Dornbusch, S. M. (1991). Authoritative parenting and adolescent adjustment across varied ecological niches. *Journal of Research on Adolescence, 1,* 19-36.

Stevenson, H. W., Chen, C., & Lee, S. Y. (1993). Mathematics achievement of Chinese, Japanese, and American children: Ten years later. *Science, 259,* 53-58.

Yau-Fai Ho, D. (1994). Introduction to cross-cultural psychology. In L. L. Alder & U. P. Gielen (Eds.), *Cross-cultural topics in psychology* (pp. 3-13). Westport, CT: Praeger.

Mexican Adolescents' Perceptions of Parental Behaviors and Authority as Predictors of Their Self-Esteem and Sense of Familism

Kevin Ray Bush
Andrew J. Supple
Sheryl Beaty Lash

ABSTRACT. The influences of adolescents' perceptions of parental behaviors and authority on the development of their self-esteem and sense of familism were examined among 534 youth living in Mexico. Results of hierarchical regression analyses suggest that boys' perceptions of their mothers and fathers were similar in relation to their development of self-esteem and familism. Males tended to have higher self-esteem when they perceived their parents as monitoring their behavior, granting behavioral autonomy, and having the right to exercise influence over them. For boys' sense of familism, parental influences tended to be less direct, with maternal and paternal education serving as negative predictors, while perceptions that mothers and fathers served as legitimate sources of guidance and advice were positive predictors of familism. For girls, significant predictors of familism and self-esteem varied in relation to mothers and fathers. Girls experienced higher levels of self-esteem when they perceived their mothers and fathers as facilitating connection, monitoring their behaviors, and as having the right to in-

Kevin Ray Bush, PhD, is affiliated with the University of Georgia. Andrew J. Supple, PhD, is affiliated with the University of North Carolina-Greensboro. Sheryl Beaty Lash, MA, is affiliated with the University of Georgia.

Address correspondence to: Kevin Bush, Child & Family Development, University of Georgia, Athens, GA 30602 (E-mail: krbush@uga.edu).

http://www.haworthpress.com/web/MFR
© 2004 by The Haworth Press, Inc. All rights reserved.
Digital Object Identifier: 10.1300/J002v36n01_03

fluence their behaviors and feelings. In addition, girls' perceptions of their fathers' expert authority also functioned as a significant predictor of their self-esteem. Mexican girls who perceived their mothers and fathers as having legitimate authority and as facilitating connection reported higher levels of familism. Additionally, age of adolescent, maternal education, and paternal education were significant predictors of familism for both boys and girls. *[Article copies available for a fee from The Haworth Document Delivery Service: 1-800-HAWORTH. E-mail address: <docdelivery@haworthpress.com> Website: <http://www.HaworthPress.com> © 2004 by The Haworth Press, Inc. All rights reserved.]*

KEYWORDS. Adolescent perceptions, familism, Mexican, parent authority, parent behaviors, self-esteem

INTRODUCTION

Across cultures, the family serves as a primary socialization agent in fostering socially competent outcomes in children and adolescents. There are mixed findings, however, regarding the universality of parental socialization processes and parental influence on developmental outcomes in the young for various cultural groups. Although some studies have found that parental support and control attempts are significant influences on psychosocial outcomes with few consistent differences across ethnicity or SES (e.g., Amato & Fowler, 2002), other studies suggest that these same relationships differ by cultural group (Chao, 1994; Lamborn, Mounts, Steinberg, & Dornbusch, 1991).

Several limitations are evident in the body of literature on parental influence on adolescent psychosocial competence. First, studies considering cultural variation have focused on comparisons of ethnic minority groups within the U.S., whereas few studies have considered parental socialization in Mexico (and other countries) in which families are believed to possess cultural orientations that are collectivistic in nature (Bronstein, 1994; Triandis, 1995). Collectivism is defined as a social orientation emphasizing behaviors, interactions, and values that put the good of the group (e.g., society, family) above the interest of the individual. From this perspective, individuals living in families endorsing a high degree of collectivism are often thought to value a familistic orientation (e.g., Shkodriani & Gibbons, 1995; Triandis, 1995). Moreover, a cultural orientation favoring collectivistic values may alter the nature of parental influence on adolescent development.

Secondly, despite the recognition by researchers that the inclusion of fathers in studies of parental socialization is important, most studies have only examined maternal influences (Amato & Fowler, 2002; Ruiz, Roosa, & Gonzales, 2002). This point is especially relevant in studies among families living in Mexico in which fathers are likely to be seen as the primary authority figures within families (Bronstien, 1994; Tallman, Marotoz-Baden, & Pindas, 1983).

A third limitation is that, although three main dimensions of parental behavior have been identified in the literature (e.g., parental support/connection, parental monitoring, and coercive parenting), the particular parenting influences selected for examination often vary across studies making it difficult to compare and generalize these results. Researchers call for the inclusion of other potential parental influences on adolescent development such as parental induction (i.e., reasoning), autonomy granting and authority to more accurately assess the potential universality of parental socialization processes (Amato & Fowler, 2002; Bush, Peterson, Cobas, & Supple, 2002; Peterson, Bush, & Supple, 1999). In reference to the potential importance of parental authority, research suggests that adolescents who perceive their parents as possessing a high degree of legitimate and expert authority report higher levels of social competence (Peterson, Bush, & Supple, 1999; Henry, Wilson, & Peterson, 1989). Considering the hierarchical nature of parent-child relationships among Mexican families (Frias-Armenta & McCloskey, 1998; Tallman et al., 1983), maternal and paternal authority may play a role in shaping adolescent development.

Lastly, most studies have focused on a single outcome, ignoring possible variation in relationships across adolescent outcomes (Ruiz et al., 2002). An examination of multiple adolescent outcomes with maternal and paternal influences in the same study will allow for a more complete examination of parental socialization. As a means to address the above limitations, this study examined the influence of parental behaviors and parental authority on the self-esteem and familism among Mexican adolescents. Although a few studies have examined the influence of parenting behaviors on the development of self-esteem among Mexican and Mexican American youth, the influence of parenting authority on self-esteem development has not been examined. Moreover, despite the importance of the family to Mexicans (Bronstein, 1994; Frias-Armenta & McCloskey, 1998), few studies have examined how Mexican parents foster a positive sense of familism, and no studies to date have examined parenting behaviors and parental authority as possible predictors of familism among Mexican adolescents.

Parenting Behavior and Adolescent Self-Esteem

Self-esteem is a central component to adolescent development (Gecas & Schwalbe, 1986; Harter, 1993; Owens & Stryker, 2001). Research conducted among samples of white, middle-class adolescents in the U.S. have suggested that youth with lower self-esteem are more susceptible to psychopathology, social problems, dropping out of school, and poor school performance, possibly because adolescents with low self-esteem have an increased vulnerability to negative influences (e.g., Mecca, Smelser, & Vasconcellos, 1989). In contrast, youth with high self-esteem are more likely to excel in school and are less vulnerable for delinquent involvements and psychopathology. The few studies that have examined correlates of self-esteem among youth of Mexican origin report similar findings. For example, self-esteem has been found to be positively correlated with social-emotional adjustment among adolescents in Mexico (Benjet & Hernandez-Guzman, 2001), while studies among Mexican American youth indicate that self-esteem is correlated with academic achievement (Powers & Sanchez, 1982), anxiety, and an internal locus of control (Emmite & Diaz-Guerrero, 1983).

Research using European American, middle-class samples has consistently found that positive connection with parents (i.e., warm, supportive and inductive parenting that facilitates close connected relationships), autonomy-granting, and low levels of coercive or harsh parenting are associated with higher levels of adolescent self-esteem (Amato & Fowler, 2002; Bartle, Anderson, & Sabatelli, 1989; Gecas & Schwalbe, 1986). In a recent study examining gender differences in the psychological well-being of early adolescents in Mexico, Benjet and Hernandez- Guzman (2001) reported that positive maternal and paternal affect were predictors of higher self-esteem among female Mexican adolescents, while harsh paternal control was a negative predictor. For Mexican adolescent boys, positive paternal affect was a positive predictor of self-esteem while harsh maternal control was a marginally significant negative predictor. Results from this study suggest that gender of adolescents and gender of parents are important moderators of the relationships between parental socialization and adolescent self-esteem among Mexican families. These results are consistent with a study by Ruiz, Roosa and Gonzales (2002) reporting that European and Mexican American children (8-14 years of age) perceived maternal acceptance (positive relationship), inconsistent discipline (negative relationship) and maternal rejection (negative relationship) as significant predictors of their self-esteem. This study did reveal, however, that the relationship between maternal acceptance and children's self-esteem was stronger among the European Americans than Mexican Americans. These results suggest that both culture and gender likely interact with the relationships between maternal parenting practices and children's self-esteem.

Amato and Fowler (2002), using a nationally representative sample of adolescents in the U.S., found that parental support, monitoring, and harsh discipline were related to child and adolescent outcomes in expected directions with few consistent differences across ethnic, socioeconomic, family structure, or gender (i.e., of adolescent and parent) groups. For example, parental support was a significant positive predictor of adolescent self-esteem while parents' use of harsh discipline was negatively associated with self-esteem (parental monitoring was unrelated to adolescent self-esteem) and these associations were similar for European American, African American and Mexican American adolescents.

Overall, few studies have examined the parental socialization practices of Mexican parents residing either in Mexico or the U.S. The scholarship that does exist characterizes parenting among families of Mexican origin as firm and demanding, with particular emphasis being placed on concern and conformity (Baca Zinn, 2000; Buriel, 1993; Frias-Armenta & McCloskey, 1998). In reference to the influence of parenting on adolescent self-esteem, only one study has examined parental monitoring as a potential predictor of self-esteem among adolescents of Mexican origin (i.e., Mexican Americans) and found monitoring to be unrelated (Amato & Fowler, 2002). However, other empirical and theoretical work suggests that parental support and control may be perceived differently across cultural groups (Chao, 1994; Hill, Bush, & Roosa, 2003). For example, Hill et al. (2003) reported that maternal hostile control attempts and maternal acceptance were positively correlated among Spanish-speaking Mexican American mothers, but negatively correlated among European American mothers. This finding suggests that control and concern may be conveyed simultaneously among families of Mexican origin, at least among less acculturated Mexican American families. This is consistent with recent conceptualizations of parenting among Chinese families where strict parenting is often considered to be synonymous with parental care and concern (e.g., Chao, 1994). Following this perspective, as parents ask about their activities and behaviors, youth of Mexican descent may perceive this (i.e., parental monitoring) as indications of care, concern, and support, thus facilitating positive self-evaluations.

Similarly, although researchers have not directly examined the relationship between parental autonomy-granting and self-esteem among Mexican adolescents, previous theoretical work and studies of other cultural groups suggest that Mexican adolescents who perceive their parents as granting autonomy will experience positive self-esteem. Adolescents expect more behavioral autonomy as they age, and parents who grant adolescents autonomy will be perceived as conveying that the adolescent has met desired role expectations (Peterson et al., 1999), resulting in more positive self-evaluations by adolescents. Moreover, previous research among U.S. (e.g., Bartle et al., 1989) and Chinese samples (e.g., Bush et al., 2002) has found autonomy from parents to be a positive predictor of adolescent self-esteem. Based on the above reviewed literature it is hypothesized that connection with parents, parental monitoring, and parental autonomy-granting will be positive predictors of Mexican adolescents' self-esteem. In contrast, it is hypothesized that coercive parenting will be a negative predictor of self-esteem among Mexican adolescents. This study is exploratory in nature because few studies have examined these relationships among Mexican families; therefore, no specific hypotheses will be made regarding gender differences between parenting behaviors and adolescent self-esteem.

Parenting Behavior and Adolescent Familism

Familism is considered to be a defining feature of social and personal relationships for individuals of Mexican origin (Baca Zinn, 2000; Buriel, 1993; Buriel & Rivera, 1980). Baca Zinn (2000) defines normative familism as the value that one places on family unity and solidarity. Marotz-Baden (1984) and Tallman et al. (1983) define familism in a context of commitment to social relationships over and against a competing commitment to material rewards. Certainly then, familism is a complex and multidimensional construct involving the extent to which adolescents possess a strong family orientation and assign priority to family interests over personal interests. Few studies have examined the direct connection between parenting influences and the development of a sense of familism. In an experimental study among families in Mexico and the U.S., Tallman et al. (1983) and Marotz-Baden (1984) concluded that Mexican parents tended to focus on the societal requisites for material advancement that would be required of their children, rather than focusing directly on the social affiliations incumbent in familism. Relatively affluent U.S. parents, on the other hand, were reported to focus on the development of social affiliation (e.g., familism). The findings from this study contradict the stereotypical views of U.S. families emphasizing individual goals and outcomes at the expense of family relationships and Mexican families as sacrificing individual interests for family-related goals. However, as Martoz-Baden (1984) points out, these results underscore the importance of family values in both the U.S. and Mexico. The findings of Tallman and colleagues also highlight the importance of examining outcomes that are typically considered to be differentially relevant across cultural contexts. Following this perspective, it is important to examine if and how parents in Mexico might socialize self-esteem, an outcome considered more salient to "individualistic" cultures, while examining parental socialization of familistic attitudes, a more collectivistic trait. This focus on both a collectivistic and individualistic outcome during adolescence allows a more comprehensive view of the diverse socialization strategies and goals in Mexican families.

Most comparative studies have found individuals living in Mexico to report significantly higher levels of familism and collectivist values than European Americans (e.g., Shkodriani & Gibbons, 1995). Similarly, studies have also reported that Mexican Americans tend to have more familistic and collectivist values in comparison to European Americans (Buriel & Rivera, 1980; Freeberg & Stein, 1996). Furthermore, in a recent study examining felt obligation toward parents, familism and collectivistic attitudes were related to felt obligation to parents for Mexican Americans, but not for European Americans (Freeberg & Stein, 1996). Examination of previous research findings also suggest that familism may serve as a protective factor, shielding adolescents from engaging in delinquent behaviors and substance abuse (Unger, Ritt-Olson, Teran, Huang, Hoffman, & Palmer, 2002), similar to the role self-esteem is perceived to have among U.S. middle class adolescents.

Although previous research has not specifically examined the relationship between connection in the parent-adolescent relationship and Mexican adolescents' familism, theoretical and empirical work suggests that supportive and inductive (e.g., positive reasoning) parenting will provide Mexican adolescents with close and positive connection in the parent-adolescent relationships, thus fostering a sense of familism. Research on families in the U.S. suggests that parental support and positive induction (i.e., the use of reasoning to shape behavior) are positive predictors of adolescent conformity to parental expectations and the most successful means by which parents can shape desirable behaviors from adolescents (Peterson & Hann, 1999). Moreover, research with families in Mexico has found parental warmth and support to be positively related to children's development of positive feelings towards parents and the family (Bronstein, 1994). Moreover, as previously discussed, parents of Mexican origin may convey support and control simultaneously (Hill et al., 2003), with parental monitoring being perceived by adolescents as an indication of parental care, concern, and support. Through consistent interaction and organization, parental monitoring provides adolescents with clear role expectations (Peterson & Hann, 1999). Therefore, despite the lack of direct research examining the relationship between parental monitoring and adolescent familism, it is likely that parental monitoring will convey parental caring and concern to Mexican adolescents, thus facilitating positive attitudes toward the family.

As adolescents age they expect more behavioral autonomy (Peterson et al., 1999). Moreover, Mexican American adolescents have been reported to expect behavioral autonomy at similar levels to European American adolescents (Fuligni, 1998). Following this, parents who grant autonomy to their adolescent are likely to foster positive feelings toward the family, as adolescents will perceive the granting of autonomy as positive. In previous studies, autonomy from parents has been found to be a positive predictor of prosocial adolescent outcomes in samples of European American (Bartle et al., 1989) and Chinese adolescents (Bush et al., 2002). In contrast, coercive parental behaviors toward the young person can convey rejection and a lack of respect and, thus, likely foster negative attitudes toward parents and the family. Previous research among Mexican American (Amato & Fowler, 2002) and Mexican (Benjet & Hernandez-Guzman, 2001) samples has found coercive parenting to be a negative predictor of positive adolescent outcomes. Considering the lack of empirical and theoretical literature on the socialization of familism among Mexican families, we present exploratory hypotheses. It is hypothesized that connection with parents, parental monitoring, and parental autonomy-granting will be positive predictors of Mexican adolescents' sense of familism. In contrast, it is hypothesized that coercive parenting will be a negative predictor of familism among Mexican adolescents.

Parental Authority and Adolescent Self-Esteem and Familism

For the purposes of the present study, parental authority is defined as adolescents' perceptions of parental abilities or resources to influence them (cf. Peterson Rollins, & Thomas, 1985; Smith, 1986). As adolescents and parents interact over time, social bases of perceived authority (i.e., expert, referent, legitimate, reward, and coercive power; French & Raven, 1959) are established (Peterson et al., 1985). Parental authority, then, refers to what adolescents believe mothers and fathers have the ability to do, not perceptions of parents' actual behaviors. Parenting among families in Mexico has been characterized as emphasizing conformity, obedience, respect, and parental authority (e.g., Frias-Armenta & McCloskey, 1998). Consequently, considering the importance of the family and parental authority in Mexican origin families, variables emphasizing the perceived abilities of parents should be related to adolescent development (e.g., self-esteem and familism). However, few studies have examined parental authority among Mexican families, and no studies to date have examined parental authority as predictors of adolescent self-esteem or familism. Based on recent conceptualizations of parental power and authority in studies of parent-adolescent relationships (e.g., Peterson et al., 1985) and factor analyses of the present data, three constructs of parental authority were examined in the present study (i.e., legitimate, expert, and coercive authority).

Legitimate parental authority is based in normative conceptions of credibility and refers to adolescents' perceptions that mothers and fathers have the "right" to exercise influence over them (Henry et al., 1989; Peterson et al., 1985). Expert parental authority refers to the extent to which adolescents perceive their parents as knowledgeable and reliable sources of information. Coercive authority represents adolescents' feelings of their parents' ability to bring about negative or adverse consequences as a means to influence the adolescents' behavior. Previous studies have found that adolescent perceptions of legitimate and expert authority are positive predictors of conformity and autonomy among European American adolescents (Henry et al., 1989; Peterson et al., 1985). Coercive authority, on the other hand, has been found to be positively related to adolescent conformity, but negatively related to adolescent autonomy. Researchers have argued that parents who are perceived by adolescents as being legitimate influences and reliable sources of information are likely to convey clear role expectations (Peterson et al., 1985), thus fostering positive self-evaluations, as adolescents trust and evaluate themselves against their parents' appraisals and positive feelings toward the family. Coercive authority, on the other hand, is less likely to foster positive self-esteem and familism among adolescents. Given the lack of research examining the relationships between parental authority and adolescent self-esteem and familism, the following exploratory hypotheses are proposed. Parental legitimate authority and parental expert authority will be positive predictors of Mexican adolescents' self-esteem and familism, whereas coercive parental authority will be a negative predictor of self-esteem and familism.

METHODS

Sample

Six hundred project questionnaires were distributed to students in six state-funded secondary schools in Hermosillo, Mexico, of which 543 were completed and included in the present study. Participants ranged in age from 10 to 16 with a mean age of 13.35. The sample consisted of 235 males and 299 females. In reference to socioeconomic status, the participants ranged from those whose parents had less than a grade school education to those having a college or graduate education (mean parental education was completion of high school). Although a nonprobability sampling strategy was employed, the respondents varied sufficiently across sociodemographic characteristics to be considered reasonably representative of adolescents in this area of Mexico.

Measurement

The data examined in the present study are part of a larger cross-national study of adolescent social competence including data from samples of adolescents in the U.S., China, Chile, Colombia, Ecuador, India, Kenya, Russia, South Korea, and The Czech Republic (e.g., Bush et al., 2002; Peterson et al., 1999). The questionnaire for the larger study consisted of items assessing characteristics of the participating adolescents, their parents, parent-adolescent relationships, and developmental outcomes related to adolescent social competence (i.e., self-esteem, self-efficacy, academic achievement, conformity to parents).

Sociodemographic control variables were included to control for possible confounding effects related to the age of adolescent, gender of adolescent, and parental education (in reference to both mothers and fathers). With the exception of the demographic variables, adolescents responded to each item in the questionnaire using a four-point Likert scale ranging from "Strongly Agree" (4 points) to "Strongly Disagree" (1 point). As a means of maximizing the comparability of item meanings across language, the questionnaire was translated using a back translation technique. Additionally, the questionnaire was also examined by two native Spanish speakers (a school psychologist and a college student from this area of Mexico) to address possible differences in dialect.

In the current study we relied upon adolescent self-reports of their own level of familism, self-esteem and their perceptions of each of their parents' behaviors and authority. The adolescent self-report strategy is justified based on previous research suggesting that youthful perceptions of parental behavior are more strongly predictive of the adolescents' own self-perceptions than are parents' reports of their own child-rearing behavior (Gecas & Schwalbe, 1986). Moreover, a distinct advantage to adolescent reports of parental behavior and authority is that the assessment of parental behaviors directly from parents raises the potential for response bias from parents who may attempt to conceal certain behaviors (that the parents may perceive as being socially unacceptable) and to maximize their reports of more "socially desirable" parenting behaviors (Gecas & Schwalbe, 1986; Peterson & Hann, 1999). A reasonable assumption, therefore, is that aspects of adolescents' perceptions of their self-esteem and familism would be more likely to be influenced by their own constructions of reality (i.e., their perceptions of parental behavior and authority) than would their parents' conceptions of the same phenomenon (Gecas & Schwalbe, 1986).

Familism. The Bardis Familism Scale (Bardis, 1959) was used to assess to the extent to which the young person has a strong orientation toward the family as evidenced by family interests taking precedence over personal interests related to career, residence, and friendships. Five items were used to tap into adolescent familism and included items asking, "Family responsibility should be more important than my career plans in the future." This scale demonstrated adequate reliability based on a Cronbach's alpha of .63 for girls and .61 for boys.

Self-Esteem. Adolescent self-esteem was assessed using 7 items taken from the 10-item Rosenberg Self-Esteem Scale (Rosenberg, 1979). These items were selected based on previous factor analytic studies (e.g., Peterson et al., 1985) and research using the same items in a study of Mainland Chinese adolescents (Bush et al., 2002). Five items provided positive assessments of self-issues ("I feel I have a number of good qualities"), whereas two items were derogatory in nature ("I certainly feel useless at times") and were reverse coded so that higher scores indicated higher levels of self-esteem. In this sample of Mexican adolescents the self-esteem composite measure demonstrated a Cronbach's alpha of .68 for females and .64 for male adolescents.

Parental behaviors. Measures of parental behaviors were assessed with the Parent Behavior Measure (PBM), a 34-item self-report instrument assessing adolescent perceptions of several dimensions of parenting (Peterson et al., 1985; cf. Bush et al., 2002, for a more detailed description of the PBM). Adolescents responded to items in reference to each parent.

For the present study, scale scores for parental behavior measures were constructed based on the results of two separate factor analyses (i.e., adolescents' perceptions of paternal behavior and adolescents' perceptions of maternal behaviors). In the original PBM measure, items are included to tap into unique dimensions of parental support and positive induction. Results from the factor analyses, however, suggested that these items represent a single higher order construct that we refer to as connection. In addition, the original conceptualizations of the PBM included separate dimensions for parental punitiveness (use of threats, punishments) and love withdrawal (psychological coercion). Our analyses suggested that these items should be combined into a single factor, which we have labeled as coercive parenting. For parental monitoring, factor analyses suggested that all items purported to measure parental monitoring loaded onto a distinct factor. A one-factor structure was also obtained for parental autonomy-granting, after items tapping into educational and occupational plans were removed from the analyses (these latter items tended to load on their own factor).

Parental connection was measured with eight items concerning the degree that mothers and fathers were perceived by adolescents as explaining to adolescents how their behavior affects others, and as being accepting, warm, and nurturant, thus facilitating positive connection within the parent-adolescent relationship. A sampled item included, "This parent tells me how much he/she loves me."

Six items were used to tap into youthful perceptions of parental monitoring or the extent to which adolescents felt that their mothers and fathers possess knowledge regarding their free-time activities, friends, and how the young spend their money. A sample item from the monitoring composite score was, "This parent knows where I am after school."

Coercive parenting was assessed with 12 items and assessed the extent to which adolescents perceive their mothers and fathers as using verbal and physical behaviors in a coercive, threatening, and punitive manner. A sample item for coercive parenting is: "This parent will not talk to me when I displease him/her." Cronbach's alphas for these composite parenting scores were above acceptable levels and ranged from .72 to .88 and were similar for adolescent males and females.

Autonomy-granting behavior by mothers and fathers was measured with 10 items originally derived from studies focused on the development of adolescent self-direction (Peterson et al., 1999). These items measure adolescent perceptions regarding the extent to which parents trust the adolescent's decision-making, and provide sufficient freedom in day-to-day activities. A sample item from this scale is: "This parent allows me to choose my own friends without interfering too much." The Cronbach's alpha for this scale ranged from .67 to .75 in reference to fathers and mothers, for boys and girls.

Parental authority. Adolescents responded to items assessing perceptions of coercive, legitimate, and expert parental authority in reference to each parent. These measurement strategies demonstrated good reliability with Cronbach's alpha statistics ranging from .73 to .83 for both adolescent males and females.

Coercive authority is represented by six items that assess adolescents' perceptions of their parents' abilities to deliver negative experiences to influence adolescent behavior. A sample item included, "If I did not follow this parent's advice about my classroom behavior, I would really suffer the consequences."

Legitimate parental authority was measured with 4 items tapping into adolescent perceptions of parents' right to guide or influence adolescent decision-making. A sample item from this composite measure includes the statement, "This parent has a right to give me counsel and advice about selecting an occupation."

Expert parental authority refers to adolescents' perceptions of parents as being knowledgeable and reliable sources of information. A sample item for this measure includes, "This parent knows how to help me with my school work."

ANALYSIS AND RESULTS

Hierarchical multiple regression analyses were employed to assess the magnitude and direction of relationships between the predictor variables and each criterion variable. Previous studies (e.g., Chiñas, 1993) have suggested that Mexican parents are more controlling of adolescent-aged females and provide more freedom to adolescent males. Moreover, a recent study examining the influence of parental harsh control and parental positive affect on Mexican adolescent outcomes found variations in effects by gender of parent and by gender of child (Benjet & Hernandez-Guzman, 2001). Consequently, we analyzed models separately by gender of parent and gender of adolescent to examine potential differences in the manner in which the measures of parental behavior and authority influence adolescent familism and self-esteem.

Each regression model involved a nested regression procedure with three steps in the variable-entry process. The first step in the analyses involved the entry of the sociodemographic control variables (adolescent age and parental education). Subsequently, the four parent behavior measures (connection, monitoring, autonomy-granting, and coerciveness) were entered into the model as a block. In the third step, parental authority measures (legitimate, expert, and coercive) were introduced into the model.

Descriptive statistics for the predictor, criterion, and sociodemographic control variables are presented in Table 1 for the entire sample by gender of adolescent. There were few significant gender differences in mean levels of reported parental behaviors and authority or the outcome variables. We did find, however, that adolescent females in this sample reported greater monitoring by mothers and that boys reported greater coerciveness by both fathers and mothers (see Table 1). Correlations for the paternal and maternal models are presented in Tables 2 and 3, respectively. Results of the multiple regression analyses are presented in Tables 4 and 5 for adolescents' perceptions of fathers and Tables 6 and 7 for perceptions of mothers.

In models using maternal behaviors and measures of authority, maternal educational attainment is included, whereas, for paternal models, fathers' level of education is included. The results suggested that while neither adolescent age nor parental education (either mother's or father's) were associated with adolescent self-esteem, both age and parental education (mother and father models) were negative predictors of familism. Specifically, with familism as the dependent variable, adolescent age was a negative predictor for boys ($\beta = -.32, p < .001$) and girls ($\beta = -.25, p < .001$). Moreover, paternal education was negatively associated with boys' ($\beta = -22, p < .01$) and girls' ($\beta = -.15, p < .01$) scores on the familism scale. Similar results were obtained in reference to maternal education ($\beta = -.15, p < .10$ for boys; $\beta = -.19, p < .01$ for girls; see Table 7). In analyses with self-esteem as the outcome variable, however, results suggested that neither age nor parental education was related to adolescent self-esteem.

In reference to the parenting behavior measures, the results provided mixed support for expectations regarding the positive influence of connection on both adolescent self-esteem and familism. In reference to models including measures of father behavior, connection was not found to be significantly associated with self-esteem for boys, but did demonstrate a positive association for girls ($\beta = .21, p < .01$; see Table 4). We found similar results when considering adolescent reports of familism, as paternal connection was found to be a positive predictor for girls ($\beta = .28, p < .01$; see Table 5), but was not significantly associated with familism among boys.

Results regarding connection in reference to mothers were similar to those found for fathers, with connection being a positive predictor of adolescent self-esteem among girls ($\beta = .19, p < .01$) but not among boys (see Table 6). Moreover, with adolescent familism as the outcome variable, maternal connection was positively associated with familism among female ($\beta = .30, p < .001$) but not male adolescents see Table 7).

Partial support was found for the expectation that parental monitoring would be a positive predictor of both adolescent self-esteem and familism. Specifically, monitoring by Mexican fathers was a positive predictor of self-esteem for adolescent males ($\beta = .28; p < .001$) and females ($\beta = .30, p < .001$). Consistent positive associations between maternal monitoring and adolescent self-esteem among boys ($\beta = .25, p < .01$) and girls ($\beta = .27, p < .001$) were also found. When considering models with familism as the outcome of interest we found few significant associations between parental monitoring and the outcome variables for both boys and girls. Specifically, monitoring by fathers was a positive predictor of familism for adolescent boys; however, this effect was reduced to nonsignificance after the inclusion of the authority variables (see Table 5). Moreover, paternal monitoring was not found to significantly predict familism among the adolescent girls in this sample. We found a similar pattern of results when considering monitoring by Mexican mothers. Maternal monitoring was not significantly associated with familism among the boys in this sample after including the authority measures, nor did maternal monitoring predict familism among the girls (see Table 7).

Equivocal support was found for our expectation regarding the influence of parental autonomy-granting on Mexican adolescents' self-esteem and familial orientations. Autonomy-granting behaviors by fathers demonstrated a significant positive relationship with boys' self-esteem ($\beta = .18, p < .05$); however, no comparable association for girls was found. Autonomy-granting by mothers, on the other hand, was positively associated with adolescent self-esteem for both boys ($\beta = .37, p < .001$) and girls ($\beta = .17, p < .01$), although the effect for girls was reduced to marginal significance once the parental authority variables were

TABLE 1. Descriptive Statistics of the Total Sample and Sample by Gender

	Total Sample	Male	Female
Familism	15.04 (2.89)	15.18 (3.0)	14.94 (2.8)
Self-esteem	15.92 (2.64)	16.18 (2.66)	15.74 (2.6)
Age	13.43 (1.31)	13.48 (1.37)	13.39 (1.3)
Father education	6.61 (3.49)	--	--
Mother education	5.60 (2.99)	--	--
Paternal connection	3.23 (.59)	3.18 (.61)	3.26 (.59)
Maternal connection	3.30 (.59)	3.28 (.61)	3.33 (.57)
Paternal monitoring	2.99 (.65)	2.96 (.69)	2.99 (.63)
Maternal monitoring	3.11 (.60)	3.02 (.64)	3.18* (.56)
Paternal autonomy-granting	3.07 (.54)	3.11 (.53)	3.04 (.55)
Maternal autonomy-granting	3.17 (.47)	3.17 (.42)	3.16 (.50)
Paternal coerciveness	2.21 (.63)	2.30 (.63)	2.14* (.63)
Maternal coerciveness	2.25 (.63)	2.33 (.60)	2.18* (.64)
Paternal coercive authority	2.80 (.79)	2.86 (.75)	2.76 (.82)
Maternal coercive authority	2.82 (.79)	2.86 (.74)	2.79 (.82)
Paternal expert authority	3.24 (.65)	3.23 (.57)	3.26 (.65)
Maternal expert authority	3.14 (.60)	3.15 (.61)	3.14 (.59)
Paternal legitimate authority	3.46 (.56)	3.44 (.58)	3.48 (.54)
Maternal legitimate authority	3.44 (.58)	3.39 (.63)	3.48 (.53)

Note. *p < .05 indicates a significant male-female difference. Standard deviations in parentheses.

included in the regression model. In reference to adolescent familism, results suggested that autonomy-granting either by fathers or mothers was not significantly related to adolescent familism (see Tables 5 and 7).

Contrary to previous research and our hypotheses, parental coerciveness did not predict adolescent self-esteem or familism, regardless of gender. That is, examination of the regression results suggest that both paternal and maternal coercive parenting were unrelated to either adolescent self-esteem (see Tables 4 and 6) or familism (see Tables 5 and 7).

Among the parental authority variables, the most consistent predictor of adolescent outcomes was legitimate authority. Legitimate authority from fathers was found to be a positive predictor of adolescent self-esteem for girls (β = .15, $p < .05$) and was consistently associated with higher familism among both boys ($\beta = .32, p < .001$) and girls ($\beta = .18, p < .05$). Adolescent percep-

TABLE 2. Fathers' Behaviors Predicting Adolescent Self-Esteem and Familism: Correlations by Gender of Adolescent

Variable Name	1	2	3	4	5	6	7	8	9	10	11
1. Familism	1.00	.10	-.25*	-.14*	.30*	.17*	.08	.01	.33*	.21*	.19*
2. Self-esteem	.16*	1.00	-.04	.09	.36*	.39*	.23*	-.17*	.33*	.35*	.15*
3. Age of adolescent	-.29*	-.12	1.00	-.03	-.14*	-.08	-.05	-.01	-.22*	-.22*	-.04
4. Father education	-.15*	.10	-.25*	1.00	.12	.16*	.36*	.00	.19*	.41*	.05
5. Connection	.25*	.20*	-.27*	.10	1.00	.48*	.24*	-.13*	.35*	.33*	.32*
6. Monitoring	.30*	.32*	-.17*	.00	.48*	1.00	.28*	-.07	.27*	.28*	.21*
7. Autonomy-granting	.16*	.22*	-.15*	.02	.30*	.19*	1.00	-.26*	.13*	.29*	.23*
8. Coerciveness	.04	-.03	-.13	.00	.04	.12	-.12	1.00	.02	.05	.17*
9. Legitimate authority	.41*	.27*	-.26*	.15*	.25*	.27*	.23*	-.11	1.00	.51*	.37*
10. Expert authority	.27*	.19*	-.23*	.27*	.30*	.34*	.19*	.11	.52*	1.00	.35*
11. Coercive authority	.14*	.02	-.11	.20*	.11	.10	.13	.26*	.34*	.35*	1.00

Note. *$p < .05$; Correlations for boys are under the diagonal; correlations for girls are above the diagonal.

TABLE 3. Mothers' Behaviors Predicting Adolescent Self-Esteem and Familism: Correlations by Gender of Adolescent

Variable Name	1	2	3	4	5	6	7	8	9	10	11
1. Familism	1.00	.10	-.25*	-.16*	.33*	.09	.10	.02	.35*	.23*	.21*
2. Self-esteem	.16*	1.00	-.04	.05	.38*	.42*	.37*	-.15*	.30*	.34*	.12
3. Age of adolescent	-.29*	-.12	1.00	-.05	-.17*	-.07	.00	-.06	-.16*	-.24*	.00
4. Mother education	-.07	.06	-.25*	1.00	-.03	.15*	.16*	-.02	.00	.21*	-.06
5. Connection	.23*	.19*	-.21*	.09	1.00	.39*	.46*	-.17*	.44*	.40*	.29*
6. Monitoring	.27*	.34*	-.17*	.06	.47*	1.00	.39*	-.15*	.28*	.27*	.15*
7. Autonomy-granting	.15*	.38*	-.12*	.04	.36*	.33*	1.00	-.22*	.38*	.39*	.22*
8. Coerciveness	.07	-.11	-.16*	-.06	.02	.10	-.13	1.00	-.05	.00	.16*
9. Legitimate authority	.36*	.36*	-.20*	.02	.29*	.32*	.34*	-.03	1.00	.37*	.41*
10. Expert authority	.20*	.18*	-.25*	.34*	.34*	.27*	.33*	.01	.45*	1.00	.26*
11. Coercive authority	.13*	.04	-.14	.00	.18*	.14	.13	.30*	.34*	.26*	1.00

Note. *p < .05; Correlations for boys are under the diagonal; correlations for girls are above the diagonal.

TABLE 4. Paternal Model: Fathers' Behaviors Predicting Adolescent Self-Esteem by Gender

	Boys						Girls					
	I		II		III		I		II		III	
	β	β	β	β	β	β	β	β	β	β	β	β
Demographic Controls												
Age of adolescent	−.23	−.12	−.11	−.06	−.04	−.02	−.01	−.01	.13	.06	.23	.11+
Father education	.03	.06	.02	.03	.03	.04	.04	.06	−.04	−.05	−.09	−.13+
Parental Behaviors												
Connection			.01	.00	.00	.00			.96	.21**	.70	.15*
Monitoring			1.11	.28**	.96	.25**			1.28	.30***	1.15	.27***
Autonomy-granting			.84	.18*	.81	.17*			.42	.08	.26	.05
Coerciveness			−.25	−.06	−.03	−.01			−.33	−.08	−.42	−.10
Parental Authority												
Legitimate					.78	.18+					.77	.15⁻
Expert					−.04	−.01					.95	.22**
Coercive					−.37	−.10					−.26	−.08
R^2	.02		.15		.17		.00		.23		.30	

Note. + $p < .10$, *$p < .05$, **$p < .01$, ***$p < .001$

TABLE 5. Paternal Model: Fathers' Behaviors Predicting Adolescent Familism by Gender: Unstandardized and Standardized Regression Coefficients

	Boys						Girls					
	I		II		III		I		II		III	
	β	β	β	β	β	β	β	β	β	β	β	β
Demographic Controls												
Age of adolescent	-.74	-.32***	-.64	-.27***	-.47	-.20**	-.57	-.25***	-.44	-.20**	-.37	-.17**
Father education	-.20	-.22**	-.20	-.22**	-.25	-.27***	-.13	-.15**	-.18	-.22**	-.21	-.26***
Parental Behaviors												
Connection			.22	.04	.08	.02			1.35	.28***	1.05	.22**
Monitoring			.96	.21*	.56	.12			.25	.06	.11	.02
Autonomy-granting			.19	.03	-.08	-.01			.44	.08	.30	.06
Coerciveness			-.08	-.02	.09	.02			.31	.07	.17	.04
Parental Authority												
Expert					.47	.09					.35	.08
Coercive					.12	.03					.06	.02
R^2	.12		.18		.29		.09		.19		.23	

Note. + p < .10, *p < .05, **p < .01, ***p < .001

227

TABLE 6. Maternal Model: Mothers' Behaviors Predicting Adolescent Self-Esteem by Gender: Unstandardized and Standardized Regression Coefficients

| | Boys | | | | | | Girls | | | | | |
| | I | | II | | III | | I | | II | | III | |
	β	β	β	β	β	β	β	β	β	β	β	β
Demographic Controls												
Age of adolescent	-.26	-.14+	-.20	-.10	-.16	-.09	-.07	-.04	.02	.01	.11	.05
Mother education	.03	.05	.02	.02	.03	.05	.04	.05	.04	.05	-.03	-.04
Parental Behaviors												
Connection			-.33	-.08	-.37	-.09			.88	.19**	.63	.14*
Monitoring			1.01	.25**	.93	.28**			1.26	.27***	1.21	.26***
Autonomy-granting			2.00	.37***	1.83	.31***			.86	.17**	.60	.11+
Coerciveness			-.54	-.13+	-.49	-.12			-.16	-.04	-.19	-.05
Parental Authority												
Legitimate					.70	.17*					.45	.09
Expert					-.19	-.04					.79	.17**
Coercive					.00	.00					-.19	-.06
R²		.02		.25		.27		.00		.25		.28

Note. + p < .10, *p < .05, **p < .01, ***p < .001

TABLE 7. Maternal Model: Mothers' Behaviors Predicting Adolescent Familism by Gender: Unstandardized and Standardized Regression Coefficients

	Boys						Girls					
	I		II		III		I		II		III	
	β	β	β	β	β	β	β	β	β	β	β	β
Demographic Controls												
Age of adolescent	-.65	-.28***	-.55	-.24**	-.47	.20**	-.53	-.24***	-.40	-.18**	-.34	-.16*
Mother education	-.14	-.15+	-.15	-.16*	-.14	-.15	-.19	-.19**	-.17	-.18**	-.18	-.18**
Parental Behaviors												
Connection			.55	.10	.39	.07			1.51	.30***	1.07	.21**
Monitoring			.75	.15+	.55	.11			.02	.01	-.11	-.02
Autonomy-granting			.38	.05	-.11	-.02			.11	.02	-.28	-.05
Coerciveness			.12	.03	.25	.05			.28	.06	.14	.03
Parental Authority												
Legitimate					1.35	.27**					.92	.17*
Expert					.25	.05					.50	.10
Coercive					-.14	-.03					.16	.05
R^2		.08		.13		.20		.09		.18		.22

Note. + p < .10, * p < .05, ** p < .01, *** p < .001

tions of maternal legitimate authority, however, was only found to positively predict self-esteem for boys ($\beta = .17$, $p < .05$) but was significantly associated with greater familism for both boys ($\beta = .27$, $p < .01$) and girls ($\beta = .17$, $p < .05$).

Results in reference to adolescent perceptions of parental expert authority demonstrated few significant associations with the adolescent outcomes. Paternal expert authority was positively related to girls' self-esteem ($\beta = .22$, $p < .01$); however, no comparable association was found between paternal legitimate authority and boys' self-esteem, or for familism among boys and girls. In reference to maternal expert authority, significant associations were not found between this aspect of parenting and levels of adolescent familism or self-esteem, with the exception of a positive association between maternal expert authority and self-esteem among the Mexican girls ($\beta = .17$, $p < .01$). In all models, coercive authority did not demonstrate any significant associations with either adolescent familism or self-esteem, thus none of our expectations regarding the influence of coercive authority were supported.

DISCUSSION

The purpose of this study was to examine the influence of adolescent perceptions of parental behaviors and parental authority on adolescent familism and self-esteem in a sample of adolescents in Mexico. Limitations of previous studies were addressed by examining parental socialization influence on adolescents living in a relatively collectivistic culture, including adolescent reports of father behaviors, multiple adolescent outcomes, and by also considering more intangible aspects of parental influence (e.g., adolescents' perceptions of parental authority). We hypothesized that paternal and maternal connection, monitoring and autonomy-granting would be positive predictors of adolescent familism and self-esteem, while adolescent perceptions of coercive parenting behaviors by fathers and mothers would be negative predictors. In reference to adolescent perceptions of parental authority, we hypothesized that paternal and maternal legitimate and expert authority would be positive predictors of both adolescent familism and self-esteem, while coercive authority would be a negative predictor.

Familism

In reference to adolescent familism, few of our hypotheses were supported. Adolescent familism was not associated with monitoring, autonomy-granting, coercive parenting, or expert or coercive authority. In contrast, perceptions of parents as legitimate sources of guidance and influence (i.e., legitimate authority), age of adolescent, and parental education level were significant predictors of familism across all gender dyads. Interestingly, although there were differences across mothers and fathers, significant predictors of adolescent familism were identical for each parent in reference to boys and girls (e.g., for father models, legitimate authority, adolescent age, and paternal education were significant predictors for both boys and girls). Additionally, regression analyses indicated differences in the predictors of familism by gender of adolescent, with paternal and maternal connection predicting familism for girls, but not for boys.

Several nonsignificant findings from the regression models were also noteworthy. While the results of regression models suggested that there were few significant relationships between the measures of parenting behaviors, parental authority and adolescent familism, examination of the correlation analyses indicated greater support for the hypotheses (see Tables 2 and 3). That is, although the effects were reduced to nonsignificance in the full regression models, parental monitoring (except for girls' maternal model), parental coercive authority, and parental connection were all significant positive correlates of familism. These results stress the importance of examining multiple predictors of adolescent outcomes (i.e., as guided by theory and previous research) so that the covariance among the predictor variables can be considered. Otherwise, conclusions drawn from the data will be not be based on a complete model, and, therefore, less accurate and possibly leading to inaccurate inferences. For example, it appears that connection with parents influences the development of familism for boys, but to a lesser extent compared to their perceptions that mothers and fathers have the right to exercise influence on them (i.e., once the other predictor variables are considered). For girls, in contrast, parenting that encourages connection to parents and the establishment of parents as legitimate sources of influence were of similar importance in facilitating a sense of family obligation.

In addition to parental legitimate authority, the most consistent predictors of adolescent familism across gender dyads were age of the adolescent and parental education. The significant relationships between these sociodemographic variables and adolescent familism suggest that Mexican adolescents who are younger and have less educated parents have a greater orientation toward their families. Considering the few studies that have examined these specific relationships (e.g., parental education and familism), besides variation in the conceptualization and operationalization of familism, these findings are difficult to explain. For example, Valenzuela and Dornbusch (1994) found familistic attitudes (similar to the operationalization of familism in the present study) to be to a have a weak but significant negative correlation with parental education level among a large sample of European and Mexican American adolescents. However, this relationship was no longer significant when the ethnic groups were examined separately. In contrast, findings from a cross-national study of families in Mexico and the U.S. conducted by Tallman et al. (1983) suggest that familism is more pronounced among more affluent groups, especially in the U.S. However, the definition and operationalization of familism was different and more complex, focusing on the context of commitment to social relationships over and against a competing commitment to material rewards, and measured through responses to simulated indicators of familism. Taken together, these findings underscore the importance of avoiding simplistic interpretations of the relationships between these sociodemographic variables and familism. In reality, the relationships between familism and its correlates are complex and difficult to disentangle. For example, Valenzuala and Dornbusch (1994) found that neither familistic attitudes nor parental education were significant predictors of academic achievement among Mexican American adolescents; rather, the interaction between familism and parental education served to facilitate achievement. Future research is needed to further examine, simultaneously, both the causes and consequences of adolescent familism.

The size and cross-sectional nature of the present sample prevents further exploration of potential development differences among the predictor variables and adolescents' degree of affinity with familism. However, the wide age range did allow for the detection of possible age differences in the development of a sense of familism, suggesting that youth's sense of familism may decrease with age. This negative relationship between age and familism is consistent with the increasing importance of the peer group during adolescence, and recent research highlighting the importance of autonomy among Mexican American adolescents (Fuligni, 1998).

Self-Esteem

Results from the regression analyses provided mixed support for hypotheses predicting adolescent self-esteem as connection, monitoring, autonomy-granting, legitimate authority and expert authority were all positively associated with self-esteem in at least one of the gender dyad models. Neither coercive parenting nor adolescent perceptions of coercive authority, however, were significantly related to self-esteem.

These results highlight important and intriguing gender differences in the nature of parental influence on adolescent self-esteem. For example, while monitoring by mothers and fathers was positively associated with self-esteem for both boys and girls, connection and autonomy- granting demonstrated gender-of-adolescent differences in the identified association with youthful self-esteem. Specifically, connection to fathers and mothers was associated with self-esteem for the female adolescents in this study but not for the males. Autonomy-granting, on the other hand, was found to be a positive predictor of the self-esteem of boys but not for girls. Such results suggest that for Mexican girls, supportive and inductive behaviors (i.e., connection) by parents influence positive feelings toward the self, whereas for boys, increased behavioral freedom and decreased parental interference influences self-esteem.

Parental monitoring was the only consistent predictor of self-esteem across all gender-of-parent and gender-of-adolescent dyads. These results suggest that when adolescents perceive parents as having knowledge about their adolescents' activities, there is a benefit to self-esteem, regardless of gender. That is, the extent to which boys and girls perceived their mothers and fathers as keeping track of them served as an important predictor of self-esteem. From a symbolic interactionist perspective, parental monitoring serves as a method through which parents convey clear role expectations and standards in reference to which they can evaluate themselves (Bush et al., 2002; Gecas & Schwalbe, 1986). Having clear expectations provides a better basis for positive self-esteem development in contrast to circumstances in which a person's expectations are ambiguous.

Adolescents' perception of fathers' legitimate parental authority was a positive predictor of self-esteem for both adolescent girls and boys (although marginally significant for boys), whereas maternal legitimate authority was a predictor of self-esteem in boys, but not for girls. Adolescents' perception of maternal and paternal expert authority was related to self-esteem, but only for girls. It appears, then, that self-esteem among adolescent girls in Mexico is promoted when the young female perceives her father as possessing a right to influence her life and her mother as being a reliable source of knowledge. For adolescent males, perceptions of legitimacy for both fathers and mothers were predictive of positive feelings about the self.

CONCLUSIONS

Unique patterns of parental influence were found across gender dyads and adolescent outcomes, highlighting the importance of testing for gender differences across cultures. Results in reference to parental authority indicated that adolescents' perceptions of parents' legitimate right to influence them was particularly important in fostering familistic attitudes and adolescent self-esteem (especially for boys). Moreover, perceptions of the parent as a reliable source of knowledge also positively influenced self-esteem among the girls in this sample. Autonomy-granting was of particular importance for boys' self-esteem, whereas connection was found to be an important predictor of self-esteem and familism among adolescent girls.

Taken together, the results from the present study suggest there are gender differences in the manner by which parenting practices influence developmental outcomes in adolescents from Mexico. Given arguments that boys and girls are differentially socialized in Mexican families (Benjet & Hernandez-Guzman, 2001; Chiñas, 1993), these results are not surprising. Moreover, ethnographic studies of Mexican families illuminate cultural differences in gendered expectations related to adolescent development. While Mexican adolescent boys are typically allowed more freedom from parents, adolescent girls spend more time at home in interaction with parents and are more strictly controlled (Chiñas, 1993). As a result, adolescent boys may perceive that the normative developmental trajectory during adolescence involves increased freedom from parental control and when the adolescent male experiences these behaviors from parents, there is a positive influence on self-esteem. Among Mexican adolescent girls, on the other hand, there are likely fewer expectations regarding autonomy from parents and the relatively higher amount of time they spend with parents may increase the salience of a warm and supportive connection with parents. These results are also somewhat consistent with a study by Benjet and Hernandez-Guzman (2001) in which parental positive affect (similar to parental support) by both fathers and mothers was found to predict adolescent self-esteem in Mexican females, but that among Mexican males, only affect by fathers was a positive predictor.

Our results also add to the literature on parental influence on adolescent outcomes by including measures of parental authority. Overall, adolescent perceptions of paternal and maternal legitimate authority were the most consistent predictor of both boys' and girls' self-esteem and familistic orientation. For both boys and girls, feelings that parental authority is legitimate positively predicted familism. Legitimate authority by mothers also was a positive predictor of self-esteem among the boys in this sample, but legitimate authority of fathers was only related to boys' self-esteem at the trend level. In reference to adolescent girls, legitimate and expert authority by fathers was a positive predictor of self-esteem. In general, expert and coercive authority were unrelated to self-esteem and familism, when all variables were included in the models.

In reference to understanding parental socialization of self-esteem and attitudes toward familism, therefore, these results suggest that parental authority is an important variable to consider, especially for familism and among boys. Moreover, while perceptions of legitimate authority from either mothers or fathers is associated with feelings of familism for both Mexican boys and girls, the female adolescents in this sample seemed to be influenced more (in terms of their self-esteem) by authority attributed to their fathers rather than mothers. These results point to the importance of considering adolescents' perceptions of parental authority, in addition to traditional measures of parental behaviors. In fact, legitimate parental authority, by both mothers and fathers, demonstrated the strongest positive association with male adolescents' sense of familism. These findings lend empirical support for previous suggestions of the importance of parental authority to families of Mexican origin. Moreover, they are consistent with arguments that adolescent-aged children reared in families with more collectivistic orientations (regarding individualism in families) may be more influenced by parenting strategies that are nonbehavioral and that are rooted in traditional definitions of respect for parents and families (Gorman, 1998).

Limitations

Specific limitations of this study should be considered when interpreting these findings. First, the sample for this study was drawn using a non-probability strategy from a restricted geographic area of Mexico, limiting generalizability to the entire population of Mexican adolescents, especially those residing in rural areas. Second, the data are cross-sectional and, consequently, the implied direction of influence (e.g., that parents influence adolescents) is posed for heuristic reasons only. It is equally plausible, for instance, that adolescents who have positive feelings about themselves may elicit warmth from parents (as in the case of females) or may be given more freedom by parents (for males).

The measures employed in the current study have been derived through the study of primarily white, two-parent samples of adolescents and their parents. Although the measurement items and summary variables seem to demonstrate adequate reliability and validity in a quantitative/empirical sense, we cannot be certain that the *interpretation* by Mexican adolescents accurately reflect the original intent of the items. Moreover, we likely are omitting from the analyses important elements of parenting in Mexican culture that are related to the development of self-esteem and familism.

Future studies on family process in Mexican families should include random samples from both urban and rural population, instruments tested on Mexicans, and should consider more culturally relevant and indigenous aspects of parenting. Future studies should also incorporate longitudinal models to examine bi-directional influences between parenting and adolescent outcomes with samples from Mexico.

REFERENCES

Amato, P. R., & Fowler, F. (2002). Parenting practices, child adjustment, and family diversity. *Journal of Marriage and Family, 64*, 703-716.

Baca Zinn, M. (2000). Diversity within Latino families: New lessons for family social science. In D. Demo, K. R. Allen & M. A. Fine (Eds.), *Handbook of family diversity* (pp. 252-273). New York: Oxford University Press.

Bardis, P. D. (1959). A familism scale. *Journal of Marriage and the Family, 21*, 340-341.

Bartle, S. E., Anderson, S. A., & Sabatelli, R. M. (1989). A model of parenting style, adolescent individuation and adolescent self-esteem. *Journal of Adolescent Research, 4*, 283-298.

Benjet, C., & Hernandez-Guzman, L. (2001). Gender differences in psychological well-being of Mexican early adolescents. *Adolescence, 36*, 47-65.

Bronstein, P. (1994). Patterns of parent-child interaction in Mexican families: A cross-cultural perspective. *International Journal of Behavioral Development, 17*, 423-446.

Buriel, R. (1993). Childrearing orientations in Mexican American families: The influence of generation and sociocultural factors. *Journal of Marriage and the Family, 55*, 987-1000.

Buriel, R., & Rivera, L. (1980). The relationship of locus of control to family income and familism among Anglo- and Mexican-American high school students. *The Journal of Social Psychology, 111*, 27-34.

Bush, K. R., Peterson, G. W., Cobas, J. A., & Supple, A. J. (2002). Adolescents' perceptions of parental behaviors as predictors of adolescent self-esteem in Mainland China. *Sociological Inquiry, 72*, 503-526.

Chao, R. K. (1994). Beyond parental control and authoritarian parenting style: Understanding Chinese parenting through the cultural notion of training. *Child Development, 65*, 1111-1119.

Chiñas, B. N. (1993). *The Isthmus Zapotecs: A matrifocal culture of Mexico* (2nd Ed.). Fort Worth, TX: Harcourt Brace Jovanovich College Publishers.

Emmite, P. L., & Diaz-Guerrero, R. (1983). Cross-cultural differences and similarities in coping style, anxiety, and success-failure on examinations. *Series in clinical and community psychology: Stress and anxiety*, Vol. 2 (pp. 191-206). Washington, DC: Hemisphere Publishing Corp.

Freeberg, A. L., & Stein, C. H. (1996). Felt obligation toward parents in Mexican-American and Anglo-American young adults. *Journal of Social and Personal Relationships, 13*, 457-471.

French, J. R. P., & Raven, B. (1959). The bases of social power. In D. Cartwright (Ed.), *Studies in social power* (pp. 150-167). Oxford, England: University of Michigan Press.

Frias-Armenta, M., & McCloskey, L. A. (1998). Determinants of harsh parenting in Mexico. *Journal of Abnormal Child Psychology, 26*, 129-139.

Fuligni, A. J. (1998). Authority, autonomy, and parent-adolescent conflict and cohesion: A study of adolescents from Mexican, Chinese, Filipino, and European backgrounds. *Developmental Psychology, 34*, 782-792.

Gecas, V., & Schwalbe, M. L. (1986). Parental behavior and adolescent self-esteem. *Journal of Marriage and the Family, 48*, 37-46.

Gorman, J. C. (1998). Parenting attitudes and practices of immigrant Chinese mothers of adolescents. *Family Relations, 47,* 73-80.

Harter, S. (1993). Causes and consequences of low self-esteem in children and adolescents. In R. F. Baumeister (Ed.), *Self-esteem: The puzzle of low self-regard* (pp. 66-88). New York: Plenum.

Henry, C. S., Wilson, S. M., & Peterson, G. W. (1989). Parental power bases and processes as predictors of adolescent conformity. *Journal of Adolescent Research, 4,* 15-32.

Hill, N. E., Bush, K. R., & Roosa, M. R. (2003). Parenting and family socialization strategies and children's mental health: Low income, Mexican American, and Euro-American mothers and children. *Child Development, 74,* 189-204.

Lamborn, S. D., Mounts, N. S., Steinberg, L., & Dornbusch, S. M. (1991). Patterns of competence and adjustment among adolescents from authoritative, authoritarian, indulgent, and neglectful families. *Child Development, 62,* 1049-1065.

Marotz-Baden, R. (1984). Trade-offs in satisfaction: A United States-Mexican comparison. *Journal of Marriage and the Family, 46,* 145-151.

Mecca, A. M., Smelser, N. J., & Vasconcellos, J. (1989). *The social importance of self-esteem.* Berkeley, CA: University of California.

Owens, T. J., & Stryker, S. (2001). The future of self-esteem: An introduction. In T. Owens, S. Stryker, & N. Goodman (Eds.), *Extending self-esteem theory and research: Sociological and psychological currents* (pp. 1-9). Cambridge, UK: Cambridge University Press.

Peterson, G. W., Bush, K. R., & Supple, A. J. (1999). Predicting adolescent autonomy from parents: Relationship connectedness and restrictiveness. *Sociological Inquiry, 69,* 431-457.

Peterson, G. W., & Hann, D. (1999). Socializing parents and families. In M. Sussman, S. K. Steinmetz, & G. W. Peterson (Eds.), *Handbook of marriage and the family, 2nd ed.* (pp. 327-370). New York: Plenum.

Peterson, G. W., Rollins, B. C., & Thomas, D. L. (1985). Parental influence and adolescent conformity: Compliance and internalization. *Youth and Society, 16,* 397-420.

Powers, S., & Sanchez, V. V. (1982). Correlates of self-esteem of Mexican American adolescents. *Psychological Reports, 51,* 771-774.

Rosenberg, M. (1979). *Conceiving the self.* New York: Basic Books.

Ruiz, S. Y., Roosa, M. W., & Gonzales, N. A. (2002). Predictors of self-esteem for Mexican American and European American youths: A reexamination of the influence of parenting. *Journal of Family Psychology, 16,* 70-80.

Shkodriani, G. M., & Gibbons, J. L. (1995). Individualism and collectivism among university students in Mexico and the United States. *The Journal of Social Psychology, 135,* 765-772.

Smith, T. E. (1986). Influence in parent-adolescent relationships. In G. K. Leigh & G. W. Peterson (Eds.), *Adolescents in families* (pp. 130-154). Cincinnati, OH: South-Western.

Tallman, I., Marotz-Baden, R., & Pindas, P. (1983). *Adolescent socialization in cross-cultural perspective: Planning for social change.* New York: Academic Press.

Triandis, H. C. (1995). *Individualism & collectivism.* Boulder, CO: Westview Press.

Unger, J. B., Ritt-Olson, A., Teran, L., Huang, T., Hoffman, B. R., & Palmer, P. (2002). Cultural values and substance use in a multiethnic sample of California adolescents. *Addiction Research and Theory, 10,* 257-280.

Parent-Child Contact After Divorce:
The Need to Consider
the Child's Perspective

Karl-Franz Kaltenborn

ABSTRACT. This article contains a review of research on parent-child contact after parental separation and divorce and provides a case study derived from a longitudinal study of divorce. This case study is based on a child psychiatric evaluation report of a girl aged five, on a face-to-face interview at age eleven and on autobiographical narratives of the same participant at the age of 22 years. The author advocates a "childhood research" approach aimed at improving the understanding of how children

Karl-Franz Kaltenborn has a PhD in medicine from the Eberhard-Karls University of Tübingen and a PhD in sociology from the Technical University of Darmstadt. He is a lecturer at the Medical Center for Methodology and Health Research, Institute of Medical Informatics of the Philipps-University of Marburg, Germany.

Address correspondence to: Karl-Franz Kaltenborn, MD, PhD, Philipps-University of Marburg Medical Center for Methodology and Health Research, Institute of Medical Informatics, Bunsenstraße 3, D-35033 Marburg, Germany (E-mail: kaltenbo@ mailer.uni-marburg.de).

The author wishes to express his profound gratitude to Prof. Dr. R. Lempp and Prof. Dr. G. Klosinski for their valuable support. The present article was written during his recent stay at the Australian Institute of Families Studies in Melbourne, and sincere thanks are due to the Institute staff, especially to Ruth Weston and Bruce Smyth, for their hospitality and support.

The first survey of the custody project was carried out by the author as a postgraduate PhD student at the Child and Youth Psychiatry Center, Eberhard-Karls University of Tübingen, Germany. The second survey was also a project carried out by the author at the Child and Youth Psychiatry Center in Tübingen and was partly supported by a grant from the Charles-Hosie Foundation.

http://www.haworthpress.com/web/MFR
© 2004 by The Haworth Press, Inc. All rights reserved.
Digital Object Identifier: 10.1300/J002v36n01_04

perceive, experience and cope with parental separation and divorce, especially custody and visiting issues. The article ties a critical analysis of the scientific literature and the case study to approaches and topics for future research. *[Article copies available for a fee from The Haworth Document Delivery Service: 1-800-HAWORTH. E-mail address: <docdelivery@ haworthpress.com> Website: <http://www.HaworthPress.com> © 2004 by The Haworth Press, Inc. All rights reserved.]*

KEYWORDS. Child's agency, case study, custody, divorce, visiting

INTRODUCTION

Parental separation and divorce have undergone an almost global increase in modern society. The impact of divorce on children is thus a major concern for policy makers, practitioners, and separating parents alike. While an ongoing debate exists as to the precise short- and long-term effects of divorce on children (Kelly & Emery, in press; Wallerstein, Lewis, & Blakeslee, 2000), there is mounting discussion on the importance of hearing children's voices amidst the noise, haze, and emotional turmoil that often surround family members involved in the breakdown of a parental relationship.

Secularization and individualization processes have contributed to a diminished commitment to traditional norms and values as well as to the rising divorce rate (Beck, 1992; Beck-Gernsheim, 1998; Clarke, 1996). As a consequence, since living arrangements and patterns of contact have to be regulated for a growing number of children in the wake of a divorce, contemporary Western societies are relying more on scientific knowledge and its derivatives than on customs resulting from religious or familial traditions. The relevance that scientific knowledge has gained this way creates the obligation for researchers and scientists to examine carefully and critically the quality and adequacy of their knowledge base.

Research into Parent-Child Contact After Divorce

An extensive supply of research literature[1] exists on children and divorce. For reasons of economy and empirical power, the present article focuses primarily on a number of respected meta-analytic and narrative reviews.

Amato and Rezac (1994) investigated the link between children's well-being and parent-child contact. They found that 18 out of 33 studies supported the notion that children's well-being is higher overall when frequent contact is maintained with nonresident parents; nine studies found no relation overall between the frequency of contact and children's well-being; and six revealed that the frequency of contact with the nonresident parent is associated with increased problems for children.

More recently, Amato and Gilbreth (1999) applied meta-analytic methods to 63 studies dealing with fathers' behavior patterns and children's well-being. They focused on four variables: payment of child support, frequency of contact, feelings of closeness, and authoritative parenting as influences on children. They found that payment of child support by fathers was positively related to measures of children's well-being. In contrast, the frequency of contact with nonresident fathers was not related to child outcomes in general. The variables "feelings of closeness" and "authoritative parenting" showed a positive association with children's academic success and a negative association with children's externalizing and internalizing problems.

Whiteside and Becker (2000) also carried out a meta-analytic review based on an analysis of 12 studies with a focus on younger children's post-divorce adjustment. They found several factors contributing directly or indirectly to child adjustment: pre-separation father involvement, hostility/cooperation, father-child relationship quality, frequency of father visitation, maternal warmth, and maternal depressive symptoms. On the basis of these results, they concluded that a good father-child relationship was associated with the child's well-being. In line with Amato and Gilbreth's (1999) findings, Whiteside and Becker (2000) found that the time fathers and children spent together was not important for the child's well-being, but that relationship quality was a significant contributor. They noted that "The effect on child outcomes of the amount of time the father spends with the child appears to be mediated by the quality of the father-child involvement." Thus fathers' contact can have a positive or negative influence on the child but fathers who engage in frequent contact are more likely to have high-quality relationships with their children.

Two further aspects of this study warrant mention. First, because Whiteside and Becker's data were correlational, they could not determine the causal direction of the relationships between variables. For example, fathers with good relationships with their children may be committed to spending time with them; conversely, fathers committed to spending time with their children may have had the opportunity and experience to develop a good relationship. Second, although the authors' model was complex, its ability to predict the outcome variables was only moderate.

In their recent comprehensive review of research on children and divorce, Pryor and Rodgers (2001) sought to explicate the relation between parent-child contact and child outcomes. Their conclusions largely fit with the meta-analytic reviews described. With respect to negative relationships between fathers and children, they conclude that "contact between fathers and children is not necessarily a positive experience for children *if the child does not want it* or if the relationship is negative" (Pryor & Rodgers, 2001:214, italics added).

While emphasis placed by Pryor and Rodgers (2001) on the child's wishes point to one of the most important elements of the whole parent-child contact issue, it seems that children's wishes only play a marginal role in conventional divorce research. This is the case even in areas where decisions about children's lives are made in relation to residence and/or contact orders. Amato comments on the exclusion of the child in divorce research as follows:

> Most of the literature that I have reviewed (mainly U.S. studies) does not take the child's wishes into account with respect to visitation and custody. Most reports are from the perspective of parents. Even studies that ask children about parent-child relationships following divorce do not generally ask children about their preferences. Judith Wallerstein has argued in several of her works, however, that we need to pay more attention to the views of children, and I agree. My impression is that the match (or discrepancy) between children's preferences for custody and contact, and the actual custody and visitation situation, is a good predictor of children's adjustment. But I haven't seen much work that addresses this hypothesis directly. (Personal Communication, May 29, 2002)

Smart, Neale, and Wade (2001:20), using a childhood sociology perspective, also disapprove of the way divorce research is carried out, stating:

> A striking feature of the current research on children and divorce is that very little of it is based on the views of children themselves. To date, their collective views have simply not been taken into account in the area of private family law and policy. The irony of this, we quickly discovered, is that children have a lot to say if they are given the opportunity.

However, this criticism does not stand alone. Indeed there is an increasing awareness of the importance of children's wishes as well as commensurate pleas and efforts to have them included in divorce research (Arditti & Prouty, 1999; Crossman, Powell, Principe, & Ceci, 2002; Fleming & Atkinson, 1999; Kaltenborn, 2001a; 2001b; Smart et al., 2001; Smith, Taylor, Gollop, Gaffney, Gold, & Henaghan, 1997; Wallerstein et al., 2000).

Child psychiatry in Germany had an earlier tradition of taking account of children's wishes concerning residence and visitation (Lempp, 1963; 1964; 1984; Remschmidt, 1978). This tradition has lost influence in science and society, partly because of an uncritical import of North American studies focusing primarily on structural elements and ignoring the child's voice, and partly because of gender politics.[2] However, probably as a consequence of the new Children's Act of 1998 (Kindschaftsrecht, 1998), with the introduction of a *guardian ad litem*, scientific writing focusing more on the child's wishes is currently undergoing a renaissance (e.g., Dettenborn, 2001; Dettenborn & Walter, 2002; Kindler & Schwabe-Höllein, 2002; Salgo, Zenz, Fegert, Bauer, Weber, & Zitelmann, 2002; Zitelmann, 2001).

Children can be very perceptive. They can also articulate their needs and wishes if those around them are sensitive to their voices (Arditti & Prouty, 1999; Crossman et al., 2002; Kaltenborn, 2001a; 2001b; Kaltenborn & Lempp, 1998; Kelly & Emery, in press; Murray & Hallett, 2000; Smart et al., 2001; Wallerstein et al., 2000). A case study from empirical work serves as an example of the importance of including children's voices in the divorce process. Since our custody project including the present article is in line with modern childhood research endeavors, this theoretical approach will first be briefly delineated.

Theoretical Framework

In contrast to developmental and socialization concepts presenting children only from the perspective of being immature and more or less incompetent and passive beings, new childhood research paradigms offer a different approach to children and childhood. The four most important tenets of childhood research, (1) children's agency, (2) children's rights, (3) social construction and (4) social structure of childhood, are briefly discussed below.[3]

One of the main tenets of childhood research is "a view of children as persons with agency (i.e., with the capacity to act, interact and influence their social worlds)" (Smart et al., 2001:11). Consequently, childhood research began "to explore children's agency in a variety of contexts, focusing on how children negotiate rules, roles and personal relationships; how they create autonomy and balance this with their (inter)dependence; how they operate as strategic actors in different social contexts and how they take responsibility for their own well-being and that of others" (Smart et al., 2001:12). The child's agency within the familial context can be further elaborated in terms of the model of the family as a commanding or negotiating household (Büchner, 1995; du Bois-Reymond, 1995; 2001). Based on empirical data, the authors differentiate between a commanding household with an authoritarian or modernized command style, a negotiating household with a greater or lesser degree of regulation, and an ambivalent style. Depending on the type of household, the children will enjoy a different degree of (in)dependence and participation in family decision-making. Both family climate and the kind of punishment (i.e., corporal punishment, verbal admonishing, or no punishment) are characteristics of each household type. However, in the case of divorce, with ongoing contact between children and noncustodial parents, the family constellations are much more complex. The negation tasks of children and adults demand a fairly high degree of coordination within the context of a binuclear family structure involving two-parent households, influenced to varying degrees by professionals and embedded within the family justice system and national family laws (Ahrons & Rodgers, 1987; du Bois-Reymond, 2001; Mnookin, 1979). Moreover, during the course of time, the qualities and changes of the child's personal attachments within his or her familial network in connection with the child's agency deserve scientific attention. Attachments of the child are subject to attachment theory, a perspective from developmental psychology,[4] and as Bretherton, Walsh, Lependorf and Georgeson (1997:97) outline:

> Yet attachment theory is especially well suited for helping us untangle the complexities of children's and parents' postdivorce experiences, complexities that are not well captured by labeling such families "single-parent."

Another childhood research approach is concerned with children's minority status in different societies. Childhood research in this tradition puts emphasis on the various degrees to which children are exploited on a global level. This discourse points out that children's "human rights are underexpressed and inappropriately exercised" and therefore advocates change (James, Jenks, & Prout, 1998:211; Roche, 1996). Further discourses of childhood research deal with the social construction of childhood and study childhood as a particular and distinct form of any society's social structure (James et al., 1998; Qvortrup, 2001).

From a methodological point of view, the perspective of the child is central to childhood research, which has consequences on empirical methods and study designs where the child has to be included (Büchner, 1995; du Bois-Reymond, 1995; 2001; James et al., 1998; Honig, Lange, & Leu, 1999; Smart et al., 2001).

SAMPLE AND METHODS

For the custody project, 60 evaluation reports covering 81 children (51 boys and 30 girls) performed between 1964 and 1978 by a child psychiatrist and psychologists at the Child and Youth Psychiatry Center (Eberhard-Karls University of Tübingen, Germany) were selected by theoretical sampling. For these custody cases, the corresponding court files, additional specialists' reports, and, in some cases, doctors' letters that were found in the court files or in our own patient records were analyzed. During the period 1979 to 1984, I interviewed these families, including the children when possible (Kaltenborn, 1987). A second survey was carried out by the author from 1989 to 1994. For the second survey, the following design was selected in order to allow more direct participation in our research. Since many of the children requested a copy of the subsequent scientific publication after the first interview, we sent a copy of our publication including summaries together with a questionnaire to all children. This questionnaire had five questions regarding custody and visitation issues (Kaltenborn, 2001a; 2001b). The questions on visiting were "How did your contact with the visiting parent develop in the course of time after custody evaluation?" and "What were your experiences with the legal right of noncustodial parents to visit their children?"

By analyzing the answering letters with respect to visits, the method of "comparative casuistics" (comparative case analysis), a method similar to the "grounded theory" approach, is applied (Jüttemann, 1981; 1990). Comparative case analysis presents a strategy for gathering and processing empirical data by linking it with theoretical concepts in order to generate hypotheses and develop adequate theories in social sciences. The strategy can be used to analyze and compare data from single cases as well as from a collective, allowing inter-individual comparisons (idiographic and nomothetic). The method comprises fundamentally a two-phase procedure: Based on a thorough initial examination and interpretation of an individual case, hypotheses and theories are formulated to facilitate the understanding of this single case with its characteristics; in a subsequent interindividual comparison with other cases, more comprehensive hypotheses and theories covering and explaining superindividual phenomena are constructed.

In the following, a case study derived from this longitudinal study is presented. This is Ute's story, based mostly on her reflections as a 22-year-old, but also including a psychiatric evaluation at age five, and a face-to-face interview at age 11. Ute's case has been selected for presentation because of its paradigmatic character and comprehensive nature, which allow case-specific theoretical considerations to be transcended and a more comprehensive theoretical framework to be expounded. The theoretical approach demonstrated by Ute's case is applied in our custody project and is recommended here for research on children concerning custody and visiting issues after divorce (Kaltenborn, 2001a; 2001b; 2002).

UTE'S CASE HISTORY

Early History

Brother and sister, Stephan and Ute,[5] lived with their father after their parents had separated. In the clinical evaluation conducted by a child psychiatrist and psychologist(s), the mother stated with regard to the visits that:

> it was unsettling for the children each time. Ute was happy and always hugged her as soon as they met, whereas Stephan first behaved very reservedly and eased up later on. It was only when he was brought back that he became reserved again. Ute wanted to stay with her, the mother, but Stephan was more reserved.

The child psychiatric evaluation reported on the almost five-year-old Ute:

> Ute could be enticed out of her initial shyness within a short time. She became extremely lively with well-adjusted behavior. If our conversation turned to her mother Biermann [mother's pseudonym, comment KFK], then Ute checked with easygoing chatter. She turned frequently to her brother, but was quite capable of asserting herself against him. . . . When the brother was absent, the child [Ute] talked no differently from when he was present. Ute cut her brother short when he maintained that Ute too said "Mrs. Biermann" to their mother and stated that she also said "Mummy Biermann" sometimes. However, she emphasized simultaneously that she did not like visiting her mother. Her brother was not present though when she reported that her mother cuddled her, which she [Ute] did not like. "Re" [for Regina, Ute's stepmother, comment KFK] cuddled her too, she said, but she [Ute] enjoyed it with her.

The summarizing child psychiatric interpretation states:

> The psychologically less complicated and tougher Ute has obviously adapted completely to the new family situation in the meantime and has fully accepted the second mother. However, she [Ute] is far from showing the rejection towards her biological mother that the brother expresses towards her. Ute becomes insecure when the relationship with the mother comes into focus, and separation anxieties are revealed in the psychological testing. In the conflict situation, she seeks support from her brother.

First Follow-Up

At the first follow-up, the 11-year-old Ute was very happy to be living with her father and her stepmother. She and her mother still had contact for a time after the child psychiatric evaluation, but by the first follow-up, no contact visits were taking place. At the first follow-up interview, Ute spoke out forcefully against visiting her mother.

Second Follow-Up

The following are excerpts from Ute's letter to the author on the occasion of the second follow-up (when Ute was almost 22 years old).

> I must apologize for not having answered your letter earlier. My parents forwarded your letter to me in December, and I sat down right away to answer you. It was partly a lack of time and partly reluctance to recall the last few years again that made me abandon it for a while. I find it very difficult to "dig up" my recollections again, to have to live it all over again, and to write it down. One decisive factor is certainly also the death of my brother, who plays a crucial role in all my memories. Overall I do not feel capable of giving concrete responses to your answers [what is meant are questions, KFK], since the responses to the questions would also overlap. I have tried–often with reference to my old diaries–to record my recollections concerning my parents' divorce and my current relationship with my parents and my biological mother. . . .

The autobiographical record written by Ute concerning her relationship with her mother on the occasion of the second follow-up reads as follows:

> When I was four years old, my parents divorced and the custody of my eight-year-old brother and me was awarded to my father, who married my stepmother Regina that same year. During the following years, my brother and I had to observe a judicial visiting regulation: Once a fortnight on Sundays, a visit from 10 a.m. to 7 p.m. to our biological mother, who had also married again in the meantime and was living in the same town with her second husband and two stepchildren (Egon, the same age as my brother, and Christiane, three years older). The visiting regulations also provided for two weeks of summer holidays and one week of the winter holidays to be spent with our mother's family.
> I remember that I usually found the visiting Sundays very stressful. Sunday morning: get dressed nicely and be ready at the door at 10 o'clock sharp. No matter whether a child's birthday was on the agenda, no matter whether one would have preferred to spend Sunday with the "real" family. My father and Regina always encouraged us too–after all, there was always a lot on offer with our mother's family: from ice-skat-

ing or swimming pool with artificial waves, to movies. The favorite meal was served up for Sunday lunch, there were sweets in abundance; never a ban on anything, never any rebuke.

When "skimming through" the first entries in my diary (I was about ten years old) I realize how difficult I found the to-ing and fro-ing between my family and the other Sunday family, who were "Mummy" and "Uncle Theo" to me, and how I put up more and more resistance to these Sunday visits. For a while I absolutely terrorized my mother's family. I tried to be as naughty as possible. One day I climbed over the garden fence and called my parents from the nearest phone box and asked them to pick me up.

Five years after my father had married my stepmother Regina, my stepsister Anita was born, forming an even closer bond within our family. The fact that toddler Anita is "only" my stepsister is something I can't really grasp even today. Once there were five of us, I found the visits to my mother even more difficult to tolerate.

I recall a holiday with my mother's family in Bavaria. During that holiday, I wrote to my little sister every day (I was 10 years old at the time), painted pictures, sent dried flowers and called home several times a day. Homesickness–although at least my brother was with me.

During that time we were in the care of Mr. Arendt, a Court Welfare Officer with whom we had a good relationship in the course of time. We also owed it to Mr. Arendt that the court visiting regulation was cancelled and that we could visit my mother on a voluntary basis.

As far as I recall, my brother had a fairly indifferent attitude to the visits. The actual home, the family, was most certainly my father's family for him too.

Once the visiting access (compulsory visiting) arrangement had been cancelled, my mother tried desperately to maintain the contact with Stephan and me. As I see it today, the contact was of a purely material nature. At regular intervals we received enormous presents, promises of a moped, and Stephan also of a car. Stephan kept up the contact with my mother, but mostly without telling my parents. From that time onwards, the visits were no longer encouraged by my father or Regina either.

When Stephan then had difficulties at school, failed class tests, had certain bans imposed on him by our parents, he always found refuge with his mother. When my parents said Stephan should find a holiday job during the summer holidays so that he could buy a motorbike later, he got every wish fulfilled by my mother. In any dispute with my parents, every other sentence was: "but at Monika's [the mother, comment KFK] I get it, at Monika's I'm allowed to. . . ." Everything in mother's family was more perfect, more comfortable and nicer.

In 1981 when my brother was 17 years old, it was decided that my brother should spend a "trial year" with his mother's family to find out whether everything really was so rosy there. However, Stephan was usually back with us after a short time. Actually it was perfectly clear that Stephan was to come back to us in May '82. Our mother Monika fulfilled Stephan's wish for a motorbike, which my parents considered too dangerous. In March 1982, when Stephan had had his motorbike for just three weeks, he died in a road accident for which he was not to blame.

Partly out of curiosity to get to know my biological mother better, partly from a desire to understand my dead brother better, and probably also out of sheer convenience like my brother, I re-established contact with my biological mother too. The crucial reason for this decision to visit my mother now and again was certainly her remark: "All I've got now is you." Somehow I felt obliged to keep up my contact with her. The contact with my mother was unwelcome to my father and especially to my stepmother Regina. My parents made disparaging remarks about Monika, and that may have been the very reason why, as a 15/16-year-old, I wanted to gain my own impression of the woman who was supposed to be (and wanted to be) my mother, and whom my brother had also got to know more closely. Our being together was confined to afternoon shopping expeditions and vast quantities of presents. For me, that meant back to an extreme to-ing and fro-ing between my family, which gave me support, and my mother, who spoiled me and never criticized me."

But I never toyed with the idea of deciding entirely in favor of my mother. The meetings with my mother were never forbidden by my parents, although I got the clear message–especially from my stepmother, Regina–that they were not in favor of the contact. I was often in a dilemma when my parents asked me questions about my mother. Sometimes secretly, sometimes with the knowledge of my parents, I met my mother every one or two months; in the meantime, she was living about 80 km from where my father lived. Four and a half years ago I moved to Münster to train for a job; for the past one and a half years I have been living in Italy. Up to now, I have continued to meet my mother now and again, although the contact is meanwhile maintained almost exclusively by her. However, contact with my stepmother has clearly deteriorated as a result of this, since she is afraid that my mother might have a negative influence on me. I find it difficult to give a clear-cut definition of the relationship with my mother. Overall, I tend to see her rather as an aunt.

Interpretative Comments on Ute's Case History

Ute's autobiographical narrative is an exceptionally rich, sensitive description of her contact experiences that should be briefly interpreted in accordance with the method described above. However, the following comments represent a focused, not an exhaustive interpretation, especially since this case study is such a work of "aesthetic knowledge" (Lash, 1994a; 1994b) that it is left to further reading to reveal additional aspects (e.g., the long-lasting pain associated with the parents' divorce).

In describing her and her brother's post-divorce life, Ute draws attention to several important dimensions of the children's actual experiences, including the relationship qualities, structure of visits, perspectives and wishes, educational capability of adults, and agency of people involved. The dimensions used by Ute are simultaneously tenets of new childhood research as well as topics about children and divorce in academic literature. One of the most important dimensions in Ute's case description comprises the relationship quality and dynamics in the course of time within the familial networks. Even at the time of the child psychiatric evaluation, Ute has clear preferences for the paternal family, and she expresses her distinct preference for her stepmother. She uses (probably mimicking her father) the pet name "Re" for her stepmother (Re is pronounced in German like *Reh*, which means little deer, revealing some nice associations). At the same time, she illustrates a marked detachment from her mother by calling her "Mrs. Biermann" or sometimes "Mummy Biermann." However, Ute is very exact in her reporting to the psychiatrist in that she corrects her brother and draws attention to her use of "Mummy Biermann" in some cases (whereby "Mummy Biermann" is still unusual and demonstrates detachment, albeit to a lesser extent). Cuddling with Re and with her mother are also quite different: liked in the first instance and disliked in the latter, again bringing different relationship qualities to the awareness of the evaluator.

Even at the child psychiatric evaluation stage, we learn the importance of her relationship with her brother, and all these feelings are still present when she writes her letter. The importance of this sibling relationship notwithstanding, Ute always has her own personal standpoint and perspective. As a consequence of the birth of her half-sister, the paternal family becomes emotionally even closer. However, these relationship qualities are changing. The relationship with her father and to a greater degree with her stepmother takes on a more complicated aspect when Ute, as a young adolescent, visits her mother against the wishes of her father and stepmother. The family atmosphere declines. The relationship with her mother improves a little over time, but this relationship never gains a maternal quality and her mother ends up being seen "as an aunt."

Ute carefully describes the effect of the contact structure imposed by law upon her and the changes to these arrangements over time. By relating the contact structure to Ute's wishes, one can observe that, at age five, Ute dislikes the arrangements. She illustratively describes how such a visiting arrangement impinges on her time and she cites examples, such as a child's birthday party, to communicate to us the loss of childhood time. Imposed visits to which no exception is allowed are experienced as a kind of "structural coercion." But the deep feelings about this "tyranny" presumably do not result exclusively from the structure of the visits but also from a poor mother-daughter relationship. However, there is a turning point in the contact trajectory: As a teenage girl, Ute reestablishes visits with her mother, and her detailed accounts of this process need no further explanations.

Ute also devotes considerations to the educational capabilities and the behavior of her parents. Her mother seems to be aware of her poor relationship with her children and tries fervently to change this by showering them with presents–a strategy that seems to work better with Stephan than with Ute. As a consequence, a dynamic shift affecting different dimensions occurs: (1) Stephan's orientation towards his mother (based on merely material interests), (2) the dislike of this "material orientation" by his father and stepmother, (3) Stephan's playing the mother against the paternal family, (4) the loss of parental capacity by the father and stepmother, and (5) the change of power relationships between father and stepmother on one side, and Stephan on the other. There are ongoing negotiations with the final outcome that Stephan changes his residence. However, this change makes it clear that Stephan's relationship with his mother is not sufficiently stable and that the residence at his mother's is lacking so a later change of residence is already envisioned. And, there is the tragic accident in which Stephan loses his life.

When adolescent Ute reestablishes contact with her mother, the mother again tries to strengthen the relationship by buying Ute a constant flow of presents. She also puts psychological pressure on Ute with statements such as "All I've got now is you." However, these statements also reflect the mother's solitude and sadness over the loss of her son.

Finishing our analysis with a focus on the perspective and agency of the child as central tenets of childhood research, we observe five-year-old Ute as already being quite capable of expressing her preferences in the supportive environment of the child psychiatric evaluation. As a ten-year-old girl, Ute pursues her perspective, acting within three different networks: the paternal family, the maternal family, and the family justice system. The Court Welfare Officer, Mr. Arendt, represents the family justice system on Ute's behalf and thus the link to family law. In this respect, Ute is acting in "the shadow of the law" (and in this case the law is child-friendly).

The Child's Wishes and Agency in Custody and Visiting Matters

In addition to Ute's case history, references to our custody project and other respective research findings are outlined briefly to substantiate the childhood research approach. The main findings of the custody project suggests that taking account of the child's wishes in terms of relationship and residential arrangement is in the best interests of the child's welfare. The child's wishes best represent a positive living situation with loved ones both within the family and the social environment. However, the personal relationships of the child are in no way static, but demonstrate notable dynamics as they change under the influence of internal and external factors.

A residential arrangement contrary to the child's relationships and residence preferences create a difficult situation for the child which can lead to one of three different processes: adjustment, a trajectory of suffering, or initiatives to change the living situation. The child's agency in legal custody decision-making and residence changes proved to be not just an age-related skill but a complex capability involving children's personal characteristics,[6] on the one hand and family characteristics,[7] the availability of social support, and the practice of the family justice system on the other. All of these are embedded in and influenced by societal macrosystems, especially the legal system (Kaltenborn, 2001a; 2001b; Kaltenborn & Lempp, 1998).

Concerning parent-child contact, we observed in our study a broader spectrum of relationship qualities between the child and the visiting parent and, in some cases, changes in these relationship qualities. Patterns varied from children's (sometimes changing) wishes for or against visits as well as different agency patterns with varying degrees of success or failure (Kaltenborn, 2002). In other words, the children display different and changing scores for relevant dimensions such as relationship qualities, structure of visits, perspectives, and wishes. This variability notwithstanding, the study exemplifies the universal role and importance of the child's perspective and agency in visiting issues. Considering the representative nature of Ute's case history from this point of view, though individual in its specific circumstances and trajectory, is paradigmatic in its relevance for the child's perspective, agency and different dimensions of experience.

Smart et al. (2001:21, italics added) report similar findings in their study when they discuss co-parenting, noting that "the precise structuring of arrangements for children may be less important than the way in which they are practiced and negotiated and *the extent to which children are included in the negotiations.*" Smart et al. (2001) also found that parenting styles as well as the personal and social resources available to children are important in increasing or diminishing their ability to participate successfully in decision-making, a finding that is in accordance with results described above (Kaltenborn, 2001a; 2001b; 2002).

While the importance of the child's perspective and agency is advocated in this article, it is also important to recognize that some children make discrepant statements, i.e., they declare residence preferences contrary to their true emotional tendencies during the clinical exploration or court hearing. A skillful examination is then required to expose verbal information as discrepant statements on the part of the child (Kaltenborn, 1986; Lempp, von Braunbehrens, Eichner, & Röcker, 1987; Powell & Lancaster, 2003). Such discrepant statements are often the result of pressure being exerted on the child by a parent in order to suppress what the child wants–with the goal of being granted custody or visiting access or of denying these to others. Furthermore, if the child is neglected, sexually abused or battered, the situation might be even more difficult (Powell & Lancaster, 2003; Zitelmann, 2001).

Research into Parent-Child Contact and Its Inherent Limitation

There is no doubt that divorce research has to provide information *inter alia* on basic structural aspects of contact arrangements after parental separation and divorce. Since contact structures are not independent of time and space, there is a need for ongoing research and for targeted research in different countries with different cultures, social structures, and sociodemographics.

While some researchers in the tradition of childhood sociology are averse to preoccupation with outcome-focused research (Smart et al., 2001), it is nonetheless important to always keep at least one eye on outcomes. However, there are some indications that "outcome" needs to be rethought, especially with respect to contact and residence issues.

Firstly, even if we develop sophisticated models containing a plethora of variables, their predictive power in the field of divorce research is always likely to be limited because of the complexity of the child's reality (Whiteside & Becker, 2000). What we can learn from Ute's case, and from other cases as well (Arditti & Prouty, 1999; Kaltenborn, 2002; Smart et al., 2001), is that the whole familial system is permanently in flux, the various variables interacting and influencing each other, hardly providing an opportunity to determine what is in fact an "outcome" and what is in fact a "predictor" (see the difficulties reported by Whiteside & Becker, 2000). In addition, each variable changes in the course of time in its content and relevance to the child, while one and the same variable and one and the same rating may mean very different things to different children. This means that we must concede that we are unlikely ever to be able to give exact outcome results, but rather only probabilities for the occurrence of a variety of possible outcomes.[8] In this respect, we are in neither a better nor a worse position than natural science. Heisenberg's "uncertainty principle" in the microcosm is a good analogy for this:

> The more precisely the position is determined, the less precisely the momentum is known in this instant, and vice versa. (Heisenberg, 1927:175; <http://www.aip.org/history/heisenberg/p08.htm>, retrieved 7-25-2003)

Secondly, this insight about "uncertainty" has far-reaching consequences. It is not necessarily important to give special weight to each variable, especially in cases where the child dislikes and is opposed to that particular fact (e.g., Ute's mother may be well adjusted, which favors visiting, but her adjustment status can be disregarded because of Ute's rejection). So, on the one hand, uncertainty means that we cannot predict everything; on the other hand, uncertainty opens up increased freedom with the opportunity to focus more on the child.

Thirdly, outcome is typically measured by means of various psychological tests, and a (slight) outcome difference is lauded by researchers. But certain questions have to be asked: Can small differences in test scores accurately capture meaningful outcomes for children? Does outcome need to be understood in a much broader sense? Indeed, when Pryor and Rodgers (2001:214) state that "positive contact is in itself a good outcome for children who usually want it," they apply a much broader perspective by emphasizing a judgment which includes the child's contact experiences and feelings; simultaneously they are pointing to the fact that there is no direct or simple relationship between levels of nonresidential father-child contact and child well-being. Kelly and Emery (in press) make a case for distinguishing pain or distress about parental divorce from longer-term psychological symptoms or pathology. The authors also emphasize that, even though approximately 75% of children of divorced families are functioning well on a variety of objective measures, divorce can create lingering feelings of sadness, longing, worry, and regret. Laumann-Billings and Emery (2000:683) also report on the basis of their study that "most children from divorced families are resilient, but their distress—their pain—can be significant nonetheless." While we have to recognize "the limited coverage of many of the most commonly used measures of psychological adjustment" (Laumann-Billings & Emery, 2000:683), we should reflect outcome dimensions beyond conventional test scores and focus more on the child. Such child-focused perspectives can be advanced to considerations like: Isn't it a good outcome to avoid any coercion on the child aimed at encouraging nonresidential parent-child contact in cases where the child decisively refuses visiting? Likewise, isn't it a good outcome to fulfill the child's wishes for contact?

While it is beyond the scope of this article to determine definitively what "outcome" should be, it is argued that outcome cannot be defined exclusively either by scientific discipline or by research that relies primarily on parents' reports. Outcome considerations transcend scientific prescriptions and, in order to be understood, also require the collective voices of the children concerned (see also Emery, 1999; Smart et al., 2001).

The Need to Include the Child's Perspective and Agency in Divorce Research

Childhood research as outlined above depicts children as social actors vested with specific competencies as well as rights. Therefore, a link can be made to the human rights movement, of which the United Nations Convention on the Rights of the Child is of particular relevance here. Article 12 of the UN (United Nations, 1990) Convention on the Rights of the Child states:

1. Parties shall assure to the child who is capable of forming his or her own views the right to express those views freely in all matters affecting the child, the views of the child being given due weight in accordance with the age and maturity of the child.
2. For this purpose, the child shall in particular be provided the opportunity to be heard in any judicial and administrative proceedings affecting the child, either directly, or through a representative or an appropriate body, in a manner consistent with the procedural rules of national law.

Against this backdrop of children's rights, the exclusion of the child in conventional research targeted at divorce is a significant deficit and an oversight. In contrast, drawing attention just to Ute's autobiographical narrative and to new social childhood studies about children of divorce (Arditti & Prouty, 1999; Fleming & Atkinson, 1999; Kaltenborn, 2001a; 2001b; 2002; Smart et al., 2001; Smith et al., 1997) reveals immediately how important the child's perspective and agency are for contact issues, as well as for the assessment of life trajectories and turning points. It is thus essential that the child's perspective should be central to studies concerned with contact or residence issues, and with divorce research more generally. This implies that researchers and scientists need to further develop methods to study and understand the child's perspective, difficult and challenging though this research endeavor might be, given the dependence of children's communication patterns and agency on contexts (Powell & Lancaster, 2003).

Such a research approach must be sure not to limit itself to laboratory studies but must reach out to real life and must study children's communication patterns in separating families, in courts, and in social institutions that work with children of divorce. Also, the ability of professionals working in the field as well as of parents to understand and be sensitive to children's communication patterns and preferences has to be studied and improved (Powell & Lancaster, 2003). The wider context of policy and practice, e.g., family law, legislative and social politics, gender policies, and their influence on familial microsystems, also needs to be examined. The nub of the arguments outlined here is that a framework is needed of "outreach research" that builds knowledge around children's everyday life experiences and around their journeys through childhood and adolescence in cases of parental divorce. This research matches well with the conclusions drawn by Eekelaar (1991:21) in relation to the UN Convention in which he urges us to "find ways to set up a continuing process of dialogue and communication with children and young people" and, as Harrison (1991:32) states, "to raise levels of consciousness and knowledge about children."

Returning to the issue of parent-child contact, it can be said that the task is to bring the visiting structure dimension into line with the child's perspective.[9] In other words, it is not the pattern of contact itself that is important but the match of it with the child's perspective. In relation to all other observable dimensions, the child's perspective is unique insofar as it represents the child's "summary" or "condensation" of a whole range of aspects and factors in his or her environment. Because of the changes and dynamics concerning relevant contact dimensions in the course of childhood and adolescence (see Arditti & Prouty, 1999; Kaltenborn, 2002), parent-child contact may be regarded as a long-lasting "negotiation task."

To summarize, the proposals made here imply a fundamental paradigm shift. Whereas traditional divorce research about decision-related issues such as residence and contact trusts structural thinking and statistics,[10] the approach advocated here trusts the child and his or her perspective.[11]

NOTES

1. A search of keywords related to parent-child contact after divorce [(contact or visit) and divorce and child] in the database *Psychological Abstracts* yielded 567 citations (29 October 2002).

2. Divorce research is called structure orientated if its focus is primarily on the relationship between structures (like custody structure, visiting structure, etc.) and outcome variables and if the child's perspective and his or her agency is either ignored or underrepresented. Studies with structural results such as "contact with both parents is best" or "joint custody is best" regardless of the child's perspective and the individual familial circumstances are ideally suited to being used or, rather, misused in supporting gender politics.

3. Childhood research represents an interdisciplinary approach including childhood sociology as well as related childhood studies in education, psychology, social work, social policy, etc. For a more comprehensive outline of the theoretical base of childhood research see du Bois-Reymond, Sünker, and Krüger (2001), Büchner (1995), Corsaro (1997), Honig, Lange, and Leu (1999), James, Jenks, and Prout (1998), and Smart et al. (2001).

4. This way, while our custody and visiting project adheres theoretically to childhood research, it also refers when indicated to developmental psychology, e.g., by emphasizing attachment theory (Kaltenborn, 2001a; 2001b).

5. Names of children, doctors, towns, etc., have been changed to guarantee the anonymity of those involved; however, each child retains his or her pseudonym throughout all publications related to this project.

6. e.g., age, psychological development, information and knowledge, temperament, ambivalence and loyalty conflicts, experienced parental pressure, probably the child's sex, etc.

7. e.g., power boundaries, willingness to litigate, parent's sex, information and knowledge, hostility between the parents, health status, etc.

8. Smart et al. (2001) refer to "broken home" research as a further example of uncertainty about causality despite many years of research endeavors. See also Amato (2001:366) who concludes: "Knowledge of group averages, therefore, cannot predict how a particular child will adjust to family disruption."

9. Based on their analysis, Whiteside and Becker (2000:21) conclude that "the discussion with parents needs to shift from a preoccupation with number of overnights to a more complicated assessment of the parenting environment." See also Kelly and Emery (2003).

10. Historically simple linear correlations between variables were typically applied for this work. More recently, however, more complex interactional models have been used (e.g., Whiteside & Becker, 2000).

11. Of course, such an approach could be accompanied by outcome research. Ideally, this outcome research would be like a safety net in a circus, allowing free flight while preventing casualties.

REFERENCES

Ahrons, C. R. & Rodgers, R. H. (1987). *Divorce families: A multidisciplinary developmental view.* New York: Norton.

Amato, P. R. (2001). Children of divorce in the 1990s: An update of the Amato and Keith (1991) meta-analysis. *Journal of Family Psychology, 15,* 355-370.

Amato, P. R. (2002). Personal Communication, May 29th.

Amato, P. R. & Gilbreth, J. G. (1999). Nonresident fathers and children's well-being: A meta-analysis. *Journal of Marriage and the Family, 61,* 557-573.

Amato, P. R. & Rezac, S. (1994). Contact with nonresidential parents, interparental conflict, and children's behavior. *Journal of Family Issues, 15,* 191-207.

Arditti, J. A. & Prouty, A. M. (1999). Change, disengagement, and renewal: Relationship dynamics between young adults and their fathers after divorce. *Journal of Marital and Family Therapy, 25,* 61-81.

Beck, U. (1992). *Risk society: Towards a new modernity.* London: Sage.

Beck-Gernsheim, E. (1998). *Was kommt nach der Familie? Einblicke in neue Lebensformen.* München: Beck.

Bretherton, I., Walsh, R., Lependorf, M., & Georgeson, H. (1997). Attachment networks in postdivorce families: The maternal perspective. In L. Atkinson & K. J. Zucker (Eds.), *Attachment and psychopathology* (pp. 97-134). New York: Guilford Press.

Büchner, P. (1995). The impact of social and cultural modernisation on the everyday lives of children. Theoretical and methodological framework and first results of an inter-cultural project. In M. du Bois-Reymond, R. Diekstra, K. Hurrelmann, & E. Peters (Eds.), *Childhood and youth in Germany and the Netherlands. Transitions and coping strategies of adolescents* (pp. 105-125). Berlin: de Gruyter.

Clarke, L. (1996). Demographic change and the family situation of children. In J. Brannen & M. O'Brien (Eds.), *Children in families* (pp. 66-83). London: Falmer.

Corsaro, W. A. (1997). *The sociology of childhood*. Thousand Oaks, CA: Pine Forge Press.

Crossman, A. M., Powell, M. B., Principe, G. F., & Ceci, S. J. (2002). Child testimony in custody cases: A review. *Journal of Forensic Psychology Practice, 2,* 1-32.

Dettenborn, H. (2001). *Kindeswohl und Kindeswille: psychologische und rechtliche Aspekte*. München: Reinhardt.

Dettenborn, H. & Walter, E. (2002). *Familienrechtspsychologie*. München: Reinhardt.

du Bois-Reymond, M. (1995). The modern family as a negotiating household. Parent-child relations in Western and Eastern Germany and in the Netherlands. In M. du Bois- Reymond, R. Diekstra, K. Hurrelmann, & E. Peters (Eds.), *Childhood and youth in Germany and the Netherlands. Transitions and coping strategies of adolescents* (pp. 127-160). Berlin: de Gruyter.

du Bois-Reymond, M. (2001). Negotiation families. In M. du Bois-Reymond, H. Sünker, & H.-H. Krüger (Eds.), *Childhood in Europe: Approaches, trends, findings* (pp. 63-90). New York: Lang.

du Bois-Reymond, M., Sünker, H., & Krüger, H.-H. (Eds.) (2001). *Childhood in Europe: Approaches, trends, findings*. New York: Lang.

Eekelaar, J. (1991). Why children? Why rights? In P. Alston & G. Brennan (Eds.), *The UN Children's Convention and Australia* (pp. 20-21). Sydney: The Human Rights and Equal Opportunity Commission.

Emery, R. E. (1999). Postdivorce family life for children: An overview of research and some implications for policy. In R. A. Thompson & P. R. Amato (Eds.), *The postdivorce family: Children, parenting, and society* (pp. 3-27). Thousand Oaks, CA: Sage.

Fleming, R. & Atkinson, T. (1999). *Families of a different kind: Life in the households of couples who have children from previous marriages or marriage-like relationships*. Waikanae (New Zealand): Families of Remarriage Project.

Harrison, M. (1991). Does Australia really need the convention?' In P. Alston & G. Brennan (Eds.), *The UN Children's Convention and Australia* (pp. 29-33). Sydney: The Human Rights and Equal Opportunity Commission.

Heisenberg, W. (1927). Über den anschaulichen Inhalt der quantentheoretischen Kinematik und Mechanik. *Zeitschrift für Physik, 43,* 172-198.

Honig, M-S., Lange, A., & Leu, H. R. (Eds.) (1999). *Aus der Perspektive von Kindern. Zur Methodologie der Kindheitsforschung*. Weinheim: Juventa.

James, A., Jenks, C., & Prout, A. (1998). *Theorizing childhood*. Cambridge: Polity Press.

Jüttemann, G. (1981). Komparative Kasuistik als Strategie psychologischer Forschung. *Zeitschrift für klinische Psychologie und Psychotherapie, 29,* 101-118.

Jüttemann, G. (Ed.) (1990). *Komparative Kasuistik*. Heidelberg: Asanger.

Kaltenborn, K.-F. (1986). Das kommunikative Verhalten des Scheidungskindes in der kinderpsychiatrischen Exploration. *Fragmente, Schriftenreihe zur Psychoanalyse, 22,* 149-165.

Kaltenborn, K.-F. (1987). Die personalen Beziehungen des Scheidungskindes als sorgerechtsrelevantes Entscheidungskriterium: eine katamnestische Untersuchung nach kinder- und jugendpsychiatrischer Begutachtung zur Regelung der elterlichen Sorge. *Zeitschrift für das gesamte Familienrecht, 34,* 990-1000.

Kaltenborn, K.-F. (2001a). Children's and young people's experiences in various residential arrangements: A longitudinal study to evaluate criteria for custody and residence decision making. *British Journal of Social Work, 31,* 81-117.

Kaltenborn, K.-F. (2001b). Individualization, family transitions and children's agency. *Childhood: A Global Journal of Child Research, 8,* 463-498.

Kaltenborn, K.-F. (2002). "Ich versuchte, so ungezogen wie möglich zu sein." Fallgeschichten mit autobiographischen Niederschriften: die Beziehung zum umgangsberechtigten Elternteil während der Kindheit in der Rückerinnerung von jungen Erwachsenen. *Praxis der Kinderpsychologie und Kinderpsychiatrie, 51,* 254-280.

Kaltenborn, K.-F. & Lempp, R. (1998). The welfare of the child in custody disputes after parental separation or divorce. *International Journal of Law, Policy and the Family, 12,* 74-106.

Kelly, J. B. & Emery, R. E. (in press). Children's adjustment following divorce: Risk and resilience perspectives, *Family Relations.*

Kindler, H. & Schwabe-Höllein, M. (2002). Eltern-Kind-Bindung und geäußerter Kindeswille in hochstrittigen Trennungsfamilien. *Kindschaftsrechtliche Praxis, 5,* 10-17.

Kindschaftsrecht (1998). Synopse zu den Neuerungen im Kindschaftsrecht (Teil I), *Familie, Partnerschaft, Recht. Interdisziplinäres Fachjournal für die Praxis.* FPR Service 02, 1998, pp. 1-47. Synopse zu den Neuerungen im Kindschaftsrecht (Teil II), *Familie, Partnerschaft, Recht. Interdisziplinäres Fachjournal für die Praxis.* FPR Service 03, 1998, pp. 49-104.

Lash, S. (1994a). Reflexivity and its doubles: Structures, aesthetics, community. In U. Beck, A. Giddens, & S. Lash (Eds.), *Reflexive modernization. Politics, tradition and aesthetics in the modern social order* (pp. 110-173). Cambridge: Polity Press.

Lash, S. (1994b). Expert-systems or situated interpretation? Culture and institutions in disorganized capitalism. In U. Beck, A. Giddens, & S. Lash (Eds.), *Reflexive modernization. Politics, tradition and aesthetics in the modern social order* (pp. 198-215). Cambridge: Polity Press.

Laumann-Billings, L. & Emery, R. E. (2000). Distress among young adults from divorced families. *Journal of Family Psychology, 14,* 671-687.

Lempp, R. (1963). Das Wohl des Kindes in §§ 1666 und 1671 BGB. *Neue Juristische Wochenschrift, 16,* 1659-1662.

Lempp, R. (1964). Noch einmal: Kindeswohl und Kindeswille. *Neue Juristische Wochenschrift, 17,* 440-441.

Lempp, R. (1984). Die Bindungen des Kindes und ihre Bedeutung für das Wohl des Kindes gemäß § 1671 BGB. *Zeitschrift für das gesamte Familienrecht, 31,* 741-744.

Lempp, R., von Braunbehrens, V., Eichner, E., & Röcker, D. (1987). *Die Anhörung des Kindes gemäß § 50b FGG.* Köln: Bundesanzeiger.

Mnookin, R. H. (1979). *Bargaining in the shadow of the law: The case of divorce.* Oxford University: Center for Socio-Legal Studies. Working Paper No. 3.

Murray, C. & Hallett, C. (2000). Young people's participation in decisions affecting their welfare. *Childhood: A Global Journal of Child Research, 7,* 11-25.

Powell, M. B. & Lancaster, S. (2003). Guidelines for interviewing children during child custody evaluations. *Australian Psychologist, 38,* 46-54.

Pryor, J. & Rodgers, B. (2001). *Children in changing families: Life after parental separation.* Oxford: Blackwell.

Qvortrup, J. (2001). Childhood as a social phenomenon revisited. In M. du Bois-Reymond, H. Sünker, & H. H. Krüger (Eds.), *Childhood in Europe: Approaches, trends, findings* (pp. 215-241). New York: Lang.

Remschmidt, H. (1978). Das Wohl des Kindes aus ärztlicher Sicht. *Zeitschrift für Kinder- und Jugendpsychiatrie, 6,* 409-428.

Roche, J. (1996). The politics of children's rights. In J. Brannen & M. O'Brien (Eds.), *Children in families: Research and policy* (pp. 26-40). London: Falmer.

Salgo, L., Zenz, G., Fegert, J., Bauer, A., Weber, C., & Zitelmann, M. (2002). *Verfahrenspflegschaft für Kinder und Jugendliche: ein Handbuch für die Praxis.* Köln: Bundesanzeiger.

Smart, C., Neale, B., & Wade, A. (2001). *The changing experience of childhood: Families and divorce.* Cambridge: Polity Press.

Smith, A. B., Taylor, N. J., Gollop, M., Gaffney, M., Gold, M., & Henaghan, M. (1997). *Access and other post-separation issues.* Dunedin (New Zealand): Children's Issues Centre.

United Nations (1990). *Resolutions and decisions adopted by the General Assembly during its forty-fourth session,* Volume I, 19 September-29 December 1989, Supplement No. 49 (A/44/49). New York: UN.

Wallerstein, J., Lewis, J., & Blakeslee, S. (2000). *The unexpected legacy of divorce: A 25 year landmark study.* New York: Hyperion.

Whiteside, M. F. & Becker, B. J. (2000). Parental factors and the young child's postdivorce adjustment: A meta-analysis with implications for parenting arrangements. *Journal of Family Psychology, 14,* 5-26.

Zitelmann, M. (2001). *Kindeswohl und Kindeswille im Spannungsfeld von Recht und Pädagogik.* Münster: Votum.

Familial Impacts on Adolescent Aggression and Depression in Colombia

Christine L. McClellan
Tim B. Heaton
Renata Forste
Brian K. Barber

ABSTRACT. This study examines how parental conflict and parenting influence aggression and depression by adolescents in Colombia, a country characterized by high societal violence, that provides an interesting backdrop for our analysis of familial conflict. Drawing upon socialization and parenting perspectives, we model the effects of overt and covert parental conflict on adolescent outcomes as mediated by parenting behaviors. Data were gathered by questionnaires completed by 493 high school students in Bogotá, Colombia. Findings suggest that family interaction plays a role in adolescent aggression and depression. However, rather than a strong direct effect of overt parental conflict on aggression through social learning, we find a more influential association of overt conflict with parenting, which, in turn, is related to aggression. Covert parental conflict and parental support are more directly associated with depression. Controls for gender, family structure, family socioeconomic status, and authority relations in the family are also included. *[Article copies available for a fee from The Haworth Document Delivery Service: 1-800-HAWORTH. E-mail address: <docdelivery@haworthpress.com> Website: <http://www. HaworthPress.com> © 2004 by The Haworth Press, Inc. All rights reserved.]*

Christine L. McClellan lives in Provo, UT (E-mail: christinem@byu.net). Tim B. Heaton and Renata Forste are affiliated with the Department of Sociology, Brigham Young University, 852 SWKT, Provo, UT 84602. Brian K. Barber is affiliated with the Department of Child and Family Studies, University of Tennessee, Knoxville, TN 37996.

http://www.haworthpress.com/web/MFR
© 2004 by The Haworth Press, Inc. All rights reserved.
Digital Object Identifier: 10.1300/J002v36n01_05

KEYWORDS. Adolescent aggression, adolescent depression, covert conflict, overt conflict, parental conflict

INTRODUCTION

Aggression is often viewed as a manifestation of machismo within Latin culture. Statistics from the 1990 Colombian Demographic and Health Survey indicate that domestic conflict is well entrenched in Colombian families: 65 percent of women ever in a union reported fighting with their partner at least once. Aggression is also evident in society-wide trends of violence in Colombia (Bouley & Vaughn, 1995).

The relation between conflict within the home and aggression manifested outside the home is unclear (Hotaling et al., 1990). Although conflict between parents seems to encourage aggressive behavior in their children, our understanding of the effects of domestic conflict on children is incomplete. Social learning theorists argue that aggression is a learned behavior and children replicate aggressive behaviors learned in the home (Straus, 1990). Other researchers argue that parental conflict leads to children's aggression only insofar as such conflict interferes with effective parenting (O'Keefe, 1996). Some researchers point out that family conflict is often internalized instead of externalized; instead of acting aggressively, children from conflicted homes may manifest depressive behaviors and attitudes (Buehler et al., 1998; O'Keefe, 1996). This paper examines the link between conflict in the family environment and adolescent outcomes, including aggression and depression in Bogotá, Colombia. Colombia serves as a powerful setting for such an examination in light of its high rates of both societal and familial conflict (Bouley & Vaughn, 1995; Profamilia, 1991).

Colombian Families and Aggression

As Hart and colleagues (1998:687) note, we have few studies "adding cross-cultural insights into possible antecedents of aggressive childhood behavior." Most research on aggression, and on family conflict, has been conducted within North America (Fontes, 1997; Hart et al., 1998). The existing comparative studies indicate that cultural context is a crucial aspect of aggression that must be considered (see Levinson, 1989). By studying aggressive behavior in Colombia, we contribute to a more global understanding of this problem, and we provide avenues for cross-cultural comparisons. Further, the violence prevalent in Colombian society provides a provocative setting for examining the predictors of adolescent aggression.

Little research on individual aggression or familial conflict has been conducted in Colombia; however, national patterns of violence suggest that individual aggression and its manifestation through violence is a serious problem. As Bouley and Vaughn (1995:17) note, "Colombia possesses the dubious honor of having one of the highest homicide rates in the world." Colombian adolescents are clearly affected by this disturbing pattern: among male Colombian adolescents aged 15 to 24, the principal causes of hospitalization in 1985 were injuries caused by violence (Prado et al., 1988). Further, the leading cause of death in Colombia for both male and female adolescents aged 16 to 24 is homicide (Prado et al., 1988: Vélez, 1995).

While evidence of family-level aggression in Colombia has not been empirically measured, anecdotal accounts support an image of Colombian families as often aggressive or violent. Colombian researchers often characterize their own society as violently aggressive (Uribe, 1995; Vélez, 1989). Uribe (1995:357, translation authors) explains that in Colombia, "the family medium, ideally considered as a sphere of affect, of construction of positive relations, is generally a violent medium . . . where violence is exercised as a right of the aggressor." Patterns of violence and aggression both within and outside families in Colombia lend a striking context for a study of the roots of aggressive behavior. Further, by studying adolescent aggression in Colombia, we contribute to the rare, but much-needed, research conducted in a non-United States cultural context.

In our study of adolescent aggression in Colombia we first examine the literature on parental conflict and child aggression drawing particularly on social learning theories and theories of parenting practices. We examine not only the direct link between parental conflict and child aggression through socialization, but also the indirect effect through parenting behaviors. In addition, we distinguish between overt and covert forms of parental conflict and their influence on external adolescent aggression, as well as on internal adolescent depression. Finally we highlight various background factors in the literature associated with parental conflict and adolescent problem behaviors. Following our review of the literature, we describe our data and model specifications and present the results of our analyses of the relationship between familial conflict, parenting, and adolescent problem behaviors. Finally, we discuss these results and provide suggestions for future research.

LITERATURE REVIEW

The relation between conflict within the home and aggression manifested outside the home is unclear (Hotaling, Straus, & Lincoln, 1990). Although conflict between parents seems to encourage aggressive behavior in their children, our understanding of the effects of domestic conflict on children is incomplete. This paper examines the link between conflict in the family environment and adolescent outcomes, including aggression and depression in Bogotá, Colombia. Colombia serves as a powerful setting for such an examination in light of its high rates of both societal and familial conflict (Bouley & Vaughn, 1995; Profamilia, 1991).

Parental Conflict and Child Aggression

Many popular explanations of aggressive behavior place its roots in the family of origin. The intergenerational transmission of abuse and aggression suggests that those whose parents fight are more likely to be aggressive themselves (Carroll, 1977; Egeland, 1993; Emery, 1982; MacEwen, 1994; Zaidi, Knutson, & Mehm, 1989). This effect is not limited to those who were physically abused as children; a number of studies reveal that externalizing and internalizing problems, including aggression and depression, are found among children who simply witness interparental conflict (Emery, 1989; Kalmuss, 1984; O'Keefe, 1996; Pagelow, 1981; Paschall, Ennett, & Flewelling, 1996). Further, the relation between marital discord and child behavior problems has been found in studies conducted in a variety of countries (Emery, 1982).

The extent to which the intergenerational transmission framework explains aggressive behavior is still under debate; it is clear, however, that the relationship is neither inevitable nor direct (Kaufman & Zigler, 1993). Much of what is known about the link between conflict in childhood and later aggression is based on retrospective data obtained from high-risk adult groups. Consequently, studies of children and adolescents are needed to further define the link between family conflict and child aggression.

Correlations between parental aggression levels and overall child aggression levels have been documented (Bjorkqvist & Osterman, 1992; Huesmann, Maxwell, Eron, Dahlberg, Guerra, Toler, VanAcker, & Henry, 1996). In a more extreme case, Hotaling, Straus, and Lincoln (1990) identified child abuse in the backgrounds of violent criminals and people who approve of violent behavior. Certainly, family conflict and conflict in society involve different levels of intimate interaction; however, social research must consider the broader context—that is, that children publicly act out the behaviors they learn at home.

There are different explanations as to how parental conflict leads to more aggression in children. Because of this variation, concomitantly examining multiple dimensions of this relationship can be fruitful both for theoretical development and for practice. As Miller and Wellford (1997:27) note, "Integrated or multi-level theories of intimate violence clearly reveal that the response to intimate violence must be multifaceted." To explore the relationship between parental conflict and adolescent aggression, we examine both the socialization perspective and an approach that links aggressive behaviors to parenting abilities and behaviors.

The appropriateness of theoretical integration is part of a larger debate in the field of criminology. One of the most prominent supporters of theory integration is Elliott (1985). Elliott (1985) criticizes the more conventional strategy of theory competition in criminology research and argues that its explanatory power is weak. He calls for theoretical integration to move theoretical development forward (Elliott, 1985). Other theorists, such as Vold and colleagues (1998), take a neutral position regarding integration and argue that most theories "integrate" some past material in their arguments. In contrast, Liska and colleagues (1989) are more skeptical of the integration approach and argue that for it to be successful it should point to new research agendas.

We draw upon socialization and parenting perspectives to model the relationship between parental conflict and adolescent problem behaviors in an end-to-end (sequential) strategy of integration (Liska, Krohn, & Messner, 1989). End-to-end integration refers to the ordering of causal variables and allows us to model not only the direct effect of parental conflict on adolescent aggression (socialization), but also its indirect effect via parenting behaviors (parenting perspective). Wagner and Berger (1985) argue that end-to-end theorizing is better described as theoretical elaboration rather than theoretical integration.

Socialization Perspective

The socialization perspective posits that children acquire aggressive behaviors and attitudes from observing their parents' aggression within the home. Parents' aggression may teach children how to be aggressive, or it may cause children to view aggression as legitimate (Foshee, Bauman, & Linder, 1999; O'Leary, 1988; Straus, 2001). According to social learning theory, if aggressive behavior is rewarded, viewers of the behavior will model or adopt the same aggressive patterns (Bandura, 1973). Parental aggression does not always produce positive rewards for children to observe; thus, social learning theory in its original form offers a limited explanation of child aggression (Simons, Ling, & Gordon, 1998). Even if children do not view rewarded behavior, they may believe that there are no other options than the behavior they observe in parents. As O'Leary (1988:33) interprets social learning, "We observe others and from those observations, we form ideas of how new behaviors are performed. In turn, these coded observations serve as guides for further actions." From this perspective, children who observe aggression or conflict at home are likely to model the behavior and be aggressive themselves.

Parenting Perspective

The parenting perspective focuses on how parental conflict engenders a general disruption of essential family functions, including parenting behaviors such as affection, support, and discipline. Child aggression is thus attributed not to social learning, but to the ineffective parenting that results from parental conflict. As Fauber, Forehand, Thomas, and Wieson (1990:1113) clarify, studies under this framework suggest that:

> Marital conflict influences child adjustment indirectly by altering some aspect of the parent-child relationship. The disruption in the child's adjustment and functioning is thus viewed as a direct response to the alteration in the parent-child interaction, rather than the conflict itself.

Various studies demonstrate that spouses involved in marital conflict are more likely to manifest negative parenting styles (Erel & Burman, 1995; Fagan, Stewart, & Hansen, 1983; Fauber et al., 1990; Hotaling et al., 1990; Jouriles, Pfiffner, & O'Leary, 1988). Such findings are consistent with the "spillover hypothesis": "when the quality of the marriage is poor, difficulties may spill over to the parent-child relationship" (Lindahl & Malik, 1999:320). In turn, numerous studies show that children are more likely to engage in antisocial behavior when they receive poor parenting (Barber, 1996; Barber, Olsen, & Shagle, 1994; Emery, 1982; Fauber & Long, 1991; Patterson et al., 1992; Simons et al., 1998; Simons, Wu, Conger, & Lorenz, 1994). Thus, some studies have found that parent-child relations better predict child problem behaviors than does interparental conflict (Emery, 1982). As such, the inclusion of both parenting behaviors and interparental conflict in a study of child problem behaviors can better determine the relative strength, direct, and indirect effects of varied parental influences on children. Studies incorporating both parenting and parental conflict variables in the same model are few, and they are limited to samples of children from the United States (Fauber et al., 1990; Gerard & Buehler, 1999; Margolin & John, 1997).

A number of parenting dimensions are correlated with aggression and antisocial behavior. For instance, the more supportive parents are, the less aggressive their children are likely to be. This relationship is found whether support is measured by parent-child attachment (Emery, 1982; Fincham, Grych, & Osborne, 1994; Paschall et al., 1996), parental responsiveness (Hart, Nelson, Robinson, Olsen, & McNeilly-Choque, 1998), "positive parenting" (Margolin & John, 1997), or a direct measure of parental support (Barber, 1999).

In addition, parental monitoring of adolescent behavior has been shown frequently to be negatively associated with adolescent aggression and antisocial behavior in U.S. samples of children and adolescents (see Barber, 1996; Patterson & Stouthamer-Loeber, 1984). It is evident as well that the relationship is not limited to U.S. samples. Recent work demonstrates that the link between parental monitoring and adolescent problem behaviors is evident in cultures as different from the United States as Palestine and India (Barber, 1998; Barber, 1999). The more parents know about their children's activities where they are, what they do, and whom they are with–the less likely their children are to misbehave in aggressive ways. This monitoring may be indicative of an overall discipline style; inconsistent discipline has also been linked to problems of conduct and aggression (Emery, 1982). However, it should be noted that overly restrictive or coercive parenting also appears to be related to increased aggression (Balswick & Macrides, 1975; Hart et al., 1998).

Parental Conflict and Depression

Other problem behaviors are also related to parental conflict. As Barber (1992:69) explains, "We know a great deal about individual problem behaviors but relatively little about how specific behaviors are related, or the extent to which they have similar or dissimilar social and personal antecedents." Two apparently related outcomes are aggression and depression: while some children respond to conflict in aggressive ways, others internalize these problems. Just as parental conflict and parenting are often associated with externalizing behaviors such as aggression and delinquency, they also lead at times to internalizing child outcomes such as depression and suicide ideation (see Fauber et al., 1990; Garber, Robinson, & Valentiner, 1997; Shagle & Barber, 1993). Even when controlling for factors such as age, gender, race, and socioeconomic status, witnessing family conflict predicts depression (Buehler, Krishnakumar, Stone, Anthony, Pemberton, Gerard, & Barber, 1998; O'Keefe, 1996). O'Keefe (1996), for instance, finds that witnessing interparental violence is significantly associated with levels of depressive symptomatology among a sample of high school students. On the other hand, Buehler and colleagues (1998) find that more passive types of interparental conflict are associated with internalizing problems such as depression, while more overt, aggressive conflict between parents is not.

Overt and Covert Conflict

A distinction between types of interparental conflict helps to explain how interparental conflict may be associated with aggression for some adolescents and with depression for others. Recent research distinguishes between two varieties of conflict that appear to have distinct consequences for children. Overt conflict, defined as "hostile behaviors and affect which indicate direct manifestations of negative connections between parents," seems to be linked to overtly aggressive child behaviors (Buehler et al., 1998:5). Covert conflict, which embodies passive-aggressive manners of conflict management (such as "trapping" children in the middle of fights), apparently results in more internalizing child outcomes, such as depression (Buehler et al., 1998). Buehler and colleagues (1998:121) explain this relationship by describing how both covert conflict style and youth internalizing are "fairly passive techniques, have an indirect or suppressed quality, and may reflect the absence of a strong core sense of self." Children may learn from their parents that "triangling, resentment, and unspoken tension" are valid internalizing ways of responding to stress, or they may respond to the strong emotional arousal generated by overt parental conflict by turning their feelings inward to escape them (Buehler et al., 1998:121). The distinction between conflictive patterns clarifies the ways in which parental conflict may have differing consequences for children according to its manifestation in the home.

Individual and Family Characteristics Related to Aggression

Various other individual and family characteristics have been shown to effect negative child outcomes such as aggression and depression. These include the gender of the child, the socioeconomic status of the family, the structure of the family, and authority relations within the family.

Gender influences the extent to which children are aggressive or are affected by aggressive parental behaviors. Specifically, males are often found to be more aggressive overall, and also to be influenced more by exposure to interparental aggression (Emery, 1982; Hotaling et al., 1990; Langhinrichsen-Rohling & Neidig, 1995; MacEwen, 1994; Mangold & Koski, 1990). Females tend to manifest depression more often than males do as a reaction to family conflict (Buehler et al., 1998; Emery, 1982; O'Keefe, 1996). As Kimmel and Weiner (1985:542-3) explain,

> Some research has suggested that . . . males begin at adolescence to show a preference for resolving conflict through external channels of expression, or 'acting out,' whereas females develop a preference for dealing with conflict internally, or 'acting in.'

Although the source of gender differences is unclear, since gender roles and attitudes are influenced by many societal influences, gender is certainly an important factor in predicting aggression and depression.

While low socioeconomic status has been linked to aggressive behavior in children (McNeilly-Choque, Hart, Robinson, Nelson, & Olsen, 1996), it is unclear whether this relationship is independent of socioeconomic differences in parenting styles or family structure. Various studies of spousal conflict conclude that marital violence is more likely in families with low socioeconomic status (Gelles, 1989; Gelles & Cornell, 1990; Moore, 1997) or where one or both parents are unemployed (Fagan et al., 1983; Oropesa, 1997). Some research also suggests that educational level is negatively correlated with abuse (Gelles & Cornell, 1990; Oropesa, 1997).

Although some studies find that living in a single-parent household increases the likelihood of delinquency and aggression among adolescents (Paschall et al., 1996), the effects of being raised in a single-parent home are still under debate. The consequences of both parental conflict and parenting should be influenced by whether or not both parents reside in the home. For instance, Ptacek (quoted in Miller & Wellford, 1997) suggests that aggressive behavior results from a lack of sufficiently developed interpersonal skills due to parental neglect or missing role models. Such neglect or lack of role models is more likely to occur in single-parent families. In addition, there is some evidence that parental abuse of children is more likely to occur in single-parent families (Gelles, 1989; Gelles & Cornell, 1990).

Authority relations in the family are also expected to be related to parental conflict, parenting, and child outcomes. Some studies have found that families characterized by egalitarian relationships are less conflicted than families where either the husband or wife is dominant (Gelles & Cornell, 1990). Others have found that adolescent rebellion is more likely in homes characterized by strict patriarchy (Balswick & Macrides, 1975). The limited research on how the balance of power between spouses influences their parenting is mixed. That is, while McHale (1995) finds that parents have less involvement with their children where power relations between spouses are inegalitarian, a recent study by Lindahl and Malik (1999) does not support this hypothesis. Thus, there is limited research suggesting that male dominance in family relations may reduce parental involvement with adolescents. We, therefore, include a measure of male authority in the home in our model in order to further clarify its influence on parenting and child problem behaviors.

Based on this literature, we model the effects of family conflict on aggression among adolescents living in a culture characterized by high rates of both societal and domestic conflict. Specifically, we examine parental factors influencing outcomes of physical aggression and depression among Colombian adolescents. We posit that overt and covert parental conflict and background characteristics of gender, socioeconomic status, family structure, and parental authority relations will predict parenting measures and adolescent aggression and depression.

In particular, we posit that overt parental conflict is associated with both aggression and depression in adolescents, but primarily aggression. In contrast we expect covert parental conflict to be associated with both outcomes, but the effect to be stronger on depression. In addition, we hypothesize that parental conflict will both directly influence adolescent problem behaviors and indirectly by inhibiting other positive parenting behaviors. We further anticipate that parenting will be directly associated with these negative outcomes.

RATIONALE, OBJECTIVES, AND HYPOTHESIS

Rationale

As Hart and colleagues (1998:687) note, we have few studies "adding cross-cultural insights into possible antecedents of aggressive childhood behavior." Most research on aggression, and on family conflict, has been conducted within North America (Fontes, 1997; Hart et al., 1998). The existing comparative studies indicate that cultural context is a crucial aspect of aggression that must be considered (see Levinson, 1989). By studying aggressive behavior in Colombia, we contribute to a more global understanding of this problem, and we provide avenues for cross-cultural comparisons.

Little research on individual aggression or familial conflict has been conducted in Colombia; however, national patterns of violence suggest that individual aggression and its manifestation through violence is a serious problem. As Bouley and Vaughn (1995:17) note, "Colombia possesses the dubious honor of having one of the highest homicide rates in the world." Among Colombian adolescents males aged 15 to 24, the principal causes of hospitalization in 1985 were injuries caused by violence (Prado, Singh, & Wulf, 1988), and the leading cause of death in Colombia for both male and female adolescents aged 16 to 24 is homicide (Prado et al., 1988; Vélez, 1995). The homicide rate may be attributed , in part, to the drug trade in Colombia, and may not occur within a family context; however, it does expose adolescents to violence on a regular basis.

Statistics from the 1990 Colombian Demographic and Health Survey also indicate that domestic conflict is well entrenched in Colombian families: 65 percent of women ever in a union reported fighting with their partner at least once. Aggression is at times viewed as a manifestation of machismo within Latin culture; there are both positive and negative aspects of machismo

(Mirande, 1998). Anecdotal accounts also support an image of Colombian families as often aggressive or violent. Colombian researchers often characterize their own society as violently aggressive (Uribe, 1995; Vélez, 1989). Uribe (1995:357, translation authors) explains that in Colombia, "the family medium, ideally considered as a sphere of affect, of construction of positive relations, is generally a violent medium . . . where violence is exercised as a right of the aggressor." Patterns of violence and aggression both within and outside families in Colombia lend a striking context for a study of the roots of aggressive behavior.

Objectives and Hypotheses

Based on this literature, we model the effects of family conflict on aggression among adolescents living in a culture characterized by high rates of conflict. Specifically, we examine parental factors influencing outcomes of physical aggression and depression among Colombian adolescents. We posit that overt and covert parental conflict and background characteristics of gender, socioeconomic status, family structure, and parental authority relations will predict parenting measures and adolescent aggression and depression.

In particular, we posit that overt parental conflict is associated with both aggression and depression in adolescents, but primarily aggression. In contrast, we expect covert parental conflict to be associated with both outcomes, but the effect to be stronger on depression. In addition we hypothesize that parental conflict will both directly influence adolescent problem behaviors and indirectly by inhibiting other positive parenting behaviors. We further anticipate that both parental support and monitoring will have negative effects on both aggression and depression. Further, we expect that our measures of parental conflict and male authority will have negative effects on both support and monitoring. And, based on limited past studies, we anticipate that male dominance will be associated with higher levels of parental conflict, possibly lower levels of positive parenting, and negative child outcomes.

METHOD

The Sample

Our analyses of adolescent aggression and depression are based on data from the Youth and Family Project in Colombia. These surveys were originally constructed in English for English-speaking populations; a native Spanish-speaker translated the questionnaires. We also consulted with an experienced survey researcher and his well-trained staff in Bogotá who gave input into the wording of questions in the Spanish version of the instrument. We also pre-tested and revised the survey. After receiving permission from school principals and teachers, data were collected during the classes of ninth, eleventh, and twelfth graders. One hundred percent of those in attendance participated. The questionnaire was self-administered. We surveyed a total of nine schools in Bogotá from 1997 to 1998. Schools were selected by the director of the research institute in Bogota that helped us collect the data. These included two private and seven public schools selected from a range of socio-economic neighborhoods so that the sample would reflect the diversity within the city. The sample underrepresents the poorest neighborhoods and the elite, but, according to professional researchers in the cities who contacted the schools, it does represent children from low-income and middle-class families. In addition, some older teenagers were surveyed as members of a city-wide association for youth. Surveys were administered to a total of 771 adolescents ranging from age 13 to age 18. Students took approximately one hour to complete the questionnaire detailing information on family interaction, personality, youth behavior, and peer, school, and neighborhood experiences.

Surveys were given to 771 students; however, our analyses are based on a restricted sample of 493 students (222 males and 271 females) for whom we have complete data on all questions used in our analyses. Table 2 shows descriptive statistics for both the full sample (n = 771) and the restricted sample (n = 493). The distributions for each variable are very similar in the samples indicating that missing data does not appear to have biased the restricted sample.

Model Specifications

To model the effects of family conflict and parenting behaviors on negative adolescent outcomes, we estimate the effects of four background factors and four family interaction measures on two youth outcomes: aggression and depression. We analyzed the possible items for all endogenous variables using factor analysis with Varimax rotation (SPSS 8.0). While most of the items loaded on factors that clearly represent the measures we employed, a few items loaded poorly and were excluded from the constructs. The constructs for each variable were also factor-analyzed separately, with consistent results. Further, factor loadings were obtained as part of the structural equation analysis using AMOS version 3.61 (Arbuckle, 1997). For each latent construct, the questions used and the factor loadings for each are noted in Table 1.

The first outcome we examine is aggression. Our outcome indicator of overtly aggressive behavior contains five items (alpha = .714) related to the destruction of property and fighting behaviors. Respondents choose whether such statements as "I attack people physically" and "I get involved in many fights" apply, somewhat apply, or do not apply to them (coded from 0 to 2). These items were taken from the Child-Behavior Checklist–Youth Self-Report (Achenbach & Edelbrock, 1987). A measure of aggression is one of the most basic ways to represent problem behaviors which are "acted out"–externalizing ways of dealing with emotions and stress.

As previously noted, parental conflict and certain parenting styles have been demonstrated to predict both externalizing and internalizing behavior problems. While internalizing reactions may include such problems as anxiety and eating disorders, we employ a measure of depression to represent this inward reaction to stress. A measure of depression was created from eight items: each offers three statements for respondents to choose from, such as "No one really loves me," "I'm not sure if anyone loves me," or "I am sure that someone loves me" (coded from 0 to 2). These items were selected from the 10-item Child Depression Inventory (CDI; Kovacs, 1992) on the basis of factor analysis (alpha = .778).

Four latent variables measuring parental conflict and parenting are included. Scales for overt parental conflict, covert parental conflict, maternal support, and maternal monitoring were determined through Varimax-rotated factor analysis of established items; items factoring low were omitted from the scales (Table 1). These parenting scales have also been studied in other national contexts, and the consistency of these measures has been documented cross-culturally (Barber, 1998). The measures of overt and covert parental conflict consist of seven items: three measures of overt conflict, and four of covert conflict (Buehler et al., 1998). The measure of overt conflict includes questions asking how often–never, sometimes, fairly often, or very often–the child's parents threaten, yell, or call each other names in front of the child (coded from 0 to 3).

Covert conflict is also measured with questions to which the children may respond that these situations never, sometimes, fairly often, or very often occur (coded from 0 to 2). These include questions asking how often a parent tries to get the child to take sides, how often one sends a message to the other through the child, how often the child feels trapped in the middle when parents fight, and how often the child feels divided between parents. Reliability values for overt and covert conflict are .646 and .722, respectively.

Maternal monitoring is indexed by five items (alpha = .748) asking if the mother really knows who the respondent's friends are, how he or she spends money and free time, and where she or he is after school and in the evening

TABLE 1. Survey Questions and Factor Analysis Results (AMOS 3.61) for Adolescent Perceptions of Parental Behavior and Adolescent Outcomes

Overt Conflict (alpha = .6459)		Covert Conflict (alpha = .7215)	
Parents threaten each other.	.831	Child feels trapped in middle of fights.	.660
Parents yell at each other.	.813	Child feels divided between parents.	.698
Parents call each other names.	.654	Parents try to get child to take sides.	.792
		Parents send messages through child.	.797
Maternal Support (alpha = .8604)		Maternal Monitoring (alpha = .7484)	
My mother is a person who . . .		Mother knows who your friends are.	.604
Makes me feel better after		Mother knows where you go at night.	.586
discussing my worries with her.	.623	Mother knows how you spend your money.	.601
Smiles at me often.	.623	Mother knows where you pass most of	
Enjoys doing things with me.	.716	your afternoons after school.	.653
Is a person who is easy to talk with.	.664	Mother knows what you do with your	
Is able to make me feel better		free time.	.620
when I'm angry.	.639		
Cheers me up when I'm sad.	.711		
Cares for me and gives me attention.	.583		
Often praises me.	.486		
Makes me feel like the most			
important person in her life.	.705		
Aggression (alpha = .7143)		Depression (alpha = .7781)	
I destroy my own things.	.436	I feel sad all the time.	.713
I get involved in many fights.	.634	Nothing goes well for me.	.460
I destroy other people's things.	.531	No one really loves me.	.572
I attack other people physically.	.708	I hate myself.	.403
I threaten to hurt people.	.600	I feel like crying every day.	.629
		Things irritate me all the time.	.464
		I see myself as ugly.	.439
		I feel lonely all the time.	.660
Socioeconomic Status (alpha = .568)			
Have fun like my friends.	.626		
Participate in school activities.	.659		
Pay school fees.	.700		
Buy food.	.700		

(Brown, Mounts, Lamborn, & Steinberg, 1993). Respondents state whether their mother knows a great deal, knows a little, or does not know these aspects of their lives (coded from 0 to 2). Maternal support includes nine items (alpha = .860) asking whether the mother is someone who helps the adolescent to feel better, laugh, be more enthused, or feel important. Thus, the instrument measures not what the mother actually *does*, but how the child perceives that the mother makes him or her *feel*. Measures of support are taken from the Acceptance subscale from the Child Report of Parent Behavior Inventory (CRPBI) (Schaefer, 1965; Schludermann & Schludermann, 1970). We substituted parallel measures of paternal support and monitoring to see if they had a different effect than those of the mother. While father's support seems to have a somewhat stronger effect on child aggression than does mother's support, differences are slight. Since there are substantially more missing cases for fathers than for mothers, we retained maternal measures in our analysis. Exogenous variables include dichotomous variables for gender and living with two parents versus other living arrangements. We expect that males will have higher rates of aggression, and that females will have higher rates of depression. The effects of simply being raised in a single-parent home are still under debate (Paschall et al., 1996); however, the frequency of both parental conflict and parenting practices will clearly be influenced by whether or not both parents live in the home.

Socioeconomic status is measured by four items ascertaining whether the respondent has sufficient money (yes or no) to (1) have fun like their friends do, (2) participate in school activities, (3) pay school fees, and (4) buy food. Because these four individual measures are only measured as a dichotomy, the alpha level of the socioeconomic combined measure summed across them is relatively low (alpha = .568). In initial analyses we also considered a measure of maternal education but it produced a weaker correlation with parental behavior and adolescent outcomes than the composite socioeconomic measure; therefore, only socioeconomic status is included. While low socioeconomic status has been linked to aggressive behavior in children (McNeilly-Choque et al., 1996), it is unclear whether this relationship is independent of socioeconomic differences in parenting styles or family structure.

A fourth exogenous variable, male dominance, represents the extent to which the mother's point of view is taken into consideration in the home. We include this as a global measure of authority relations in the home, realizing that it oversimplifies gender relations. We also note that actual gender relations are not measured, but instead, the adolescents' perception of such relations. However, we consider that the adolescents' perceptions are what will influence their own attitudes and behavior. Responses are grouped into one variable with three categories: (0) the mother's view has the same weight as the father's or "other"; (1) the mother's opinion receives less weight than the father's; and (2) the mother's opinion is not considered at all. The "other" category was one of the response options in the survey. Initial analyses indicated that adolescents checking the "other" category were most likely to live in one-parent households and to be similar to the "equal weight as father's" respondents on the dependent variables. We therefore included the "other" responses with "mother's view has same weight as father's" category (0). Although past studies of the relationship between authority relations in the family and parental and adolescent behaviors are few, we include a measure of male dominance in an effort to shed light on previous mixed results in the literature.

RESULTS

Statistical Procedures

The model to be estimated has two particular features that require estimation with structural equation modeling. First, several of the variables have multiple indicators. Second, correlations between the two adolescent outcomes are assumed to be large enough that failure to take these correlations into account would lead to biased estimates of structural relationships. We account for these relationships by allowing error terms for these outcomes to be correlated. By estimating the entire model, we can include both the measurement model for latent constructs and correlations among error terms. Linear structural equation analysis (AMOS 3.61; Arbuckle, 1997) is used to estimate the parameters of the model (the statistical program AMOS calculates results equal to those estimated by LISREL).

Descriptive Analysis

Descriptive statistics are presented in Table 2 (correlations are available from authors). Categories of variables are grouped to show major distinctions based on our more detailed examination of distributions. A large majority of the sample (89%) comes from two-parent homes including those living in stepfamilies or extended family. Those living in single-parent families are much more likely to be living with their mothers (90%) than with their fathers (6%).

A few of the adolescents report not having enough money for basic participation, but two-thirds report sufficient money for fun, school activities, and food. Two-thirds of the adolescents report that their parents' points of view have equal weight in their homes; the stereotype of male-dominant Latin American families fits only a minority of families among this sample. However, approximately 15% of the respondents note that their mother's point of view has less weight in their homes than does their father's. Ten percent of the adolescents report that their mother's point of view is not even considered when family decisions are made. A small percentage said "other" (10%). As noted previously, the "other" respondents are more likely to live in one-parent households and are most like the category "equal weight as father's" on the dependent variables. We thus combined these groups in multivariate analyses.

While parental conflict is hardly all-pervasive, a number of the respondents report that their parents engage in overt or covert conflict. The scales in Table 2 represent the frequency of conflictive behaviors between parents; the higher the number, the more conflict in the home. A more specific look at individual measures reveals that 71% of the children witness their parents yelling at each other at least once in a while, with 27% of them witnessing such conflict on a regular basis. Over half of all the teenagers report that, at times, they feel trapped in the middle during parental conflicts.

Perceptions of maternal support vary by respondent, but most of the teenagers report at least somewhat supportive relationships with their mothers (mean 13.2 on 18-point scale). For instance, three-fourths of the adolescents report that their mothers take care of them a great deal and give them much attention. These mothers tend to monitor their children's behavior as well (mean 7.4 on 10-point scale): over 90% of them are reported to know where their children spend their afternoons and evenings, and over 90% are reported to know who their children's friends are.

The adolescents' own reported actions and attitudes are revealing. When aggressive behaviors are scaled, the average score is quite low (1.2 on a scale from zero to ten). However, a fair amount of both boys and girls demonstrate aggressive traits: 31% of the males and 20% of the females report that the statement, "I get involved in many fights," applies to them. Also, 27% of the males and 14% of the females report that they attack people physically. Signs of depression emerge among some of the respondents, with females scoring higher on the scale than males. Twenty percent of the sample feels sad either often or always, and 45% of the teenagers feel alone either often or always. One-fourth of the respondents are not sure if anyone loves them. There are no notably large differences in the total sample and the restricted sample, implying that the restricted sample is not misrepresentative of the complete sample.

Structural Model

Results of the structural equation analysis are shown in Table 3. The restricted sample included 493 cases. Some of the hypothesized relationships between parental behavior and child outcomes prove not to be statistically significant in our study. In particular, neither overt nor covert conflict among parents is significantly associated with adolescent aggression (.205 and −.112, respectively). The direct association of overt conflict with children's depression is also not statistically significant (−.149). However, the relation of covert conflict

TABLE 2. Background Characteristics, Parenting Behaviors, and Child Outcomes for Colombian Adolescents (Percentages)

			Restricted Sample		
Background Characteristics		Total	Total	Male	Female
Socioeconomic Status:					
Low (0,1)		5	4	4	4
Mod low (2)		10	8	10	6
Mod high (3)		22	25	25	24
High (4)		62	63	61	66
Family Structure:					
Two-parent family		89	89	90	89
One-parent family		11	11	10	11
Male Dominance (Mother's Opinion):					
Equal weight as father's		64	66	66	66
Less weight than father's		14	15	18	13
Not considered at all		11	10	9	10
Other		11	10	8	11
Parenting Behaviors					
Overt Conflict:	Mean	1.82	1.91		
	(Stddev)	(1.85)	(1.89)		
Low (0-2)		73	72	78	67
High (3-6)		27	28	22	33
Covert Conflict:	Mean	2.63	2.62		
	(Stddev)	(2.62)	(2.56)		
Low (0-3)		71	71	77	66
Medium (4-7)		23	24	20	27
High (8-12)		6	5	3	7
Maternal Support:	Mean	13.2	13.2		
	(Stddev)	(4.1)	(4.2)		
Low (0-5)		6	6	5	7
Medium (6-11)		22	21	19	23
High (12-18)		72	73	76	70
Maternal Monitoring:	Mean	7.4	7.4		
	(Stddev)	(2.3)	(2.4)		
Low (0-3)		8	8	10	8
Medium (4-6)		22	22	28	17
High (7-10)		70	70	62	76
Child Outcomes					
Aggression:	Mean	1.2	1.2		
	(Stddev)	(1.8)	(1.7)		
Low (0-2)		81	82	79	85
Medium (3-6)		17	16	18	14
High (7-10)		2	2	3	1
Depression:	Mean	2.7	2.7		
	(Stddev)	(2.4)	(2.6)		
Low (0-4)		81	80	87	75
Medium (5-10)		18	18	12	23
High (11-16)		1	1	1	2
[N]		[771]	[493]	[222]	[271]

to children's depression is significant: as expected, the greater the covert conflict between parents, the more likely their children are to be depressed (.420).

As the direct effects of overt conflict on negative child outcomes are somewhat weak, so too are the indirect effects of overt parental conflict. Conflict between parents appears to reduce the mother's ability to monitor children's behavior ($-.263$, $p < .06$), which in turn is related to children's aggression ($-.292$, $p < .05$). Covert conflict is also somewhat associated with reduced levels of support ($-.186$), although this relationship is not statistically significant. Thus, there is some evidence to suggest that conflict between spouses reduces mothers' effectiveness as a parent. In turn, parenting measures are associated with the aggression and depression of the adolescents in the study. When mothers are supportive, their children are less likely to exhibit depressed traits ($-.341$). Further, when mothers keep tabs on their children, their teenagers are significantly less likely to engage in aggressive behaviors ($-.292$).

Consistent with our expectations, different types of parental conflict are associated with different types of adolescent problem behaviors. Overt conflict is positively associated with aggression whereas covert conflict is positively associated with depression. In fact, the effects of overt conflict on depression and covert conflict on aggression are small and negative. The total effect (direct and indirect) of covert conflict on aggression is $-.110$, and its total effect on depression is .479. The total effect of overt conflict on adolescent aggression is .300, and its total effect on depression is $-.129$.

The background characteristics of the teen's family (exogenous variables) influence both parenting behaviors and teen outcomes in various ways. Our measure of male dominance within the home proved influential. The more husbands control family decisions, the more overt (.132) and covert (.138) conflict there is likely to be in their marriages. And, as wives have less influence on decision-making, they are less likely to be supportive of their children ($-.127$). The higher the socioeconomic status of the family, the lower the levels of overt ($-.305$) and covert ($-.273$) conflict. In addition, higher socioeconomic status is linked to higher maternal support and monitoring. Thus, its effect on adolescent outcomes is indirect, working through decreased parental conflict and increased positive parenting. As with most studies, our analysis shows that males are somewhat more likely to engage in aggressive behaviors ($-.156$) than are females. Also as expected, females are more likely than males to be depressed (.137). Females also more often report that their mothers monitor their behavior (.179), which in turn predicts less aggression. It is perplexing to note that males and females report significantly different rates of overt and covert parental conflict in their homes (.194 and .196, respectively), with females reporting more conflict.

DISCUSSION

By including parental conflict and parenting behaviors in an end- to-end integrated model we had hoped to better understand the relation that family characteristics and parenting behaviors have with adolescent aggression and depression. Our findings suggest that overt parental conflict plays, at most, a modest role in adolescent aggression, but that covert conflict does increase depression. There is also very limited support for the hypothesis that the influence of conflict on aggression works indirectly via mother's monitoring. This

TABLE 3. Standardized Regression Coefficients from Structural Equation Analysis of Parental Conflict, Parenting Behaviors, and Background Factors Related to Aggression and Depression of Male and Female Adolescents in Colombia (n = 493)

Independent Variables		Parental Conflict, Parenting Behavior, and Adolescent Outcomes					
		Overt Conflict	Covert Conflict	Mother's Support	Mother's Monitoring	Aggression	Depression
Sex		.194*	.196*	−.040	.179*	−.156*	.137*
Socioeconomic Status		−.305*	−.273*	.237*	.220*	−.019	−.055
Family Structure		−.029	−.135	−.141*	−.116*	.020	.146*
Male Dominance		.132*	.138*	−.127*	−.081	−.013	−.071
Overt Conflict				−.041	−.263	.205	−.149
Covert Conflict				−.186	.067	−.112	.420*
Mother's Support						−.114	−.341*
Mother's Monitoring						−.292*	−.059
R-squared		.141	.140	.169	.158	.215	.364
Chi-square	1234.36						
(df)	738						
GFI	0.89						
RMR	0.017						
* = significant at .05 level							

result provides only weak support for the parenting perspective, i.e., overt conflict influences adolescent aggression indirectly by decreasing maternal monitoring. Nor do we find a direct effect between overt conflict and aggression, as would be suggested by the socialization perspective. In contrast, covert parental conflict seems to more directly influence depression, supporting Buehler and colleagues' (1998) conclusion that covert conflict is associated with internalized problems among adolescents–a finding which was not predicted by either the socialization or the parenting perspectives.

At least two explanations might be advanced for failure to find strong support for either of these models. First, a measurement in other cultures is problematic. Even with help from trained researchers and interviewers from the culture and reasonable psychometric scales, we cannot be certain we are measuring precisely the same constructs. Second, exposure to high levels of public violence may alter youth's perceptions of familial interaction. Adolescents in Bogotá see armed soldiers in the streets every day, and the news is replete with stories of executions, assassinations, and murders. This greater exposure may dampen the impact of domestic conflict.

Failure to find strong support for either model does not mean that results are trivial. We do find specialized effects for types of conflict when we distinguish between overt and covert. For instance, when conflict measures are combined into one global measure of parental conflict, the perceived direct association of conflict with depression is significant. Since this effect is due primarily to covert conflict, the influence of overt conflict is overestimated when overt and covert conflict are not measured separately. Similarly, a global measure of parental conflict appears to have a much greater association with maternal support and maternal monitoring than the low association indicated by separating the two types of conflict. These findings highlight the importance of clearly specifying the types of marital conflict in future research (as indicated by Buehler et al., 1998).

In addition to documenting the influence of parenting practices on aggression and depression, our analysis reveals gender differences with males being more aggressive and females scoring higher on depression. Our measures of aggression, however, are limited to questions about hitting and destroying things, which are more likely to be reported by males than females. In contrast other studies suggest that females are more likely to express aggression in terms of relationships–that is creating jealousy or undermining relationships (McNeilly-Choque et al., 1996). Thus, more detailed measures of conflict would likely clarify gender differences in our analyses. The inclusion of experienced family violence in addition to witnessed family violence may also yield more refined results. Further, separate variations of overt aggression may fruitfully be examined: instrumental, in which physical hostility is oriented toward the purpose of obtaining an object or privilege; and bullying, in which aggression is employed with the intent of intimidating a victim (McNeilly-Choque et al., 1996).

We note that our findings regarding the relationship between parental conflict, parenting, and teen outcomes are tentative given some of the limitations of our data. Our survey of parental conflict and parenting behaviors are only from the perspective of the adolescent; responses from parents would likely further define these relationships. In addition, our data are cross-sectional as opposed to longitudinal and the generalizability of our results is uncertain. We are unable to distinguish the causal ordering between parental behaviors and adolescent outcomes. It may be that in some cases adolescent aggression or depression influences parental monitoring or support.

Despite these limitations, our results do shed light on adolescent aggressive behaviors and depression. Although factors such as broader political and economic trends contribute to societal trends in violence, the specific interactions and conflicts occurring within families may also help explain the aggression of individuals in Colombia. As Colombian researcher Uribe (1995:361, translation authors) explains,

> Today we understand with greater clarity that these multiple violences transcend the subjective and individual space, since in many ways they form the invisible fabric that sustains the other violences that scourge our country.

Perhaps the greatest contribution of this study, however, is its focus on a context outside of the United States. The expected findings of a relation between covert conflict and depression, and between parenting and negative child outcomes, show how standard findings based on a United States sample may or may not generalize to a very different culture. As the frequency of either parental conflict or adolescent aggression may vary across cultures (as comparative researchers such as Levinson [1989] suggest), so may the relations between parenting, aggression, and depression.

REFERENCES

Achenbach, T. M. & Edelbrock, C. (1987). *Manual for the youth self-report and profile*. Burlington, VT: University of Vermont, Department of Psychiatry.

Arbuckle, J. L. (1997). AMOS 3.61 [Computer software]. Chicago, IL: SPSS, Inc.

Balswick, J. O. & Macrides, C. (1975). Parental stimulus for adolescent rebellion. *Adolescence, 10,* 253-266.

Bandura, A. (1973). *Aggression: A social learning analysis.* Englewood Cliffs, NJ: Prentice Hall.

Barber, B. K. (1992). Family, personality, and adolescent problem behaviors. *Journal of Marriage and the Family, 54,* 69-79.

Barber, B. K. (1996). Parental psychological control: Revisiting a neglected construct. *Child Development, 67,* 3296-3319.

Barber, B. K. (1998). A multi-national model of parent-adolescent relations. Paper 5 presented at the International Society for the Study of Behavioral Development, Berne, Switzerland.

Barber, B. K. (1999). Political violence, family relations, and Palestinian child functioning. *Journal of Adolescent Research, 14,* 206-230.

Barber, B. K., Olsen, J. E., & Shagle, S. C. (1994). Associations between parental psychological and behavioral control and youth internalized and externalized behavior. *Child Development, 65,* 1120-1136.

Bjorkqvist, K. & Osterman, K. (1992). Parental influence on children's self-estimated aggressiveness. *Aggressive Behavior, 18,* 411-423.

Bouley, E. E. & Vaughn, M. S. (1995). Violent crime and modernization in Colombia. *Crime, Law & Social Change, 23,* 17-40.

Brown, B. B., Mounts, N., Lamborn, S. D., & Steinberg, L. (1993). Parenting practices and peer group affiliation in adolescence. *Child Development, 63,* 391-400.

Buehler, C., Krishnakumar, A., Stone, G., Anthony, C., Pemberton, S., Gerard, J., & Barber, B. (1998). Interparental conflict styles and youth problem behaviors: A two-sample replication study. *Journal of Marriage and the Family, 60,* 119-132.

Carroll, J. C. (1977). The intergenerational transmission of family violence: The long term effects of aggressive behavior. *Aggressive Behavior, 3,* 289-299.

Egeland, B. (1993). A history of abuse is a major risk factor for abusing the next generation. In R. J. Gelles & D. R. Loseke (Eds.), *Current controversies on family violence* (pp. 197-208). Newbury Park, CA: Sage.

Elliott, D. S. (1985). The assumption that theories can be combined with increased explanatory power: Theoretical integrations. In R. F. Meier (Ed.), *Theoretical methods in criminology* (pp.123-149). Beverly Hills, CA: Sage Publications.

Emery, R. E. (1982). Interparental conflict and the children of discord and divorce. *Psychological Bulletin, 92,* 310-330.

Emery, R. E. (1989). Family violence. *American Psychologist, 64,* 321-328.

Erel, O. & Burman, B. (1995). Interrelatedness of marital relations and parent-child relations: A meta-analytic review. *Psychological Bulletin, 118,* 108-132.

Fagan, J. A., Stewart, D. K., & Hansen, K. V. (1983). Violent men or violent husbands? Background factors and situational correlates. In D. Finkelhor, R. J. Gelles, G. T. Hotaling, & M. A. Straus (Eds.), *The dark side of families: Current family violence research* (pp. 48-67). Beverly Hills, CA: Sage.

Fauber, R. L., Forehand, R., Thomas, A. M., & Wierson, M. (1990). A mediational model of the impact of marital conflict on adolescent adjustment in intact and divorced families: The role of disrupted parenting. *Child Development, 61,* 1112-1123.

Fauber, R. L. & Long, N. (1991). Children in context: The role of the family in child psychotherapy. *Journal of Consulting and Clinical Psychology, 59,* 813-820.

Fincham, F. D., Grych, J. H., & Osborne, L. N. (1994). Does marital conflict cause child maladjustment? Directions and challenges for longitudinal research. *Journal of Family Psychology, 8,* 128-140.

Fontes, L. A. (1997). Conducting ethical cross-cultural research on family violence. In G. Kaufman Kantor & J. L. Jasinski (Eds.), *Out of the darkness: Contemporary perspectives on family violence* (pp. 296-312). Thousand Oaks, CA: Sage Publications.

Foshee, V. A., Bauman, K. E., & Linder, G. F. (1999). Family violence and the perpetration of adolescent dating violence: Examining social learning and social control processes. *Journal of Marriage and the Family, 61,* 331-342.

Garber, J., Robinson, N. S., & Valentiner, D. (1997). The relation between parenting and adolescent depression: Self-worth as a mediator. *Journal of Adolescent Research, 12,* 12-33.

Gelles, R. J. (1989). Child abuse and violence in single-parent families: Parent absence and economic deprivation. *American Journal of Orthopsychiatry, 59,* 492-501.

Gelles, R. J. & Cornell, C. P. (1990). *Intimate violence in families.* Newbury Park, CA: Sage.

Gerard, J. M. & Buehler, C. (1999). Multiple risk factors in the family environment and youth problem behaviors. *Journal of Marriage and the Family, 61,* 343-361.

Hart, C. H., Nelson, D., Robinson, C., Olsen, S., & McNeilly-Choque, M. (1998). Overt and relational aggression in Russian nursery-school-age children: Parenting style and marital linkages. *Developmental Psychology, 34,* 687-697.

Hotaling, G. R., Straus, M. A., & Lincoln, A. J. (1990). Intrafamily violence and crime and violence outside the family. In M. A. Straus (Ed.), *Physical violence in American families: Risk factors and adaptations to violence in 8,145 families* (pp. 431-470). New Brunswick, NJ: Transaction Publishers.

Huesmann, L. R., Maxwell, C. D., Eron, L. D., Dahlberg, L. L., Guerra, N. G., Toler, P. H., VanAcker, R., & Henry, D. (1996). Evaluating a cognitive/ecological program for the prevention of aggression among urban children. *American Journal of Preventive Medicine, 12 (supplement),* 120-128.

Jouriles, E. N., Pfiffner, L. J., & O'Leary, K. D. (1988). Marital conflict, parenting, and toddler conduct problems. *Journal of Abnormal Child Psychology, 16,* 197-206.

Kalmuss, D. (1984). The intergenerational transmission of marital aggression. *Journal of Marriage and the Family, 46,* 11-19.

Kaufman, J. & Zigler, E. (1993). The intergenerational transmission of abuse is overstated. In R. J. Gelles & D. R. Loseke (Eds.), *Current controversies on family violence* (pp. 209-221). Newbury Park, CA: Sage Publications.

Kimmel, D. C., & Weiner, I. B. (1985). *Adolescence: A developmental transition.* Hillsdale, NJ: Lawrence Erlbaum Associates.

Kovacs, M. (1992). *Children's depression inventory.* Niagara Falls, NY: Multi-Health Systems.

Langhinrichsen-Rohling, J. & Neidig, P. (1995). Violent backgrounds of economically disadvantaged youth: Risk factors for perpetrating violence? *Journal of Family Violence, 10,* 379-397.

Levinson, D. (1989). *Family violence in cross-cultural perspective.* Newbury Park, CA: Sage.

Lindahl, K. M. & Malik, N. M. (1997). Observations of marital conflict and power: Relations with parenting in the triad. *Journal of Marriage and the Family, 61,* 320-330.

Liska, A. E., Krohn, M. D., & Messner, S. F. (1989). Strategies and requisites for theoretical integration in the study of crime and deviance. In S. F. Messner, M. D. Krohn, & A. E. Liska (Eds.), *Theoretical integration in the study of deviance and crime: Problems and prospects* (pp. 1-19). Albany: State University of New York Press.

MacEwen, K. E. (1994). Refining the intergenerational transmission hypothesis. *Journal of Interpersonal Violence, 9,* 350-365.

Mangold, W. D. & Koski, P. R. (1990). Gender comparisons in the relationship between parental and sibling violence and nonfamily violence. *Journal of Family Violence, 5,* 225-235.

Margolin, G. & John, R. S. (1997). Children's exposure to marital aggression: Direct and mediated effects. In G. Kaufman Kantor & J. L. Jasinski (Eds.), *Out of the darkness: Contemporary perspectives on family violence* (pp. 90-104). Thousand Oaks, CA: Sage Publications.

McHale, J. P. (1995). Co-parenting and triadic interactions during infancy: The roles of marital distress and child gender. *Developmental Psychology, 31,* 985-996.

McNeilly-Choque, M. K., Hart, C. H., Robinson, C. C., Nelson, L. J., & Olsen, S. F. (1996). Overt and relational aggression on the playground: Correspondence among different informants. *Journal of Research in Childhood Education, 11,* 47-67.

Miller, S. L. & Wellford, C. F. (1997). Patterns and correlates of interpersonal violence. In A. P. Cardarelli (Ed.), *Violence between intimate partners: Patterns, causes, and effects* (pp. 16-28). Boston: Allyn and Bacon.

Mirande, A. (1998). *Hombres y machos: Masculinity and Latino culture.* Boulder, CO: Westview Press.

Moore, A. M. (1997). Intimate violence: Does socioeconomic status matter? In A. P. Cardarelli (Ed.), *Violence between intimate partners: Patterns, causes, and effects* (pp. 90-100). Boston: Allyn and Bacon.

O'Keefe, M. (1996). The differential effects of family violence on adolescent adjustment. *Child and Adolescent Social Work Journal, 13,* 51-68.

O'Leary, K. D. (1988). Physical aggression between spouses: A social learning theory perspective. In V. B. Van Hasselt, R. L. Morrison, A. S. Bellack, & M. Hersen (Eds.), *Handbook of family violence* (pp. 31-48). New York: Plenum.

Oropesa, R. S. (1997). Development and marital power in Mexico. *Social Forces, 75,* 1291-1317.

Pagelow, M. D. (1981). *Woman-battering: Victims and their experiences.* Beverly Hills, CA: Sage.

Paschall, M. J., Ennett, S. T., & Flewelling, R. L. (1996). Relationships among family characteristics and violent behavior by black and white male adolescents. *Journal of Youth and Adolescence, 25,* 177-197.

Patterson, G. R., Reid, J. B., & Dishion, T. J. (1992). *Antisocial boys.* Eugene, OR: Castalia.

Patterson, G. R. & Stouthamer-Loeber, M. (1984). The correlation of family management practices and delinquency. *Child Development, 55,* 1299-1307.

Prado, E., Singh, S., & Wulf, D. (1988). *Adolescentes de hoy, padres del manana: Colombia. [Today's adolescents, tomorrow's parents: Colombia]*. New York: The Alan Guttmacher Institute.

Profamilia. (1991). *Encuesta de Prevalencia, Demografia y Salud, 1990, Colombia. [Demographic and Health Survey, 1990, Colombia]*. Bogota, Colombia: Asociacion Pro-Bienestar de la Familia Colombiana, and Columbia, Maryland, USA: Institute for Resource Development/Macro International.

Schaefer, E. S. (1965). A configurational analysis of children's reports of parent behavior. *Journal of Consulting Psychology, 29,* 552-557.

Schludermann, E. & Schludermann, S. (1970). Replicability of factors in children's report of parent behavior (CRPBI). *Journal of Psychology, 76,* 239-249.

Shagle, S. & Barber, B. K. (1993). Effects of family, marital, and parent-child conflict on adolescent self-derogation and suicidal ideation. *Journal of Marriage and the Family, 55,* 964-974.

Simons, R. L., Ling, K., & Gordon, L. C. (1998). Socialization in the family of origin and male dating violence: A prospective study. *Journal of Marriage and the Family, 60,* 467-478.

Simons, R. L., Wu, C., Conger, R. D., & Lorenz, F. O. (1994). Two routes to delinquency: Differences between early and late starters in the impact of parenting and deviant peers. *Criminology, 32,* 247-276.

Straus, M. A. (2001). *Beating the devil out of them*. New Brunswick, NJ: Transaction.

Uribe, M. L. (1995). Mujeres y violencia: Una historia que no termina [Women and violence: A history that doesn't end]. In M. V. Toro, C. Cardenas & P. Jimenez (Eds.), *Las mujeres en la historia de Colombia* (pp. 403-420). Santa Fe de Bogot, Colombia: Editorial Presencia.

Vélez, A. L. (1989). Poder y democracia en la familia [Power and democracy in the family]. In C. Mejia de Restrepo (Ed.), *Familia y cambio en Colombia* (pp. 175-180). Medellin, Colombia: Editorial Lito-dos.

Vélez, A. L. (1995). Las mujeres y la salud [Women and health]. In M. V. Toro, C. Cardenas, & P. Jimenez (Eds.), *Las mujeres en la historia de Colombia* (pp. 403-420). Santa Fe de Bogot, Colombia: Editorial Presencia.

Wagner, D. & Berger, J. (1985). Do sociological theories grow? *American Journal of Sociology, 90,* 697-728.

Zaidi, L. Y., Knutson, J. F., & Mehm, J. G. (1989). Transgenerational patterns of abusive parenting. *Aggressive Behavior, 15,* 137-152.

Chinese Adolescents' Decision-Making, Parent-Adolescent Communication and Relationships

Yan R. Xia
Xiaolin Xie
Zhi Zhou
John DeFrain
William H. Meredith
Raedene Combs

ABSTRACT. The present study described Mainland Chinese adolescents' decision-making, and examined the relationship among their decision-making involvement, parent-adolescent communication and relationship variables by using Structural Equation Modeling. Results demonstrated that Chinese parents appeared to be less authoritarian than the prevailing literature had described. Chinese adolescents experienced a passage of autonomy development similar to that of their American counterparts. Good parent-adolescent communication was positively associated with cohesion and negatively associated with conflict. It also mediated the relationship between adolescent age and parent-adolescent conflict. The

Yan R. Xia is affiliated with the University of Nebraska-Lincoln. Xiaolin Xie is affiliated with Northern Illinois University. Zhi Zhou is affiliated with First Data Corporation. John DeFrain is affiliated with the University of Nebraska-Lincoln. William H. Meredith is affiliated with Kansas State University. Raedene Combs is affiliated with the University of Nebraska-Lincoln.

Address correspondence to: Yan R. Xia, Family and Consumer Sciences, University of Nebraska-Lincoln (Omaha campus), 105c Ash 60th & Dodge, Omaha, NE 68128-0214.

This paper is a contribution of the University of Nebraska Agricultural Research Division, Lincoln, NE 68583, Journal Series No. 13993.

http://www.haworthpress.com/web/MFR
© 2004 by The Haworth Press, Inc. All rights reserved.
Digital Object Identifier: 10.1300/J002v36n01_06

287

relationships between parent-adolescent communication and cohesion as well as the relationship between adolescents' age and decision involvement were significantly different for boys and girls. *[Article copies available for a fee from The Haworth Document Delivery Service: 1-800-HAWORTH. E-mail address: <docdelivery@haworthpress.com> Website: <http://www.HaworthPress.com>* © *2004 by The Haworth Press, Inc. All rights reserved.]*

KEYWORDS. Chinese adolescents, decision-making, parent-adolescent communication, parent-adolescent relationships

INTRODUCTION

China has the world's largest youth population, but little is known about Chinese adolescents' involvement in decision-making in the family, the strength of parent-child relationships, and parent-adolescent communication. Chinese tradition places value on children's obedience to their parents (Ho, Sprinks, & Yeung, 1989), with young people being discouraged from disagreeing and negotiating with their parents. Compared to Western societies, less emphasis is believed to be placed on the development of individual autonomy as a central task in adolescence.

With rapid economic development in China in the last two decades, however, this tradition has faced considerable challenge (Yau & Smetana, 1996). In addition, the endorsement of the One Child Family Policy is believed to have influenced the manner in which parents raise their children (Xia, Lin, Xie, Zhou, & DeFrain, 1998). This study is an effort to delineate current Chinese adolescent participation in the decision-making processes, and how this relates to parent-adolescent communication and adolescents' perceptions of their relationships with parents. The present study is unique in that it focuses on Mainland Chinese adolescents and uses decision-making processes as a key aspect of family interaction to examine associations among adolescents' decision-making, communication, and relationship.

THEORETICAL PERSPECTIVE

This study uses family systems theory and the ecological perspective as its theoretical framework. Adolescents grow through constant interactions with the family and the larger social systems. The implication of family systems theory for this study is to focus not only on the individuals that compose families but also on the patterns and interactions of family members. The ecological perspective (Bronfenbrenner & Morris, 1998) provides a framework that allows examination of associations among adolescents' decision-making, parent-adolescent communication, and larger social contexts. The contexts include the familial, societal, and global environment, as well as the changes in these social environments due to their interaction and mutual influences. Studies of contemporary families that embrace a broad, multicultural perspective (Smith & Ingoldsby, 1992) enable us to understand Chinese adolescents and their family relations that may well be affected by the outside changing world.

LITERATURE REVIEW

Family and Adolescents' Decision-Making

When family members make decisions, they operate within a shared system that governs the boundaries, role expectations, and the ways that they should interact with each other (Reiss, 1981). Family decision-making processes can be influenced by each member's role in the family, by their goals, values, and beliefs. Decision-making can be seen as a process of solving problems that result from the conflicts in obligation, expectation, and beliefs among family members. Decision-making in such a context needs to deal with the problem through integrating formerly opposed responsibilities and feelings, and modifying or transforming the relationships among the decision-makers (Diesing, 1962). Dornbusch, Ritter, Mont-Reynaund, and Chen (1990) found, in their study, that parents and adolescents might have different views of their roles in decision-making. Rettig noted, "These processes are often intensely emotional because of value and standard conflicts" (Rettig, 1993, p. 196).

Teenage children were found to have the greatest influence on deciding whether to buy the things that directly affected themselves, less on decisions about family vacations, and little on any other family matters (Belch, Geresino, & Belch, 1985). Adolescents were expected to have more input as they grow older.

How much responsibility an adolescent can assume in decision-making is an indicator of parental recognition of the adolescent's competence, especially in decision-making and problem-solving. Involving adolescents in making decisions is viewed as a critical component that is indicative of how adolescents are parented, with the family decision-making style being reflective of the parenting style used. It is often assumed, for example, that authoritarian parents often grant their children little freedom for making decisions on their own, whereas permissive parents may grant children excessive autonomy without proper monitoring (Baumrind, 1967).

Past literature provides support for these assumptions. Adolescent involvement in decision-making processes was found to be associated with outcome behaviors. One study showed that violent adolescent children did not have as much input in decision-making processes as did normal functioning adolescents, after controlling for the influences of external family structure, e.g., divorce, desertion, family size, and so forth (Harbin & Madden, 1983). However, excessive involvement in decision-making may not necessarily produce positive outcomes, especially for early adolescents. Individual autonomy in decision-making at too early an age was associated with low effort by adolescents in school and low school achievement. Lack of parental supervision and involvement in the younger youth's decision-making did not prompt them to excel at school (Dornbusch et al., 1990).

Parent-Adolescent Relationships

Studies of parent-child relationships during the adolescent period repeatedly show that the transition into adolescence accompanies some levels of tension between parents and their children, and disruption in the family (Collins & Russell, 1991; Fuligni, 1998; Paikoff & Brooks-Gunn, 1991). Parent-child conflict and emotional distancing are perceived predominantly as a function of the development of the adolescent's autonomy. Adolescents redefine their roles in decision-making that used to be their parents' domain, and seek an equalitarian parent-child relationship. The growing sense of autonomy and independence prompts adolescents to exercise more control over their activities, and to be more critical of their parents' values and beliefs. Conflicts occur when parents are reluctant to accommodate the change, and when there is not an agreement in role expectations between parents and children (Smetana, 1988). The level of conflict between parents and adolescents decreases after early or middle adolescence (Laursen & Collins, 1994). A reasonable degree of independence and supportive parent-child relationship are seen to be the healthiest to adolescent development (Grotevant & Cooper, 1985). Troubled relationships are reported more likely to occur between adjudicated adolescents and their parents (Smith & Kerpelman, 2002).

The fact that conflict is often seen as a synonym for adolescence does not suggest that conflict only has negative implications for adolescent growth (Collins & Laursen, 1992; Paikoff & Brooks-Gunn, 1991; Peterson, Wilson, Bush, & Zhao, 2002; Steinberg, 1990). Psychoanalytic theorists believe that conflict encourages individuation; developmental psychologists assert that conflict redefines interpersonal roles; and social exchange theorists suggest that conflict provides a context for monitoring the relationship between rewards and costs. They all believe conflict is important in fostering development (Laursen & Koplas, 1995).

Parent-Adolescent Communication and Interaction

Good parent-adolescent relationships can hardly be sustained without open and healthy communication between parents and adolescent children. Parent-adolescent communication plays an essential role in family functioning throughout adolescence (Collins, 1990; Gecas & Seff, 1990; Noller, 1994; Scabini, 1995; Sroufe, 1991; Youniss & Smollar, 1985). Communication among family members is one of the most crucial facets of interpersonal relationships and the key to understanding the dynamics underlying family relations (Clark & Shields, 1997). Within the family system, family members constantly define and adjust their relationships through patterns of communication (Watzlawick, Beavin, & Johnson, 1967). Understanding communication patterns makes it possible to better understand cohesion, decision-making processes, and family rules and role expectations (Clark & Shields, 1997).

Families with a good communication style help the adolescent develop a clearer sense of self (Barnes & Olson, 1985). Effective communication at home helps clarify the role of adolescents within families and helps them develop the skill of empathy so that their personal identity effectively balances feelings of both individuality and connectedness (Grotevant & Cooper, 1985). Good communication improves adolescents' social skills that are positively correlated with self-esteem, well-being, coping, and social support (Bijstra, Bosma, & Jackson, 1994). Adequate communication between parents and adolescents (being able to freely express opinions and feelings) can effectively mediate the stress that adolescents experience. They will be less likely to feel lonely and suffocated in the external world when they know they are encouraged, supported, and always have somebody to count on at home (Marta, 1997).

Communication facilitates the process of family cohesion and adaptability development. Good communication between parents and adolescent children leads to closer family relationships and helps them to be more loving and flexible in solving family problems (Barnes & Olson, 1985). Open communication with parents has a strong positive correlation with family satisfaction (Jackson, Bijstra, Oostra, & Bosma, 1998).

Chinese Parent-Adolescent Communication and Relationships

In traditional Chinese culture, nonconfrontational communication among people is valued in order to prevent them from losing face or dignity (Hong,

1989). Nonconfrontational communication refers to expressing one's thoughts and feelings in an indirect, and implicit manner, particularly when people disagree. This pattern of communication is evident among family members, not only to preserve an individual's dignity, but also to protect family harmony and family ties. Children are obligated to obey their parents and take care of them when the parents get old (filial piety), as their parents are obligated to nurture and raise them while the children grow up.

Most of the studies on current Chinese parent-adolescent relationships have been conducted in Hong Kong. Yau and Smetana (1996) examined adolescent-parent conflict in Hong Kong families of lower economic status. They reported that moderate conflicts were observed primarily between adolescents and mothers over daily issues of family life. Hong Kong adolescents wanted more independence in decision-making than the parents granted them. They perceived fathers as relatively less demanding, less concerned, more restrictive, and harsher than mothers, and adolescent girls perceived mothers as more demanding but less harsh (Shek, 1998; 1995). Hong Kong parents were perceived as moderately warm and relatively controlling. Other studies in Hong Kong showed that better relationships with parents were linked to higher self-concepts, better school performance, social skills, and physical ability, while poorer relationships with parents were reported to relate to more misconduct and delinquency, as well as more psychological symptoms (Lau & Leung, 1992; Shek, 1997).

In comparison with Australian and American youth, Chinese adolescents in Hong Kong had expectations for independence at a later age, and put less emphasis on individualism (Feldman & Rosenthal, 1991). However, a similar pattern of association with family environment was identified across the three groups. Expectations for later autonomy were related to adolescents' perceptions of parental monitoring, a demanding family environment, and authoritarian parents. Fuligni (1998) reported in his comparative study that Chinese American youth had later expectations for autonomy, and girls showed later expectations than boys across all ethnic groups, including Caucasian.

In studies conducted in China, Taiwan, and the U.S., researchers found that Chinese and Chinese-American parents appeared to be controlling, to encourage independence, and to emphasize achievement (Lin & Fu, 1990; Peterson et al., 2002). These findings seemed contradictory to the prevailing literature about Chinese parents' views of children's autonomy development. To explain their findings, Lin and Fu pointed out, "A distinction should be made between family interdependence and individual independence. Although Chinese people tend to value interdependence and minimize the development of individuality within families, individual independence is not necessarily discouraged" (Xu, Shen, Wan, Li, Mussen, & Cao, 1991, p. 432).

Traditional Chinese Family Values

Confucianism is the dominant philosophy that influences Chinese family values. Confucianism emphasizes social and family harmony, and family hierarchy (Ho, 1981; Hsu, 1985). The only way to achieve social harmony is to achieve family harmony by respecting family authority, namely, by conforming to and obeying people in authority. Chinese families are described as highly cohesive, partially due to a high cultural emphasis on harmony and mutual obligations and low value on overt expression of affection and disapproval. The families tend to suppress conflicts because obedience and respect for elders are valued (Liang, 1974). Even though China is undergoing rapid social change and westernization, filial piety remains one of the most important moral standards that guide the behaviors of family members and regulates the relationship between parents and older children (Goodwin & Tang, 1996).

Few studies on adolescents' decision-making and parent-adolescent communication have focused on Chinese families in Mainland China. Research on the parent-adolescent relationship in a Chinese cultural context has been conducted in Chinese families in Hong Kong and Chinese-American families in the United States. Research is needed to understand the relationship between parents and adolescents in Mainland China.

Besides, Chinese families have been traditionally characterized as emphasizing absolute parental authority and valuing collective interest more than individual autonomy. Does this characterization of Chinese families still remain a fairly accurate picture of the current families on the mainland? If parent-adolescent relationships (i.e., cohesion and conflict) were a function of autonomy development, would it occur within Chinese families in which children are expected to obey their parents? If Chinese parent-adolescent communication were still marked by indirectness, would open communication exert an impact on the adolescents' relationships with their parents? This study was aimed at addressing the first question through describing how much Chinese adolescents were involved in decision-making processes, and the latter two questions through testing a theoretical model.

METHODOLOGY

Sample

Participants were students from the seventh to twelfth grade in two metropolitan high schools, and freshmen at a state university in Baoding, Hebei, P.R. China. Baoding is a middle-sized city by Chinese standards, with a population close to one million. It is approximately one hundred miles to the south of Beijing. The economic reform that began in 1978 has significantly improved living conditions. The city has a history dating back more than 2,300 years. Baoding residents are known for their longevity. The average life expectancy of 77.8 is 6.4 years longer than the nation's average lifespan in 2000 (Embassy of P.R. China in the U.S., 2002). Three schools in Baoding were contacted, and two schools agreed to participate.

All the enrolled students at the two high schools were invited to participate in the study. Eighth and ninth graders at one school were on a field trip and could not participate. The remaining students completed self-report questionnaires administered to them in class in the spring of 2000. A total of 660 students returned the questionnaire, and the response rate was 94%. The questionnaires were also distributed at an English language class to college freshmen in the departments of biology and economics; 143 of these students responded, representing about 90% of first-year students in these two departments. In total, 803 students returned questionnaires, and 768 of these were regarded as valid for the study. The percentage of missing data is below 4%.

Sixty-four percent of the participants were female and 34.2% were male. Their ages ranged from 12 to 19 with a mean of 16.19 and standard deviation of 2.48. Among the total 768 adolescents, 83% came from nuclear families, 7.6% from extended families, 3.5% from single-parent families, 1% from stepfamilies, and 4.8% were living apart from their parents. Nearly 59% were the only children in the family, 33.7% had one sibling, and about 7.7% had two siblings. It is not clear why the only children accounted for only 59% of the total participants who were all born after the One Child Family Planning Policy was implemented in 1979. The first possible explanation could be that the policy was not strictly reinforced, in particular, in rural areas. One of the participating schools was a vocational school, which had some students from the families in the rural areas. Chinese farmers do not have pensions and usually rely on their children financially and physically in their old age. Because of that, the amendment to the One Child Family Planning Policy permits farmer families who have a daughter to petition to have another child. Second, the One Child Policy stipulates that minority families, and families with a disabled or chronically ill child could have more than one child.

Regarding parents' education, 53.8% of the mothers and 54.8% of the fathers of the adolescent participants had a high-school diploma. Fathers had a higher percentage of degrees than did mothers across all levels of education, but the discrepancy was not large. Fifteen percent of the fathers did not finish high school, while a little over 23% of the mothers did not finish high school. Overall, about 26% of the fathers had received an associate or higher degree, while 20% of the mothers had the same level of education.

Measures

Adolescent's Involvement in Decision-Making. Chinese adolescents' perceptions of their involvement in decision-making were measured by a self-report questionnaire developed by the researcher for this study. It consisted of 11 areas of decision-making on issues relevant to adolescents in the age range studied (e.g., hair style, clothes style, making friends, dating, curfew time, spending allowance, leisure activities, time of doing homework, going to college or not, choosing college major). The participants were asked to indicate who made most of the decisions (e.g., mother, father, yourself, all together). The raw score for adolescent's involvement in decision-making was computed by summing all the areas to which the adolescents perceived that they contributed most in making decisions. Then the raw score was weighted on the total number of the decisions relevant to adolescents.

Parent-Adolescent Communication. The Parent-Adolescent Communication Scale was used to assess Chinese parent-adolescent communication (Olson, McCubbin, Barnes, Larsen, Muxen, & Wilson, 1992). Each adolescent was asked to complete both The Adolescent and Mother Form and The Adolescent and Father Form of the Parent-Adolescent Communication Scale. The instrument is a 5-point Likert-type scale, and consists of 20 items of which 10 items measure each of two subscales (i.e., Open and Problems communication). The Open communication subscale includes items such as "I find it easy to discuss problems with my mother/father," "My mother/father is always a good listener," "If I were in trouble I could tell my mother/father," "My mother/father can tell how I'm feeling without asking." The Problems communication subscale includes items such as "My mother/father has a tendency to say things to me which would be better left unsaid," "When we are having problems, I often give my mother/father the silent treatment," "I am sometimes afraid to ask my mother/father for what I want," "I'm careful about what I say to my mother/father" (Olson et al., 1992). The greater value of the raw scores indicates a higher degree of openness and more problems. For the current study, the two indicators for parent-adolescent communication factor are the total scores of each subscale. Prior to data analysis, raw scores on the Problems subscale are recoded with the greater value indicating fewer problems. Scores of both mother-adolescent and father-adolescent communication reported by the adolescent child were obtained for each adolescent.

The Parent-Adolescent Communication Scale demonstrates some construct validity when applied in different cultural contexts (Conoley, 1995). The internal consistency (Cronbach's Alpha) is .87 for the Openness subscale, .78 for the Problems subscale, and .88 for the total scale. The correlation (r) of test-retest is .78. The Cronbach's Alphas for these three scales with the present

Chinese sample were .84, .72, and .84 for mothers, .88, .76, and .87 for fathers, and .84, .72, and .84 for the total sample, respectively.

Parent-Adolescent Relationship

The Chinese parent-adolescent relationship scale consisted of two subscales: cohesion and conflict. The 10-item cohesion subscale of the Family Adaptability and Cohesion Evaluation Scales (FACES II) was used to assess parent-adolescent cohesion, and the 5-item accord/conflict subscale of The Family Strengths Scale was used to assess parent-adolescent conflict (Olson et al., 1992). After an initial Confirmatory Factor Analysis with cohesion and conflict as latent variables, six indicators on the parent-adolescent relationship scale with factor loadings below .40 were dropped off. Five indicators for cohesion and four indicators for conflict were retained. The five cohesion indicators included supporting each other during difficult times, doing things together, feeling very close to each other, going along with what the family decided to do, and liking to spend free time together. The four conflict indicators included many conflicts, difficulty of accomplishing things, inability to solve the problem, and being critical of each other. The greater value of cohesion indicated higher cohesion, and the greater value of conflict indicated more conflicts. Cronbach's alphas for Cohesion, Adaptability, and Total Scale are .87, .78, and .90 for FACES II (Olson et al., 1992). FACES II is also reported having a correlation with other instruments measuring constructs similar to cohesion and adaptability (Hampson, Hulgus, & Beavers, 1991). The Cronbach's Alphas with the present Chinese sample are .69 (cohesion), .68 (conflict), and .76 (total). The low internal consistency is acceptable as this study is exploratory.

DEMOGRAPHIC INFORMATION

Demographic information included family structure, parents' gender and education, and adolescents' age and gender. Parents' education was measured in ordinal form that consists of school, not finishing high school, finishing high school, having an associated degree, a Bachelor's degree, an MA/MS, or a PhD. Measurement equivalency is an essential issue in such cross-cultural studies as the present one, which used scenario-based instrumentation outside of the country of origin. The back translation technique was used to reduce nonequivalent measurements in the instrument (Rose, 1985; Riordan & Vandenberg, 1994). After one translator translated the questionnaire into Chinese, another bilingual person translated the Chinese version back into English. Then the two translators compared the original and translated English versions. If there was a discrepancy, adjustment followed when agreement was reached after discussion.

DATA ANALYSIS

Structural Equation Modeling (SEM) was employed to analyze the data in this study by using *AMOS* 4.0 (Arbuckle & Wothke, 1999). A check on multivariate normality of the data showed the multivariate normality assumption was not seriously violated. Evidence suggests that the maximum likelihood method is reasonably robust to modest violation of the normality assumption (Hu & Bentler, 1995). Maximum likelihood method was chosen as the method of estimation. The cut-off values of the fit indices for the present study are .95 for the Normed Fit Index (NFI), Tucker-Lewis Index/ Non-Normed Fit Index (TLI/NNFI), and the Comparative Fit Index (CFI), and the Root Mean Square Error of Approximation (RMSEA) is lower than .08 (.05 indicates a close fit).

The Measurement Model

The overall measurement model for the present study consisted of four latent variables, two observed variables, and thirteen observed indicators. The latent variables were cohesion (5 indicators), conflict (4 indicators), communication (2 indicators), and parent education (2 indicators). One observed exogenous variable was adolescent age, and another observed variable, adolescent involvement in decision-making, was specified as both an exogenous and endogenous variable. This model was tested twice with the data of adolescent perceived communication with mother and father separately.

The Structural Model

The structural model was first tested without differentiating the group differences between boys and girls (see Figure 1). It was also tested twice with the data of adolescent perceived communication with mother and father separately. The following relationships were examined through testing the structural model:

1. Parent-adolescent communication and parent-adolescent cohesion;
2. Parent-adolescent communication and parent-adolescent conflict;
3. Age and parent-adolescent communication;
4. Age and parent-adolescent conflict;
5. Age and adolescent involvement in decision-making;
6. Adolescent involvement in decision-making and parent-adolescent cohesion;

7. Adolescent involvement in decision-making and parent-adolescent conflict; and
8. Parent education and adolescent involvement in decision-making.

Although a structural model was specified, cause-and-effect relationships cannot be inferred because all the data were collected at the same time.

Mediating Effects of Adolescents' Decision Involvement and Communication. The researchers followed the three criteria, suggested by Baron and Kenny (1986) which need to be met for a significant mediating effect: (1) the predictor is significantly linked to the criterion variable; (2) the predictor and the mediator are significantly associated; and (3) the mediator and criterion are significantly associated. They note that the mediating effect "accounts for the relations between the predictor and the criterion" (p. 1176), and explains how a significant relationship occurs. The structural model was specified in a way that allows the following mediating effects to be examined: the mediating effects of parent-adolescent communication on the age-conflict relationship, adolescents' involvement on the age-conflict relationship, and adolescents' involvement on the association of parent-adolescent communication and relationships (i.e., cohesion and conflict).

Moderating Effect of Gender. A moderating effect exists when a significant relationship occurs depending on the condition specified by the moderator. In our study, there would be a moderating effect of gender if a significant path existed for one gender group but not for the other, or a path coefficient was significantly different between boys and girls. Multi-group analysis was used to test if each path coefficient in the adolescent boys' group was different from the corresponding coefficient in the girls' group. Prior to comparing the differences on the path coefficients between boys and girls, it was examined whether the factor loadings for latent variables differed significantly between the groups. If the latent variables were not defined consistently across the groups, the path coefficients from the structural model would not be comparable. This analysis was accomplished by testing three nested models: baseline/unconstrained, factor loading constrained, and factor loading and path coefficient constrained. Then a Chi-square difference test was done to determine whether the model with paths constrained was not significantly less fit than the less or unconstrained models.

RESULTS

Adolescent Involvement in the Decision-Making Processes

The adolescent participants were asked who made the decision in their families on issues such as curfew, making friends, dating, hair style, clothes,

FIGURE 1. The Full Model

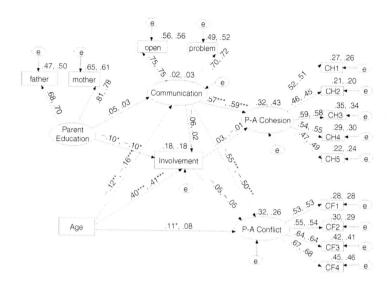

Note: The first set of parameter estimates is based on mother-adolescent communication, and the second set is based on father-adolescent communication.
All the factor loadings are significant at p < .001.
Parameter estimates above endogenous variables are R-squares.

spending allowance, leisure activities, doing school assignment, and college education. Results demonstrated that the adolescent participants had the highest input in deciding when they should do their homework. Nearly 89% of them made this decision on their own. The next highest input in decision-making they had was over how to spend their allowance. The adolescents reported that they had least power in deciding how late they could stay out (31%), and whether they could attend parties at night (25.4%). Less than one-third of them indicated that they made decisions over these issues by themselves.

Parents made most joint decisions about their adolescent children over curfews (29.3%), dating (27.1%) and attending parties (34.6%). Parents involved their adolescent children most in deciding the highest education degree their children should pursue (36.5%), and the college major they should choose (34%) by engaging them in making joint decisions. Mothers were most involved in making decisions over their children's clothing styles (20.1%) and curfew time (19.1%), while fathers were most involved in decisions over level of education and curfews.

The Measurement Model

Results of the Confirmatory Factor Analysis (CFA) indicated that the model fit both father-adolescent and mother-adolescent data well (for both sets of data: NFI, TLI/NNFI, and CFI = .99; Re: mother, $\chi^2[77] = 152.32$, $p < .01$; Re: father, $\chi^2[77] = 162.82$, $p < .01$). RMSEA was .036 with RMSEALO = .027, RMSEAHI = .044, and PCLOSE = .998 for both models. The factor loadings of the 13 indicators ranged between .45 and .84 with $p < .001$. Correlation estimates among factors from the measurement model are presented in Table 1.

The Structural Model

The structural model was estimated twice using the data of father-adolescent communication and mother-adolescent communication, respectively. Results indicated that the model fit both data well (for both sets of data: NFI, NNFI/TLI, and CFI = .99; Re: mother, $\chi^2[82] = 179.24$, $p < .05$, $\chi^2/df = 2.2$; Re: father, $\chi^2[82] = 189.95$, $p < .05$, $\chi^2/df = 2.3$). RMSEA was .034 with RMSEALO = .028, RMSEAHI = .040, and PCLOSE = 1.000 for the mother's model, and RMSEA was .032 with RMSEALO = .026, RMSEAHI = .038, and PCLOSE = 1.000 for the father's model. The factor loadings of all the indicators were statistically significant at $p < .001$ (see Figure 1).

Relationships Among the Constructs and Variables. The structural parameter estimates–path coefficients from the model with mother-adolescent communication and the model with father-adolescent communication are presented in Figure 1. Results indicated that as adolescents were growing older, father- or mother-adolescent communication became less open and more problematic, and mother-adolescent relationship experienced more conflict. Adolescent age was a strong predictor of decision involvement. Parents' education was not observed to have a significant link to parent-adolescent communication. Better mother-adolescent communication was observed to be strongly associated with higher cohesion and less conflict. The more adolescents were involved in decision-making, the less conflict between mother and son or daughter. Father-adolescent communication was found to be a strong predictor of cohesion and conflict as was mother-adolescent communication.

Mediating Effects. Both father- and mother-adolescent communication had a significant mediating effect on the relationship between age and conflict. The older the adolescent was, the poorer parent-adolescent communication (Re: father, $\gamma = -.16$, p < .001; Re: mother, $\gamma = -.12$, p < .01). In turn, the poorer parent-adolescent communication, the more conflict there was between parents and adolescent children (Re: father, $\gamma = -.50$, p < .001; Re: mother, $\gamma = -.55$, p < .001). No significant path coefficients were observed from either father- or mother-adolescent communication to decision involvement (Re: father, $\gamma = .02$, p > .10; Re: mother, $\gamma = -.06$, p > .10). Nor were the paths from decision involvement to cohesion (Re: father, $\gamma = -.01$, p > .05; Re: mother, $\gamma = .03$, p > .10). Therefore, decision involvement did not have any mediating effect on the relationship between parent-adolescent communication and cohesion. Decision involvement was observed to have a mediating effect on the relationship between age and conflict in the model with mother communication data. More involvement of older adolescent in decision-making appeared to decrease parent-adolescent conflict (age-involvement: $\gamma = .40$, p < .001; involvement-conflict: $\gamma = -.09$, p < .05).

The Moderating Effect of Gender. Multi-group analysis was conducted to examine the moderating effect of gender. In addition to the unconstrained model (baseline model), two constrained models were tested in sequence. The first was a model with each factor loading set to be equal between the groups of boys and girls, but with error variances and path coefficients free. The second was a model with invariant factor loadings and path coefficients. The fit indexes for the nested models are presented in Table 2.

Compared to the baseline model, the model with constrained factor loadings had $\Delta\chi^2$ (Δdf) = 6.57(9), p > .10 for mother-adolescent communication data, and had $\Delta\chi^2$ (Δdf) = 6.12 (9), p > .10 for the father-adolescent communication data, indicating the constrained model did not appear to be significantly

TABLE 1. Correlation Estimates from the Measurement Model

	Conflict	Cohesion	Communication	Education	Age	Involvement
Conflict	--	−.25***	−.57***	−.06	.14***	.01
Cohesion	−.25***	--	.58***	.10	−.08	.04
Communication	−.52***	.60***	--	.06	−.13**	−.11**
Education	−.04	.09	.01	--	−.20***	−.18***
Age	.14***	−.06	−.18***	−.20***	--	.41***
Involvement	.01	−.04	−.06	−.18***	.42***	--

Note: The communication in the upper diagonal is father-adolescent communication, and that in the lower diagonal is mother-adolescent communication.
** p < .01, *** p < .001.

less fit than the unconstrained one. Therefore, the latent variables are not defined differently across the gender groups. Further comparison between the models with only factor loadings constrained and with both factor loading and path coefficients constrained revealed a significant Chi-square reduction in the model with mother- adolescent communication data ($\Delta\chi^2$ (Δdf) = 23.39(10), $p < .01$), but not with father-adolescent communication data ($\Delta\chi^2$ (Δdf) = 10.02(10), $p > .05$). The results indicated that there was a moderating effect of gender. Inspection of critical ratios for parameter differences showed that the path coefficients from mother-adolescent communication to cohesion and conflict were significantly different between the gender groups (for cohesion, t = 2.33, $p < .05$; for conflict, t = 3.27, $p < .01$). Gender also accounts for the associations between adolescent age and decision involvement (t = -2.05, $p < .05$), age and father-adolescent communication (t = -10.07, $p < .001$), and father-adolescent communication and cohesion (t = 7.74, $p < .001$).

DISCUSSION

Chinese Adolescents' Involvement in Decision-Making

In literature, Chinese parents are often reported as controlling and authoritarian (Ho, 1981; Shek, 1999, 2000), and Chinese teenagers are not believed to have much autonomy. The results from this study seem to suggest that present Chinese parents listen more to their children than has been previously believed. Counting the input that Chinese adolescents made in joint decisions with parents, the percentage of adolescent involvement in making decisions over the 11 issues ranged from 44.3% to 90.5%. Over 60% of the adolescents reported that they had input in decisions in 9 out of 11 issues surveyed in this study. Chinese teenagers seemed to be most likely either to decide by themselves or to have some input in the decisions about issues like making friends, going for entertainment, choosing a college major, doing homework, and having an allowance. Chinese parents appeared to retain their power over issues like curfews and attending parties. Parents and children made most joint decisions on children's education, such as choosing a college major and pursuing higher education. These results showed that the Chinese parent participants allowed their children to have input into decision-making, and the majority of them made shared decisions with their children. The finding seems to shed some new light on the parenting style of contemporary Mainland Chinese parents. The information gained from the present survey questions the popular image of authoritarian Chinese parents who have absolute power over their children. It supports the research findings from Lin and Fu (1990), and from Xu and his colleagues (1991) that Chinese parents may encourage both individuation and family connection.

This empirical data may suggest that the authoritarian Chinese parent is not an accurate stereotype or/and there is a change in Chinese parenting style. Allowing children to make decisions on their own shows parents' recognition of children as an individual rather than their possessions. A recent study documents that Chinese parents' values of raising children has shifted from emphasizing filial piety and obedience to emotional satisfaction (Xia et al., 1998). All the adolescent participants of this present study were born after 1979, the year when the One Child Family Planning Policy was implemented. Only children are frequently referred to as "little emperor or empress" in the media as well as by the public. These are the children who get away with unacceptable behaviors at home, and whose parents surrender their leadership in the family. Chinese parents are observed to be more doting, and more involved when choice of births is limited (Fablo & Boston, 1994; Guo, 2001). The less controlling image of Chinese parents may mirror the impact of One Child Family Planning Policy upon Chinese parenting style.

The present study has found that adolescents' decision-making is strongly age-related. This finding is consistent with results from studies in Western cul-

TABLE 2. Fit Indices for Nested Models in Multi-Group Analysis

Model	X^2	NFI	NNFI	CFI	ΔX^2	Δdf	ΔNFI
Re: mother							
1. Baseline/free parameters	306.20	.989	.992	.995			
2. Constrained factor loadings	312.77	.989	.993	.995			
Model 2 & Model 1					6.57	9	.000
3. Constrained factor loadings & path coefficients	336.06	.988	.993	.995			
Model 3 & Model 2					23.29**	10	.001
Re: father							
1. Baseline/free parameters	291.84	.989	.993	.995			
2. Constrained factor loadings	297.96	.989	.994	.995			
Model 2 & Model 1					6.12	9	.000
3. Constrained factor loadings & path coefficients	308.18	.989	.994	.995			
Model 3 & Model 2					10.02	10	.000

Note: NFI = Normed Fit Index, TLI/NNFI = Tucker-Lewis Index/Non-Normed Fit Index, and CFI = Comparative Fit Index. ** $p < .01$

tural environments (Bosma, Jackson, Zijsling, Zani, Cicognani, Xerri, Honess, & Charman, 1996; Liprie, 1993). Adolescents enjoy more power of decision-making as they grow older. The study does not reveal a significant link between adolescents' decision involvement and high family cohesion and good parent-adolescent communication, although a weak relationship between communication and decision-making is reported in another study that also uses the Parent-Adolescent Communication Scale (Jackson et al., 1998). However, less involvement is significantly related to more parent-adolescent conflict. The detected linkage to conflict is in agreement with findings reported by Australian researchers (Brown & Mann, 1990), and supports that conflicts occur when adolescents want more independence in decision-making than their parents grant. It shows that Chinese adolescents experience the same passage of autonomy development as their Australian counterparts. As to why significant associations of adolescent involvement with parent-child cohesion and communication were not detected in this sample, one explanation may be that the adolescent decision-making involvement in this study was more a measure of frequency of making decisions rather than competence in decision- making. Good decision-making and communication skills can enhance each other and foster cohesion. Further research should examine the relationships between adolescent competence in decision-making and parent-adolescent communication and relationships.

Parent-Adolescent Communication and Parent-Adolescent Relationships

The present study has observed a strong positive link from parent-adolescent communication to parent-adolescent cohesion, and a strong negative link to parent-adolescent conflicts. This finding adds to the existing literature that positive parent-adolescent communication leads to closer family relationships, helping them to be more loving and flexible in solving family problems.

Parent-adolescent conflict and emotional distancing are documented repeatedly as a function of the development of adolescents' autonomy in Western studies (Fuligni, 1998; Collins & Russell, 1991; Paikoff & Brooks-Gunn, 1991). Results from the present study demonstrate the distancing effect of autonomy development of Chinese adolescents. The results may imply that Chinese adolescents go through a similar passage of struggle for autonomy and transformation of their communications and relationships with their parents as their American counterparts.

The present study has also found that positive mother-adolescent communication may reduce the conflicts that occur as adolescent children are growing up. Good parent-adolescent communication improves adolescents' social skills that lead to not only closeness in the parent-adolescent relationship, but also positive psychological outcomes such as high self-esteem, adequate coping and social support network (Bijstra et al., 1994). Other positive outcomes of family support and adequate communication are adolescents' individual and social adjustment and absence of deviant or delinquent attitudes (Hess, 1995; Marta, 1997; Noller, 1994), and the reduced risk of youth substance abuse and other delinquent behaviors (Clark & Shields, 1997; Hirschi, 1969; Kafka & London, 1991). Although the present study does not test the association of parent-adolescent relationships and communication with the physical and psychological outcomes of Chinese adolescents, the findings from research in Hong Kong and the U.S. have shown that parent-adolescent communication plays an essential role in this relationship (Lau & Leung, 1992; Shek, 1997; Smith & Kerpelman, 2002).

Gender Differences

The significant differences in the direct effect of age on involvement indicated that Chinese adolescent age is related differently to boys and girls in their involvement in decision-making. Age is a less strong predictor for adolescent girls' involvement than for adolescent boys'. That is, for both Chinese adolescent boys and girls, the older they are, the more involved they are. Furthermore, boys are more likely than girls to be involved if they are of the same age. Fuligni's (1998) study reported that Chinese American girls had a later expectation for autonomy. This may explain why the variable girls' age in this study was not linked to girls' involvement in decision-making as strong as was boys' age linked to boys' involvement. Moreover, Chinese males are expected to play a more active role in making family decisions than Chinese females (Ho, 1989). The different role expectations for boys and girls in Chinese culture may also explain this gender difference.

Chinese adolescent girls studied in this research report increased conflicts with parents but this is not the case for boys. The present finding is different from the literature in the U.S indicating that both American adolescent boys and girls experience increased conflicts with parents as they age (Collins & Russell, 1991; Laursen & Collins, 1994; Steinberg, 1990). This suggests that Chinese parents may be more controlling of daughters and may not negotiate with them as much as commonly occurs with sons. It may also reflect the girls' increasing voice of seeking autonomy.

Adolescent boys and girls are differently related to their fathers in both Western and Chinese cultures (Marta, 1997; Noller & Callan, 1991; Shek, 1999, 2000; Youniss & Smollar, 1985). Communication between Chinese fathers and mothers and adolescents appear to be associated strongly with parent-adolescent cohesion and conflict. For both boys and girls, the more open and less demeaning communication they have with parents, the closer they feel to their parents. In addition, girls were more likely than boys to experience a closer and less conflicting relationships with their parents when daughters and sons communicate equally well with them. When compared with girls, boys have a less open and more negative communication with their fathers when they are of the same age. The difference is not evident in adolescent-mother communication. Cultural factors may explain this difference. "A man should drop blood rather than tears" is a popular saying in Chinese culture (Shek, 2000). Males are not socialized with emotion and are not encouraged to talk about feelings. Mothers are regarded by most teens, particularly girls, as more understanding and accepting. Fathers are generally seen as more judgmental, authoritarian, and less willing to discuss emotional or personal issues (Youniss & Smollar, 1985). This may also explain why fathers are not as responsive as mothers to their children's emotional needs and why adolescents go to mothers more than fathers for emotional comfort.

A strength of the present study is the use of Structural Equation Modeling. The advantage of this approach is that the inclusion of measurement errors as explicit parameters in a model allows reliability of variables to be estimated. When measurement errors are taken into account in the analysis, there is an increased "probability of detecting association and obtaining estimates of free parameters close to their population values" (Hoyle, 1995, p. 14). The present study is unique in that it has provided new literature on Mainland Chinese adolescents' decision-making process, and its association with parent-adolescent communication and relationships.

Future Directions

The differences in levels of development in economy and social reform may have an impact on the results of the study. People from more developed areas may have different beliefs and values about parenting, family relationship, and family communication when compared to those from less developed areas. Families from rural areas may have different values from those from urban areas. Children from nuclear families may be expected to participate differently in the decision-making processes from those from extended families, stepfamilies, or single-parent families. Small, rural, and inland areas are not as well developed as large, urban and coastal areas, with the result being that traditional values may be retained. The results of this study may be limited by the nature of its sample, and future studies should acquire samples that are more representative in terms of location, family structure, and social economic status. Another limitation of the study is that it only examines parent-adolescent communication and relationship variables perceived by adolescents. Parents' perspectives should be included in the future investigation.

Applied Implications

Parent-adolescent communication patterns have demonstrated relationships with parent-adolescent relationships, family functioning, youth's self-esteem, depression, competence in decision-making, school performance, and delinquent behaviors in American populations. The findings from this study have significant implications for practice in China where parenting or communication skills training has not been a common practice of prevention or intervention. Programs that are created to help Chinese parents and adolescents develop communication and problem-solving skills may not only help parents with parenting skills, but may also help adolescents become capable of making responsible choices, develop confidence and competence in making decisions, gain self-esteem, and stay free from high-risk behaviors. The results of this study point to the need for the implementation of family life education and programs of communication and problem-solving skills training in China.

REFERENCES

Arbuckle, J. L., & Wothke, W. (1999). *AMOS 4.0 user's guide*. Chicago, IL: SmallWaters Corporation.

Barnes, H. L., & Olson, D. H. (1985). Parent-adolescent communication and the circumplex model. *Child Development, 56*, 438-447.

Baron, R. M., & Kenny, D. A. (1986). The moderator-mediator variable distinction in social psychological research: Conceptual, strategic, and statistical considerations. *Journal of Personality and Social Psychology, 51*(6), 1173-1182.

Baumrind, D. (1967). Childcare practices anteceding three patterns of preschool behavior. *Genetic Psychology Monograph, 75*, 43-88.

Belch, G. E., Geresino, G., & Belch, M. A. (1985). Parental and teenager child influences in family decision-making. *Journal of Business Research, 13*, 163-176.

Bijstra, J. O., Bosma, H. A., & Jackson, A. E. (1994). The relationship between social skills and psychosocial functioning in early adolescence. *Personality and Individual Differences, 16*, 767-776.

Bosma, H. A., Jackson, S., Zijsling, D. H., Zani, B., Cicognani, E., Xerri, M. L., Honess, T. M., & Charman, L. (1996). Who has the final say? Decisions on adolescent behavior within the family. *Journal of Adolescence, 19*, 277-291.

Bronfenbrenner, U., & Morris, P. A. (1998). The ecology of developmental processes. In W. Damon (Series Ed.) & R. M. Lerner (Vol. Ed.), *Handbook of child psychol-*

ogy: Vol. 1. Theoretical models of human development (5th ed., pp. 993-1028). New York: Wiley.

Brown, J. E., & Mann, L. (1990). The relationship between family structure and process variables and adolescent decision-making. *Journal of Adolescence, 13,* 25-37.

Clark, R. D., & Shields, G. (1997). Family communication and delinquency. *Adolescence, 32*(125), 81-92.

Collins, W. A. (1990). Parent-child relationships in the transition to adolescence: Continuity and change in interaction, affect, and cognition. In R. Montemayor, G. R. Adams, & P. Gullotta (Eds.), *Advances in adolescent development: Vol. 2. From childhood to adolescence: A transitional period?* (pp. 85-106). Newbury Park, CA: Sage.

Collins, W. A., & Laursen, B. (1992). Conflict and relationships during adolescence. In C. U. Shantz & W. W. Hartup. (Eds.), *Conflict in child and adolescent development* (pp. 216-241). New York: Cambridge University Press.

Collins, W. A., & Russell, G. (1991). Mother-child and father-child relationships in middle childhood and adolescence: A developmental analysis. *Developmental Review, 11,* 99-136.

Conoley, J. C. (1995). Multicultural family assessment. In J. C. Conoley & E. B. Werth (Eds.), *Family assessment* (pp. 103-129). Lincoln, NE: Buros Institute of Mental Measurements.

Diesing, P. (1962). Reason in society: Five types of decisions and their social conditions. Westport, CT: Greenwood Press.

Dornbusch, S. M., Ritter, P. L., Mont-Reynaund, R., & Chen, Z. Y. (1990). Family decision-making and academic performance in a diverse high school population. *Journal of Adolescent Research, 5*(2), 143-160.

Embassy of P.R. China in the United States. (2002, September 17). Changes of Chinese people's lives: Facts and figures (No. 0217). Retrieved October 28, 2002, from *http://www.china.org/eng/35247.html.*

Fablo, T., & Boston, Jr., D. L. (1994). The academic, personality, and physical outcome of only children in China. *Child Development, 64*(1), 18-35.

Feldman, S. S., & Rosenthal, D. A. (1991). Age expectations of behavioral autonomy in Hong Kong Australian and American youth: The influence of family variables and adolescents' values. *International Journal of Psychology, 26*(1), 1-23.

Fuligni, A. J. (1998). Authority, autonomy, and parent-adolescent conflict and cohesion: A study of adolescents from Mexican, Chinese, Filipino, and European backgrounds. *Developmental Psychology, 34*(4), 782-792.

Gecas, V., & Seff, M. A. (1990). Families and adolescents: A review of the 1980s. *Journal of Marriage and the Family, 52,* 941-958.

Goodwin, R., & Tang, C. (1996). Chinese personal relationships. In M. H. Bond (Ed.), *The handbook of Chinese psychology* (pp. 294-308). Hong Kong: Oxford University Press.

Grotevant, H. D., & Cooper, C. R. (1985). Patterns of interaction in family relationships and the development of identity exploration in adolescence. *Child Development, 56,* 415-428.

Guo, H. (2001). The "little emperors grow up." *Psychology Today, 33,* 10.

Hampson, R. B., Hulgus, Y. F., & Beavers, W. R. (1991). Comparison of self-report measures of the Beavers Systems Model and Olson's Circumplex Model. *Journal of Family Psychology, 4*(3), 326-340.

Harbin, H. T., & Madden, D. J. (1983). Assaultive adolescents: Family decision-making parameters. *Family Process, 22,* 109-118.

Hess, L. (1995). Changing family patterns in West Europe: Opportunities and risk factors for adolescent development. In M. Rutter & D. Smith (Eds.), *Psychosocial disorder in young people* (pp. 104-119). Chichester: Wiley.

Hirschi, T. (1969). *Causes of delinquency.* Berkeley, CA: University of California Press.

Ho, D. Y. F. (1981). Traditional patterns of socialization in Chinese society. *Acta Psychologica Taiwanica, 23,* 81-95.

Ho, D. Y. F., Spinks, J. A., & Yeung, C. S. H. (Eds.). (1989). *Chinese patterns of behavior: A sourcebook of psychological and psychiatric studies.* New York: Praeger.

Hong, G. K. (1989). An application of cultural and environmental issues in family therapy with immigrant Chinese Americans. *Journal of Strategic and Systemic Therapies, 8,* 14-21.

Hoyle, R. H. (1995). *Structural equation modeling: Concepts, issues, and applications.* Thousand Oaks: Sage.

Hsu, J. (1985). The Chinese family: Relations, problems and therapy. In W. Tseng & D. Y. H. Wu (Eds.), *Chinese culture and mental health* (pp. 95-112). Orlando, FL: Academic Press.

Hu, L., & Bentler, P. M. (1995). Evaluating model fit. In R. H. Hoyle (Ed.), *Structural equation modeling: Concepts, issues, and applications* (pp. 76-99). Thousand Oaks: Sage.

Jackson, S., Bijstra, J., Oostra, L., & Bosma, H. (1998). Adolescents' perceptions of communication with parents relative to specific aspects of relationships with parents and personal development. *Journal of Adolescence, 21,* 305-322.

Kafka, R. R., & London, P. (1991). Communication in relationships and adolescent substance use: The influence of parents and friends. *Adolescence, 26*(103), 587-598.

Lau, S., & Leung, K. (1992). Relations with parents and school and Chinese adolescents' self-concept, delinquency, and academic performance. *British Journal of Educational Psychology, 62,* 193-202.

Laursen, B., & Collins, W. A. (1994). Interpersonal conflict during adolescence. *Psychological Bulletin, 115*(2), 197-209.

Laursen, B., & Koplas, A. L. (1995). What's important about important conflicts? Adolescents' perceptions of daily disagreements. *Merrill-Palmer Quarterly, 41*(4), 536-553.

Liang, S. M. (1974). *The essential features of Chinese culture.* Hong Kong: Chi-Cheng T'u-Shu Kung Shu.

Lin, C. Y. C., & Fu, V. R. (1990). A comparison of child rearing practices among Chinese, immigrant Chinese, and Caucasian-American parents. *Child Development, 61,* 429-433.

Liprie, M. L. (1993). Adolescents' contributions to family decision-making. *Marriage & Family Review, 18*(3/4), 241-253.

Marta, E. (1997). Parent-adolescent interactions and psychosocial risk in adolescents: An analysis of communication, support and gender. *Journal of Adolescence, 20,* 473-487.

Noller, P. (1994). Relationships with parents in adolescence: Process and outcome. In R. Montemayor, G. Adams, & T. Gullotta (Eds.), *Personal relationships during adolescence* (pp. 37-77). London: Sage.

Noller, P., & Callan, V. (1991). *The adolescent in the family.* London: Routledge.

Olson, D. H., McCubbin, H. I., Barnes, H., Larsen, A., Muxen, M., & Wilson, M. (1992). *Family inventories* (2nd revision). St Paul, MN: Family Social Science, University of Minnesota.

Paikoff, R. L., & Brooks-Gunn, J. (1991). Do parent-child relationships change during puberty? *Psychological Bulletin, 110*(1), 47-66.

Peterson, G. W., Wilson, S. M., Bush, K. R., & Zhao, B. (2002). Strengths in the Chinese parent-adolescent relationship: Socializing adolescent self-esteem and prosocial behavior. Presentation at the International Family Strengths Conference, Shanghai, P.R. China.

Reiss, D. (1981). *The family's construction of reality.* Cambridge, MA: Harvard University Press.

Rettig, K. D. (1993). Problem solving and decision-making as central processes of family life: An ecological framework for family relations and family resource management. *Marriage & Family Review, 18*(3/4), 187-222.

Riordan, C. M., & Vandenberg, R. J. (1994). A central question in cross-cultural research: Do employees of different cultures interpret work-related measures in an equivalent manner? *Journal of Management, 20,* 643-671.

Rose, M. G. (1985). Back-translating to recover form. *International Journal of Translation, 31*(1), 6-11.

Scabini, E. (1995). *Psicologia sociale della famiglia* [The social psychology of the family]. Torino: Bollati Boringhieri.

Shek, D. T. L. (1995). Chinese adolescents' perceptions of parenting styles of fathers and mothers. *The Journal of Genetic Psychology, 156*(2), 175-190.

Shek, D. T. L. (1997). The relation of family functioning to adolescent psychological well-being, school adjustment, and problem behavior. *The Journal of Genetic Psychology, 158*(4), 467-479.

Shek, D. T. L. (1998). Adolescents' perceptions of parental and maternal parenting styles in a Chinese context. *The Journal of Psychology, 132*(5), 527-537.

Shek, D. T. L. (1999). Paternal and maternal influences on the psychological well-being of Chinese adolescents. *Genetic, Social & General Psychology Monographs, 125,* 269-296.

Shek, D. T. L. (2000). Differences between fathers and mothers in the treatment of, and relationship with, their teenage children: Perceptions of Chinese adolescents. *Adolescence, 35,* 135-144.

Smetana, J. G. (1988). Concepts of self and social convention: Adolescents and parents' reasoning about hypothetical and actual family conflicts. In M. R. Gunnar & W. A. Collins (Eds.), *Minnesota symposia on child psychology* (Vol. 21, pp. 79-122). Hillsdale, NJ: Erlbaum.

Smith, S., & Ingoldsby, B. (1992). Multicultural family studies: Educating students for diversity. *Family Relations, 41*(1), 25-30.

Smith, S. L., & Kerpelman, J. L. (2002). Adjudicated adolescent girls and their mothers: Examining relationship quality and communication styles. *Journal of Addictions to Offender Counseling, 23,* 15-29.

Sroufe, J. W. (1991). Assessment of parent-adolescent relationships: Implications for adolescent development. *Journal of Family Psychology, 5,* 21-45.

Steinberg, L. (1990). Autonomy, conflict, and harmony in the family relationship. In S. Feldman & G. Elliott (Eds.), *At the threshold: The developing adolescent* (pp. 255-276). Cambridge, MA: Harvard University Press.

Watzlawick, P., Beavin, J., & Johnson, D. (1967). Pragmatics of human communication: A study of interactional patterns, pathologies, and paradoxes. New York: Norton.

Xia, Y., Lin, S., Xie, X. L., Zhou, Z., & DeFrain, J. (1998). One child family policy in China and its impact on Chinese parents' perception of children's values. Presentation at National Conference on Family Relations Annual Meeting, Milwaukee, WI.

Xu, Z., Shen, J. X., Wan, C. W., Li, C. M., Mussen, P., & Cao, Z. F. (1991). Family socialization and children's behavior and personality development in China. *Journal of Genetic Psychology, 152*(2), 239-253.

Yau, J., & Smetana, J. G. (1996). Adolescent-parent conflict among Chinese adolescents in Hong Kong. *Child Development, 67,* 1262-1275.

Youniss, J., & Smollar, J. (1985). *Adolescent relations with mothers, fathers, and friends.* Chicago: University of Chicago Press.

Predicting Korean Adolescents' Sexual Behavior: Individual, Relationship, Family, and Extra-Family Factors

Gyung Ja Yoon

ABSTRACT. Using data from 370 adolescent males and 390 adolescent females, this study investigates factors associated with Korean adolescents' sexual behavior. The data showed that sixteen percent of the sample reported some type of intimate sexual behavior. The results from regression analyses indicate that alcohol use, dating mood, love for partner, similarity of sexual attitude between partners, and interaction between respondents' attitude on sex and alcohol use were significant predictors of Korean adolescents' sexual behavior with adjusted R^2 of .61. The factors significant for adolescents' sexual behavior differed by gender. The factors significant for adolescent males and adolescent females accounted for 65% and 61% of the explained variance for adolescent males' and adolescent females' sexual behavior, respectively. In both cases, dating mood was a strong predictor of adolescents' sexual behavior. Contrary to expectations specified, neither parental factors nor sibling influence was significant. *[Article copies available for a fee from The Haworth Document Delivery Service: 1-800-HAWORTH. E-mail address: <docdelivery@haworthpress.com> Website: <http://www.HaworthPress.com> © 2004 by The Haworth Press, Inc. All rights reserved.]*

Gyung Ja Yoon is affiliated with the Department of Child Development and Family Environments, Dongeui University, Pusanjin-gu Gaya-dong 24, Pusan, South Korea (E-mail: gjyoon@dongeui.ac.kr).

The author thanks Dr. Walter Schumm and anonymous reviewers for their valuable comments on earlier drafts of the paper.

http://www.haworthpress.com/web/MFR
© 2004 by The Haworth Press, Inc. All rights reserved.
Digital Object Identifier: 10.1300/J002v36n01_07

KEYWORDS. Adolescent, alcohol use, dating mood, risk factors, sexual behavior

INTRODUCTION

During the past few years, Korean adolescents' sexual behavior has been rapidly changing. The incidences of adolescent pregnancies and sexual activities have received considerable public attention in recent years (Chung & Lee, 1999; Choi & Kim, 2001). Korean society has been experiencing great turmoil about traditional sex values with a rapid increase in adolescent female prostitutes. It is estimated that 42.9% of illegally employed girls in the 'service industries,' such as karaoke singers and barmaids, are minors and many of them get involved in prostitution (Chung, 1999). With the rapid increase in adolescent sexual experience, age at first sexual intercourse is younger. The majority (76.5%) of unmarried pregnant women experienced their first sexual intercourse while still in their teens (www.prolife.or.kr), and the recent profile of Korean pregnant adolescents has changed from an average of 18-19 to 15-16 years old (*The Women's News*, 1998).

However, there has not been much research to explore the prevalence of adolescents' sexual problems and social attention in Korea. This is unfortunate, for as Repke (1990) found, adolescents' sexual behavior is a predictor of a high dropout rate from school, abortion, delinquency, and a high divorce rate. Although adolescents' sexual behavior has been associated with numerous serious long-term effects, there has been little research available in spite of the level and scope of changes in Korean adolescents' sexual behavior. Research on adolescent sex in Korea has mainly focused on classifying adolescent sex as a deviant behavior that is part of social problems rather than identifying its related variables (e.g., Kim, 1989; Lee, 1994; Shon, 1995). In addition, although a few studies have attempted to investigate antecedents of sexual behavior using samples in their twenties (e.g., Kim, Kim, & Yoon, 2001; Park, Lee, Park, & Jeoung, 1995; Yoon, 1995), treating teenagers as active agents of sex rather than objects of sexual violence has remained mostly an unexplored arena. This may be derived from the social taboo against open discussion of sexuality and premarital sex.

Attempting to understand why certain adolescents engage in sexual activity is a complex task. Although sexual practice is generally influenced by holistic synthesis of individual, relational, and family level aspects, much of research on adolescents' sexual behavior has focused on only part of these aspects (e.g., East, Felice, & Morgan, 1993; Jaccard, Dittus, & Gordon, 1996; Pick & Palos, 1995; Udry & Billy, 1987; Widmir, 1997; Zabin, Smith, Hirsch, & Hardy, 1986). In other words, associations between variables reported to be strongly related in some studies may not even be statistically significant because additional significant variables are included in multivariate analyses (Miller, 1998). Our understanding of adolescents' sexual behavior is complicated because of such methodological limitations.

Literature reviews about adolescents' sexual behavior have identified characteristics of both adolescents and their families as significant predictors of adolescents' sexual behavior. However, factors significant in some studies (e.g., parental support, gender of adolescent child, relationship with parents, parental monitoring, siblings' influence, communication with parents, parental attitude, siblings' attitude and sexual behavior, peers, and religiosity) are often not significant in other studies. A few factors, namely, number of partners, alcohol use, and age were consistently significant.

Although traditional Korean culture has been influenced by Confucianism, Korea has undergone extensive social change due to rapid industrialization in the past four decades. This has inevitably brought about changes in traditional norms and values of family life, including relationships between parents and children, and has resulted in weakening parental influence upon children. For example, the parent generation showed much more traditional values than their offspring on attitudes about sex and marriage (Kim, 1998; Yang, 1996), expectations about their children (Park, 1986), and filial responsibility (Sung, 1995). Kim (1998) found the 'generation gap' about views of child and sex roles was significantly more obvious between the parent-adolescent child generation than between the parent-grandparent generation. How much power do parents exert today on their adolescent children's sexual activity in Korea? This question remains yet unanswered.

In addition to examining influential factors on adolescents' sexual behavior, the present study attempts to explore the impact of a neglected variable from previous research. Little evidence has been presented on how dating mood affects adolescent sexual activity, although it may be a powerful explanatory variable on adolescents' sexual behavior when considering how sexual interactions occur. Past research on adolescents' sexual behavior has tended to neglect the dating situation itself. Dating mood may have a great impact empirically on whether an adolescent becomes involved sexually. Yoon's study with a sample of university students (1995) showed that dating mood was an influential factor affecting both male and female university students' sexual behavior.

THEORETICAL BACKGROUND

To explore factors predicting Korean adolescents' sexual behavior, this study employs an ecological perspective (Bronfenbrenner, 1986). Bronfenbrenner proposed that intrafamilial processes are affected by extra-familial conditions, with intrafamilial processes, in turn, affecting each family member. This framework has been used to examine adolescents' sexual activity, implying that risk factors at the individual level and at environmental levels are related to the greater risk of sexual behavior (Small & Luster, 1994; Perkins, Luster, Villarruel, & Small, 1998). The present study utilizes variables from the individual level, the relationship level, the family level, and the extra-family level in order to investigate Korean adolescents' sexual behavior.

Individual Factors

Alcohol use has been consistently identified with the increased risk of sexual behavior (Elliott & Morese, 1989; Ensminger, 1990; Santelli, Brenner, Lowry, Bhatt, & Zabin, 1998; Small & Luster, 1994; Smith, 1997), especially for males (Small & Luster, 1994). Although alcohol use has been considered to be one of the most influential risk factors for adolescent sexual behavior in studies from a western culture, it has not been well investigated in the studies of Korean adolescents' sexual behavior, except in the cases of nonconsensual sexual behavior (Yoon, 2002a).

Age was associated with adolescents' sexual behavior (Davis, 1989; Santelli et al., 1998). Santelli et al. (1998) reported that younger age at first intercourse was related to the increased number of multiple sexual partners. Age at first consensual sex for female students was significantly related to subsequent problematic sexual behavior such as unwanted sex (Himelein, Vogel, & Wachowiak, 1994). The younger a female was at the time of initial sexual experience, the more the likely it was for her to become a victim of nonconsensual sex.

The influence of respondents' sexual attitudes on sexual behavior has been demonstrated in the research literature (e.g., Plotnick, 1992; Sack, Keller, & Hinkle, 1984; Winslow, Franzini, & Hwang, 1992). Respondents' permissive sexual attitudes were more likely associated with greater involvement in sexual behavior. Yoon (2002b) also found that a respondent's sexual attitude distinguished less sexually experienced girls from more sexually experienced girls.

In addition, religiosity plays an important role in the involvement of sexual behavior, though results have not been consistent. A number of research studies found religiosity (measured by religious participation) to be either an influential factor (Bock, Beeghley, & Mixon, 1983; Day, 1992) or the most significant factor on adolescent sexual involvement (Werner-Wilson, 1998). However, other studies found that the effect differed by gender in that only male university students were affected (Yoon, 1995) whereas there was little or no effect on girls' sexual experience (Yoon, 2002b).

Relationship Factors

Although both males and females engage in premarital sexual relations, love for the partner has been a more influential factor for females. For example, females report the need for more strict standards in sexual activities (Cohen & Shotland, 1996), more commitment because women are viewed as more relational than their male counterparts (Bettor, Hendrick, & Hendrick, 1995; Hynie, Lydon, Cote, & Weiner, 1998), and love for partner as the factor determining whether a female respondent will engage in sex (Yoon, 2002b). Moreover, both male and female university students view the status of the relationship as the primary basis for women's sexual desire (Regan & Berscheid, 1995).

Research on the similarity of sexual attitude between partners show that dating and married partners seem to hold more congruent sexual attitudes and regard a partner with similar attitudes as more desirable (Cupach & Metts, 1995; Smith, Becker, Byrne, & Przybyla, 1993; Stuart, Rau, Fuhrer, & Hillebrand, 1996). Investigators of one study (Sprecher, Regan, McKenney, Maxwell, & Wazienski, 1997) found that sexually experienced women prefer partners with either moderate or high levels of sexual experience to partners with restricted sexual experience. This tendency was not found for men and the present study will test this issues again with a sample of adolescents.

The number of reported sexual partners for adolescents and casual sex has increased in recent years (Santelli et al., 1998), implying that adolescents engage in unplanned and sporadic sex (Chilman, 1986). It was found in a recent study, for example, that girls were affected by dating mood, regardless of their level of sexual experience (Yoon, 2002b). Dating mood, a neglected variable in the literature of adolescent sex, may explain and tap the unexplored part of adolescent sexual behavior.

Family Factors

Research on adolescents' communication about sex with parents demonstrate that adolescents who report having good personal talks with a parent are more likely to communicate about sexual matters as well (Raffaelli, Bogenschneider, & Flood, 1998). Unless a teenager perceives understanding and support from a parent, he/she may not communicate with a parent about more difficult issues related to sex. However, results from prior studies are complex and inconsistent on the effect of parent-child communication. Some studies report positive effects on the prevention of children's sexual intercourse (Handelsman, Cabral, & Weisfeld, 1987; Pick & Palos, 1995) whereas other studies report no relationship between parent-child communication and sexual behavior (Hovell, Sipan, Blumberg, Atkins, Hofstetter, & Kreitner, 1994) or are related to more active sexual behavior (Widmer, 1997).

The effect of parental monitoring on adolescent sex is not consistent. Some studies show that it is related to lower level of adolescent sexual behavior (Abrahamse, Morrison, & Waite, 1988; Moore, Peterson, & Furstenberg, 1986; Schreck, 1999), whereas other studies reported that parental supervision or rules had no effect on daughters' sexual behavior (East, 1996; Smith, 1997). In the specific case of a sample of Korean middle school students, however, Park and Doh (2001) found that mothers' monitoring was related to a lower degree of externalizing problem behavior.

Several studies of parental attitudes about sex indicate that parents' sexual attitude was positively related to adolescents' postponement of sexual intercourse (Luster & Small, 1994; Small & Luster, 1994). Conservative parental sexual attitudes and parental disapproval of premarital sex had a strong negative effect on adolescent sex. However, Inman- Amos, Hendrick, and Hendrick (1994) also found that parental love attitudes were not related to children's attitudes about love.

The quality of relationship between adolescents and parents has been documented as being related positively to a later onset of first intercourse (Danziger, 1995) and to a diminished frequency of intercourse (Jaccard et al., 1996). The quality of parent-adolescent relationships seems to mediate the effect of parent-adolescent interactions on sexual behavior (Whitbeck, Hoyt, Miller, & Kao, 1992).

Older siblings' attitudes about sex usually have been related to younger siblings' intercourse (East, 1996) or early onset of intercourse (Widmer, 1997). Cicirelli (1994; 1995) reported that the sexual behavior of older siblings had a significant impact on the timing of younger siblings' initiation of sexual intercourse. Siblings influence younger siblings through communication and emotional support (Cicirelli, 1994; 1995; Widmer, 1997). Younger siblings, especially, report greater admiration for older siblings and imitate their older siblings more than vice versa (Buhrmester, 1992; cited in Widmer, 1997).

Extra-Family Factor

Peer influence as a reference group (Benda & DiBlasio, 1994; Boyer, Tschann, & Shafer, 1999; Herold & Goodwin, 1981; Kinsman, Romer, Furstenberg, & Schwarz, 1998; Sack et al., 1984; Smith, 1997) has been related to adolescents' sexual behavior. Adolescents associated with similar norms of peers are more likely to experience sexual behavior.

The present study investigates multiple influences on Korean adolescents' sexual behavior and explores how individual, relational, family, and extra-family characteristics are related to the occurrence of Korean adolescents' sexual behavior. Nevertheless, this study does not attempt to include all predictors; rather, this study examines salient factors for adolescents' sexual behavior. This study is timely because little research has investigated Korean adolescents' sexual behavior despite recent increases in adolescent pregnancy and higher frequencies of adolescent girls being featured in the sex industry. These social problems in Korea demand investigation and intervention.

METHOD

The data for this study are provided by 769 adolescent males and females selected from 14 junior high schools and high schools in Pusan, Korea. Thirteen schools were contacted and nine schools agreed to participate in the study. Seven hundred sixty-nine (769) of the 800 students who initially were given the questionnaire returned the instrument. The questionnaire was administered anonymously during regular classes to students who agreed to participate. The survey was conducted in December 2000.

Sample

Subjects were 370 unmarried adolescent males and 390 unmarried females ranging in age from 12 to 19 years, with an average age of 15.9 years (SD = 1.6). The majority lived with both parents (94.3%), with 3.4% residing with a single parent, 0.8% with a stepparent, and 0.1% having no parent. More than half of the respondents (55.6%) designated their religious affiliation as Buddhism (33.2%), Protestant (12.0%), Roman Catholics (9.0%), and other religions (2.2%). Approximately 57% (57.2%) of the respondents' parents were dual-employed couples, which is slightly higher than the 47.9% reported for the 2000 Census in Korea (National Statistical Office, 2000). Although a majority of the respondents' fathers (76.8%) had at least a high school education (college education 26.7%), some had either an elementary (4.2%) or junior high school education (10.9%), with only a few having graduate school education (5.9%). Similarly, most mothers of the respondents had a high school education (59.7%) or a junior high school education (17.3%). Although a few had an elementary education (4.6%), over 10% (13.8%) of the mothers had a college education, with 2.1% having a graduate degree. Total annual family income was combined in three levels: below $10,285 (26.6%), $10,286 to $24,857 (47.1%), and $24,858 or more (13.1%).

Measures

Sexual behavior. The dependent variable for this study was adolescents' sexual behavior. This was created in order to assess the likely sequence of sexual experiences, rather than dichotomous variables, such as sexual intercourse versus no sexual intercourse, as Hovel and associates (1994) have noted. Adolescents were asked a series of yes/no questions regarding their sexual activity experiences on a shorter form of the Sexual Activity Scale (Table 1) (Hovel et al., 1994). Each item of the scale was recoded and added to show higher scores indicating higher level of sexual activity. Each questionnaire item of the scale was scored as 1 if a respondent reported being sexually experienced, whereas the inexperienced was scored as 0. The scale ranges from 0 to 4. The internal consistency reliability of the scale was high with Cronbach's $\alpha = 0.89$.

For the purpose of this explorative study on adolescents' sexual behavior, plausible predictors, including an extra-family variable, family variables, relational variables, as well as individual level variables were computed.

Individual Variables

Alcohol use. Alcohol use was measured by one item asking that how the respondent perceived his/her alcohol consumption related to sexual activity. The response scale for this item ranged from 1 (strongly agree) to 5 (strongly disagree) and was reverse scored.

Respondent's attitude about sex. This scale is based on a 5-point Likert scale developed by Yoon (1995) (10 items, $\alpha = .86$) that asked about the respondent's attitude about: (1) his/her future marital partner's virginity at the time of marriage; (2) sexual relationship between partners in love with each other before marriage; (3) feeling guilty if he/she has sexual intercourse before engagement or marriage; (4) his/her intention to remain a virgin before marriage; (5) sexual intercourse with someone you don't know very well; (6) woman's virginity before marriage; (7) man's virginity before marriage; (8) sexual intercourse for a woman before marriage; (9) sexual intercourse for a man before marriage; and (10) immorality of sexual intercourse before marriage. Item scores range from 1 (strongly agree) to 5 (strongly disagree) and recoded so that higher score indicated a more conservative attitude about sex.

Religiosity. Religiosity was assessed by the frequency of religious worship attendance. Scores range from 1 (not at all or never) to 6 (more than four times a week).

Relationship Variables

Dating mood. A respondent rated the degree to which he/she felt in a romantic and intimate mood during a dating relationship before becoming in-

TABLE 1. A Shorter Form of the Sexual Activity Scale*

Scale	Frequencies (%)
No sexual activity	600 (79.9)
Kissing	120 (15.7)
Petting above the waist	70 (9.2)
Petting below the waist	40 (5.3)
Intercourse	35 (4.6)

* Note: Respondents checked more than one category. Therefore, the percentage exceeds 100 percent.

volved in a sexual relationship. The single-item measure asked, "The dating mood was romantic." Scores range from 1 (strongly disagree) to 5 (strongly agree).

Love for partner. Two items assess the degree to which a respondent was in love with his/her dating partner, either in the present relationship or in the previous relationship(s). The 5-point Likert scale responses for these items ranged from 1 (strongly agree) to 5 (strongly disagree) and were reverse scored ($\alpha = .72$).

Similarity of sexual attitude between partners. A respondent assessed his/her attitude about sex to the degree he/she felt similar to his/her present partner by answering the item, "My attitude about sex is similar to that of my partner." A 5-point Likert scale was used, ranging from 1 (strongly agree) to 5 (strongly disagree) and was reverse scored.

Family Variables

Communication with parent. Respondents were asked to rate the degree to which they communicate with their parents about each of the following issues: (1) sex, (2) sexual problems, and (3) important matters (three items, Cronbach's $\alpha = .58$). Scores range from 1 (strongly agree) to 5 (strongly disagree) and were reverse scored.

Similarity of sexual attitudes with siblings. Respondents assessed their overall perception of similar attitudes with their siblings (two items, Cronbach's $\alpha = .50$). Scores range from 1 (strongly agree) to 5 (strongly disagree) and were reverse scored.

Parental monitoring. Parental monitoring was adopted from Small and Eastman's work (1991), with higher scores indicating adolescents' perceptions of higher parental supervision (three items, Cronbach's $\alpha = .76$). Items included parents' awareness of (1) the respondent's close friends, (2) the respondent's plans with friends, and (3) respondent's spending time. Scores range from 1 (strongly agree) to 5 (strongly disagree) and were reverse scored.

Parental attitude about sex. Two items measure each parent's acceptance of premarital sex of their child, as perceived by the respondent (Cronbach's α = .93).

Parental premarital sexual behavior. The respondent assessed his/her awareness of each parent's premarital sexual behavior (two items, Cronbach's α = .99). The 5-point Likert scale ranged from 1 (strongly agree) to 5 (strongly disagree) and was reverse scored.

Relationship with parents. Two items assessed a respondent's overall perception of the relationship with his/her parent. The items included "I have a good relationship with my father." A similar question was asked about the relationship with the mother. The items were rated on a 5-point Likert scale ranging from 1 (strongly agree) to 5 (strongly disagree) and were reverse scored (Cronbach's α = .63).

Extra-Family Variable

Peer influence. A measure of peer influence consisted of four items (α = .80). Respondents were asked about the similarity of their sexual experience with that of close friend(s), the similarity of their sexual experience with that of peers, friends' empathy about a respondent's sexual behavior, and the similarity of a respondent's sexual attitude with close friend(s). Item scores range from 1 (very much) to 5 (not at all) and recoded to show higher scores indicating higher influence.

RESULTS

Analysis

The effects of predictors on Korean adolescents' sexual behavior are assessed through a series of stepwise regression models. Model 1 assesses extra-family variables, and additional models address added explanation of individual variables, relationship variables, and family variables, respectively. Four potential interaction effects are also examined.

Table 1 shows the frequencies for adolescents' involvement in sexual activities. While the majority of the respondents (79.9%) had no sexual experience, a considerable proportion of adolescents had some sexual experience. Although the proportion of each category of sexual activities seems relatively low compared to that of American counterparts (e.g., Irwin & Shafer, 1992; Kahn, Kalsbeek, & Hofferth, 1988; Smith, 1997), this result deserves attention since there is little, if any, comparable empirical data available regarding Korean adolescents' sexual activity.

To explore factors related to Korean adolescents' sexual behavior, stepwise regression analyses were conducted (Table 2), with each model testing variables from the levels of an ecological perspective in addition to variables at inner boundaries (Bronfenbrenner, 1986). An overview of models shows that Model 2 is the best model for Korean adolescent sex. Compared to Model 2, neither Model 3 (with added family variables) nor Model 4 (with added family and extra-family variables) show that improvement in adjusted R^2. Contrary to expectations, the adjusted R^2 in Model 3 was not improved.

Individual Variables

Alcohol use was a strong predictor that played an important role in adolescents' sexual experience. The effect was consistently significant even after the influence of other factors was taken into account (in Model 4, Beta = .87, $p <$ .00005). Adolescents who were under the influence of alcohol in a dating situation experienced more sexual behavior. A key finding of this study, therefore, is consistent with the prior research, with alcohol use being a very important risk factor influencing Korean adolescents' sexual behavior.

Age also had a significant effect on adolescent sex (Model 1) though the effect was not strong and diminishes to nonsignificance in subsequent models in which other variables are included. Previous studies indicated that age at first intercourse was related to sexual experience (Santelli et al., 1998). This finding suggests that biological age itself cannot explain the range or depth of sexual experience when other variables are included in the model. Older adolescents in Korea may have more sexual experience than younger adolescents, but the effect of age is not an explanatory factor once other relationship variables are included.

The more respondents had conservative sexual attitudes, the less sexual experience was indicated in Model 1 of Table 2. Sexual attitude, however, diminished to nonsignificance when other predictors were added to the equations. For Korean adolescents in general, whether a sexual attitude was permissive or conservative was not a powerful predictor when other predictors beyond individual factors were taken into account.

Religiosity did not have any significant impact on adolescent sex, a finding that is consistent with results from a study on university students (Yoon, 1995). Findings from this study and prior research, therefore, imply that religiosity seldom plays a significant role in the development of adolescents' sexual life today. Previous findings demonstrating a significant impact for religiosity

TABLE 2. Standardized Multiple Regression Coefficients Predicting Korean Adolescent Sexual Behavior

Variable	Model 1	Model 2	Model 3	Model 4
Individual variables				
Alcohol use	1.24***	.88***	.85***	.87***
Respondent's attitude	−.09**	−.05	−.05	−.05
Religiosity	.02	−.02	−.02	−.02
Age	.06*	.05	.05	.05
Interaction 1	−.61***	−.71***	−.66***	−.68***
Interaction 2	.01	−.03	−.03	−.03
Relationship variables				
Dating mood		.51***	.51***	.50***
Love for partner		.08*	.07*	.07*
Similarity of sexual attitude between partners		.09**	.09**	.09**
Family variables				
Communication with parents			−.04	−.04
Parental monitoring			4.169E-04	−.00
Parental attitude on sex			2.03E-04	−6.876E-04
Sexual attitude similar to siblings			−.05	−.05
Parental premarital sexual behavior			−.01	−.01
Relationship with parents			−.05	−.05
Interaction 3			−.06	−.06
Interaction 4			−.11	.11
Extra-family variables				
Peer influence				.01
Adjusted R^2	.53	.61	.61	.61

Note: Interaction 1 = (Respondent's attitude) × (Alcohol use); Interaction 2 = (Respondent's attitude) × (Religiosity); Interaction 3 = (Parental monitoring) × (Alcohol use); Interaction 4 = (Parental attitude about sex) × (Alcohol use).
*p < .05,   **p < .005,   ***p < .00005

were based on the studies in the early 1980s (e.g., Bock et al., 1983; Herold & Goodwin, 1981; Singh, 1980; Young, 1982).

Factors from the individual sphere, therefore, indicate that high-risk adolescents were more likely to have sexual experiences when they were involved in alcohol use and maintained permissive sexual attitudes.

Relationship Variables

In Model 2, each of the relationship variables significantly predicted adolescent sex, in addition to the variables from individual factors. Together these explained 61% of Korean adolescent sexual involvement. Dating mood was the variable that contributed most to the explained variance, with multiple R of .73. Dating mood is the most influential factor in explaining Korean adolescents' sexual behavior by solely explaining 54% of the variance ($F = 680.28$, $p < .00005$). Although, the effect of dating mood was reduced with other variables in the equation (Beta = .51, $p < .00005$), the F value for this variable was still the largest. However, the possibility of multicollinearity was found only in Model 1 in Table 2 (by the standard suggested in SPSS Base 8.0) (SPSS Base 8.0, 1998, p. 230).

Korean adolescents were greatly influenced by dating mood, that is, the more their mood was romantic, the more adolescents' sexual behavior was reported. This finding implies that adolescents may engage in impetuous sex rather than planned sex. This finding also suggests that, although an adolescent may not have planned to have sex while dating, he/she is more likely to engage in a sexual relationship if the mood or timing 'fit.' Thus, it may be more difficult to predict occurrences of adolescent sex in a dating situation than previously thought.

Love for partner was also a significant predictor of sexual experiences, though it showed that the relationship was not very strong (Betas = .07 ~ .08, $p < .05$). Adolescents who were in love with their partners showed some tendency to have a sexual experience with them.

The similarity of the adolescent's attitudes about sex with those of one's partner was a significant predictor (Beta = .09, $p < .005$) of sexual involvement. Thus, adolescents who had similar attitudes, presumably permissive attitudes, about sex with their partners tended to be more sexually involved.

Family Variables

None of the family variables emerged as significant predictors of sexual behavior among Korean adolescents, though the quality of their relationships with parents and having sexual attitudes similar to their siblings approached significance ($p = .0666$, $p = .0555$, respectively). Those who engaged in sexual activities were not likely to be influenced by communication with parents, the attitude of parents, parental monitoring, or parental premarital sexual behavior. Although the betas of all family variables showed a weak, negative influence on adolescents' sexual behavior, none of them achieved statistical significance.

Extra-Family Variable

Peer influence did not have a significant impact on Korean adolescents' sexual behavior. The effect of peer influence did not attain statistical significance as a predictor of adolescent sexual involvement.

Interactions and Sexual Behavior

The present study includes factors from individual, relational, family, and extra-family levels, and an analysis of prior studies raises the possibility that some factors may interact with each other in ways that may affect their influence on sexual behavior. Alcohol use, for example, may vary in combination with sexual attitude. For example, male students may interpret females' alcohol use as a willingness to get involved sexually on a date (Abbey & Harnish, 1995; George, Cue, Lopez, Crowe, & Norris, 1995). The results of this study show that the interaction between the respondent's attitude and alcohol use consistently had a significant impact on Korean adolescent sexual involvement (Betas = $-.61$, $-.71$, $-.66$, $-.68$, $p < .00005$) (Table 2). That is, adolescents with permissive sexual attitudes used more alcohol, and the combined effect functioned to increase the likelihood of engaging in sexual experiences.

Also, religious people usually hold a conservative sexual attitude, though, in this case, the interaction was not significant (see Table 2). A number of explanations are possible, with one being that religiosity may not function for adolescents as it does for persons at later stages of the life cycle.

Adolescents' alcohol use may vary by parental monitoring and also may differ by parental attitudes about sex. The use of alcohol also varied by gender (Tables 3 and 4) for Korean adolescents as a whole, but no significant interactions involving parental monitoring and parental attitude emerged. Overall, Interaction 1 was a significant predictor, which may reveal the general tendency for Korean adolescents' sexual experiences to be more strongly affected by individual and intimate factors than by other kinds of factors.

Gender Difference:
Individual Variables and Relationship Variables

To further investigate risk factors related to gender difference, stepwise regression analyses were conducted separately by gender. Dating mood, love for partner, similarity of sexual attitude between partners, alcohol use, and the interaction between parental attitude and alcohol use accounted for 65% of the variance for boys' sexual behavior in Model 4 (Table 3). The strongest predictor was dating mood, followed by alcohol use, the interaction between parental monitoring and alcohol use, love for partner, and similarity of sexual attitudes between partners. Dating mood had the strongest effect, solely explaining 57% of adolescent males' sexual behavior ($F = 367.52, p < .00005$). The beta for this predictor was reduced somewhat when other predictors were added, but the F value for dating mood was still the greatest. The possibility of moderate multicollinearity was not found in Models 2, 3 or 4.

As shown in Table 4, dating mood, alcohol use, and the interaction between parental attitude and alcohol use had similar effects for Korean female adolescents' sexual behavior. However, a respondent's attitude about sex and the interaction between respondent's attitude and alcohol use were factors salient only for females. Both of these predictors explained 61% of the variance for the sexual behavior of adolescent females. Dating mood explained 49% of the sexual behavior of adolescent females, though the beta was a bit reduced when other factors were included. In Models 2 and 3, a possibility existed for moderate multicollinearity to be an issue, though the condition indices are much lower than 30, the standard for serious collinearity concerns (see SPSS Base 8.0, 1998, p. 230). For both Korean male and female adolescents, dating mood was the most powerful predictor of sexual engagement.

Alcohol use was another strong significant predictor of the sexual behavior for both Korean adolescent males and females. Both Korean boys and girls who used alcohol, therefore, were equally more likely to be sexually experienced.

In Table 3, the interaction between respondent's attitude and alcohol use significantly affected Korean boys' sexual experience (Models 1, 2 in Table 3). However, its predictive power became insignificant with effects of family variables (Models 3, 4). On the contrary, in Table 4, the interaction had a consistently negative effect on females' sexual behavior. Korean adolescent girls' alcohol use changes much with their own sexual attitude.

Another gender difference was found in the respondent's attitude. While it had a consistent negative effect on females' sexual behavior, it consistently had no effect on males' sexual behavior. Female adolescents who held conservative attitudes about sex engaged in less sexual behavior than their male counterparts. Moreover, girls who had conservative sexual attitudes were significantly different from those who had permissive sexual attitudes in reference to sexual behavior ($F = 5.61, p < .05$). Such a finding suggests that girls who have conservative sexual attitudes may limit their opportunities to get involved in sexual relationships.

All of the relationship factors significantly predicted adolescent males' sexual behavior (Table 3), with dating mood being the strongest predictor for both males and females. In addition to dating mood, love for partner was a significant predictor of male adolescents' sexual experience, though, for females,

TABLE 3. Standardized Multiple Regression Coefficients Predicting Adolescent Males' Sexual Behavior

Variable	Model 1	Model 2	Model 3	Model 4
Individual variables				
Alcohol use	1.10****	.67****	.61****	.61****
Respondent's attitude	−.05	−.01	−.02	−.02
Religiosity	.03	5.433E-04	.01	.01
Age	.10**	.06	.07	.07
Interaction 1	−.40***	−.50****	−.21	−.21
Interaction 2	.01	−.00	.00	.01
Relationship variables				
Dating mood		.53****	.58****	.57****
Love for partner		.10*	.10*	.10*
Similarity of sexual attitude between partners		.11**	.09*	.10*
Family variables				
Communication with parents			−.00	−4.952E-04
Parental monitoring			−5.247E-04	−.00
Parental attitude on sex			−.03	−.03
Sexual attitude similar to siblings			−.00	−.00
Parental premarital sexual behavior			−.01	−.01
Relationship with parents			−.06	−.06
Interaction 3			−.15	−.15
Interaction 4			−.48****	−.48****
Extra-family variables				
Peer influence				−.01
Adjusted R^2	.55	.64	.65	.65

Note: Interaction 1 = (Respondent's attitude) × (Alcohol use); Interaction 2 = (Respondent's attitude) × (Religiosity); Interaction 3 = (Parental monitoring) × (Alcohol use); Interaction 4 = (Parental attitude about sex) × (Alcohol use).
*$p < .05$, **$p < .01$, ***$p < .005$, ****$p < .00005$

this variable did not quite reach statistical significance ($p = .0504$). Frequently, love has been considered a legitimate rationale for sexual involvement for girls in both Asian (Althaus, 1997; Yoon, 1995, results from university students) and Western cultures (Flores, Eyre, & Millstein, 1998). However, this factor was not as strong a predictor of sexual behavior by Korean adolescent females in this study as in other Western research.

Finally, the more that partners have similar sexual attitudes, the greater the likelihood that sexual experiences will result (Beta = .10, $p < .05$ for males;

TABLE 4. Standardized Multiple Regression Coefficients Predicting Adolescent Females' Sexual Behavior

Variable	Model 1	Model 2	Model 3	Model 4
Individual variables				
Alcohol use	1.74****	1.31****	.89****	.96****
Respondent's attitude[1]	−.13***	−.09*	−.10*	−.10*
Religiosity	−.00	−.02	−9.344E-04	.01
Age	.02	.02	.04	.04
Interaction 1	−1.17****	−1.12****	−.98****	−1.02****
Interaction 2	−.00	−.02	.00	.01
Relationship variables				
Dating mood[1]		.44****	.46****	.43****
Love for partner		.08*	.07	.08
Similarity of sexual attitude between partners		.03	.05	.05*
Family variables				
Communication with parents			−.04	−.04
Parental monitoring			−.00	−.00
Parental attitude on sex			.01	.01
Sexual attitude similar to siblings			−.07	−.07
Parental premarital sexual behavior			.01	.01
Relationship with parents			−.03	−.03
Interaction 3			.08	−.07
Interaction 4			.33***	.32**
Extra-family variable				
Peer influence				.03
Adjusted R^2	.53	.60	.61	.61

Note: Interaction 1 = (Respondent's attitude) × (Alcohol use); Interaction 2 = (Respondent's attitude) × (Religiosity); Interaction 3 = (Parental monitoring) × (Alcohol use); Interaction 4 = (Parental attitude on sex) × (Alcohol use).
*$p < .05$, **$p < .01$, ***$p < .005$, ****$p < .00005$
[1]Reported in Yoon, 2002b.

Beta = .05, $p < .05$ for females). This presumes, of course, that similarity in permissive sexual attitudes occurs, which inclines them to engage in sexual behavior.

Family and Extra-Family Variable

Family variables had only an indirect influence on both boys' and girls' sexual behavior through interaction effects. Although the interaction between alcohol use and parental attitude was a significant negative predictor of boys' sexual experience, this variable functioned as a positive predictor of girls' sexual experience. For example, when a Korean male adolescent who used alcohol had parents with a conservative sexual attitude, he was less likely to have sexual experience, whereas a Korean female adolescent was more likely to have sexual experience. The interpretation is complicated since girls whose parents' attitudes were more conservative were more active sexually. This result might be caused by the reaction against overly conservative parents.

For Korean adolescent females, holding a similar attitude on sex as their siblings had the effect of reducing sexual activity ($F = 3.05, p < .10$). Although it was not statistically significant at $p < .05$ level, it is worth noting the result that none of the family factors, except the interactions, were significant when additional factors were included in the analysis. Similarly, peer influence was not found to be as significant for males' or females' sexual behavior.

In sum, boys who had less sexual experience were less likely to be in a romantic mood during dating, less likely to love their partners, and less likely to use alcohol–three factors that influence the intimate sexual conduct of dating adolescents. Adolescent females with more sexual experience were more likely to be affected by dating mood and to use alcohol, whereas adolescent females having conservative sexual attitude were less likely to engage in sexual practices.

DISCUSSION

The present study explored factors that were potential predictors of Korean adolescents' sexual behavior, with the major result being that relationship and individual variables are better predictors of adolescents' sexual behavior than were family variables. Of particular interest is the influence of dating mood, which proved to be a substantial influence on the sexual behavior of Korean adolescents. The most sexually experienced boys and girls were more likely to have experienced romantic dating moods, thereby increasing the risk of being sexually involved. Surprisingly, boys were as likely as girls to be subject to dating mood.

One of most distinctive findings from the present study is that Korean adolescents were more likely to engage in sexual practices because of romantic dating mood, a neglected variable in previous research on adolescents' sexual behavior. The fact that dating mood explained 57% and 49% of the explained variance for boys' and girls' sexual behavior, respectively, may indirectly explain the nature of Korean adolescents' sexual interactions. Consistent with research in Western culture, adolescents' sexual behavior is unplanned

(Chilman, 1986) and is greatly influenced by the dating mood, rather than planning and commitment.

It has been suggested that high risk girls often begin solo dating considerably earlier than other peers (Pawlby, Mills, Taylor, & Quinton, 1997). Consistent with this result, the present findings indicate that Korean adolescent females at high risk were more likely to engage in sexual behavior when experiencing romantic dating moods, solo dating, and even when not being in love with their dating partners. Traeen and Kvalem's study (1996) reported that adolescents who had intercourse with their partners only once often engaged in intercourse unexpectedly, saying "it just turned out that way."

Love for partner in this study was significant only for adolescent males. Because previous research indicates that love plays an important role for adolescent females' sexual involvement (Traeen & Kvalem, 1996), the present results may reflect changing norms about sexual involvement for female adolescents today. Perhaps, for many Korean adolescent females, love may no longer be necessary to justify their sexual behavior. Girls who become sexually active may be inclined to do so regardless of being in love with their partners. Moreover, high risk females were more likely to be sexually involved when experiencing romantic moods and having sexually permissive attitudes.

The present findings which indicate that family variables do not encourage or inhibit adolescents' sexual behavior in Korea are surprising. Although frequently thought to be distinctive by its family-oriented and conservative sexual norms, these findings suggest that Korea may be rapidly changing. As Park (1986) shows, views held about the family by the younger generation of Korea seem to be different from those of the older generation. Moreover, the nature of parent-child relationships appears to be changing, with parents being less powerful agents in the transmission of family norms about sex to their adolescent offspring. Adolescents may not communicate with parents about issues related to sex, regardless of their level of sexual involvement. Not surprisingly, only 2.3% of adolescents in this study report that they had frequent communication about sexual issues with their parents. Adolescents of this generation tended to perceive that they discuss sexual issues with their mothers less than mothers perceive such discussions to occur (Jaccard, Dittus, & Gordon, 2000).

Although none of the family factors were significant predictors of Korean adolescents' sexual behavior, it is possible that parental influence may operate indirectly through various means, rather than directly through either communication or monitoring. In particular, the interaction between parental attitude and alcohol significantly affected the sexual behavior of both Korean adolescent males and females. For males, the interaction between parents' conservative sexual attitudes and alcohol use had a strong impact on reducing sexual behavior. Since alcohol use was a very influential predictor of adolescent males' sexual behavior, parents could exert parental values of sex indirectly, yet powerfully, on their adolescent child by disapproving of alcohol use. However, the interaction effect influenced adolescent females differently. The influence had the effect of increasing adolescent females' sexual activity. This result implies that a very conservative parental attitude on premarital sex functions negatively for adolescent females. When they perceive parental sexual attitude is too rigid or too strict, they may react to it in negative ways such as engaging in sexual behavior.

The contrasting results of the present study suggest that adolescents in Korea are using family norms and the traditional culture for making decisions about premarital sex less than in past times. Instead, adolescents are using their own and their partner's experience to guide their sexual experience while relying less on their parents' influence.

In terms of intervention implications, these findings suggest that sex education for children would be more effective and preventive if provided before the young reach their teenage years. Sex education during adolescence may less effective than it could be at an earlier age. Such an intervention approach is supported by the finding that adolescent females having conservative sexual attitudes were less likely to engage in sexual activity. The fact that adolescents' own sexual attitudes influenced their sexual behavior suggests that Korean sex education should focus on fostering conservative attitudes, both at early ages and during adolescence.

Another implication is that family influences and ties in Korea, especially those between parents and adolescents, seem to be waning. Korean parents should recognize this normative change that they, as parents, have less influence over their offspring's sexual behavior than in past times and take increased responsibility. As Korea undergoes rapid changes in sexual norms, it will require a lot of adjustment for parents as well as for adolescents.

Consistent with studies in the United States (Elliott & Morse, 1989; Ensminger, 1990; Larimer, Lydum, Anderson, & Turner, 1999), the present study found that male and female Korean adolescents who were using alcohol also tended to engage in more sexual activity. Adolescents who were under the influence of alcohol were more likely to experience sexual involvement, which was often linked to sexual assault (Abbey, McAuslan, & Ross, 1998; Muehlenhard & Linton, 1987).

The present study reveals two major findings that have potential implications for further research. The first is that none of the family and peer influences emerged as significant predictors of adolescent sexual behavior, especially in the presence other predictors that are tested simultaneously (Miller, 1998). Although this finding contradicts the common belief in Korea in which family concerns have priority over individual or social concerns, this finding is not surprising when the modern reality of family life in Korea is considered. What is obvious is that no longer do parents and family factors exert much influence on sexual behavior, at least for sexually active adolescents.

Another point is that although adolescent sexual behavior has been extensively studied in the United States, our understanding of how adolescents' sexual behavior occurs is still limited. The present study reveals that there is a strong association between dating mood and adolescents' sexual behavior for both males and females. The strongest influence of dating mood on adolescents' sexual behavior may be on the adolescents' perception of sexual encounter, namely, what the sexual encounter implies. Is it the beginning of a commitment relationship or just sex for the sake of pleasure (Traeen and Kvalem, 1996)? Obviously romantic dating mood, as the strongest predictor in this study, provides compelling sexual involvement of adolescents even when not being in love with the partner and should be considered in future research.

This study investigated factors associated with Korean adolescents' sexual activity. Given the dearth of available data in Korea, the present study identified factors, including a neglected variable, related to sexual behavior of Korean adolescents. Identifying what factors are associated with high sexual behavior, hence facilitating prevention of its occurrence, would be valuable to researchers and practitioners. Despite these strengths, there are limitations in this study. One limitation is that the nature of sex norm and behavior is culture-based, which makes it difficult to draw universal conclusions about the present study variables. Sex norms and sexual behavior cannot be interpreted separately from possible cultural variations. Another limitation is the possible social desirability of the sample. Given the sensitive issues of this study, it is possible that adolescents' sexual behavior could be somewhat underreported and that the actual occurrence is greater than reported.

However, these agendas are not limited to the present study but apply to studies of its kind. Nowadays adolescents' sexual behavior has become a universal phenomenon throughout the world and adolescents are so fast to take to modernized norms and culture that there is considerable convergence in adolescents' sexual behavior in Korean and Western societies. The present study explored factors related to sexual behavior among Korean adolescents. Our understanding of this phenomenon is still limited. More future studies are needed to delineate internal relations of factors related to Korean adolescents' sexual behavior.

REFERENCES

Abby, A. & Harnish, R. J. (1995). Perception of sexual intent: The role of gender, alcohol consumption and rape supportive attitudes. *Sex Roles, 32,* 297-313.

Abbey, A., McAuslan, P., & Ross, L. T. (1998). Sexual assault perpetration by college men: The role of alcohol, misperception of sexual intent, and sexual beliefs and experiences. *Journal of Social and Clinical Psychology, 17,* 167-195.

Abrahamse, A. F., Morrison, P. A., & Waite, C. J. (1988). Teenagers' willingness to consider single Japanese students do not have intercourse until after adolescence. *Family Planning Perspectives, 29,* 145-146.

Althaus, F. (1997). Most Japanese students do not have intercourse until after adolescence. *Family Planning Perspectives, 29,* 145-146.

Benda, B. B. & DiBlasio, F. A. (1994). An integration theory: Adolescent sexual contacts. *Journal of Youth and Adolescence, 23,* 403-420.

Bettor, L., Hendrick, S. S., & Hendrick, C. (1995). Gender and sexual standards in dating relationships. *Personal Relationships, 2,* 359-369.

Bock, E. W., Beeghley, L., & Mixon, A. J. (1983). Religion, socioeconomic status, and sexual morality: An application of reference group theory. *Sociological Quarterly, 24,* 545-559.

Boyer, C. B., Tschann, J. M., & Schafer, M. (1999). Predictors of risk for sexually transmitted diseases in ninth grade urban high school students. *Journal of Adolescent Research, 14,* 448-465.

Bronfenbrenner, U. (1986). Ecology of the family as a context for human development: Research perspectives. *Developmental Psychology, 22,* 723-742.

Buhrmester, D. (1992). The development courses of sibling and peer relationships. In F. Boer & J. Dunn (Eds.), *Children's sibling relationships: Developmental and clinical issues* (pp. 19-40). Hillsdale, NJ: Erlbaum.

Chilman, C. S. (1986). Some psychosocial aspects of adolescent sexual and contraceptive behaviors in a changing American society. In J. Lancaster & B. Hamburg (Eds.), *School-age pregnancy and parenthood: Biosocial dimensions* (pp. 191-218). New York: Aldine de Gruyter.

Choi, J. H. & Kim, M. G. (2001, February 23). The ruined adolescents (Second). *The Chosun Ilbo,* p. 31.

Chung, B. S. (1999, September 3). Bribe of drinking . . . prostitution . . . Bars that illegally employ minors are expanding their business. *The Choson Ilbo,* p. 31.

Chung, B. S. & Lee, G. S. (1999, September 4). Girls in uncontrolled service industries (2). *The Chosun Ilbo,* p. 33.

Cicirelli, V. G. (1994). Sibling relationships in cross-cultural perspective. *Journal of Marriage and the Family, 56,* 7-20.

Cicirelli, V. G. (1995). *Sibling relationships across the life span.* New York: Plenum.

Cohen, L. L. & Shotland, R. L. (1996). Timing of first sexual intercourse in a relationship: Expectations, experiences, and perceptions of others. *The Journal of Sex Research, 33,* 291-299.

Cupach, W. R. & Metts, S. (1995). The role of sexual attitude similarity in romantic heterosexual relationships. *Personal Relationships, 2,* 287-300.

Danziger, S. K. (1995). Family life and teenage pregnancy in the inner-city: Experiences of African-American youth. *Children and Youth Services Review, 17,* 183-202.

Davis, S. (1989). Pregnancy in adolescents. *Pediatric Clinics of North America, 36,* 665-680.

Day, R. D. (1992). The transition to first intercourse among racially and culturally diverse youth. *Journal of Marriage and the Family, 54,* 749-762.

East, P. L. (1996). The younger sisters of childbearing adolescents: Their attitudes, expectations, and behaviors. *Child Development, 67,* 267-282.

East, P. L., Felice, M. E., & Morgan, M. C. (1993). Sisters' and girlfriends' sexual and childbearing behavior: Effects on early adolescent girls' sexual outcomes. *Journal of Marriage and the Family, 55,* 953-963.

Elliott, D. B. & Morse, B. J. (1989). Delinquency and drug use as risk factors in teenage sexual activity. *Youth and Society, 21,* 32-60.

Ensminger, M. (1990). Sexual activity and problem behavior among black urban adolescents. *Child Development, 61,* 2032-2046.

Flores, E., Eyre, S. L., & Millstein, S. G. (1998). Sociocultural beliefs related to sex among Mexican American adolescents. *Hispanic Journal of Behavioral Sciences, 20*(1), 62-82.

George, W. H., Cue, K. L., Lopez, P. A., Crowe, L. C., & Norris, J. (1995). Self-report alcohol expectancies and postdrinking sexual inferences about women. *Journal of Applied Social Psychology, 25,* 164-186.

Handelsman, C. D., Cabral, R. J., & Weisfeld, G. E. (1987). Sources of information and adolescent sexual knowledge and behavior. *Journal of Adolescent Research, 2,* 455-463.

Herold, E. S. & Goodwin, M. S. (1981). Adamant virgins, potential non-virgins, and non-virgins. *Journal of Sex Research, 17,* 97-113.

Himelein, M. J., Vogel, R. E., & Wachowiak, D. G. (1994). Nonconsensual sexual experiences in precollege women: Prevalence and risk factors. *Journal of Counseling and Development, 72,* 411-415.

Hovel, M., Sipan, C., Blumberg, E., Atkins, C., Hofstetter, C. R., & Kreitner, S. (1994). Family influences on Latino and Anglo adolescents' sexual behavior. *Journal of Marriage and the Family, 56,* 973-986.

Hynie, M., Lydon, J. E., Cote, S., & Weiner, S. (1998). Relational sexual scripts and women's condom use: The importance of internalized norms. *The Journal of Sex Research, 35,* 370-380.

Inman-Amos, J., Hendrick, S. S., & Hendrick, C. (1994). Love attitudes: Similarities between parents and children. *Family Relations, 43,* 456-461.

Irwin, C. E., Jr. & Shafer, M. A. (1992). Adolescent sexuality: Negative outcomes of a normative behavior. In D. E. Rogers & E. Ginzberg (Eds.), *Adolescent at risk: Medical and social perspectives* (pp. 35-79). Boulder, CO: Westview Press.

Jaccard, J., Dittus, P. J., & Gordon, V. V. (1996). Maternal correlates of adolescent sexual and contraceptive behavior. *Family Planning Perspectives, 28,* 159-165, 185.

Jaccard, J., Dittus, P. J., & Gordon, V. V. (2000). Parent-teen communication about premarital sex: Factors associated with the extent of communication. *Journal of Adolescent Research, 15,* 187-208.

Kahn, J., Kalsbeek, W., & Hofferth, S. (1988). National estimates of teenage sexual activity: Evaluating the comparability of three national surveys. *Demography, 25,* 189-204.

Kim, K. S. (1998). The family value orientations among adolescent, middle, and old generation. *Journal of Korean Home Economics Association, 36,* 145-160.

Kim, K., Kim, O., & Yoon, S. (2001). Gender differences in the conception of love, sexual attitudes, and mate conditions of unmarried men and women. *Journal of Korean Home Economics Association, 35*, 15-30.

Kim, Y. H. (1989). Interrelationship between the juvenile delinquency and the couple relationship, parent-adolescent communication, and family functioning. Unpublished doctoral dissertation, Sookmyung Women's University, Seoul, South Korea.

Kinsman, S. B., Romer, D., Furstenberg, F. F., & Schwarz, D. F. (1998). Early sexual initiation: The role of peer norms. *Pediatrics, 102*, 1185-1192.

Larimer, M. E., Lydum, A. R., Anderson, B. K., & Turner, A. P. (1999). Male and female recipients of unwanted sexual contact in college student sample: Prevalence rates, alcohol use, & depression symptoms. *Sex Roles, 40*, 295-308.

Lee, I. S. (1994). A study on knowledge, attitude, experience in sex and the needs of sex education for college students. Unpublished master's thesis, Yonsei University, Seoul, South Korea.

Luster, T. & Small, S. A. (1994). Factors associated with sexual risk-taking behaviors among adolescents. *Journal of Marriage and the Family, 56*, 622-632.

Miller, B. (1998). *Families matter: A research synthesis of family influences on adolescent pregnancy.* Washington, D.C.: The National Campaign to Prevent Teen Pregnancy.

Moore, K. A., Peterson, J. L., & Furstenberg, F. F. (1986). Parental attitudes and the occurrence of early sexual activity. *Journal of Marriage and the Family, 48*, 777-782.

Muehlenhard, C. L. & Linton, M. A. (1987). Date rape and sexual aggression in dating situations: Incidence and risk factors. *Journal of Counseling Psychology, 34*, 186-196.

National Statistical Office (2000). *Annual report on the economically active population survey.* Seoul, Korea. National Statistical Office.

Park, H. S., Lee, J. S., Park, C. A., & Jeoung, M. J. (1995). Premarital sexual attitudes and behavior among the youth. *Journal of Korean Home Economics Association, 33*, 11-23.

Park, J. K. & Doh, H. S. (2001). The effects of maternal monitoring and information sources of maternal knowledge on externalizing and internalizing behaviors of adolescents. *Journal of Korean Home Economics Association, 39*, 129-140.

Park, S. Y. (1986). Relationships between mothers and daughters. *Journal of Korean Home Economics Association, 24*, 189-197.

Pawlby, S. J., Mills, A., Taylor, A., & Quinton, D. (1997). Adolescent friendships mediating childhood adversity and adult outcome. *Journal of Adolescence, 20*, 633-644.

Perkins, D. F., Luster, T., Villarruel, F. A., & Small, S. (1998). An ecological, risk-factor examination of adolescents' sexual activity in three ethnic groups. *Journal of Marriage and the Family, 60*, 660-673.

Pick, S. & Palos, P. A. (1995). Impact of the family on the sex lives of adolescents. *Adolescence, 30*, 667-675.

Plotnick, R. O. (1992). The effects of attitudes on teenage premarital pregnancy and its resolution. *American Sociological Review, 57*, 800-811.

Raffaelli, M., Bogenschneider, K., & Flood, M. F. (1998). Parent-teen communication about sexual topics. *Journal of Family Issues, 19*, 315-333.

Regan, P. C. & Berscheid, E. (1995). Gender differences in beliefs about the causes of male and female sexual desire. *Personal Relationships, 2*, 345-358.

Repke, J. T. (1990). Book reviews: Pediatric and adolescent gynecology. *The New England Journal of Medicine, 323*, 1213.

Sack, A. R., Keller, J. F., & Hinke, D. E. (1984). Premarital sexual intercourse: A test of the effects of peer group, religiosity, and sexual guilt. *The Journal of Sex Research, 20*, 168-185.

Santelli, J. S., Brener, N. D., Lowry, R., Bhatt, A., & Zabin, L. S. (1998). Multiple sexual partners among U.S. adolescents and young adults. *Family Planning Perspectives, 30*, 271-275.

Schreck, L. (1999). Adolescent sexual activity is affected more by mothers' attitudes and behavior than by family structure. *Family Planning Perspectives, 31*, 200-201.

Shon, H. S. (1995). A study on the main causes and prevention policy of unwed mother from the home-welfare view. *Journal of Korean Home Economics Association, 33*, 51-62.

Singh, B. K. (1980). Trends and attitudes toward premarital sexual relations. *Journal of Marriage and the Family, 42*, 387-393.

Small, S. A. & Eastman, G. (1991). Rearing adolescents in contemporary society: A conceptual framework for understanding the responsibilities and needs of parents. *Family Relations, 40*, 455-462.

Small, S. & Luster, T. (1994). Adolescent sexual activity: An ecological, risk-factor approach. *Journal of Marriage and the Family, 56*, 181-192.

Smith, C. A. (1997). Factors associated with early sexual activity among urban adolescents. *Social Work, 42*, 334-346.

Smith, E. R., Becker, M. A., Byrne, D., & Przybyla, D. P. J. (1993). Sexual attitudes of males and females as predictors of interpersonal attraction and marital compatibility. *Journal of Applied Social Psychology, 23*, 1011-1034.

Sprecher, S., Regan, P., McKenney, K., Maxwell, K., & Wazienski, R. (1997). Preferred level of sexual experience in a date or mate: The merger of two methodologies. *The Journal of Sex Research, 34*, 327-337.

SPSS (1998). *SPSS Base 8.0 Applications Guide.* Chicago, IL: SPSS, Inc.

Stuart, B., Rau, H., Fuhrer, N., & Hillebrand, H. (1996). Traditional ideology as an inhibitor of sexual behavior. *The Journal of Psychology, 130*, 615-626.

Sung, K. T. (1995). Korean's willingness to practice filial piety and generation gaps. *Journal of Korean Gerontological Society, 15*, 1-14.

Traeen, B. & Kvalem, I. L. (1996). Sexual socialization and motives for intercourse among Norwegian adolescents. *Archives of Sexual Behavior, 25*, 289-302.

Udry, J. R. & Billy, J. O. B. (1987). Initiation of coitus in early adolescence. *American Sociological Review, 52*, 841-855.

Werner-Wilson, R. J. (1998). Gender differences in adolescent sexual attitudes: The influence of individual and family factors. *Adolescence, 33*, 519-531.

Whitbeck, L., Hoyt, D., Miller, M., & Kao, M. (1992). Parental support, depressed affect, and sexual experiences among adolescents. *Youth and Society, 24*, 166-177.

Widmer, E. D. (1997). Influence of older siblings on initiation of sexual intercourse. *Journal of Marriage and the Family, 59*, 928-938.

Winslow, R. W., Franzini, L. R., & Hwang, J. (1992). Perceived peer norms, casual sex, and AIDS risk prevention. *Journal of Applied Social Psychology, 22,* 1809-1827.

The Women's News (1998, December 12). Rapid increase of unwed teenage pregnancy, *506,* 21.

Yang, M. (1996). A study on the values of marriage, child and sex role between male and female college students. *Journal of Korean Home Economics Association, 34,* 167-181.

Yoon, G. J. (1995). Factors related to sexual permissiveness among university students in Korea. *Journal of Korean Home Economics Association, 33,* 251-263.

Yoon, G. J. (2002a). The incidence and risk factors of adolescents' unwanted sexual behavior. *Journal of Korean Home Economics Association, 40,* 179-194.

Yoon, G. J. (2002b). The risk factors associated with adolescent females' sexual behavior. *Journal of Korean Home Economics Association, 40,* 107-121.

Young, M. (1982). Religiosity, sexual behavior, and contraceptive use of college females. *Journal of American College Health, 30,* 216-220.

Zabin, L. S., Smith, E. A., Hirsch, M. B., & Hardy, J. B. (1986). Ages of physical maturation and first intercourse in black teenage males and females. *Demography, 23,* 595-605.

Willingness and Expectations: Intergenerational Differences in Attitudes Toward Filial Responsibility in China

Heying Jenny Zhan

ABSTRACT. This paper explores intergenerational differences in attitudes toward willingness to and expectations for parent care based on survey data collected during 1997-1999 with 777 one-child generation students and 110 current familial caregivers. Findings suggest that current caregivers have very low expectations for their children's provision of elder care in the future. Children from one-child families experienced high levels of obligation to provide help although they expressed lower levels of willingness to co-reside with parents than did children from multiple-child families. Socialization factors, such as close contacts with grandparents, were negatively associated with one-child generation respondents' levels of personal obligation for parent care in the future. Structural factors, such as family income and respondents' educational levels, were important factors predicting student respondents' attitudes toward filial responsibility. The author argues that the culture of *xiao* is not declining; rather, the structural changes due to the one-child policy, increasing educational opportunity, and greater geographic mobility are going to have a greater effect on future elder care in China. *[Article copies available for a fee from The Haworth Document Delivery Service: 1-800-HAWORTH. E-mail address: <docdelivery@haworthpress.com> Website: <http://www.HaworthPress.com> © 2004 by The Haworth Press, Inc. All rights reserved.]*

Heying Jenny Zhan, PhD, is affiliated with the Department of Sociology, Georgia State University, 38 Peachtree Center Avenue, General Classroom Building 1041, Atlanta, GA 30303 (E-mail: sochjz@langate.gsu.edu).

http://www.haworthpress.com/web/MFR
© 2004 by The Haworth Press, Inc. All rights reserved.
Digital Object Identifier: 10.1300/J002v36n01_08

KEYWORDS. China, expectations, filial responsibility, willingness, one-child policy

INTRODUCTION AND BACKGROUND

The one-child policy in China, implemented in 1979, has been described as one of the "most significant and ambitious social experiments ever attempted in human history" (Ching, 1982; Falbo, Poston, Jiao, Jing, Wang, Yin, & Liu, 1989: 483). Despite its laudable goals of population control and raising per-capita living standards, unintended consequences of the policy have begun to emerge. The policy has exerted strains throughout China's social system, such as altering the family structure to a 4-2-1 (four grandparents, two parents, one child) inverted pyramid. This new family structure threatens a rupture of the tradition of filial piety crucial to familial elder care, imposes a daunting array of obligations upon the one-child generation, and raises questions even about the character and filial piety (*xiao*) of "only children." At the turn of the 21st century, as the first cohort of the one-child generation enter adulthood, many of their parents are caring for their dependent elderly grandparents. This paper explores familial and structural factors that influence the attitudes of filial responsibility between two generations: the middle-aged caregiver generation or the Chinese baby-boomers and the first maturing cohort of the one-child generation.

Studies About the Only Children

Ever since the implementation of the one-child policy, there has been great concern about any negative impact the policy might have on the development of only children (Bian, 1987; Chow & Zhou, 1996; Feng, 1992; Poston & Yu, 1985). However, there is a paucity of research on the implications for elder care and filial responsibility. On the one hand, studies concerning consequences of being an only child have mostly drawn samples from preschool or kindergarten children and have not addressed the adult issue of filial responsibility because the research subjects were too young (Chow & Zhao, 1996; Falbo & Poston, 1996; Poston & Falbo, 1990; Wu, 1996). On the other hand, studies of socialization and Chinese culture have yet to take into account the recent but widespread phenomenon of being an only child in contemporary urban China and any implications for familial elder care (Berndt, Cheung, Lau, Hau, & Lew, 1993; Ho 1989; 1994; Harwood, Giles, Ota, Pierson, Gallois, Ny, Lim, & Somera, 1996; Kelly & Tseng, 1992; Zhang & Bond, 1998).

As the only children mature and begin to face adult concerns, they also enter currents of rapid economic changes in China. Economic restructuring has increased income disparity in urban China. Having only one child has increased many urban families' financial well-being. Parents of the only children are found to be more eager to invest in children's education (Chow & Zhao, 1996). More and more children, especially those who are the only child in the family, are going to college and often moving out of their hometowns. Even girls in urban China are increasingly gaining equal access to higher education (Tsui & Rich, 2002). Increased family well-being and higher educational achievements of the only children, however, are not necessarily a positive factor for the future of elder care. As this first cohort of one-child generation reaches midlife, most will face the dilemmas of work and parental care. Having no siblings to assist them, a married couple (of two only children) might have to care for four elderly parents, possibly several grandparents, along with one or more of their own children. At present, as these only children come of age, their attitudes toward filial duties are influencing decisions about where to live and work. Their willingness as regards such responsibilities can help illuminate the future prospects for elder care in China. This study pioneers a consideration of how social and familial structural factors influence only children's attitudes toward filial responsibility. These factors include one-child status, family income, and educational levels.

Link Between Contacts with Elders and Attitudes Toward Elder Care

Although young adults' attitudes toward filial responsibility do not necessarily determine their actual commitment toward parental care in the future, research in the West, however, has shown evidence that contacts with grandparents in childhood can influence individuals' attitudes toward aging, elder care, and public policy on aging. Silverstein and Parrott (1997), in their study of attitudes toward public support of the elderly, found that greater childhood contact with grandparents had the effect of reducing young adults' opposition to aging policies, thus moderating age-group tension.

Several studies have found that young adults' knowledge of aging is positively related to their attitudes toward aging (Palmore, 1988; Duerson, Chang, & Stevens, 1992). However, Cummings, Kropt, and DeWeaver (2000: 87) suggest an opposite result, stating that "increased exposure due to caregiving demands may highlight the disabling effects of the aging process." Women who had "lived experience in dealing with their own ill older relatives" in particular tended to experience higher levels of anxiety and apprehension than men. Whether it is through knowledge, family contact, personal experience, and early exposure to grandparents in the family or other elders, more knowledge and contact with elders have been found to have an impact on a person's attitude toward aging and elder care in later life.

Early research on only children in China has consistently found that only children tend to live in urban areas where they generally do not live with their grandparents in the same household (Bain, 1987; Feng, 1992; Chow & Zhou, 1996; Poston & Yu, 1985). Does this lack of contact with grandparents among only children suggest a weakening socialization process in terms of filial responsibility? Do only children express lower levels of willingness to provide parental care due to their reduced contact with grandparents? The goal of this article is to explore the relationship between children's contact with grandparents and their attitudes toward filial responsibility in the Chinese context. Findings from this study will shed light on the importance of cultural socialization in shaping children's attitudes toward filial responsibilities among the first maturing cohorts of the only children.

Parents' Expectations in Relation to Children's Willingness in China

In a survey on elder care in Beijing, Xu (1994) found that few current caregivers expected that children would take care of them in their old age. They were already aware that it was somewhat unrealistic for them to hold on to such expectation as an absolute or dependable outcome. Only 10% of current caregivers interviewed expressed the desire to rely solely on children's support. The survey offered striking evidence that many current Chinese care givers have a bleak outlook as to their future elder care possibilities. Of those who were married, 24% actually marked euthanasia as a viable option, and among those already widowed, 41% gave a similar indication.

Treas and Wang (1993) found that there was an association between parents' expectations for filial responsibility and their description of children's actual filial behavior. They noted that elder parents who had higher expectations for support from their children reported their children providing more assistance, even when untrue. This finding offered an astounding example of the suggestibility of current care recipients or at least their concern with "saving face."

When the above finding is applied to the future of current caregivers as care recipients of care from the one-child generation, it points to a rather linear negative premise: When current caregivers have repeatedly expressed low expectations regarding their own elder care, their children, having heard these remarks, are likely to internalize them, thereby developing a lowered sense of obligation for providing parental care. Has the one-child generation in effect retained or lost the essential willingness to commit to and carry out filial responsibilities, especially in the face of the staggering challenges ahead? Or, have the prevalent social changes in economy, society, and family begun to irretrievably upset the social order so as to make the traditions of filiality and familial elder care less viable, less efficacious, and less likely? These have been some of the major questions that this study has tried to explore.

RESEARCH METHODS

Research Questions and Hypotheses

The central research questions addressed in this study are: Do current caregivers and the first cohort of one-child generation differ in their attitudes toward filial responsibilities? If so, what are the major familial and structural factors that explain the intergenerational differences? Specifically, is the one-child policy affecting the attitudes of these two generations in their attitudes toward parent care? Five conceptually different groups of hypotheses were formulated to explore the differences and their explanations. Each group of hypotheses contains an overarching hypothesis. The first hypothesis addresses the issue of intergenerational differences in attitudes toward filial responsibilities.

Hypothesis 1: There is a generational difference in attitudes toward parental care: Current caregiver respondents express lower expectations than one-child generation respondents in their willingness to accept filial responsibilities.

Among the one-child generational respondents, one would expect that all respondents would continue to express a similar level of filial respect since filial piety continues to be stressed in the family and the state and familial elder care continues to be the only option for parent care. However, the one-child status could influence respondents' attitudes toward more explicit parent care duties. One would expect, for example, being the only child can lead to greater pressure for them to work in order to make a living. Only child status can also possibly reduce levels of willingness to co-reside with parents, whether due to self-centeredness as some researchers claimed or due to increasing geographic mobility. Being an only child could lead her/him to become more aware of filial responsibilities earlier, thus feeling more obligated to take parent care responsibilities. Based on these understandings, the second hypothesis is proposed:

Hypothesis 2: There is a difference in attitudes toward filial responsibility between respondents from one-child and multiple-child families. Specifically, four aspects of this difference are explored: (a) There is no difference in the general attitude of filial respect between children from only-child and multiple-child families. (b) Respondents from one-child families express lower levels of willingness to sacrifice work for care than those from multiple-child families. (c) Respondents from one-child families express lower levels of willingness to co-reside with parents in the future than those from multiple-child families. (d) Respondents from only-child families repress higher levels of personal obligation to provide parent care than those from multiple-child families.

As the one-child policy was implemented at roughly the same time as economic reforms, one would expect income disparity and differing educational levels start to affect the maturing cohorts of the only children. The disparity between urban and rural residence is particularly evident in current China. The third hypothesis explores the impact of structural factors on different attitudes between only children and children with siblings. These factors include family income, respondents' educational level, and respondents' rural or urban residence.

Hypothesis 3: Structural conditions influence respondents' attitudes toward filial responsibility. Specifically, (a) respondents with higher educational level express lower levels of willingness to sacrifice career for parent care. (b) Respondents from higher income families show a greater willingness to make job and care adjustment. (c) Urban respondents express lower levels of willingness to co-reside with parents in the future.

In explaining the potential influences in only children's attitudes, co-residence with grandparents can be understood as one of the major family socialization factors; it may exert positive or negative influence in early childhood in their attitudes toward future filial responsibility. The fourth hypothesis explores the relationship between contacts with grandparents and attitudes toward parent care.

Hypothesis 4: More contacts with grandparents positively influence respondents' attitudes toward filial responsibilities. Specifically, (a) co-residence with grandparents enhances young adults' sense of obligation for parental care: Those who lived with grandparents express higher levels of personal obligation for parent care. (b) Those who lived with grandparents express greater willingness to co-reside with parents when their parents become older and dependent. (c) Those who had dependent grandparents in the household express higher levels of personal obligation for parent care. (d) Respondents who have more grandparents living in the same city or geographic area express higher levels of willingness to co-reside with parents in the future.

The actual co-residence between caregivers and care recipients could lead caregivers to similar expectations for their future care. One can assume that caregivers who provided more personal care for parents must have juggled work and care; therefore, they would also expect their own children to be willing to do the same for them. The next hypothesis explores the association between caregivers' behavior and their expectation for their own future care.

Hypothesis 5: Caregivers who are more involved in parent care express higher levels of expectation for their future care. Specifically, four aspects of the caregiving behavior are examined in relation to their care expectations: (a) Caregivers who lived with care recipients expressed higher levels of expectation for filial respect. (b) Caregivers who lived with their care recipients express higher levels of expectation for their future co-residence with their own children. (c) Caregivers who performed more personal care for their parents express higher expectations for their children to sacrifice work for care. (d) Caregivers who performed more personal care also express higher levels of personal obligation for parent care.

To explore these hypothetical questions, two sample data are used. Sample selection process and sample characteristics are described below.

METHODOLOGY

Data Collection Process

Structured survey interviews with 110 caregivers were administered in Chinese by the author during the fall of 1997 and 1998. To qualify for the study, caregivers had to be providing financial, physical, or emotional assistance to parents or parents-in-law on a regular basis, and the care recipients had to be in need of assistance with one or more activities of daily living (ADL) or instrumental activities of daily living (IADL). A snowball sampling method was used to identify the caregivers in Yiyang City, Hunan Province, and Baoding City, Hebei Province.

Most of the interviews were conducted in the caregivers' homes, although a few were conducted in the caregiver's workplace during lunch break or in an agreed-upon public meeting place. Each participant was given a questionnaire written in Chinese and asked to either complete the questionnaire or allow the investigator to read the questions and complete the form for the participant. Only 18 caregivers chose to complete the form themselves in the researcher's presence. Information collected through the interview process included basic demographic data, the health and functional status of the elder and the caregiver, caregivers' attitudes and beliefs about caregiving responsibilities, and the type and extent of assistance that the caregiver was providing to the parent or parent-in-law.

Data from 777 maturing one-child generation students were also collected during the same time period. All high school students were recruited from the same cities where caregivers were recruited. University students were found in colleges and universities located in these two provinces.[1] Structured survey questionnaires were distributed in 36 classrooms in 12 high schools, occupational schools, and universities. The researcher generally gave a brief self-introduction and a general description of the research before each survey. The response rate was 95%. Although the researcher stressed that students were free to leave anytime during the survey, few students actually did so, partially due to their curiosity about the survey, partially out of their respect toward the teacher who introduced the researcher. Twelve incomplete surveys were not analyzed.

Both Yiyang and Baoding are medium-sized cities located in the interior of China. These two cities were selected because they are smaller interior cites, which are not often studied but are representative of the locations where the majority of the interior urban population reside and work. It is in cities like these that the majority of Chinese who have experienced economic reforms and vigorous one-child family implementation still live in a relatively "traditional" style and where cultural norms and practices of elder care are more likely to remain relatively stable. Hence these samples provide an excellent opportunity to assess the influence of the one-child policy and economic reforms on the changing attitudes between the generations toward filial responsibilities.

Within the context of available resources it was not possible to obtain representative samples of either caregivers or students. However, an effort was made to select a sample that was sufficiently diverse in terms of the key independent variables for both samples. To maximize the variation of class status within the sample, the snowball process for caregivers and locations of high schools for students were initiated in four districts: factories, government, residential, and college/university localities. As most families still lived in apartments assigned by work units, though purchased by employees in the mid-1990s, this method facilitated the inclusion of respondents with very diverse backgrounds. There was little variation in ethnicity because the vast majority of urban dwellers in these cites are Han Chinese, as is true for most Chinese cities.[2]

Caregiver Characteristics

The demographic characteristics for both the elders and the caregivers included in the sample are shown in Table 1. The majority (68%) of caregivers in the sample were female. The caregivers ranged in age from 27 to 60 with the vast majority (86%) being between the ages of 30 and 49. All but seven of the caregivers were married. Fifty-six of the caregivers were daughters assisting parents, nineteen were daughters-in-law assisting parents-in-law, Thirty-three were sons assisting their parents, and two sons-in-law were primary caregivers for fathers-in-law.

Co-residence with parents or parents-in-law in this sample did not occur as frequently as in other studies, which have reported rates above 80 percent (Lavely & Ren, 1992). Nearly half of caregivers (46%) did not live with their care recipients. About a third (31%) of the caregivers lived with parents while 23 percent lived with parents-in-law. One of the major reasons for this difference in patterns of co-residence was that caregivers in this sample resided in urban interior China where elders were more likely to own apartments and live by themselves than is the case among rural elders.

The large majority (86%) of caregivers had at least a middle school education and the mean income was between 200 to 300 yuan (or $25-$35) per month. Nearly half (43.6%) of the interviewees reported that they were not working full-time. Most of these caregivers were laid off; however, a few reported going to the former workplace to register their presence but rarely obtained work. While most caregivers (66.4%) received no reimbursement for medical expenses or doctor visits, some reported that their hospitalization would be paid by the insurance company under the new insurance program.

Elder Characteristics

Different from the United States where most elders do not become physically dependent until after age 80, a large majority of Chinese elders in this sample (87.4% were physically dependent between ages 50-79. Just over half of the elders were married (54%), forty-seven (43%) were widowed, and the remaining four (4%) care recipients were divorced. However, three of the divorced elders were remarried. Nearly half (47.3%) of the care recipients had no formal education. The mean income for care recipients was between 100 to 200 yuan (or $15-$25) per month, which was generally lower than that of caregivers due to the lack of pensions. Almost two-thirds (63.6%) reported having no medical coverage. In most cases, even those elders who had medical coverage relied on their children for medicines, doctor visits, and/or hospitalization due to their own meager coverage.

One-Child Generation Student Sample

Among 777 students, 395 (50.8%) were male. There were 266 (34.2%) respondents from one-child families. Approximately one-quarter (23.7%) of respondents described themselves as the oldest child in the family.

TABLE 1. Characteristics of Elders and Caregivers (n = 110)

Variables	Elders		Caregivers	
	N	%	N	%
Sex				
Men	32	29.1	35	31.8
Women	78	70.9	75	68.2
Age				
20-29			3	2.8
30-39			47	43.1
40-49			47	43.1
50-59	4	3.6	11	10
60-69	46	41.9	1	.9
70-79	46	41.9		
80-89	13	11.8		
90 and above	1	.9		
Marital status				
Married	59	53.6	104	94.5
Widowed	47	42.7	1	.9
Divorced	4	3.6	4	3.6
Other (never married)			2	1.8
Relationship between caregiver and care recipient				
Daughters caring for parents			56	50.9
Daughters-in-law caring for parents-in-law			19	17.3
Sons caring for parents			33	30
Sons caring for fathers-in-law			2	1.8
Living arrangements				
With parents			34	30.9
With parents-in-law			25	22.7
Elders by themselves or alone			51	46.4
Individual income*				
None	36	33	5	7.4
Less than 200 yuan	28	25.5	23	21.5
201-400 yuan	28	25.5	39	35.5
401-600 yuan	17	15.5	41	37.3
Above 600 yuan	4	5.9	4	3.6
Educational levels				
No formal education	52	47.3	2	1.5
5 years or less	21	19.1	14	12.7
Middle school	10	9.1	34	30.9
High school	12	10.9	52	47.3
College	1	1.5	6	5.5
Beyond college	1	1.5	2	1.8
Medical bills reimbursed				
None	70	63.6	73	66.4
Some	40	36.4	37	33.6
Full-time employment				
Yes			61	55.5
No			48	43.6

*At the current rate, 100 yuan equals roughly $12.

Respondents' age in the sample ranged from 16-25 (see Table 2). There were 328 (42.2%) students from high schools or occupational and technical schools. The remainder were university students. This sample excluded non-students of this cohort because of difficult access. However, students from high schools, occupational schools, and universities represented above 90% of this cohort population in urban China. The drop-out rates from junior high schools were relatively low, for example, between 3-8% in Yiyang in 1997. Although the sample is mostly urban (81.6%), it did include 142 students from rural backgrounds.

The majority (66.3%) of the respondents had no grandparents living in the same household. Around one-third (33.7%) of the students reported sharing the same household with their grandparents. Only children in this study did not live with their grandparents in the same household as often as the multiple children. While nearly 40% of children from multiple-child families had grandparents living in the same household, only 23% of only children shared the same household with their grandparents.

Instruments

The measurements of filial responsibility, which were used as predictor variables, were built on the work of Harwood et al. (1996) and Ho (1994). Their measures have been applied in eight countries in the Pacific Rim. Measures used in this sample consisted of 11 items representing 4 different aspects of respondents' attitudes toward filial responsibility: filial respect (5 items), job and care conflict (2 items), co-residence (1 item), and personal obligation (3 items). For the first three measures, respondents in the student sample were asked the lead-in sentence, "When your parents become older and physically dependent, are you willing to. . . ." For current caregivers, they were asked, "When you become older and physically dependent, do you expect your child[ren] to. . . ." Personal obligation measures consisted of three items, testing the respondents' extent of internalization of social norms as personal obligations. Respondents used a 5-point response set ranging from strongly disagree (= 1) to strongly agree (= 5) with 3 being ambiguous.

Factor analysis with varimax rotation was used to examine the dimensionality of the measures. Reliability levels of these measures in the student sample were .68 for filial respect, .72 for job and care conflict, and .68 for personal obligation. Reliability levels for the caregiver sample were .76, .62, and .74, respectively. The measure for co-residence was a straightforward question, asking the respondent whether they were willing/expect to live in the same house with their parents/children.

TABLE 2. Characteristics of School Children

Variables	N	%*
Age		
Born in or after 1979	411	53.8
Born before 1979	353	44.5
Gender		
Male	395	50.8
Female	378	48.6
The only child in the family		
Yes	266	34.2
No	511	65.8
Number of siblings in the family		
None	266	34.2
One	167	21.5
Two	199	25.6
Three	106	13.6
Four	28	3.6
Five or more	9	1.2
Number of grandparents in the same household		
None	515	66.3
One	133	17.1
Two	104	13.4
Three	11	1.4
Four	12	1.5
Number of grandparents in the same city		
None	227	29.2
One	118	15.2
Two	175	22.5
Three	64	8.2
Four	186	23.9
Number of grandparents who are physically dependent		
None	590	75.9
One	133	17.1
Two	37	4.8
Three	7	.9
Four	9	1.2
Educational level		
Second year in high school	114	14.7
Third year in high school	214	27.5
First year in college	290	37.3
Second year in college	151	19.4
Parents' per capita monthly income		
0-200 yuan	83	10.7
201-400 yuan	149	19.2
401-600 yuan	205	26.4
601-800 yuan	150	19.3
801-1000 or above	74	9.5
Above 1000	102	13.1
Area of study or interest		
Science/engineering	434	56.4
Liberal arts and humanities	336	43.6
Being urban or rural		
Urban	625	81.6
Rural	141	18.4

*Percentages may not sum to 100% due to missing data.

Compository independent variables in the caregiver sample included caregiver's personal care, instrumental care, and monetary assistance. The measure of personal care captured the frequency with which a caregiver assisted an elder with six tasks: bathing, shaving, changing, daily laundry, toilet usage, and handling daily bills. Caregivers used a 5-point response set that ranged from once a month to everyday to respond to these items. The six-item composite score had an internal reliability score of .91.

Instrumental care was measured with 5 items, including assistance with visiting friends and families, finding maids or home care services, changing bandages or cleaning wounds, going to the hospital, and going to drug stores. The reliability level for these items was .88.

Level of financial assistance was measured by the amount of money caregivers spent on food, clothing, medicine, doctor's visits, home care, and hospitalization for one's relative. Respondents used a five-point response set ranging from "the elder pays it all" to "we pay it all" to answer these questions. The Cronbach's alpha for financial assistance was .98.

Data Analysis

Two t-tests were used to test mean differences between only children and non-only children in their attitudes and between student respondents and caregiver respondents. To understand factors that associate with these differing attitudes, bivariate analyses were conducted to examine the correlations among all the variables used in the study (these tables are not included in this paper due to space limitations). Finally, statistically significant and theoretically important factors were selected for multivariant regression analyses to explore factors that influence respondents' attitudes toward filial responsibility.

FINDINGS

Differences in Attitudes Between the Generations

Data on intergenerational differences in attitudes toward filial responsibility are shown in Table 3. In every category, caregivers are shown to express lower levels of expectations than the one-child generation respondents' expression of willingness. This finding supports Hypothesis 1.

Differences in Attitudes Between Children from One- and Multiple-Child Families

In comparing the levels of expressed willingness between children from one-child and multiple-child families, only children were not found to express lower levels of willingness toward general levels of filial respect. This finding supports Hypothesis 2a.

Only children were not found to express lower levels of willingness to sacrifice job for parent care. This result rejects Hypothesis 2b. Only children, however, did express lower levels of willingness to co-reside with parents. This research result supports Hypothesis 2c.

Only children also expressed higher levels of personal obligation for parent care. This finding supports Hypothesis 2d.

Overall, there are differences in attitudes toward filial responsibility between children from one- and multiple-child families. These differences are shown in their felt sense of obligation and their levels of willingness to co-reside with parents in the future. These findings support Hypothesis 2.

Explaining Attitudinal Differences: Structural Factors

Among the three structural factors, educational level was found to be an important factor negatively associated with student respondents' level of willingness toward job and care conflict and co-residence, but positively associated with filial respect (see Table 4). In other words, although student respondents with higher educational level expressed higher levels of willingness to fulfill general duties of filial respect, they scored lower on levels of willingness to sacrifice work for care and to live under the same roof with parents. These findings support Hypothesis 3a.

Parents' income was found to be positively associated with both measures of filial respect and job and care conflict. Respondents from families with higher incomes expressed higher levels of willingness to accept general levels of filial responsibility and to juggle work and care in the future. These findings support Hypothesis 3b.

There is no difference found between urban and rural respondents in their attitudes toward filial responsibilities. Hypothesis 3c is rejected.

Overall, structural factors, particularly income and educational levels, are found to be important in predicting student respondents' attitudes toward future commitment of elder care. These findings support Hypothesis 3.

Explaining Attitudinal Differences: Socialization

Contacts with grandparents are often viewed as major socialization factors in instilling traditional attitudes of filial piety. In this study, co-residence with grandparents was negatively associated with student respondents' expression of personal obligation toward filial responsibility: Respondents who lived with grandparents scored lower in their obligation

TABLE 3. Test of Mean Differences Between Generations and Between Only and Non-Only Children

Variables	Current Caregivers		One-Child Generation Students				Only Children		Non-Only Children		
	Mean	S.D.	Mean	S.D.	d.f.	t-value	Mean	S.D.	Mean	S.D.	d.f.	t-test
Filial respect	3.61	3.32	4.10	3.02	880	−7.8***	4.15	2.96	4.09	3.11	775	1.23
Job and care conflict	1.89	1.40	2.85	2.05	884	−9.48***	2.79	2.02	2.88	2.07	774	1.25
Co-residence	2.84	1.15	3.37	1.06	882	−4.878***	3.21	1.95	3.45	1.05	772	−2.90**
Personal obligation	4.14	1.69	4.51	1.77	883	−6.14***	4.61	1.70	4.46	1.79	774	3.45***

***p < .001; **p < .01. Coded as: Current caregivers = 1; one-child generation students = 0; only children = 1; non-only children = 0

scales. This finding rejects Hypothesis 4a. Interestingly, having grandparents residing in the same household was not statistically significant in its association with respondents' willingness to co-reside with parents. This finding rejects Hypothesis 4b.

Student respondents who had dependent grandparents in the same household expressed lower levels of personal obligation toward parent care. This finding rejects Hypothesis 4c. Having more grandparents living in the same city was found to be positively related to respondents' levels of willingness to co-reside with parents. This finding supports Hypothesis 4d.

Contrary to socialization theory, findings in this study indicate that more direct contacts with grandparents were negatively associated with young adult respondents' attitudes toward filial responsibilities. Relatively distant and irregular contact, such as having more grandparents living in the same city or geographic district, seem to have positive effect on young adults' level of willingness to co-reside with parents.

Caregivers' Care Involvement and Expectations

Table 5 shows the multiple regression results of current caregivers' attitude toward filial responsibility. The goal is to explore the association between current care involvement and expectations for future care.

Current caregivers who lived with their parents did express higher expectations for filial respect from their own children. This finding supports Hypothesis 5a. Caregivers who co-resided with their elder parents did not express higher levels of expectations for their future co-residence with their own children; this finding rejects Hypothesis 5b. Caregivers who performed more personal care for physically dependent parents were found to express higher expectations for their own children's willingness to sacrifice work for parent care. This finding supports Hypothesis 5c. Finally, caregivers who performed more personal care were not expressing higher levels of personal obligation for parent care; rather, they expressed lower levels of personal obligation. This finding rejects Hypothesis 5d.

Overall, findings in this study indicate that caregivers' greater involvement in parent care is positively associated with their greater expectations for future elder care only in general aspects. Few current caregivers expected to co-reside with their children in the future whether or not they currently co-resided with their care recipients or were heavily involved in personal care activities. These findings only partially support Hypothesis 5.

TABLE 4. Standardized Regression Analysis of One-Child Generation Students' Attitude Toward Filial Responsibilities

Variables (N = 777)	(A) Filial Respect				(B) Job-Care Conflict				(C) Co-Residence				(D) Obligation			
	Step 1	2	3	4	1	2	3	4	1	2	3	4	1	2	3	4
Only-child	.04	.03	.05	.07	-.07	-.07	-.09*	.01	-.11**	-.11**	-.13**	-.06	.09*	.09*	.11*	.14*
Being female	.04	.03	.03	.03	.05	.06	.05	.05	-.02	-.01	-.01	-.01	.08*	.08*	.08*	.07
Educational level	.09	.09*	.09*	.10*	-.15***	-.15***	-.15***	-.17***	-.13***	-.12**	-.16**	-.17**	.07	.07	.07	.09
Parents' income	.08	.08*	.09*	.09*	.15***	.15***	.15***	.15***	-.05	-.05	-.05	-.05	-.00	-.00	-.00	-.00
Urban area	-.00	-.01	-.01	-.01	-.02	-.01	-.01	-.01	.02	.04	.04	.04	.04	.04	.04	.04
Major	.01	.01	.01	.01	-.02	-.02	-.02	-.02	.02	.02	.01	.02	-.05	-.05	-.05	-.05
Share house w/ GP		-.04	-.03	-.03		.05	.03	.03		.05	.02	.02		-.16	-.14***	-.14***
Same city w/ GP		.02	.02	.02		.01	.02	.01		.08*	.09*	.09*		.06	.06	.06
No. of dependent GP		.02	.01	.01		.05	.05	.04		-.03	-.03	-.03		-.11	-.11**	-.11**
Only child X co-residence			-.03	-.03			.05	.05			.06	.06			.04	.04
Born in/after 1979				.04				.03				-.03				.05
Only child X born in/after 1979				-.04				-.14*				-.10				-.05
R square	.020	.022	.022	.023	.047	.052	.054	.060	.03	.04	.04	.05	.026	.064	.065	.066
R square change		.002	.000	.001		.005	.002	.006		.01	.00	.01		.038	.001	.001

***p < .001; **p < .01; †p < .05

355

DISCUSSIONS

Intergenerational Differences: Is the Culture of Filiality Declining?

Data in this study show significant differences in attitudes toward filial responsibilities between the two generations. It can be argued that current caregivers may express low expectations for their own care due to their personal experience of the demand and strain of such care; young adults are more likely to express high levels of willingness because parent care is still a distant concept and they have no specific knowledge of what care may entail. However, the reverse can also be argued: Current caregivers may express high levels of expectations from their own children due to the fact they are performing such care for their own parents. The logic goes, if we can do it for our parents, they can do it for us. And young adults may express low levels of willingness because they are too young to take the issue seriously. These speculations obviously are too general to make sense without specific cultural and social contexts.

In the cultural specific context of China, the cultural norm of *xiao* may be the major explanation for parent elder care. The argument, then, would be: If *xiao* is properly maintained, the young will fulfill the filial duties in the same way as their parents' generation. The implication of this argument is that if the young do not express a similar level of filial responsibility, then, it must be due to the decline of the culture because of socialization or social change. Data in this study showed that the young generation expressed higher levels of willingness to accept filial responsibility than the current caregivers' expectations in all categories ($p < .001$). These findings suggest that the culture of *xiao* is not declining; rather, the one-child generation youth still firmly uphold the tradition. The average mean scores for one-child generation respondents' levels of willingness to show filial respect and personal obligation are 4.10 and 4.51, respectively, compared to 3.61 and 4.10 for the caregivers in their expectations. One-child generation respondents also expressed higher levels of willingness in sacrificing job for care and in co-residence (2.85 and 3.37) compared to the caregivers' expectations (1.89 and 2.84), although these scores were lower for both groups in comparison to the attitudes toward general cultural norms, such as filial respect and personal obligations. Together, these results suggest that cultural indoctrination of filial responsibilities is not declining from one generation to the other. Instead, one-child generation youth continue to hold onto the cultural norms and obligations.

The question arises, then: Do all one-child generation students share similar attitudes toward cultural norms and obligations? Is there any difference between children from one-child and multiple-child families in their attitudes

TABLE 5. Standardized Regression Analysis of Caregivers' Attitude of Filial Responsibility on Family Background and Care Tasks

Variables	(A) Filial Respect			(B) Job-Care Conflict			(C) Co-Residence			(D) Obligation		
	1	2	3	1	2	3	1	2	3	1	2	3
Family Background Variables												
Elder's gender (female)	-.33	-.27	-.27	-.02	-.06	-.13	-.13	-.16	-.13	-.21*	-.24	-.17
Caregivers' gender (female)	.18	.18	.16	-.04	.02	.03	.05	.08	.07	.20*	.17	.16
Elders' marital status (widowed)	.23*	.22*	.16	.04	-.01	.05	.11	.08	.08	-.05	-.01	-.07
Co-reside with parents	.26**	.22*	.26**	.30**	.25*	.23*	.09	.06	.06	.07	.14	.16
Family Structural Resources												
Caregivers' educational level		-.20*	-.16		-.19	-.15		-.11	-.10		.26*	.23*
Caregivers' monthly income		.020	.04		.11	.02		.05	.08		-.09	.00
Elders' monthly pension		.080	.09		-.03	.04		-.02	-.09		-.03	-.11
Number of care assistance		-.14	-.16		.15	.14		.10	.11		.05	.07
Care Task Performance												
Personal care			-.13			.28*			-.05			-.26*
Instrumental care			.23*			-.11			.15			.17
Monetary assistance			.13			.04			-.10			-.06
R square	.18	.24	.30	.10	.16	.22	.03	.05	.07	.08	.14	.21
R square change		.06	.06		.06	.06		.02	.02		.06	.07

*p < .05; **p < .01

357

toward their future filial responsibility? If so, what are the differences and why?

One-Child Status and Attitudes Toward Filial Responsibilities

As shown in the t-test of mean difference in attitudes toward filial responsibilities between only and non-only children, no statistically significant difference was found in their expressions of filial respect and willingness to sacrifice work for care. Only children, however, were found to express higher levels of personal obligation for parent care, yet lower levels of willingness to co-reside with parents.

When controlling for other familial background variables, although the negative association between only children and co-residence was no longer significant, only-child status continues to be a statistically significant factor in the expression of personal obligation toward filial responsibilities. Also, only children born after the one-child policy imple- mentation expressed lower levels of willingness to adjust jobs for parent care. These results may suggest that only children in general are not necessarily less culturally indoctrinated about their filial responsibilities in parent care than children from multiple-child families. They expressed similarly high levels of willingness in filial respect. However, their expression of higher levels of obligation may suggest that only children have already felt the eventual pressure of financial and physical provision for their parents. Being the only child in the family, they may indeed feel more obligated to take care of their parents; and yet, they, especially those born after the one-child policy, cannot afford giving up their jobs in order to support themselves as well as their family. These only children seem to be expressing a clear understanding of the pressures to be placed upon them at both social and familial levels.

Explaining Attitudinal Differences: Structural Factors

The negative associations between educational level and job-care conflict as well as co-residence are rather troubling. As more Chinese youth are going to colleges or even graduate schools, their commitment to parent care is likely to become secondary to their career. Especially when girls in one-child families gain increasing access to higher education in urban China, as found in a recent study (Tsui & Rich, 2002), the gendered cultural expectation for daughters or daughters-in-law to take care of dependent parents may be expected to change. As more and more urban women choose to pursue careers, they may well become physically or geographically unavailable for parent care in the future.

der care, then, comes down to redefinitions of "familial" or "filial" responsibilities.

Such a redefinition should probably be multitiered. The process should involve a major increase in various service options for elder care, government provision of a basic safety net for the elders, and financial compensation for familial elder care. Service options would allow only-child families to purchase care for physically dependent older parents. Government provision of a safety net allows elders more independence and relieves some of the burden from the younger generation. Financial compensation for familial elder care will allow one-child families to continue the care for parents while sustain a living wage. These measures would allow familial and filial responsibilities to adapt to the pressures of social change in China, while maintaining an important semblance of essential cultural integrity.

NOTES

1. These two cities have only junior colleges and occupational schools (like small-town colleges in the United States); there are certainly enough students in number, but these students probably have little variance in their "willingness" and "obligation," and probably have few opportunities to work outside the same city after graduation. Therefore, I chose to select students in the larger geographic location although in the same province in order to provide greater diversity.

2. Han Chinese are the vast majority (above 90%) of the Chinese population. Because they represent the largest ethnic group, typically the adjective "Han" is not noted. Other ethnic groups include the Tibetans, Mongols, and Manchus.

REFERENCES

Berndt, T. J., Cheung, P. C., Lau, S., Hau, K. T., & Lew, W. (1993). Perceptions of parenting in mainland China, Taiwan, and Hong Kong: Sex differences and social differences. *Developmental Psychology, 29,* 156-164.

Bian, Y. (1987). A preliminary analysis of the basic features of the lifestyles of China's single child families. *Social Science in China, 2,* 189-209. [in Chinese].

Ching, C. C. (1982). The one-child family in China: The need for psychosocial research. *Study of Family Planning, 13,* 208-214.

Chow, E. N. & Zhao, S. M. (1996). The impact of one-child policy on parent-child relations in the People's Republic of China. *The International Journal of Sociology and Social Policy, 16,* 35-62.

Cummings, S. M., Kropf, N. P., & DeWeaver, K. L. (2000). Knowledge of and attitudes toward aging among non-elders: Gender and race differences. *Journal of Women and Aging, 12,* 77-91.

Duerson, M., Thomas, J. W., Chang, J., & Stevens, C. B. (1992). Medical students' knowledge and misconceptions about aging: Response to Palmore's facts on aging quizzes. *The Gerontologist, 32,* 171-174.

Falbo, T. & Poston D. L. (Eds.). (1996). *Zhongguo Dushen Zinu Yanjiu (Research on Single Children in China)*. Shanghai: Huandong Shifan Daxue Chubanshe (East China Normal University Press).

Falbo, T., Poston, D.L., Ji, G., Jiao, S., Jing, S., Wang, G., Gu, H., Yin, H., & Liu, Y. (1989). Physical, achievements, and personality characteristics of Chinese children. *Journal of Biosocial Science, 21*, 483-495.

Feng, X. T. (1992). Social characteristics of single-child families in urban China. *Sociological Studies, 1*, 108-116. [in Chinese].

Harwood, J., Giles, H., Ota, H., Pierson, H. D., Gallois, C., Ny, S. H., Lim, T. S., & Somera, L. (1996). College students' trait ratings of three age groups around the Pacific Rim. *Journal of Cross-Cultural Gerontology, 11*, 1-11.

Ho, D. Y. F. (1994). Filial piety, authoritarian moralism, and cognitive conservatism in Chinese societies. *Genetic, Social, and General Psychology Monographs, 120*, 347-365.

Ho, D. (1989). Continuity and variation in Chinese patterns of socialization. *Journal of Marriage and Family, 51*, 149-163.

Kelly, M. L. & Tseng, H. M. (1992), Cultural differences in child rearing: A comparison of immigrant Chinese and Caucasian American mothers. *Journal of Cross-Cultural Psychology, 23*, 444-455.

Lavely, W. & Ren, X. (1992). Patrilocality and early marital co-residence in rural China, 1955-1985. *The China Quarterly, 127*, 594-615.

Palmore, E. B. (1988). *The facts on aging quiz*. New York: Springer Publishing Company.

Poston, D. L. & Falbo, T. (1990). Academic performance and personality traits of Chinese Children: 'Onlics versus others.' *American Journal of Sociology, 96*, 433-51.

Poston, D. L. & Yu, M. Y. (1985). Quality of life, intellectual development and behavioral characteristics of only children in China: Evidence from a 1980 survey in Changsha, Hunan Province. *Journal of Biosocial Science, 17*, 127-136.

Silverstein, M. & Parrott, T. (1997) Attitudes toward public support of the elderly: Does early involvement with grandparents moderate generational tensions? *Research on Aging, 19*, 108-132.

Treas, J. & Wang, W. (1993). Of deeds and contracts: Filial piety perceived in contemporary Shanghai (pp. 87-98). In V. L. Bengtson & W.A. Achenbaum (Eds.), *The changing contract across generations*. New York: Aldine De Gruyter.

Tsui, Ming & Rich, L. (2002). The only child and educational opportunity for girls in urban China. *Gender and Society, 16*, 74-92.

Wu, D. Y. H. (1996). Parental control: Psychocultural interpretations of Chinese patterns of socialization (pp. 1-28). In S. Lao (Ed.), *Growing up the Chinese way: Chinese child and adolescent development*. Hong Kong: The Chinese University Press.

Xu, Q. (1994). Status quo and problems of old age support by youth and adult within the family. *Sociological Research, 4*, 80-84.

Zhang, J. & Bond, M. H. (1998). Personality and filial piety among college students in two Chinese societies: The added value of indigenous construct. *Journal of Cross-Cultural Psychology, 29*, 402-417.

PART III

MACRO-LEVEL INFLUENCES ON PARENT-YOUTH RELATIONS

Introduction:
Macro-Level Influences
on Parent-Youth Relations

Gary W. Peterson
Suzanne K. Steinmetz
Stephan M. Wilson

The articles in this final section tend to examine how macro-level societal variables from different cultural traditions may have socialization consequences for parents and youth within families. As in previous sections, the articles in this collection originate from a diversity of societies. Characteristic of this selection, however, is a focus on the consequences of economic, political, and social belief systems from different societies that may shape the dynamics and consequences of the parent-youth relationship. Some societies, for example, are characterized by policies, economic practices, and cultural belief systems that are consistent with and encourage individualism, which is typical of the United States and, perhaps to a lesser extent, Mexico. Other societies represented in the papers of this section are characterized by a broader range of centrally developed policies and a focus on collectivism such as Cuba, or the kibbutzim in Israel. Finally, other studies examine samples from countries, such as China, that appear to be in transition from collectivism to a more individualistic or globalized system of cultural values for guiding socialization processes.

Esteinou, in her article "Parenting in Mexican Society," notes that the family has been of central significance to Mexican society, but ironically has received little formal scholarly attention by Mexican scholars. This pattern is even more evident in the paucity of work on Mexican parent-child/adolescent relations. Esteinou argues that the recent revival of interest in studying the Mexican family and parent-youth relations reflects the growing realization by

http://www.haworthpress.com/web/MFR
© 2004 by The Haworth Press, Inc. All rights reserved.
Digital Object Identifier: 10.1300/J002v36n03_01

Mexican scholars of the substantial socio-demographic changes that are occurring within Mexico. Specifically, she describes how substantial economic forces, labor market restructuring, demographic changes, and social-cultural transitions associated with modernization and globalization may be contributing to substantial change in Mexican families and parent-child relationships. These changes in macro-level forces have resulted in a growing emphasis on individualism which, in turn, may be altering family structures and processes in the direction of more democratic childrearing patterns, with fathers taking a more active role in parenting. Esteinou also shows how these macro-level forces of societal change may have differential influence on various Mexican sub-populations that vary in the extent to which they are responding to the forces of change or maintaining traditional patterns.

Noack and Buhl in their article entitled "Relations with Parents and Friends During Adolescence and Early Adulthood" examine conflict, power and intimacy among German high school (*Gymnasium*) students and their mothers, fathers, and best friends. Major findings of this study consist of age-graded patterns suggesting increases in the relative power of young people within families accompanied by comparably low rates of conflict. Likewise, the postulated differences between parent and peer relations were confirmed by their analyses. In particular, the balanced distribution of power between same-age friends provided a sharp contrast with the more hierarchical situation within the adolescents' families. These patterns were consistent with a strong societal emphasis on individualism and displayed considerable similarities with research on students in the U.S. Overall, the results of this study were consistent with individuation theory, the perspective providing the basis for the study's hypotheses.

In their article "Korean-American Mothers' Experiences in Facilitating Academic Success for Their Adolescents," Yang and Rettig examine how Korean-American mothers adapt traditional Korean values to contemporary American values about academic success for their children. For these mothers, their traditional values led them to identify admission to an Ivy league university in the U.S. as a primary indicator of being a successful parent. Using a qualitative research strategy, the authors demonstrate how this Korean ideal of academic success is in conflict with both the American definitions of academic success and the more democratic childrearing strategies used to encourage this ideal. Specifically, European-American parents tend to support a more integrative definition of academic success involving a balance of cognitive achievement and participation in school activities. This study demonstrates how Korean mothers eventually came to terms with these expectations and made adjustments to the majority culture by accepting the child's new standards for performance and changed their socialization approaches to acknowledge this.

In "Sex Differences and Conjugal Interdependence on Parenthood Stress and Adjustment: A Dyadic Longitudinal Chinese Study," Lu explores sex differences and conjugal interdependence in the stress and adjustment of young Chinese fathers and mothers during the transition to parenthood. The results show that (a) wives report heightened stress, worse health, and lower marital satisfaction than husbands during the transition to parenthood. Moreover, a substantial degree of conjugal interdependence was revealed by significant correlations of health and marital satisfaction between partners. Finally, conjugal discrepancies in stress had an adverse impact on the personal well-being and marital satisfaction of wives. These results are interpreted in terms of the cultural milieu of modern Taiwanese society in which both traditional (collectivistic) and modern (individualistic) values coexist as a result of societal modernization and Western cultural influences. The once rigid gender role division of men as providers and women as homemakers is becoming more flexible, with corresponding changes occurring in the expectations for parental and marital roles.

Lavee, Katz, and Ben-Dror examine the links between Israeli parent-child relationships in childhood and adulthood and the marital quality of adult children in their article entitled "Parent-Child Relationships in Childhood and Adulthood and Their Effect on Marital Quality." This study also tested the hypothesis that these associations are moderated by residential proximity and frequency of contact between the two generations. Central to the study is the comparison of children who remained on the Kibbutz, a collectivist subculture, with those who moved away into the larger, more individualistic sectors of Israeli society. Findings indicated a strong association between family experiences during childhood (family cohesion, parental marital happiness, and parent-child relationships) and the emotional as well as contact solidarity of parents during adulthood. Marital quality was found to be associated with parent-child relations only for those who remained in the collectivistic Kibbutz but not for those who transitioned into the more individualistic society of Israel.

Two of the studies from this section specifically examine parenting and youth outcomes in societies that were formerly communist but have since undergone extensive transition toward capitalist-democratic systems. The first of these is the article by Walper, Kruse, Noack and Schwarz entitled "Parental Separation and Adolescents' Felt Insecurity with Mothers: Effects of Financial Hardship, Interparental Conflict, and Maternal Parenting in East and West Germany." This study investigates comparative effects of living in nuclear, separated single mother, or stepfather families on adolescents' relationship to their mothers. Although no simple association between family type and adolescents' experience of insecurity was found, tests confirmed that interparental conflict, impaired parenting, mothers' pressure to side against the father, and adolescents' feelings of being caught in the middle serve to link family type to adolescents' relationship to their mothers. Despite some regional variations in maternal strategies to draw their children into an alliance against the father, adolescents' feelings of being caught in loyalty conflicts between parents emerges as a common reason for their lack of security in relation to the mother in both West and East Germany. This study provides important information about the socialization experiences of adolescents in a society making the transition from one political economic system to another.

The second article that addresses changes in parenting after the fall of communism is the article by Wejnert and Djumabaeva entitled "From Patriarchy to Egalitarianism: Parenting Roles in Democratizing Poland and Kyrgyzstan." The purpose in this article is to provide insights into the effects of the fall of Soviet communism on parent-youth socialization within two different societies, Poland and Kyrgyzstan. Two tendencies are observed in these countries: (a) a move towards Western democratic values, including the idea of egalitarianism and small nuclear families, and (b) a revival of cultural traditions relating to family life and marital relationships. Although families in both societies have now become solely responsible for how they choose to organize themselves, whether in the spirit of Western values and egalitarian roles (i.e., individualism), or in the spirit of traditional patriarchy, this paper posits that recent democratization and diffusion of Western, egalitarian models of family relationships have a stronger effect on parenting roles than does religious traditionalism.

Peterson and colleagues in their article "Parent-Youth Relationships and the Self-Esteem of Chinese Adolescents: Collectivism versus Individualism" explore how several child-rearing behaviors within the Chinese parent-adolescent relationship were predictive of youthful self-esteem. The investigators test a theoretical model intended to show whether adolescent self-esteem is influenced in Chinese families through general socialization approaches characterized as either collectivistic or individualistic patterns. Theoretically based relationships are tested with structural equation modeling to examine whether dimensions of parental behavior (i.e., support, reasoning, monitoring, and punitiveness) influenced the self-esteem of Chinese adolescents through the mediating influences of either conformity (i.e., collectivism) or autonomy (i.e., individualism) in reference to parents. The sample consisted of adolescents from Beijing, China, who responded to self-report questionnaires administered in school classrooms. Results provided support for parental behaviors as predictors of self-esteem development through individualistic patterns of socialization. Although collectivistic parent-adolescent patterns did not predict the self-esteem of Chinese adolescents, several results also supported a collectivistic conception of socialization through significant relationships involving parental behaviors as predictors of adolescent conformity to parents. Consequently, this overall pattern of mixed results suggests that a combination of individualistic and collectivistic patterns, referred to as interdependence, may be what is emerging within Chinese socialization processes.

Steinmetz, in her article entitled "Parental versus Government Guided Policies: A Comparison of Youth Outcomes in Cuba and the United States," examines a variety of outcomes for youth and families who live in Cuba and the United States. These two societies are characterized by distinct political systems, one a communist and the other a capitalist system. Although both societies claim to be child-centered, Steinmetz demonstrates that the value placed on health care, education, and the percentage of the governmental budget allocated to support children is greater in Cuba than in the United States. Specifically, in many cases, the circumstances of Cuban children were found to equal and/or exceed U.S children on a variety of measures such as infant mortality, low birthweight data, levels of health care, literacy, educational attainment, and quality of life. Data from this study demonstrate the Cuban youth and that parents in both countries were found to be quite similar in the methods they selected to discipline their children. These accomplishments for Cuban youth are truly remarkable, especially when one realizes that Cuba is a "developing" country with a struggling economy. Moreover, although the United States is a major world power and leader in technological and medical advances, few differences exist in the indicators of many life quality dimensions for children and families.

The final article in this collection, "Persisting Issues in Cultural and Cross-Cultural Parent-Youth Relations" by Peterson, Steinmetz and Wilson, examines some needed areas of research. The issues of particular importance in this article consist of the need (1) for more research based on more complex models of socialization, (2) for scholarship that captures a more complex conception of culture, (3) to recognize dilemmas about cultural universals in the parent-child relationship, (4) to address conceptual and cross-cultural problems with parental styles or typologies, (5) to expand beyond parental styles and behaviors as disproportionate preoccupations over other parental attributes and (6) to assess the impact of shifting cultural, economic and political paradigms on values and attitudes regarding childrearing. The authors address these issues as a means of charting directions for future scholarship that addresses patterns of cross-cultural diversity and commonality in the most elementary of human associations, the parent-youth relationship.

Parenting in Mexican Society

Rosario Esteinou

ABSTRACT. Parenting is a topic that has received little attention in Mexican scholarship. In the field of family studies, Mexican parenting has not been treated directly or received sufficient status to deserve a lot of specific study. In this article I interpret the existing knowledge through a review of the works that do exist and that I have grouped in four fields: (1) studies focused on the construction of the self or the individual; (2) anthropological and sociological studies that describe parental practices related to the construction of gender differences and the sexual division of labour; (3) sociological studies that describe the resources used in parenting; and, (4) studies that do not deal with parenting but with parent-child relationships. *[Article copies available for a fee from The Haworth Document Delivery Service: 1-800-HAWORTH. E-mail address: <docdelivery@haworthpress.com> Website: <http://www.HaworthPress.com> © 2004 by The Haworth Press, Inc. All rights reserved.]*

KEYWORDS. Parenting, Mexican families, parental practices, rearing practices, resources in parenting, parent-child relationships

INTRODUCTION

Mexican scholarship has characterized by a paucity of research on parenting. In the field of family studies, Mexican parenting has not been treated directly or received sufficient status to be granted a lot of specific study. With the exception of a few psychological studies, parenting has been

---

Rosario Esteinou is affiliated with Centro de Investigaciones y Estudios Superiores en Antropología Social (CIESAS), Juárez 87, Tlalpan, 14000, México D. F., México (E-mail: esteinou@juarez.ciesas.edu.mx).

http://www.haworthpress.com/web/MFR
© 2004 by The Haworth Press, Inc. All rights reserved.
Digital Object Identifier: 10.1300/J002v36n03_02

addressed indirectly and in partial ways, either as a result or as an aspect of other issues. Anthropological studies, for example, have described parent education and child-rearing practices in terms of gender and age differences among different ethnic groups, but frequently these are presented as "customs" that are part of group traditions and not as a topic for distinctive study (INI, 1995). Without disregarding these findings for understanding parenting, the focus of ethnographic work in anthropology has not specifically addressed issues related to parenting. In another area of scholarship, gender studies, parenting has been examined in the seventies and eighties as an aspect of focusing on motherhood. Specifically, motherhood became an object of attention to examine the forms of women's subjugation and assignment to traditional roles, the unequal power relationships between men and women, and the diminished social positions occupied by women—among them, it was assumed, the family (De Barbieri, 1984).

From another perspective, we can also say that this indirect study of parents and parenting are simply reflections of the fact that the field of family studies had little separate identification in Mexico. Ironically, however, the family has been such an important reality in Mexican society that the need for studying it has simply been taken for granted and seldom acted upon. This implicit "empirical fact" and prominence of the family gave it unquestionable efficacy to solve its own problems without the need for intervention by scientific professionals. The emergence of scientific approaches dedicated explicitly to examining families has been a very recent phenomenon and, accordingly, the development of scholarship on Mexican parenting is only just emerging. This new focus on families and parenting can be explained, in part, as resulting from various changes experienced by Mexican society during the last three decades. The changes in economic, demographic, and sociocultural patterns have had substantial impact on family structure and relations (Esteinou, 1999), particular aspects of which are parenting practices and styles. The study of parenting practices and styles will be very important in subsequent years to develop a comprehensive view of the Mexican family, including the challenges that public policy and clinical practice should address.

Since parenting has been largely absent as a primary topic of research in Mexico, my plan is to interpret the existing knowledge through a review of the works that do exist. It is important to note that after conducting a bibliographic search through a library service (i.e., a service covering all the journals, reviews, and periodicals in Latin America) at the Universidad Nacional Autónoma de México, only three articles were found that explicitly dealt with parenting, with only one of these being scientific in its focus.

Another type of literature exists about Mexican parenting, represented mainly by manuals about how to parent or how to raise and deal with children.

These sources are largely translations from other countries, especially from the United States. The literature found in these sources deals largely with the following topics: (1) Studies focused on the construction of the self or the individual. These studies are psychological in focus and deal with parenting through the study of child-rearing practices or styles. (2) Anthropological and sociological studies that describe parental practices related to the construction of gender differences and the sexual division of labour. (3) Sociological studies that describe the resources used in parenting. (4) Studies that do not deal with parenting but with parent-child relationships. The present article is intended to focus on these topics with the addition of an initial section on recent societal changes in Mexico and their impact on the family. It is also important to observe that the ideas reviewed here come from different disciplines, distinctive perspectives, and vary in other ways. Some of the sources refer to children, adolescents, or parents. Some are psychological in nature, whereas others are based in anthropological or sociological perspectives. Although this may suggest a fragmented view and may sacrifice some coherence as to a central theme, I chose this interdisciplinary approach with the intention of showing the range of what is available in the current literature.

SOCIETAL CHANGES AND THEIR IMPACT ON THE FAMILY

Mexico has experienced, particularly in the last three decades, a set of important changes in areas that have had an impact on individual and family life. These changes include economic crisis, labor market restructuring, demographic alterations, and accelerated social-cultural transition toward modernization and globalization. From an economic point of view, an abundant literature exists that describe and documents, from different approaches, the arrangements, strategies and responses developed by households and families to manage their resources. The challenge for families and households is to face the challenges of monetary income deterioration and changes in labor markets so they can overcome the difficult socioeconomic conditions and changes in their standard of living (Cortés, 1995; García & de Oliveira, 1994).

An important means of responding to difficult economic circumstances has been the increased involvement of other family members, such as women, children, and the elderly, in labor markets. Of particular note has been the growing participation of women in labor markets, with women's participation in economic activity doubling between 1970 and 1995 from 17% to 35% (CONAPO, 1998). Besides increases in female economic participation, a relatively new and important trend is the consistent increase of married women and married women with small children in the labor force (García & de

Oliveira, 1994). In 1995, for example, nearly 30% of married, 69% of divorced and 73% of separated women were participating in the labor force (López, 1998: 31).

The most relevant consequence is that roles are changing within the families, and new family forms, such as dual career families, are emerging in greater proportions. Dual career families, an alternative family arrangement, differ substantially from what is conventionally understood as the nuclear family. Specifically, nuclear families are composed of biologically related parents and their offspring who reside with them. Moreover, nuclear families are guided by specific sets of norms and values such as those that prescribe that adult women should be dedicated to housework and child-rearing, whereas adult males are cast in breadwinner roles. Although emerging new family forms, such as dual career families, may have a nuclear structure on the surface, the relationships within these families imply different forms of organization and value orientations. Alternative family forms may distribute child care activities, deal with educational issues, and assign parental roles differently than nuclear families. There is a great need to examine aspects of these emerging families more extensively in the future.

Another set of changes has taken place in the demographic area, with some of these changes contributing to individualism and greater possibilities for family members. In contrast, other changes reveal points of tension and conflict that can lead to increased separation and divorce. Among the most important trends impacting family life has been a declining birth rate per woman from 6.11 to 2.4 children between 1974 and 1999 (CONAPO, 1999). Since women now have more time to engage in other activities (i.e., besides childcare), this has been a benefit to them in terms of greater levels of personal freedom and control over their lives. Some estimates indicate that, with the birth rate or fecundity of 1976, women devoted about 18 years of their lives to rearing children, whereas in recent years they spend only about 13 years engaged in this activity (Gómez de León, 1998). Another important change is the increased life expectancy of Mexican family members that reached 72 for men and 77 for women in 1999 (CONAPO, 1999). Thus, reduction in the number of years that women devote to child-rearing and the expansion of life expectancy can result in a greater personal freedom, expansion in the number of years that individuals can live as couples, and expansion of personal horizons. By virtue of greater flexibility and cultural diversity in Mexican society, both individuals and families are exposed more extensively today than 30 years ago to a diversity of cultural models and to stressful experiences associated with individualism. These changes provide options in life, but, on the other hand, burdens are placed on family relations to reconcile individual interests with the values of couples and the family group. This greater cultural diversity, combined with an extended life expectancy, is weakening the nuclear family's traditional institutional base as a symbolic point of reference. Similar to such alterations in nuclear families, in turn, traditional models of parenting and parent-child relationships are also changing.

Signs of this transition process in Mexican families is evident if we consider some of the changes in family patterns and trends toward more dissolution of relationships. Cohabitation, for example, is a growing pattern that, by 1996, had reached 26% of relationships in Mexico (CONAPO, 1999). This type of relationship involves the formation of coresident relationships by men and women without being either legally or religiously sanctioned. Divorce is also more common today than in the past and has become a reality in an estimated 14.5% of relationships in recent years. Although comparatively low in Mexico in contrast to other countries like the USA, it has been growing rapidly in the last decade (CONAPO, 1999). Because of the growing frequency of divorce and separation, we are witnessing the emergence of other family forms and the reconstitution of current families. Single parent families are increasingly evident and especially those which are headed by women. Remarriage and stepfamily patterns are becoming more prevalent in the Mexican population. Consistent with these changes and the emergence of new family forms, we can assume that parenting also is changing, a development that we need to examine and understand more thoroughly.

Demographic data can provide us with some understanding of the changes in Mexican family life. This is particularly true if we combine demographic data with sociocultural insights, another set of changes that I have introduced above. For centuries, Mexico has been a country marked by cultural diversity that comes from different ethnic, Spanish, and Mestizo cultures. Thus, diversity in itself is not new, but during the last decades, Mexico has experienced a significant modernization process, not only in the economic sphere but also within sociocultural dimensions. As experienced in many other countries, differentiation and multiplication of sociocultural subsystems have developed and coexist with the process of globalization. Although less evident than in other advanced industrial societies, we can observe the development of some of these features in Mexico. For example, a national survey about the Mexican attitudes and values (Beltrán, Castaños, Flores, Meyenberg & Del Pozo, 1996) indicated that, in 1996, along with the traditional base of native cultural values, significant development has occurred in values associated with a market economy, formal democracy, and individualism.

Besides growing tolerance for value and attitude differences, however, there is substantial continuity in the deeply rooted conceptions of (1) nepotism and the dominance of family relationships over social mobility, (2) linkages of sexual and gender roles with one's biological nature, and (3) the importance of family priorities prevailing over individual interests. The impact of these co-existing processes, of course, varies substantially across the different regions, social classes, and ethnic groups of Mexico.

Important changes worth mentioning in Mexican family life are associated with transitions occurring at the economic and demographic levels of society. Specifically, this refers to changes in the meanings of mother, housewife, father, and breadwinner roles that result from increased expectations and trends for women to occupy employment roles outside the family. Although Mexican society has experienced diversity in sociocultural practices for a long time, there are some aspects of Mexican culture that have been persistent across time. Mexican culture, for example, has placed strong emphasis on family life and has a long tradition of valuing and worshipping the role of being a mother. Motherhood is believed to be a major aspect of personal development and role performance that is socially recognized as commonly assigned to women. Although many women are involved in some sort of economic activity, it is symptomatic of continuing values that, when they were asked their occupation, their answers were "housework" and "child-rearing." A popular belief existed that they were "the queens of the house," a statement that recognizes the place of women in many sectors of family and society.

This maintenance of the traditional roles of mother and housewife was reinforced by mechanisms of social control through negative sanctions displayed by other kin members or friends when women became employed outside the home. Expressions such as "This man is supported by his woman." or "Look, he put his wife to work!" function to sanction the "failure" of men to be breadwinners but also inhibit the tendency for women to participate in the labor market. Other sanctions were specifically directed at women who were employed with statements such as "she is neglecting her kids," or "she is selfish; her duty is first with her children." Only when women found themselves in more unusual circumstances (i.e., when they were abandoned, separated or widowed) were their roles in the labor market accepted. Women's involvement in the labor market was seen as role inversion for the genders that defied normative and value standards. The value of being a mother was not viewed as compatible with that of labor involvement, nor was it viewed as an area of priority for women. The highly valued status of the maternal role and the normatively intertwined role of housewife often function to delimit the life horizons and the social status of adult women. Moreover, the Catholic religion was an important social force that reinforced this set of norms and values.

This strong linkage between the roles of housework and child-rearing has been eroding and it is part of a process that is weakening the traditional nuclear family as a symbolic referent. As indicated by recent studies, in contrast to 30 years ago, women's employment, and particularly mothers' employment outside the home, is becoming a more general expectation and value orientation (Beltrán, Castaños, Flores, Meyenbers, Del Pozo, 1996; Esteinou, 1996). The potential horizons for women's employment have become increasingly diversified. Women's economic contribution to family well-being is being increasingly accepted, not only for economic necessity, but also for providing personal and professional development for women.

The changes I have described have had considerable impact on family structure and on family relationships. New family forms, individualistic belief systems, increasing emphasis on rational solutions, as well as new expectations and value orientations have emerged and become more prominent. These sociocultural changes are subsequently affecting practices and styles of parenting as well as relationships between parents and their children. In fact, such changes seem similar to those conceptualized by Parsons and Bales (1955) in which authoritarian and rigid role divisions of traditional family systems are giving way to more flexible and democratic models. In spite of these changes, however, it is important to observe that family cohesion is still high in Mexico and that Mexicans continue to be a substantially family-oriented populace.

THE CONSTRUCTION OF THE INDIVIDUAL

As indicated previously, the literature on Mexican parenting is very limited. One particular theme about which some information exists, however, is literature on child-rearing styles and practices. These studies are conceptualized from a psychological perspective and focus on the relationship between child-rearing practices and styles as well as the construction of the self or one's sense of individuality. The study of child-rearing styles or practices has been important because of the belief that these behaviors contribute to the development and performance of the individual within the social environment. As the existing research establishes, certain optimal conditions are necessary for the individual to develop a positive concept of self, feel competent, demonstrate independence or autonomy, establish affective interpersonal relationships, and develop effective problem-solving skills (Baumrind, 1967, 1971). Child-rearing practices have been conceptualized mainly by popular beliefs and sometimes reduced to such issues as basic behaviors and nurturing practices used during meals, feeding, and dressing. However, several authors in other societies have provided classifications of child-rearing styles, taking into account several dimensions such as affection, hostility, permissiveness, restriction, indulgence, and democracy (Baldwin, 1949; Baumrind, 1967, 1973; Hoffman, 1994).

A study by Osorio Román and Sánchez Mejía (1996), for example, entitled "Rearing Styles in Mexico: An Epidemiological Study," considers adolescents' perceptions of their parents' behavior and analyses some of the child-rearing dimensions mentioned above. The study was conducted on 3432 female and male adolescents who attended public high schools located in fourteen geographic zones of Mexico City. The participants' ages ranged from 15 to 18 years old and they were from either medium-low, medium, or medium-high socioeconomic levels. The study used the Health, Life Styles, and Behavioral Inventory composed of 204 questionnaire items with five point response options that measured psychological health, child-rearing styles, and family interaction. Factor analysis was used to validate the questionnaire scales and additional descriptive analyses of the data were conducted.

According to this study, a predominantly supportive relationship was found between adolescents and their father figures, particularly in regard to evidence of affection, support, interest, communication, as well as the fathers' conception of their adolescents. However, as Baumrind (1967) has indicated, although a good relationship appears to exist between adolescents and fathers, some of the young report low tendencies to confide in their fathers, a finding that suggests lower levels of certain types of communication between fathers and children. Communication among parents and children is an important dimension of effective psychosocial adaptation.

The relationship of adolescents with their mothers appears to be largely positive, with a great percentage of adolescents indicating that they have received support, interest, affection, and confidence from their mothers. Their relationships also were characterized by mothers' expressing confidence in their children and reporting that effective communication exists between adolescents and their mothers. Comparing the relationships of adolescents with mothers versus fathers revealed that a stronger bond existed with mothers than with fathers. This finding is consistent with a study by Elder (1962), which indicated that adolescents perceived their mothers as being more comprehensive in their parenting, expressive of their affection, and as expressing more interest than fathers. This stronger bond with mothers is because children's primary needs for feeding, care, and affection are provided by mothers, whereas fathers tend to be more detached from the family life.

Besides parent-child relationships, Osorio Roman and Sanchez Mejia (1996) considered couple relationships between the parents as well as the more general family relationships and the family environment. Couple relationships in their sample tend to be good, with the frequency of physical violence and threats of divorce being quite low. An interesting finding is that the incidence of verbal violence (i.e., discussions in front of the children) is low but present. Nevertheless, signs of love and affection are more frequent than negative relationships. It is clear, according to Osorio Roman and Sanchez Mejia (1996), that adolescents' perceptions of good relationships between their parents leads to optimal emotional, social, and intellectual development in the young. This evidence of youthful competence, in turn, provides feedback to couples about their abilities as parents and the quality of their child-rearing practices. Regarding family relationships, it was observed that family integration is good and the majority of families were characterized by the presence of both parents.

In general, the results of this research project indicate that adolescents have positive perceptions of their families and their parents. Such positive views of one's family circumstances are commonly consistent with effective emotional, social, and intellectual adaptation. As part of the relationships that adolescents have with their parents and families, some of the literature from other countries seeks to identify and classify variables and parent behaviors. Although Osorio Roman and Sanchez Mejia (1996) do not specifically attempt to classify different styles of child-rearing, they do observe that expressions of confidence, affection, love, interest, support, and a family environment without tensions are components of democratic (Baumrind, 1967), egalitarian (Elder, 1962), or permissive-affective (Becker, 1964) styles of parenting. These styles, in turn, are associated with adaptive functioning as was evident in the majority of households of the individuals who were studied.

Consistent with these themes, a study by Roberto Oropeza Tena (1995) focuses on the influence of child-rearing practices on the development of self-concept. A common finding has been that the self-concept explains, predicts, and controls adaptative behavior and emotional stability. One's concept of self is central to organizing, forming, and developing an individual's personality. Self-concept has been defined as the perceptions, feelings, images, attributions, beliefs, attitudes, and evaluations of individuals about themselves as well as their relationships with others. The study followed a methodology quite similar to the investigation by Osorio Roman and Sanchez Mejia (1996).

The goal of the study was to identify how child-rearing practices predict the self-evaluative part of the adolescent self-concept, to identify gender differences in these predictions, and to estimate the status of self-evaluation in a sample of healthy adolescents. The study involved 2909 adolescents as participants who were students in 14 public high schools in Mexico City. The ages of these adolescents ranged between 15 and 20 years of age. Results of this study demonstrated that relatively specific child-rearing practices and family relationships functioned as predictors of adolescents' devalued self-concept and self-esteem, with several individual and social implications associated with such outcomes. Specifically, the association between child-rearing practices and self-devaluation and despair was examined. Relationships that generated self-devaluation in males were circumstances in which there was involvement with an abusive, alcoholic father or those where the individual did not have good relationships with their brothers and sisters. In the case of women's parenting, mothers in whom the young expressed little confidence and who showed little interest in their children were significant contributors to feelings of self-devaluation by the adolescents.

The results also demonstrate that, among the child-rearing practices that generate despair, low expressions of affection by mothers are particularly relevant to the despair of males. The same result appears for women when they are frequent recipients of offensive orders by their mothers. In fact, significant gender differences existed, with some variables affecting one gender over the other. The results for males, for example, demonstrated more connected relationships with their fathers, whereas females were more connected to their mothers. Self-devaluation in males was associated with fathers who made negative comparisons of their young with others, used physical punishment, and engaged in excessive alcohol consumption. In contrast, females were more affected when their mothers punished them, showed little interest in them, did not provide support, and failed to have confidence in them. Similar results were obtained by Sánchez-Sosa and Hernández (1992) in the sense that fathers may mistreat sons more than daughters, which may be one reason for fathers' greater effects on males.

Another aspect of self-devaluation affecting males more than females was demonstrated when bad relationships were evident with their siblings (Oropeza Tena, 1995; Sánchez Sosa & Hernández, 1992). Moreover, fathers' physical punishment had some role in fostering despair in males, but not in females. These inadequate child-rearing practices generated feelings of self-devaluation and despair, which may have had maladaptive consequences for distorted body images, problems conforming and forming one's personal identity, feelings of insecurity, deficits in social relationships, diminished personal capabilities, school failure, depression, anxiety, as well as other problems.

Other studies exist on the child-rearing practices or styles of Mexican parents, but these studies tend to be focused on urban samples and on other issues such as pregnancy, health problems, and practical issues about nurturance (Barrón, 2002; Becerril, 1996; Castellanos, 1997; Cuevas, 2001; Moreno, 1996). In contrast, an interesting and unique study by Aguilar, Vallejo and Valencia (2002) examined parenting styles in Mexico, but, in this case, within a rural, ethnic group, the Totonacas in Veracruz. They analysed relationships between adolescents' perceptions of parental styles and the promotion of psychological autonomy by Totonacan parents, with additional attention being given to age differences. Two hundred eighty-three adolescents, who ranged from 12 to 18 years of age, provided their perceptions of both maternal and paternal styles as well *as* the degree of psychological autonomy that was fostered. Significant differences were found for the associations between different parental styles and psychological autonomy, with no significant age differences being found for these relationships.

Considering the four parenting styles defined by Baumrind (1971, 1991), the authoritative, authoritarian, permissive, and neglected styles, the authors found that significant differences for males existed. Specifically, psychological autonomy for males was associated more strongly with the authoritative style than either the authoritarian or neglected styles. Among female adolescents, though the statistical means for authoritative parenting were higher, significant differences between authoritative and both authoritarian and neglecting parental styles did not result. Significant differences were evident for how the permissive and the neglected parenting styles were associated with psychological autonomy, with the *highest* mean values being demonstrated for the permissive style (Aguilar et al., 2002).

For the association between autonomy and the *adolescents'* age, it was observed that autonomy was promoted both in male and female adolescents (mainly by the mother), but without age being an important contributor to differences in the development of autonomy. Instead, it is rather the parental style that influences autonomy, or a particular way of thinking about the development of children and choice of the appropriate child-rearing behavior This research demonstrated that mothers are more sensitive in promoting autonomy, with male youth being perceived as facing greater promotion of autonomy than female youth. In contrast, females are socialized for greater dependency on their parents than are males, a finding consistent with other studies on this rural ethnic group (Vallejo, Aguilar, & Valencia, 2000).

These results also indicated that the prevailing child-rearing approach used by fathers and mothers is the authoritative style, followed by the neglectful strategy. This is an interesting result that contradicts the generalized belief that rural ethnic groups, such as the Totonacas, are traditionalistic and strongly hierarchical in their approach to parenting. Instead of the expected authoritarian style, this study on a rural Mexican parental style as well as other work on urban samples suggest a tendency toward the diffusion of more democratic styles. Further analyses are needed in both contexts to explore the tentative findings about these trends.

PARENTAL PRACTICES AND THE CONSTRUCTION OF GENDER DIFFERENCES

Some scholarly literature exists that deals with parental practices and the construction of gender differences, including studies we just reviewed in previous sections. Evidence exists, for example, that fathers may mistreat their sons more than their daughters, whereas mothers promoted psychological autonomy in their sons rather than their daughters (Sánchez Sosa & Hernández, 1992; Aguilar et al., 2002). Other qualitative and ethnographic studies describe how certain parental practices are clearly oriented to the socialization of gender behavior. Because these studies are from an anthropological perspective, the focus is usually on rural ethnic groups (INI, 1995; Pozas, 1977).

Many of the ethnographic descriptions by anthropologists refer to Mesoamerican people, a group of diverse ethnic groups located in rural areas ranging from central Mexico to the Yucatan and Chiapas states (Kirchhoff, 1968). These groups often demonstrate differences in language and culture, but also have some customs and traditions in common. Among these ethnic groups, the cultural standards and norms of the nuclear family have not been the primary basis for family formation in terms of either structure or internal relationships. Because the idea of family as we know it does not apply within these ethnic groups, the expectation is that parenting within these contexts will also have different forms and distinctive goals. That is, the idea of children having economic value in the labor force has prevailed over the idea that children have emotional value. This does not mean, however, that parents fail to care for or love their children, but only that it is a matter of assigning differential priorities to cultural values. Anthropological accounts describe how the division of labor, based on gender, begins at a very early age, often when the young are 10 or 11 years old. Boys go to the fields with their fathers, helping them with daily duties in the crafts, painting, or agriculture, whereas daughters remain at home with their mothers to help with their activities. Specifically, females learn to grind corn, to weave, and to make tortillas. Although boys and girls are involved in work at early ages, they are also under close supervision by their parents through a strict hierarchical model of authority and through relationships that tend to be authoritarian. Parents, adult kinship members, and other adults must be respected and children must obey their parents and grandparents. Education and socialization are provided mainly through authoritarian means and children are not asked their opinions, but simply are taught in a dominant manner. Parents are in charge of the young and decide what is most convenient for them. These practices have prevailed for generations but now appear to be moving toward a more flexible pattern (INI, 1995; Lara, Gómez & Fuentes 1992).

At the same time, however, relationships in these ethnic groups can be characterized as permissive or indifferent because parenting is conceived as having few responsibilities and tasks (INI, 1995; Pozas, 1977). The responsibilities of parents are defined largely through giving material support, as it appears that in these ethnic groups managing children's lives is not a central concern. The cultural ethos, including the definition of parenting, parental roles, and the prevailing view of childhood, is linked substantially to a way of life centered on the importance of the land. Such a traditional perspective, however, has undergone substantial change as opportunities for making a living from the land have diminished and entire families, or some of their family members, have migrated to cities and to the USA in search of better economic opportunities. Migration has been so prevalent that towns now exist where most of the men are gone and the towns are inhabited mainly by children, women, and the elderly. These migrations have also meant that cultural contact has increased, which has become a vehicle of social change within family life (Mummert, 1999).

From the available ethnographical descriptions on rural samples, some of the features about how parenting is conducted become evident, though more studies with deeper insight are needed. For example, you are not able to identify the prevailing parenting style among Mesoamerican people. Consequently, an important need in this research is to establish the role of traditional culture, or one that encourages authoritarian parenting practices.

In the case of urban samples, parental practices also reveal gender differences but not as markedly as in samples from rural areas (CONAPO 2000). In rural samples, gender differences encompass all spheres of action, whereas in urban samples gender differences are low in certain aspects of the parent-child relationship. Getting an education is an important area that demonstrates the growing equality between men and women. Acquiring an education is viewed by females as a way to develop themselves personally in professional careers, the traditional domain of males. Becoming educated, in turn, used to be a social domain marked by gender differences in rural areas, with parents often emphasizing the importance of school for boys but not for girls. Today, Mexican girls increasingly attend school in rural areas and, in urban contexts, both genders commonly go to school and become educated (CONAPO 2000). Urban parents are particularly aware of the inequalities and sufferings that gender differences may cause and desire to correct these disparities (Mier y Terán & Rabell 2001).

Studies conducted in urban contexts also indicate that gender differences exist in the way that parental roles are performed. These studies tend to have a sociological perspective and are qualitative in nature (Esteinou, 1996; in press). In my own work, for example, I have conducted research analysing some of the features of parenting in an urban, middle class population (Esteinou, in press). Thirty men and women, whose ages ranged from 25 to 35 years of age, were asked about how their parents raised them and how they raise their own children. Consequently, the study sought information about two generations, the first with an age range between 50 and 60 and the second generation with the previously specified 25-35 age range. An important goal of the study was to identify resources used by both generations in their parental roles. The first generation had children in the 1960s and early 1970s, a time when some of the previously mentioned social changes were beginning. The second generation, on the other hand, had lived through all of these changes.

A previous proposal was made that the nuclear family has not been an important source of norms for families living in rural areas, but in urban areas the cultural ethos of the nuclear family has been a compelling model for family life in Mexico. It is important to observe that this conception of the family is similar to that conceptualized by Parsons and Bales (1955) for the United States in the 1950s. It implied a gender-based division of labor established along the axis of expressive/instrumental role distinctions, with females performing the expressive roles of mother and housewife, while males centered upon the instrumental roles of father and breadwinner.

In general, role structures during the first generation of families followed a traditional and rigid path, with mothers being responsible for childcare and child-rearing, while fathers' participation in these activities was low. Mothers were in charge of preparing meals, supervising homework, tending to bath times, monitoring bedtimes, and being responsible for healthcare. Among the second generation, the expectation still prevails that mothers should be primarily responsible for these activities, but compared to previous times, fathers participate more frequently in some of these activities, including supervising homework, bedtimes, caretaking activities during some afternoons. Because mothers must increasingly work or study, this circumstance has contributed to new dynamics that can be referred to as "taking turns" within couples, a circumstance that is commonly supervised by the mothers. For example, "today is your turn to take Maria to her piano lesson," or "today is your turn to stay with the girls and see that they do their homework because I must go out later." Family networks (i.e., grandmothers in particular) and childcare institutions are other important resources that parents must use to take care of their children.

The study also deals with the resources used in managing relationships and authority through which we conceptualize the presence and changes in expressive/instrumental role divisions. Some aspects of the study concerned the establishment of rules and limits, dealing with conflict, and the structure of authority in couple relationships. During the first generation, mothers established the limits and routines for their children. It is interesting to note that when the interviewers were asked about how many hours they spent with mothers compared to fathers the difference was 3 times higher for mothers. Although the number of hours in itself does not tell us much about the quality of time spent, what was clear from the answers was that Mexican mothers had primary responsibility for the role of childcare and child-rearing. The time fathers spent with their children was relatively small, prior to school, during meals, and at nights.

Parenting role structure for the interviewees was rigid and followed gender role divisions. Relationships in terms of authority had a similar pattern, with the central authority figures in an overall sense being the fathers, while mothers' authority was rooted in everyday life, face to face relationships, and most issues relating to education and child-rearing. Two spheres of authority appeared in reference to asking parents for permission. Mothers of the first generation were asked to give their consent when children were younger in such areas as making messes, inviting friends home, going out to play, and doing anything inside the domestic space. In fact, at an early age, it was sufficient for children to ask permission from their mothers.

Fathers' authority, in turn, became more prevalent as children become older, such as during the preadolescent phase of development. The fathers' consent was essential for any matter that implied an important change in children's routine, the beginning of a transition, or situations believed to be risky and important. Examples of such circumstances include the first time their sons and daughters desired to go to a discotheque, go to parties, travel, go out alone, get home late, or ask for more money. Frequently, daughters made use of a strategy in which they first asked for mother's consent and then both of them subsequently tried to "convince" or "cheat" fathers to get their permission. Two spheres of maternal and paternal authority also appeared when issues about education were analyzed.

An interesting finding is that, although mothers were generally in charge of discipline in everyday life, fathers were identified by children as having primary responsibility for discipline. This was in spite of the fact that fathers were identified in only secondary ways as being responsible for supervising and reinforcing values. Mothers, in contrast, were identified as the primary person who instilled values, provided care and affection, but were also perceived as being the less demanding parent. According to their children, mothers managed relationships and conflicts between brothers and sisters. Fathers of the first generation tended to have instrumental authority directed at requirements that children would be expected to fulfill in the larger society, whereas mothers represented a more emotional, affective, and practical form of authority.

Among representatives of the second generation, important but not radical changes are evident. Compared to fathers, the majority of mothers continue to spend much more time with their children, which means that the traditional gender role divisions remain prevalent. There are also some cases in which practically no change has occurred. However, if first and second generation mothers are compared in terms of the quantity of time spent with children, second generation mothers spend less time with children due to their employment roles. In fact, a surprising finding was that approximately one-third of second generation fathers actually spend more time than mothers with their children. Overall, in contrast to first generation parents, there are increased tendencies for second generation mothers to spend less time with children and for fathers to spend more. Such findings suggest that changes are taking place in traditional parenting roles in the form of moderate but significant slides and shifts.

Regarding authority, the traditional structure tends to be maintained as a main point of reference, but in practice, we see some signs of growing flexibility. Permissions or consent to children tend to be given by both parents, with mothers being more independent to decide matters that in the traditional model were decided by fathers. Nevertheless, fathers still continue to be identified as being the primary authority to administer discipline and to have overall responsibility, whereas mothers are responsible for the everyday process of instilling values, providing care, and giving affection.

Recent studies have demonstrated, therefore, how parenting practices differ, depending upon the gender of the parent, and promote gender differences in the young. Other patterns of findings indicate that the nuclear family's expressive/instrumental role divisions have had considerable influence on the responsibilities of Mexican parents, but that change is also occurring in reference to these traditional gender role assignments.

THE RESOURCES USED IN PARENTING

My own study on urban middle-class families also addressed the quality and resources used by these two generations in their parental role performance and on educating their children. The information gathered from this study indicated that the main concerns of first generation parents were to provide the following to their children: (1) material support and security, (2) formal education as a form of capital and means of social mobility, as well as (3) the socialization of individuals who are capable of economic and social integration (Esteinou, in press).

The practice of "giving orders" was an important means of communication and type of child-rearing approach with the young. First generation parents made primary use of orders to get desired behaviors from the young. In the second place, they made frequent use of scolding and, in the third place, advice-giving (Esteinou, in press). Orders were so important as a child-rearing strategy that the logical outcome in children, obedience to parents, was considered a requirement in the socialization of children. Questioning orders was not encouraged and strict rules were imposed, with little option being available for negotiation. Orders and obedience were strictly associated and constituted a central resource in the socialization process. Scolding and punishment were corrective measures to get desired conduct and also to discipline behaviors. Advice-giving was another resource for first generation parents to transmit experiences, ways of thinking and strategies for problem-solving as well as for conveying a strong moral orientation. Advice-giving dealt with four main issues: (1) caring about one's physical image, cleaning, encouraging order, and fostering conformity to family and social norms. Examples of advice given by first generation parents to their children includes comments to "behave well," "be polite to people," and "obey and respect adults"; (2) achieve economic self-sufficiency, success, and social prestige through education. Advice-giving about studying was very important; (3) the importance of the family as a core value or a "good" orientation, especially when contrasted with the dangers represented by external forces. Some parental advice cultivated mistrust and fear of failure, especially in regard to associating with peer groups. For example, a mother would say: "there is advice that friends give that can blind you and cause you to fail; look for the help of someone who loves you, look for your family." Through this and other forms of advice, family bonds are portrayed as the primary source of connection characterized by affection and sound values, and as not being contaminated; (4) Much advice was oriented toward the development of youth who adhered to an ethical point of view, with certain values being conceived as fundamental ingredients of success for a person's life. Along these lines, parents provided a lot of advice that praised such values as honesty, effort, responsibility, study, obedience, and respect for adults.

Some shifts in these patterns are observed when an examination is made of the resources used by second generation parents in the education of their children. One-third of these parents demonstrated qualities that essentially reproduced many of the elements of the traditional pattern. Giving orders was considered to be the main resource in children's education and a disciplinary measure that molds "character" for success in the future. These parents indicate considerable interest in being strong authority figures by sustaining relationships between parents and children that are rather vertical in nature. Some of these second generation parents, however, try to introduce other resources, such as communication, that may lead to closer relationships with their children. Such an approach may be due to new social and cultural conditions emphasizing more flexible and less vertical relationships between parents and children.

The other two-thirds of the new parents mentioned that orders are not used as the main resource, but, instead, as means to mark limits. Great interest and concern exists among these parents to establish communication, flexibility, and closeness in relationships with their children. Although concern exists to function as authority figures, substantial interest exists to encourage communication. Obedience is still a very important expectation, but more emphasis is placed on negotiation, making requests, and being flexible to achieve this outcome. Moreover, children are given opportunities to question things when they are asked or even ordered to do something, which means that relationships tend to be less vertical in terms of authority.

The result is that a shift has occurred from the use of orders to that of greater communication as a main resource for socializing the young. Thus, the use of advice is much more prevalent and there is more frequent use of open communication about such matters as sexuality and emotions. In fact, emotional communication represents an important change, particularly for male youth. This is especially true compared to first generation fathers who tended to be distant, express limited affection, and to restrict their emotionality. In contrast, second generation fathers are much more expressive, not only verbally, but also through physical contact.

The overall pattern of these results indicates that parenting among first generation parents was clearly authoritarian, whereas among second generation parents a shift had occurred in the direction of more democratic or authoritative styles characterized by greater flexibity and expressiveness (Esteinou, in press). The first generation pattern of parenting was focused on providing material support, security, and moral education consistent with the Catholic religion and other traditional social standards. For second generation parents, material support and security were still very important, but greater attention to communication introduced new issues that have modified the approach between parents and children.

Changes also have occurred in the type of values that were encouraged. One of the most important shifts was the new emphasis on the child as an individual who has a lot more needs. Individualism was promoted more than in the past and unquestioned values about showing deference and respect to adults and older people are receiving less emphasis. Children are now allowed to express their opinions and show emotions in reference to their parents, grandparents, kinship members, and adults in general.

Another interesting pattern was the tendency of first generation parents to express more confidence in the knowledge based in tradition or that transmitted by their parents and relatives. In contrast, second generation parents indicated that they make greater use of knowledge provided by specialists (doctors, pediatricians, etc.) and from literature on parenting.

PARENT-CHILD RELATIONSHIPS

Another literature provides information specifically about parent-child relationships, though not necessarily about parenting (ENJ, 2000). Previous sections of this article have dealt with this topic in the form of child-rearing styles and the construction of the individual, the development of gender differences, and through resources that parents use to educate and socialize their children.

An important national survey about the youth (ENJ, 2000), developed in the year 2000, provides some information about aspects of parent-child relationships and confirms some of the findings provided in studies reviewed above. The survey analysed the condition and needs of youth as well as the processes by which young individuals are prepared for Mexican society. Individuals between the ages of 12 and 29 years were included in this study of youth. Nearly two-thirds of the youth live with both parents, while approximately a third had left home and were living on their own. Although the age span is quite wide in this study, many of the results are of interest for our purposes here.

Young individuals report that they have little influence on their families' decision-making processes, with parents tending to make most of the decisions. Overall, a restricted range of issues exists within which youth exercise decision making about their choices. The majority of all respondents can decide to have a girl/boyfriend and how to dress themselves, but parents have strong influence and control over the remaining issues. In general, boys have greater autonomy than girls.

Parents tend to use more conversation than punishment and the majority talked primarily with their mothers about problems. Almost half of these youth talked about their problems with their mothers on a regular basis, while at least half talked to her occasionally. The young seldom talked to their fathers, with only one of five reporting that they always talked to them and one-third indicating that they never talked to their fathers. The themes they talk about most often with fathers were school and work issues, whereas sex and politics were themes they talked about very little with them. The young people talked with their mothers a lot, with the most common themes being school, work, religion, politics and their feelings. Overall, girls talk about sex a lot with their mothers but boys do not.

Such results about gender differences as to which parent the young talk to also seem consistent with the idea, as proposed earlier in this article, that the nuclear family and its associated ideas has had considerable impact on contemporary Mexican family life. Mothers seem to focus on the expressive function in the couple relationship by being in charge of managing relationships, giving comfort, as well as hearing and supporting children, whereas fathers appear to be the instrumental members who are more emotionally distant and primarily in charge of providing economic and material resources to the family. Beyond this basic model, however, signs of democratization are evident in the tendency for communication to become more important than punishment. The young have a positive evaluation of their families because they find solidarity and support in these relationships. They view their families as a social means to socialize responsible, productive workers, but they also choose to spend most of their free time with their families.

These results demonstrate that young individuals in Mexico are very family oriented. Parents have a lot of control over decision-making about their activities, though the young report growing flexibility and democratization through the growth of communication within the parent-child relationship. Mothers continue to perform important socialization roles and expressive functions as they emphasize listening to feelings and talking more to their children. Such results are consistent with the previously reviewed study by Osorio Roman and Sanchez Mejia (1996).

CONCLUDING REMARKS

The studies reviewed in this paper have examined some of the features that are characteristic of parenting in Mexican society, though many more issues remain unexplored. Serious consideration must be given to fostering more empirical research about Mexican parenting styles, with one possibility being to apply the classifications used in other societies (i.e., such as in the USA) to the Mexican circumstance. Based on existing empirical studies, our second task is to engage in a theoretical discussion about the relationship between traditional and modern assets and contexts. We need to determine how traditional traits remain dominant in reference to individual and family behaviors.

Mexico appears to be a society experiencing change from one of tradition in which rigid gender/parental roles were performed and parent-child relationships are mainly hierarchical in authority structure. Instead, greater flexibility in the normative structure and a growing emphasis on individualism are beginning to play significant roles in structuring individual and family behavior. These transitions are progressing both in rural and urban areas of Mexican society.

More studies are needed to precisely examine the changes in Mexican parenting, with particular focus on the emerging traits of parenting. Such transitions include changes from authoritarian styles of parenting to more democratic patterns in which expectations are more flexible and with somewhat diminished emphasis on parental dominance. Related to this is the growth of communication as part of parenting styles and the increasing participation of fathers in the domestic sphere. Fathers not only spend more time with their children but also are becoming somewhat more expressive as part of their family role.

The study of parenting styles has been based largely in particular societies with specific characteristics. An implicit assumption exists that democratic styles of parenting are associated with individualism and autonomy, which, in turn, are characteristics commonly believed to be associated with modern societies. In contrast, traditional societies are presumed to be associated with authoritarianism and to exclude individualism. Mexican society used to be authoritarian but in recent times has become more democratic in a manner that includes traditional traits in some ways but very modern ones in others. According to a national survey of Mexican youth, individualism is not very prevalent in some groups but more so in sectors of society that identify with modern values and individualism. It seems possible, therefore, to identify two kinds of developing democratic styles, the first in which collectivism or familism is very strong and another form in which individualism prevails. Complicated conceptions of this kind are needed when trying to examine the nature of parenting in Mexican society.

REFERENCES

Aguilar, J., Vallejo, A & Valencia, A. (2002). Estilos de paternidad en padres totonacas y promoción de autonomía psicológica hacia los hijos adolescentes. *Revista Psicología y Salud, 12,* 101-107. Enero-junio. Jalapa, México: Universidad Veracruzana.

Baldwin, A. L. (1949). The effect of home environment on nursery school behavior. *Child Development, 20,* 49-62.

Barrón, P. B. (2000). *Los estilos de crianza y su vínculo con el rendimiento académico,* Tesis de licenciatura en psicología. Facultad de Psicología. México: Universidad Nacional Autónoma de México.

Baumrind, D. (1967). Child care practices anteceding three patterns of preschool behavior. *Genetic Psychology Behavior, 75,* 43-88.

Baumrind, D. (1971). Current patterns of parental authority. *Developmental Psychology Monographs, 4.*

Baumrind, D. (1973). The development of instrumental competence through socialization. In A. D. Pick (ed.). *Minnesota simposium child psychology, 7,* 3-46. Minneapolis: University of Minnesota Press.

Baumrind, D. (1991). Parenting styles and adolescent development. Brooks, J., Gunn, R., Lerner, A., Petersen, L. (eds.). *The Encyclopedia of Adolescence.* New York: Garland.

Becerril, M. D. (1996). *La disciplina y los estilos de crianza su efecto en la autoestima.* Tesis de licenciatura en Psicología. Facultad de Psicología. México: Universidad Nacional Autónoma de México.

Becker, W.C. (1964). Consequences of different kinds of parental discipline. Hoffman M. L. & Hoffman L. W. (eds.). *Child Development, 1*, New York.

Beltrán, U., Castaños, F., Flores, J., Meyenbers, G., & Del Pozo, T. (1996). *Los mexicanos de los noventa.* México: Instituto de Investigaciones Sociales, UNAM.

Castellanos, T. A. (1997). *Interacción familiar y estilos de crianza como predictores del embarazo adolescente.* Tesis de licenciatura en psicología, Facultad de Psicología. México: Universidad Nacional Autónoma de México.

CONAPO. (1998). *La situación demográfica en México.* México: Consejo Nacional de Población.

CONAPO. (1999). *La situación demográfica en México.* México: Consejo Nacional de Población.

CONAPO. (2000). *La situación demográfica en México.* México: Consejo Nacional de Población.

Cortés, F. (1995). El ingreso de los hogares en contextos de crisis, ajuste y estabilización: un análisis de su distribución en México. *Estudios Sociológicos, XIII*, 37, 91-108. Enero-abril. México: El Colegio de México.

Cuevas, C.L. (2001). *Análisis retrospectivo: estilos de crianza.* Tesis de licenciatura en Psicología, Facultad de Psicología. México: Universidad Nacional Autónoma de México.

De Barbieri, T. (1984). *Mujeres y vida cotidiana.* México D. F.: Fondo de Cultura Económica/Secretaría de Educacion Pública.

De la Peña, Guillermo, Agustin Escobar et al. (comps.), 1990, Crisis, Conflicto y Sobrevivencia: Estudios Sobre la Sociedad Urbana de México, Universidad de Guadalajara/CIESAS. Guadalajara, México.

Elder, G. H. Jr. (1962). Structural variations in the child-rearing relationship. *Sociometry, 25*, 241-262.

ENJ. (2000). *Encuesta Nacional de Juventud. Resultados generales.* México: Secretaría de Educación Pública/Instituto Mexicano de la Juventud.

Esteinou, R. (1996). *Familias de sectores medios: perfiles organizativos y socioculturales.* México: CIESAS.

Esteinou, R. (1999). Fragilidad y recomposición de las relaciones familiares. *Desacatos, 2*, 11-25.

Esteinou, R. (in press). La parentalidad en la familia: cambios y continuidades. In Ariza M., De Oliveira O. (eds.). *Imágenes de la familia en el cambio de siglo. Universo familiar y procesos demográficos contemporáneos*, México D. F.: Instituto de Investigaciones Sociales, Universidad Nacional Autónoma de México.

García, B. & de Oliveira, O. (1994). *Trabajo y vida familiar en México.* México: El Colegio de México.

Gómez de León, J. (1998). Fenómenos sociales y familiares emergentes. DIF. *La familia mexicana en el tercer milenio*, (pp. 10-26). México: Sistema Nacional para el Desarrollo Integral de la Familia.

Hoffman, M. (1994). Discipline and internalization. *Developmental Psychology, 30*, 1, 26-28.

INI. (1995). *Etnografía contemporánea de los pueblos indígenas de México.* 6 vol. México D. F.: Instituto Nacional Indigenista.

Kirchhoff, P. (1968). Mesoamerica: its geographic limits, ethnic composition and cultural characteristics. In Tax, S. (ed.). *Heritage of conquest. The ethnology of middle America* (pp. 17-30). New York: Cooper Square Publishers Inc.

Lara, T. L., Gómez, P. & Fuentes, R. (1992). Cambios socioculturales en los conceptos de obediencia y respeto en la familia mexicana: un estudio en relación con el cambio social. *Revista Mexicana de Psicología, 90,* 21-26.

López, M. P. (1998). Genero y familia. *La familia mexicana en el tercer milenio* (pp. 27-40). México: Sistema Nacional para el Desarrollo Integral de la Familia.

Mier y Terán, M. & Rabell C. (2001). Condiciones de vida de los niños en México, 1960-1995. In Gómez de León J. & Rabell C. (coords.). *La población de México* (pp.759-834). México D. F.: Fondo de Cultura Económica/Consejo Nacional de Población.

Moreno, C. A. (1996). *Relación entre quejas de hijos, las percibidas por sus madres y estilos de crianza en somatización gastrointestinal: estudio exploratorio en el estado de Sonora.* Tesis de licenciatura en psicología, Facultad de Psicología. México: Universidad Nacional Autónoma de México.

Mummert, G. (1999). "Juntos o desapartados": migración transnacional y la fundación del hogar. In Mummert G. (ed.). *Fronteras fragmentadas* (pp. 451-470). México: El Colegio de Michoacán/Centro de Investigación y Desarrollo del Estado de Michoacán.

Oropeza Tena, T. R. (1995). *Estilos de crianza y autoconcepto en adolescentes.* Tesis de Licenciatura en psicología, Facultad de Psicología. México: UNAM.

Osorio Roman, S. A. & Sánchez Mejía, S. (1996). *Estilos de crianza en México: estudio epidemiológico.* Tesis de licenciatura en psicología, Facultad de Psicología. México: Universidad Nacional Autónoma de México.

Parsons, T. & Bales, R. F. (1955). *Family socialization and interaction process.* Illinois: The Free Press, Glencoe.

Pozas, R. (1977). *Chamula.* México: Instituto Nacional Indigenista.

Vallejo, A. Aguilar, J. & Valencia A. (2001). Estilos de paternidad en familias totonacas con hijos adolescentes que viven en el medio rural. *Enseñanza e Investigación en Psicología, 6,* 37-48.

Sánchez Sosa, J. & Hernández G. L. (1992). La relación del padre como factor de riesgo psicológico en México. *Revista Mexicana de Psicología. 9,* 27-34.

Relations with Parents and Friends During Adolescence and Early Adulthood

Peter Noack
Heike M. Buhl

ABSTRACT. Relative power, conflict, and intimacy in adolescents' and young adults' relations with mothers, fathers, and best friends were examined. Two hundred eighty-five students from German high-track (i.e., university bound schools 6th, 9th, 12th grade), undergraduate and graduate students completed the respective scales of the Network of Relationships Inventory (Furman & Buhrmester, 1985). Relations with friends were more symmetrical and had a better socio-emotional quality than relations with parents. Still, increases in relative power in relations with parents were accompanied by low absolute levels of conflict. A symmetrical distribution of power in the family was not reached before the end of the third decade of life. To explore the influence of the entry into worklife on close relations, an additional subsample of 55 working young adults was compared with the participating university students. Despite slight differences in age-related patterns of intimacy, similarities prevailed. Overall, findings mostly converge with observations in U.S. samples of high school and college

Peter Noack and Heike M. Buhl are affiliated with the University of Jena.

Address correspondence to: Peter Noack, Department of Psychology, University of Jena, Humboldtstr. 27, D-07743 Jena, Germany (E-mail: S7NOPE@RZ.UNI-JENA.DE).

The authors thank Linda Juang, who greatly helped in the editing of the manuscript.

This research was supported by a grant from the Johann Jacobs Foundation. The authors are grateful to Michael Fingerle, Christine Krettek, and Sabine Walper for their assistance in the data collection and to the adolescents and young adults who were involved with the project.

http://www.haworthpress.com/web/MFR
© 2004 by The Haworth Press, Inc. All rights reserved.
Digital Object Identifier: 10.1300/J002v36n03_03

students and point to a more general process of relationship development as suggested by individuation theory. *[Article copies available for a fee from The Haworth Document Delivery Service: 1-800-HAWORTH. E-mail address: <docdelivery@haworthpress.com> Website: <http://www.HaworthPress.com> © 2004 by The Haworth Press, Inc. All rights reserved.]*

KEYWORDS. Early adulthood, parent-child relations, peer relation, adolescent-parent relations

Across the lifespan, personal relationships provide an important context for individual well-being and development. Although it is clear that relationships differ in their specific contributions to individual growth, there is no doubt concerning the outstanding role that parents and same-sex friends play throughout the course of development (Laursen & Bukowski, 1997). The quality of relationships with parents and friends and its age-related changes has been investigated most extensively for young people in their childhood and adolescent years (e.g., Collins, 1990; Grotevant & Cooper, 1985; Noack & Kracke, 1998; van Aken & Asendorpf, 1997). In these studies, particular interest was paid to changes in close relationships during adolescence initiated by pubertal maturation (Montemayor, Eberly & Flannery, 1993; Papini & Sebby, 1987; Steinberg, 1987). Clearly, less is known concerning the quality of relationships with mothers, fathers, and friends during the third decade of life which, only recently, has attracted more systematic interest of developmental scholars (Galambos & Leadbeater, 2000).

The present cross-sectional study is a replication and extension of earlier work conducted by Furman and Buhrmester (1985, 1992) and Buhrmester and Furman (1987). Our primary goal was descriptive, aiming at the analysis of variations in perceptions of parent and friend relationships depending on age and sex. The study includes age-graded subsamples covering the second and third decade of the lifespan which allow us to examine the quality of close relationships beyond the transition to adulthood. Moreover, a comparison of early adult subsamples from campus and community settings helps to elucidate variations in the quality of close relationships depending on the step into worklife that is considered a prominent aspect of the transition to adulthood (Bynner & Roberts, 1991; Hamilton, 1990; Vondracek, Lerner & Schulenberg, 1986; cf. Super, 1980). Even though the study we present is not cross-cultural in nature, the fact that our data were collected in Germany allows for a tentative comparison with earlier findings which are largely based on North American samples. Thus, we expected some first insights into the general or culture-specific quality of age-graded differences of young people's close relationships (Claes, 1998).

The following discussion of earlier research is organized into three sections. Taking the work of Furman and Buhrmester as the point of departure, we first summarize findings on adolescents' close relationships. Then, we turn to the more scattered studies focusing on early adulthood. In the final paragraphs, we provide some background information on Germany as the cultural context of our study.

THE NETWORK OF ADOLESCENTS' CLOSE RELATIONSHIPS

A major research program investigating the quality of relationships between children and their parents as well as further significant others has been conducted by Buhrmester and Furman (1987). Studying young people between fourth grade and college, that is, roughly from age 9 to 19, Furman and Buhrmester (1992) could show that adolescents describe their relationships with fathers and mothers in quite favorable terms. While reported levels of parental support remained above the scale midpoint in all age groups the opposite was true of perceived conflict with parents. Age-graded patterns, however, followed u-shaped curves, suggesting heightened levels of tension around mid-adolescence which could be interpreted as indicating intensified negotiations of roles, rights, and duties in the family. At the same time, adolescents' subjective power in their parent relationships also showed a u-shaped pattern as a function of age. While fourth-graders felt comparably more powerful vis-à-vis their parents than did sons and daughters in early and mid-adolescence, the age-graded pattern suggests an increase of relative power as adolescents approach majority. While children in the youngest group might simply overestimate the extent of their self-direction and of their influence on their parents, it could also be that a decrease of subjective power results from more active attempts on the part of parents to stay in control when adolescents start to push more strongly for autonomy (cf., Youniss & Smollar, 1985).

Furman and Buhrmester's findings correspond to claims of individuation theory (Grotevant & Cooper, 1986; Youniss & Smollar, 1985). According to this perspective, relationships between parents and their offspring change from hierarchical and unilateral to more egalitarian and reciprocal patterns in the course of adolescence. Abandoning core assumptions of earlier theorizing (e.g., Blos, 1979; Hall, 1904; Kroh, 1958; Steinberg, 1990), a major tenet of individuation theory is that adolescents do not become more autonomous by turning away from their parents. Rather, a high level of connectedness is seen as the necessary basis for structural changes of the relationship resulting in reciprocity and mutual acceptance as self-directed individuals, that is, individuality in the relationship. Considerable evidence supports this view suggesting, for example, that most parent-adolescent relationships are characterized by sound emotional bonds in absolute terms despite a modest peak in conflicts and a low in harmony between parents and their sons and daughters around mid-adolescence (Montemayor, 1983; Noack, Oepke, & Sassenberg, 1998; Steinberg, 1990). Even irritations in family relationships linked to pubertal maturation seem to be minor in size (Laursen, Coy, & Collins, 1998). At the same time, an increase of reciprocity and egalitarian interchanges was observed during the second half of adolescence (Hunter, 1984; Noack & Kracke, 1998; Wintre, Yaffe, & Crowley, 1995).

The quality of relationships with friends contrasts with parent-adolescent relationships (Laursen & Bukowski, 1997). In line with theoretical accounts of peer relations as–in principle–egalitarian and reciprocal (Krappmann, 1998; cf., Piaget, 1973; Sullivan, 1953), Furman and Buhrmester (1992) observed a balanced distribution of power among friends as opposed to the unilateral power constellation characterizing the relationships with parents. At the same time, the socio-emotional quality of same-sex friendships equalled or even exceeded the quality of family bonds. While these findings as well those from other studies (e.g., Clark-Lempers, Lempers, & Ho, 1991; Hunter, 1984; Noack & Fingerle, 1994) correspond to expectations of individuation theory concerning adolescent friendship relations, the more far-reaching claim that experiences of reciprocity in same-sex friendships systematically contribute to the initiation of changes in the family system (Youniss, 1980) remains speculative.

Sex differences in subjective relationship quality vary depending on the specific type of relationship as well as on the relationship aspect which is analyzed. In general, female adolescents experience more support in several of their relationships than do young males, namely in their mother- and same-sex friendship relationships (Furman & Buhrmester, 1992; Noller & Callan, 1990; Sharabany, Gershoni, & Hofman, 1981; Youniss & Smollar, 1985). Positive socio-emotional bonds linking girls and their mothers, however, seem to reflect the closeness typical of relationships with the same-sex parent, as boys report on comparably more support on the part of their fathers (Noack, 1995; Richardson, Galambos, Schulenberg, & Petersen, 1984). Concerning relative power, imbalances are generally less pronounced in young males' relationships while adolescent girls tend to describe their relationships as slightly more unilateral.

It seems plausible to assume that patterns of relationship development as suggested by the findings reported up to this point do not reach a stable plateau by the age of majority. Addressing parent-child relationships, statements of individuation theory are somewhat vague in this respect. The findings reported by Furman and Buhrmester (1992) show that even college students experienced more relative power exerted by their parents as compared to their own power. If their parent relationships are to eventually assume a peer-like character (Smollar & Youniss, 1989), further changes of these relationships can be expected to take place during early adulthood.

PARENT-CHILD AND FRIEND RELATIONSHIPS DURING EARLY ADULTHOOD

Young adults' close relationships have not been a major focus of developmental research. Data available typically address the transition to college and the years directly subsequent to this step. Little is known about family and friendship relationships of young people in the second half of their 20s. Despite the marked changes of several aspects of life that the transition to college entails, the quality of family relationships shows a remarkable stability, indicated by longitudinal correlations (e.g., Rice & Mulkeen, 1995; Schneewind & Ruppert, 1995; Tubman & Lerner, 1994). It may not come as a total surprise, however, that the entry into college goes along with a systematic improvement of the socio-emotional quality of relationships with parents if this transition is linked with a move out of the family home (cf., Golish, 2000; Larose & Boivin, 1998; Takahashi & Majima, 1994). After all, not sharing the same home brings an end to many everyday conflicts related to the distribution of chores, duties, and mutual consideration (Papastefanou, 1997). At the same time, the ecological transition from school to college goes along with an increase of relative power in the relationships with fathers and mothers (Furman & Buhrmester, 1992; Pipp, Shaver, Jennings, Lamborn, & Fischer, 1985). However, it is less clear whether and at which age these relationships reach a state of power symmetry.

The change from school to college is but one of several life transitions on the way to adulthood. In most instances, it does not bring young people's dependence on their parents to an end. In this respect, the entry into worklife can be considered more decisive as it may result in financial independence which, in turn, facilitates autonomous decision-making in various aspects of life (Arnett & Taber, 1994). However, Scabini and Galimberti (1995) report that the transition of sons and daughters into worklife goes along with an increased level of tension within the family. When interpreting these findings, the different cultural contexts of young adult life i.e., U.S. vs. Italy, have to be considered. In general, only scattered evidence presently informs us about possible changes of relationships with parents when young people start to work.

Likewise, little is known about the course that same-sex friendship relationships take during early adulthood. Furman and Buhrmester (1992) report a stable level of relative power as well as of conflict from 10th grade to college age and a decrease in support, while findings from other studies addressing the beginning of early adulthood point to stability or even an increase in the level of intimacy (Clark-Lempers et al., 1991; Rice & Mulkeen, 1995). The socio-emotional quality of friendship, however, seems to depend particularly on the living arrangement of the young adults (Takahashi & Majima, 1994).

CLOSE RELATIONSHIPS IN THE GERMAN CONTEXT

In the present study, we examine parent and friend relationships of adolescents and young adults in Germany. In our review of the relevant literature, most of the research we referred to is based on data from North American samples. Given the scarcity of studies which directly compare close relationships of young people in North America and Germany, predictions concerning differences and similarities are difficult.

Findings from a study including subsamples from the United States, East and West Germany (Rippl & Boehnke, 1995) suggest somewhat higher levels of acceptance of parental authority among young North Americans than in the participating German groups. Even though the observed difference was small in absolute terms, it might deviate from commonly held expectations. However, Lederer (1982) taking a more general approach to attitudes towards authority came to similar conclusions. In her study covering several decades after World War II, (West) German respondents showed markedly stronger orientations towards authority during the time shortly after the war than did U.S. participants (cf., Devereux, Bronfenbrenner & Suci, 1962). In more recent assessments, attitudes among samples from both countries had become quite similar with slightly less authoritarian views stated in Germany. Of course, it is an open question whether and to which extent the attitudinal context translates into aspects of close relationships (cf., Laursen, Wilder, Noack, & Williams, 2000).

Turning to the socio-emotional closeness in close relationships, a study conducted by Claes (1998) may provide some indirect information. The comparison of adolescents' closeness with parents, siblings, and friends based on data from Canada, Belgium, and Italy yielded comparably higher similarities between adolescents from the countries in North America and Northwest Europe as compared to the Southern Europeans who reported more closeness in their relationships (cf., Georgas, Christakopoulou, Poortinga, Angleitner,

Goodwin & Charalambous, 1997). Again, it remains quite speculative to extrapolate these findings to young people in the United States and Germany and to predict levels of socio-emotional quality in the parent and friend relationships in our data that parallel the findings reported by Furman and Buhrmester (1992). Addressing the focal aspect of intimacy in a general way, Lewin's (1936) writings from the first half of the 20th century suggest that Germans show lower levels of self-disclosure as compared to people in the United States. As is the case with power and authority in relationships, however, these differences may have leveled during the subsequent decades.

Moreover, it has to be kept in mind that the interest of the present study is not in absolute levels of relationship qualities. Rather, our major objective is to examine age-graded patterns of structural and socio-emotional aspects of close relationships as well as gender-specific variations. In this respect, we are not aware of strong evidence suggesting differences between samples from Western industrial democracies. As far as previous research addressing our questions is available, we base our hypotheses on earlier findings. Consequently, a consistently symmetrical power structure is expected concerning young people's friendships as opposed to hierarchical patterns in the family which slowly give way to a balance of relative power in the course of the second and third decade of life. Moreover, young males are expected to report more relative power in their relationships as compared to young females. Concerning conflict and intimacy, we assume that young people experience their friendship relationships more favorably than their parent relationships. In the light of earlier research, we expect a relative low in closeness with parents around mid-adolescence, whereas little change or slight improvements are expected with regard to friendship relationships. At the same time, young females should experience less conflict and more intimacy vis-à-vis their mothers and their friends, whereas males should report more positive perceptions with regard to their father-relationship.

Given the prominent role of the entry into work life in the course of the transition to adulthood, we further explore differences in parent- and friendship relationships between university students and working young adults. We expect a more positive socio-emotional quality of parent relationships among the latter as well as a more egalitarian distribution of power between working sons and daughters and their parents. However, the limited evidence available from earlier studies renders this part of the study exploratory.

METHOD

Sample

A total of 285 young people participated in this study. Participants were 48 sixth-grade (25 males, 23 females; *M* age = 12.0 years), 44 ninth-grade (14 males, 30 females; *M* age = 14.7), 36 12th-grade (18 males, 18 females; *M* age = 17.8), 85 undergraduate (24 males, 61 females; *M* age = 21.8), and 72 graduate students (37 males, 35 females; *M* age = 26.9). All participants were of German origin living in a medium or large size city in the southern part of Germany. Given the structure of the German school system the three adolescent subsamples were confined to students attending high-track schools (*Gymnasium*) which provide a university-bound education. Only a minority of them can be expected not to go on to university after completing their school education. Even though data were also collected in low- and middle track schools, we decided on this limitation for the purpose of the present study, as only high-track schools have late-adolescent students while young people in other tracks leave school earlier and enter a variety of different educational and occupational trajectories. Thus, the majority of our participants–including university students–came from middle- to upper-middle-class families.

The high-school students were contacted in their schools which were selected on a voluntary basis. As the questionnaires were completed in class, the response rate approached 100% with only those excluded who did not get parental permissions to participate. Moreover, a lottery of *compact discs* served as a further incentive for participation in the study with names placed in the lottery only of those adolescents who completed the questionnaire. The university students were asked to participate during lectures, completed the questionnaire at home, and returned them to us using the free university mail service. No further incentives were offered to these young adults. Even though almost all questionnaires handed out were returned, the system of distribution does not allow for a reliable estimate of the initial return rate.

In our exploratory analyses focusing on early adulthood, two further groups of young adults who were working on a regular full-time basis were included in addition to the two university student subsamples. The younger group of working participants was comprised of 32 subjects (17 males, 15 females; *M* age = 22.4 years), and the older group was comprised of 23 subjects (10 males, 13 females; *M* age = 26.6). These young people held a variety of different jobs, most of which did not require a university-bound school education. None of them had attended the university. When interpreting the findings, it has to be kept in mind that work-status is thus confounded with educational experience. Moreover, the share of working young adults living away from their family's home is larger than the one among university students, even though the majority of the latter also did not live together with their parents. University students and working adults did not differ with regard to involvement in romantic relationships or parenthood.

Procedure and Measure

A German adaptation of Furman and Buhrmester's (1985) Network of Relationships Inventory (NRI) was employed in the classroom assessments conducted in the adolescents' schools as well as in the individual assessments of the young adults. The original items were translated into German and the equivalence was checked by way of back translation. Several studies administering the NRI in German samples suggest the applicability of the measures to this cultural context (Buhl, 2000; Gödde, Schwarz & Walper, 1996; Seiffge-Krenke, 2001). Subjects rated the quality of their relationships with their mother (or stepmother), their father (or stepfather), and their closest same-sex friend.

Guided by the conceptual focus of our research questions addressing the structural and socio-emotional quality of relationships with parents and friends, three NRI scales were considered in the following analyses: *Relative power* (of the subject and the other person in the relationship) was included to tap the power structure in a given relationship. The *conflict* scale captures a central facet of the socio-emotional quality of the relationship. The third scale that was included addresses *intimacy*. Even though the construct also taps the socio-emotional quality of a relationship, it has to be distinguished conceptually from warmth or affection (MacDonald, 1992). It rather captures closeness in a relationship as expressed by open communication and self disclosure (e.g., "How much do you share your secrets and private feelings with this person?" cf. Rotenberg, 1995). Each relationship quality was assessed by three items. Subjects were asked to rate how much a relationship quality occurred in a given relationship using five-point rating scales. Means of the responses to each set of three items were used as scale scores ranging from 1 to 5 with a midpoint of 3. Given the shortness of scales, internal consistencies with alphas ranging between .70 and .82 can be considered satisfactory. Alphas did not vary as a function of age.

RESULTS

Age and Sex Differences in Relationship Quality in Adolescence and Early Adulthood

In an initial step, a multivariate repeated-measures analysis of variance with grade and sex as independent variables, relationship type (mother, father, friend), and relationship quality (relative power, conflict, and intimacy) as within-subject factors was conducted. Significant effects were found for relationship type, relationship quality, sex x relationship type, grade x relationship quality, sex x relationship quality, relationship type x relationship quality, grade x relationship type x relationship quality, and gender x relationship type x relationship quality (all p's(F) < .05). Based on the substantial interaction effects including relationship quality, further analyses served to examine variations depending on relationship type, grade, and sex separately for the three relationship qualities studied. F-values are presented in Table 1. Newman-Keuls tests and t-Tests for dependent samples were then conducted to follow up significant effects.

Relative Power. Considerable differences concerning the relative power that young people experience in their relationships with parents and friends were hypothesized. Furthermore, it was expected that relative power increases with age, namely, in the relationships with fathers and mothers. Finally, we predicted higher levels of perceived relative power among males than females. An analysis of variance with grade and sex as independent variables and relationship type as between-subjects factor yielded highly significant main effects of grade and relationship type (p's(F) > .001), and a significant sex-effect ($p(F)$ > .05). In addition, we found significant interactions between grade and sex ($p(F)$ > .05) as well as between grade and relationship type ($p(F)$ > .001). Confirming our expectation, relative power vis-à-vis both parents was lower than in the friendship relationships. While concerning friends, the scores slightly exceeded the scale midpoint indicating a symmetrical structure, young people's relative power in the family was mostly lower despite in-

TABLE 1. Effects of Grade, Sex, and Relationship Type on Relationship Qualities (F-Scores)

	Relative Power	Conflict	Intimacy
Grade	15.12***	2.47*	3.71**
Sex	5.52*	.02	4.37*
Relationship Type	126.55***	42.95***	171.51***
Grade x Sex	2.99*	.48	1.44
Grade x Relationship Type	9.37***	1.90+	4.14***
Sex x Relationship Type	.17	.87	6.07
Grade x Sex x Relationship Type	1.74+	.48	.77

Note. *** p < .001, ** p < .01, * p < .05, + p < .10

creases with age. It should be noted that a subjective equality of power of parents and children was not reached until graduate age. Significant increases in relative power in the mother relationship were observed from grade 9 to grade 12 as well as from grade 12 to graduate school. In the father relationship, relative power significantly increased from grade 9 to grade 12, and between undergraduate and graduate school. The differential pace of change resulted in a significant difference concerning the two parent relationships in the undergraduate group, while in all other groups relative power in the relationships with mothers and fathers did not differ. Mean scores at each grade level are presented in Table 2.

In line with our hypothesis, sex differences resulted from females' perceptions of less relative power in their relationships. While, in the follow-up tests, the difference was significant concerning the friendship relationship, variations between sexes with regard to the parent relationships were only marginal. For all three types of relationships age-graded patterns for females suggest a steady increase of relative power. For males, on the other hand, age-specific variations similar to the findings reported by Furman and Buhrmester (1992) suggest a decrease of perceived power in early adolescence followed by an increase in the subsequent age groups. It should be noted, however, that in the Furman and Buhrmester study the youngest age group consisted of 9-year-olds and that their 7th-graders were only about a half a year older than the youngest subsample in our study. In general, mean scores for comparable age groups in the North American sample were slightly lower than the ones we observed among German adolescents.

Conflict. In our analyses of conflict in close relationships, we found only two significant effects, namely, the main effects of grade ($p(F) > .05$), and relationship type ($p(F) > .001$). While mean scores for both parent relationships suggest a peak of conflict in mid-adolescence, follow-up tests revealed a significant grade difference only for relationships with mothers. As can be seen in Table 2, sixth-graders reported less conflict with their mothers than did students attending ninth grade. Despite this differential finding the ranking of relationships according to conflict did not change across age-graded subsamples, with conflict in friendships being clearly lower than conflict in relationships with both parents. It should be pointed out, however, that the absolute level of conflict with parents also constantly remained below the scale midpoint, suggesting low to moderate tension in the families. This finding slightly diverges from the inverted u-shape pattern depending on age as reported by Furman and Buhrmester (1992).

Intimacy. Perceived intimacy in relationships varied significantly depending on grade ($p(F) > .01$), sex ($p(F) > .05$), and relationship type ($p(F) > .001$).

TABLE 2. Means and Standard Deviations of Ratings by Grade and Relationship Type

	Grade				
	6	9	12	U	G
Relative Power					
Mother	2.21[1,a]	2.24[1,a]	2.56[1,b]	2.77[2,b,c]	3.01[1,c]
	(.68)	(.64)	(.54)	(.60)	(.70)
Father	2.06[1,a]	2.05[1,a]	2.47[1,b]	2.56[1,b]	2.93[1,c]
	(.67)	(.58)	(.70)	(.75)	(.82)
Same-Sex Friend	3.06[2,a]	3.20[2,a]	3.11[2,a]	3.15[3,a]	3.12[1,a]
	(.46)	(.45)	(.53)	(.43)	(.59)
Conflict					
Mother	2.01[2,a]	2.64[2,b]	2.55[2,b]	2.47[2,b]	2.33[2,b]
	(.62)	(.86)	(1.12)	(.94)	(.77)
Father	2.05[2,a]	2.54[2,a]	2.15[2,a]	2.37[2,a]	2.32[2,a]
	(.71)	(.99)	(.88)	(.85)	(.97)
Same-Sex Friend	1.78[1,a]	1.70[1,a]	1.77[1,a]	1.85[1,a]	1.89[1,a]
	(.62)	(.54)	(.81)	(.65)	(.64)
Intimacy					
Mother	2.97[2,b]	2.56[2,a,b]	2.61[2,a,b]	2.75[2,a,b]	2.24[2,a]
	(1.12)	(1.00)	(1.04)	(1.13)	(.99)
Father	2.56[1,b]	1.79[1,a]	1.85[1,a]	1.96[1,a]	1.66[1,a]
	(1.08)	(.74)	(.85)	(.83)	(.59)
Same-Sex Friend	3.21[2,a]	3.75[3,a]	3.73[3,a]	3.66[3,a]	3.46[3,a]
	(1.10)	(1.22)	(.94)	(1.00)	(1.06)

Note. U = undergraduate, G = graduate. Numbers in parentheses are standard deviations. The numbers in superscripts indicate significant differences in means between types of relationships within a given grade level. The letters in superscript indicate significant differences in means between grade levels within types of relationship.

In addition, we found significant interaction effects of relationship type with grade ($p(F) > .001$), and sex ($p(F) > .01$). An inspection of the mean scores presented in Table 2 shows that intimacy with both parents followed a u-shaped pattern from sixth grade to undergraduate school to reach another low point in the graduate subsample. Follow-up analyses, however, yielded a significant difference for reports on relationships with mothers only between the sixth grade and graduate subsamples. Concerning relationships with fathers, sixth graders' intimacy scores were significantly higher than in all other groups. While the age-graded pattern observed for intimacy in same-sex friendships was almost a perfect mirror image of the one for intimacy with parents, individual comparisons were not significant. The ranking of relationships according to intimacy was the same from ninth grade to graduate school. Intimacy with friends was highest and intimacy reported for the relationship with fathers was lowest while the relationship with mothers held a middle rank. Scores for relationships with both parents did not differ significantly except in the youngest group.

In line with our expectation, follow-up analyses of sex differences pointed to females' more intimate relationships with same-sex friends and mothers. In contrast, males perceived more intimacy in their paternal relationship than females which was, however, only a marginally significant difference. Still, this finding underscores the peculiar character of relationships with the same-sex parent as reported in our review of earlier research.

Comparison of University Students and Working Young Adults

As in our main analyses, we first conducted a multivariate repeated measures analysis of variance as an initial screening test in which age group, sex, and work status (university student, working young adult) were independent variables, and relationship type and relationship quality were within-subject factors. Guided by our specific research question, we confined ourselves to effects involving the work status variable when examining the findings. The interaction of work status, relationship type, and relationship quality as well as the four-way interaction including these three variables and sex were significant (both p's$(F) < .05$). Subsequent analyses of variance conducted separately for each relationship quality yielded a significant interaction of age group and work status concerning perceptions of intimacy, while this was not the case for relative power and conflict in relationships. These analyses did not help to elucidate the multivariate four-way interaction including sex.

Age-graded differences in *intimacy* in the relationships of university students and working young adults show reverse patterns as can be seen in Figure 1. Students reported lower levels of intimacy in graduate school than in undergraduate school which were significant in follow-up tests for both parental relationships. Conversely, scores for young adults who had already entered worklife suggest a slight, albeit insignificant increase of intimacy in their close relationships. Thus, higher intimacy in the relationships of students among the

FIGURE 1. Intimacy in Three Relationship Types as Rated by Young Adults Depending on Work Status and Age Group

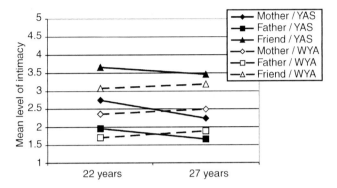

Note. YAS = Young adult students; WYA = Working young adults. To denote the respective subsamples among the student and working participants, mean ages are used instead of grade levels which we consider less instructive concerning young adults.

two younger subsamples gave way to the opposite picture in the two older groups concerning relationships with parents, while the difference in intimacy characterizing friendships decreased.

DISCUSSION

In this investigation of relations with mothers, fathers, and same-sex friends across adolescence and early adulthood, a major objective was to examine variations depending on age and work status. Our findings of age-graded patterns that suggest increases in relative power of young people in the family accompanied by comparably low rates of conflict are in line with our expectations. Likewise, the postulated differences between parent and peer relations were confirmed by our analyses. In particular, the balanced distribution of power between same-age friends sharply contrasts with the more hierarchical situation in the family. Our findings thus mostly correspond with the observations of Furman and Buhrmester (1992) who studied age groups up until the college years. The u-shaped pattern of age-graded variation which Furman and Buhrmester observed is due to the fourth-graders included in their study and could be a peculiarity of this age group. Findings for parallel age groups in the North American sample and in the groups we studied are basically parallel.

In absolute terms, young people in our German sample experienced more relative power in their relations than adolescents in the Furman and Buhrmester (1992) study. While differences are negligible concerning young people's friendships, they range between approximately one-third of a standard deviation and half a standard deviation when comparing reports on parent relationships. Differences between findings from the two studies should, however, be interpreted with caution. It has to be considered that the samples are not identical, for instance, concerning age. Still, a direct comparison of data from sixth and ninth graders participating in our study with data based on parallel assessments conducted in the U.S. (Wilder, 1995) points to a certain validity of the observed differences in relationship power. They correspond to recent findings of systematic, albeit small variations in general orientations toward authority (Rippl & Boehnke, 1995) as well as to data from a large-scale international youth study conducted in Europe and the United States (Nurmi, Liiceanu & Liberska, 1999) suggesting stronger normative orientations toward institutions such as one's parents and one's country among adolescents in the United States than among their agemates in Germany and other Western European countries such as Switzerland, Finland, and France.

Results of a comparison are less clear when it comes to conflict and intimacy in relations. Both studies point to a better socio-emotional quality of friendships as compared to relations with parents. However, the age-graded decrease of conflict rates as reported by Furman and Buhrmester (1992) was only found on the absolute level in our data on parent-adolescent relationships but failed to reach significance. Moreover, we observed higher levels of intimacy between parents and their offspring in the younger age groups paralleling a trend reported by Furman and Buhrmester. However, it has to be acknowledged that a direct comparison is not possible as in the earlier study analyses included a composite measure of social support which considered intimacy and additional provisions of support while we solely focused on the intimacy scale.

Gender differences pointed out by our analyses, again, correspond to Furman and Buhrmester's (1992) findings. For example, young males experienced more power in their relationships than did young females. At the same time, female respondents described their relationships as being more intimate than did males.

In general, slight differences such as in the level of relationship power are less instructive than the overall similarities between German and U.S. samples. This is particularly true of age-graded patterns which are suggestive of a more general course of transformation of family relations during adolescence as posited by individuation theory (Youniss & Smollar, 1985). At the same time, our data clearly show that this process is not completed by the age of majority. A rough balance of power between young people and their parents seems not to be reached before the end of the third decade of life. Still, popular views stating that "parents will always remain parents" seem not to be true with regard to the distribution of power. In this respect, the situation is described as symmetrical by sons and daughters who have reached their late 20s. On the other hand, the overall picture is complex. Higher conflict rates and lower levels of intimacy in young adults' interactions with parents as compared to friendship conflict and intimacy speak against a fully peer-like character of family relations in early adulthood. Further research is needed to arrive at a better understanding of the differentiated character of relations between parents and their adult sons and daughters.

Our comparison of university students and working young adults could only partly elucidate conditions shaping close relations in early adulthood. Even though a decrease of intimacy in relations with parents and friends was only observed in the student subsample, the differential age-related pattern is difficult to interpret. Focusing on the structural meaning of intimacy, a strong tendency toward self-disclosure vis-à-vis parents could be seen as an indication of dependency. Reversely, higher levels of intimacy could also be indicative of a more relaxed stance assumed by working young adults who might feel less need to affirm their privacy (cf., Altman, 1976) and to keep up informational boundaries between themselves and their parents. In the latter case, it could be speculated that the situation of university students is a continued moratorium which allows for further identity development while working young adults have already moved beyond this stage. However, respondents from the university setting might also simply indulge in the intensity of student life and not see their parents as prime addressees of their private thoughts and concerns.

It should be noted that we cannot rule out the possibility that differences in intimacy between university students and working young adults just reflect differences of socio-economic status. While working young adults certainly have more money available for personal use than the average university student, students' educational status is superior and their family backgrounds are more advantaged in an educational as well as material respect. There is some evidence that socio-economic status and, in particular, the level of education is associated with the intensity of verbal exchange between parents and their sons and daughters (Galland, 1997; Lye, 1996). Still, the discussion of a particular difference should not obscure the fact that similarities between the two groups prevailed. Despite the considerable differences in conditions of everyday life, close relations of students and working young adults were similar concerning levels of conflict and the balance of power.

Despite the advantages of confining our main analyses to a homogeneous sample (i.e., high-track students), this decision sets limits to the generalization of our findings. A further limitation of this study results from the cross-sectional character of the data. With almost two decades separating the birth dates of our oldest and youngest subsamples, we cannot discard the possibility that age-related differences observed in the study are partly due to cohort-specific variation (cf. Steinberg, 1996; Schneewind & Ruppert, 1995). Findings from longitudinal studies, however, which covered far shorter time intervals (Noack & Kracke, 1998; Noack, Oepke, & Sassenberg, 1998; Powers & Welsh, 1993), provide some support for an interpretation of the reported age-group differences in terms of change across time. Longitudinal studies that provide comparable information on relationship development well into early adulthood still remain a desideratum for future research.

It should also be noted that we focused on aspects of close relationships as perceived by adolescents and young adults while not considering the perspectives of their relationship partners. Subjective relationship quality as seen by the different partners involved are indeed only moderately correlated (e.g., Noack, 1991). Even though it is not plausible to assume that we would arrive at different findings in the case of friendships as seen by friends, this is less obvious for descriptive analyses of family relations based on parental reports. Direct comparisons of family members' perceptions of their relations typically point to systematic perceiver effects (e.g., Branje, van Aken & van Lieshout, 2002; Lanz, 2000). Data from our own studies suggest, for instance, that mothers systematically provide more positive accounts concerning their families than do their adolescent sons and daughters. It is open to question how far mean level differences between partners' perspectives also affect age-graded patterns. Even though subjective experiences as captured in our assessments can be assumed to provide more instructive descriptions of family and friendship relations as developmental contexts, further analyses are needed to clarify this question.

At the same time, our findings based on the multi-age subsamples in this study covering almost two decades of life as well as our analyses comparing young adults in the university and in worklife who face quite different contextual conditions have yielded instructive insights. Moreover, the parallel methodology employed in our study and earlier research conducted in the United States allows for tentative comparisons which could stimulate future investigations into cultural similarities and differences in the development of close relationships.

REFERENCES

Altman, I. (1976). Privacy. A conceptual analysis. *Environment and Behavior*, 8, 7-29.

Arnett, J., & Taber, S. (1994). Adolescence terminable and interminable: When does adolescence end? *Journal of Youth and Adolescence*, 23, 517-537.

Blos, P. (1979). *The adolescent passage*. New York: International Universities Press.

Branje, van Aken, M. & van Lieshout, C. (2002). Relational support in families with adolescents. *Journal of Family Psychology*, 16, 351-362.

Buhl, H. (2000). Biographische Übergänge und Alter als Determinanten der Eltern-Kind-Beziehung im Erwachsenenalter. [Life transitions and age as determinants of parent-child relations during adulthood] *Zeitschrift für Soziologie der Erziehung und Sozialisation*, 4, 391-409.

Buhrmester, D., & Furman, W. (1987). The development of companionship and intimacy. *Child Development*, 58, 1101-1113.

Bynner, J., & Roberts, K. (Eds.) (1991). *Youth and work: Transition to employment in England and Germany*. London. Anglo-German Foundation for the Study of Industrial Society.

Claes, M. (1998). Adolescents' closeness with parents, siblings, and friends in three countries: Canada, Belgium, and Italy. *Journal of Youth and Adolescence*, 27, 165-184.

Clark-Lempers, D., Lempers, J., & Ho, C. (1991). Early, middle, and late adolescents' perceptions of their relationships with significant others. *Journal of Adolescent Research*, 6, 296-315.

Collins, W.A. (1990). Parent-child relationships in the transition to adolescence. In R. Montemayor, G.R. Adams & T.P. Gulotta (Eds.), *From childhood to adolescence* (pp. 85-106). Newbury Park: Sage.

Devereux, E.C., Bronfenbrenner, U., & Suci, G.J. (1962). Patterns of present behavior in the United States of America and the Federal Republic of Germany: A cross-national comparison. *International Social Science Journal*, 14, 488-506.

Furman, W. & Buhrmester, D. (1985). Children's perceptions of the personal relationships in their social networks. *Developmental Psychology*, 21, 1016-1024.

Furman, W. & Buhrmester, D. (1992). Age and sex differences in perceptions of networks of personal relationships. *Child Development*, 63, 103-115.

Galambos, N.L., & Leadbeater, B.J. (2000). Trends in adolescent research for the new millennium. *International Journal of Behavioral Development*, 24, 289-294.

Galland, O. (1997). Leaving home and family relations in France. *Journal of Family Issues*, 18, 645-670.

Georgas, J., Christakopoulou, S., Poortinga, Y.H., Angleitner, A., Goodwin, R., & Charalambous, N. (1997). The relationship of family bonds to family structure and function across cultures. *Journal of Cross-Cultural Psychology*, 28, 303-320.

Gödde, M., Schwarz, B., & Walper, S. (1996). Adaptation und erprobung des Network of Relationship Inventory (NRI). [Adaptation and psychometric analysis of the Network of Relationship Inventory (NRI)] *Berichte aus der Arbeitsgruppe "Familienentwicklung nach der Trennung #10*. Munich: Ludwig Maximilians University.

Golish, T.D. (2000). Changes in closeness between adult children and their parents: A turning point analysis. *Communication Reports, 13*, 79-98.

Grotevant, H.D., & Cooper, C.R. (1985). Patterns of interaction in family relationships and the development of identity exploration in adolescence. *Child Development, 56*, 415-428.

Grotevant, H.D., & Cooper, C.R. (1986). Individuation in family relationships. *Human Development, 29*, 82-100.

Hall, G.S. (1904). *Adolescence*. New York: Appleton.

Hamilton, S.F. (1990). *Apprenticeship for adulthood: Preparing youth for the future*. New York: Free Press.

Hunter, F.T. (1984). Socializing procedures in parent-child and friendship relations during adolescence. *Developmental Psychology, 20*, 1092-1099.

Krappmann, L. (1998). Sozialisation in der Gruppe der Gleichaltrigen. [Socialization in the peergroup]. In K. Hurrelmann & D. Ulich (Eds.), *Handbuch der Sozialisationsforschung* (5th ed., pp. 355-375). Weinheim: Beltz.

Kroh, O. (1958). *Entwicklungspsychologie des Grundschulkindes. Teil 1: Die Phasen der Jugendentwicklung* [Developmental psychology of the elementary school child: Part 1: Phases of adolescent development]. Weinheim: Beltz.

Lanz, M. (2000). From adolescence to young adulthood: A family transition. In C. Violato, E. Oddone-Paolucci & M. Genius (Eds.), *The changing family and child development* (pp. 132-146). Aldershot: Ashgate.

Larose, S., & Boivin, M. (1998). Attachment to parents, social support expectations, and socioemotional adjustment during the high school-college transition. *Journal of Research on Adolescence, 8*, 1-27.

Laursen, B., & Bukowski, W.M. (1997). A developmental guide to the organization of close relationships. *International Journal of Behavioral Development, 21*, 747-770.

Laursen, B., Coy, C., & Collins, W.A. (1998). Reconsidering changes in parent-child conflict across adolescence: A meta-analysis. *Child Development, 69*, 817-832.

Laursen, B., Wilder, D., Noack, P., & Williams, V. (2000). Adolescent perceptions of reciprocity, authority, and closeness in relationships with mothers, fathers, and friends. *International Journal of Behavioral Development, 24*, 464-471.

Lederer, G. (1982). Trends in authoritarianism: A study of adolescents in West Germany and the United States since 1945. *Journal of Cross-Cultural Psychology, 13*, 299-314.

Lewin, K. (1936). Some social-psychological differences between the United States and Germany. *Character & Personality, 4*, 265-293.

Lye, D.N. (1996). Adult child-parent relationships. *Annual Review of Sociology, 22*, 79-102.

MacDonald, K. (1992). Warmth as a developmental construct: An evolutionary analysis. *Child Development, 63*, 753-773.

Montemayor, R. (1983). Parents and adolescents in conflict: All families some of the time and some families most of the time. *Journal of Early Adolescence, 3*, 83-103.

Montemayor, R., Eberly, M., & Flannery, D.J. (1993). Effects of pubertal status and conversation topic on parents' and adolescent affective expression. *Journal of Early Adolescence, 13*, 431-447.

Noack. P. (1991). *"Soziale Interaktion und Selbstkonzept im Jugendalter"–Zwischenbericht an die Deutsche Forschungsgemeinsschaft* ["Social interaction and self concept in adolescence"–Intermediate report to the German Research Council]. Unpublished manuscript. University of Mannheim.

Noack. P. (1995). *Entwicklung naher beziehungen im jugendalter* [Development of close relations in adolescence]. Unpublished habilitation thesis, University of Mannheim. Mannheim, Germany.

Noack. P., & Fingerle. M. (1994). Gespräche jugendlicher mit eltern und gleichaltrigen freunden [Conversations of adolescents with parents and same-age friends]. *Zeitschrift für Entwicklungspsychologie und Pädagogische Psychologie, 26,* 331-349.

Noack. P., & Kracke. B. (1998). Continuity and change in family interactions across adolescence. In M. Hofer, J. Youniss & P. Noack (Eds.), *Verbal interaction and development in families with adolescents* (pp. 65-81). Stamford: Ablex.

Noack. P., Oepke. M., & Sassenberg. K. (1998). Individuation in familien mit jugendlichen nach der deutschen Vereinigung [Individuation in families with adolescents after German unification]. *Zeitschrift für Sozialisationsforschung und Erziehungssoziologie, 2. Beiheft,* 199-214.

Noller, P., & Callan, V. (1990). Adolescents' perceptions of the nature of their communication with their parents. *Journal of Youth and Adolescence, 19,* 349-362.

Nurmi. J.-E., Liicenu, A., & Liberska, H. (1999). Future-oriented interests. In F.D. Alsaker & A. Flammer (Eds.), *The adolescent experience.* (pp. 85-98). Mahwah: Erlbaum.

Papastefanou, C. (1997). *Auszug aus dem elternhaus* [Moving out of the family home]. Weinheim: Juventa.

Papini, D.R., & Sebby, R.A. (1987). Adolescent pubertal status and affective family relationships: A multivariate assessment. *Journal of Youth and Adolescence, 16,* 1-15.

Piaget. J. (1973). *Das moralische urteil beim kinde.* [The moral judgment of the child] Frankfurt/M.: Suhrkamp.

Pipp, S., Shaver, P., Jennings, S., Lamborn, S., & Fischer, K.W. (1985). Adolescents' theories about the development of their relationships with parents. *Journal of Personality and Social Psychology, 4,* 991-1001.

Powers, S.I., & Welsh, D. (1993, March). *Changes in family interaction from middle to late adolescence.* Paper presented at the Biennial Meeting of the Society for Research in Child Development; New Orleans, LA.

Rice, K.G., & Mulkeen, P. (1995). Relationships with parents and peers: A longitudinal study of adolescent intimacy. *Journal of Adolescent Research, 10,* 338-357.

Richardson, R.A., Galambos, N.L., Schulenberg, J.E., & Petersen, A.C. (1984). Young adolescents' perceptions of the family environment. *Journal of Early Adolescence, 4,* 131-153.

Rippl, S., & Boehnke, K. (1995). Authoritarianism: Adolescents from East and West Germany and the United States compared. *New Directions for Child Development, 70,* 57-70.

Rotenberg, K.J. (Ed.) (1995). *Disclosure processes in children and adolescents.* New York: Cambridge University Press.

Scabini, E., & Galimberti, C. (1995). Adolescents and young adults: A transition in the family. *Journal of Adolescence, 18*, 593-606.

Schneewind, K.A., & Ruppert, S. (1995). *Familien gestern und heute: Ein Generationenvergleich über 16 Jahre* [Families yesterday and today: A 16 year generational comparison]. München: Quintessenz.

Seiffge-Krenke, I. (2001). Beziehungserfahrungen in der adoleszenz: Welchen stellenwert haben sie zur vorhersage von romantischen beziehungen im jungen erwachsenenalter? [Experiences in relationships during adolescence: Their relevance to the prediction of romantic relationships during young adulthood] *Zeitschrift für Entwicklungspsychologie und Pädagogische Psychologie, 33*, 112-123.

Sharabany, R., Gershoni, R., & Hofman, J. (1981). Girlfriend, boyfriend: Age and sex differences in intimate friendship. *Developmental Psychology, 17*, 800-808.

Smollar, J., & Youniss, J. (1989). Transformations of adolescents' perceptions of parents. *International Journal of Behavioral Development, 12*, 71-84.

Steinberg, L. (1987). The impact of puberty on family relations: Effects of pubertal status and pubertal timing. *Developmental Psychology, 23*, 451-460.

Steinberg, L. (1990). Autonomy, conflict, and harmony in the family relationship. In S.S. Feldman & G.R. Elliott (Eds.), *At the threshold* (pp. 255-276). Cambridge: Harvard University Press.

Steinberg, L. (1996). *Adolescence* (4th ed.). New York: McGraw-Hill.

Sullivan, H.S. (1953). *The interpersonal theory of psychiatry.* New York: Norton.

Super, D.E. (1980). A life-span, life-space approach to career development. *Journal of Vocational Behavior, 16*, 282-298.

Takahashi, K., & Majima, N. (1994). Transition from home to college dormitory: The role of preestablished affective relationships in adjustment to a new life. *Journal of Research on Adolescence, 4*, 367-384.

Tubman, J.G., & Lerner, R.M. (1994). Affective experiences of parents and their children from adolescence to young adulthood: Stability of affective experiences. *Journal of Adolescence, 17*, 81-98.

van Aken, M.A.G., & Asendorpf, J.B. (1997). Support by parents, classmates, friends, and siblings in preadolescence: Covariation and compensation across relationships. *Journal of Social and Personal Relationships, 14*, 79-93.

Vondracek, F.W., Lerner, R.M., & Schulenberg, J.E. (1986). *Career-development: A life-span developmental approach.* Hillsdale: Erlbaum.

Wilder, D. (1995). *Changes in relationship closeness, reciprocity, and authority during adolescence.* Unpublished masters thesis, Florida Atlantic University, Boca Raton, Florida..

Wintre, M.G., Yaffe, M., & Crowley, J. (1995). Perception of parental reciprocity scale (POPRS): Development and validation with adolescents and young adults. *Social Development, 4*, 129-148.

Youniss, J. (1980). *Parents and peers in social development: A Piaget-Sullivan perspective.* Chicago: University of Chicago Press.

Youniss, J., & Smollar, J. (1985). *Adolescent relations with mothers, fathers, and friends.* Chicago: University of Chicago Press.

Korean-American Mothers' Experiences in Facilitating Academic Success for Their Adolescents

Sungeun Yang
Kathryn D. Rettig

ABSTRACT. The study reported a phenomenological analysis of interviews with 17 Korean-born mothers raising adolescents in the United States. The two research questions were: What does academic success mean to Korean-American mothers? What do they experience in facilitating the academic success of their adolescents? Results indicated that academic success meant admission to an Ivy League University by studying well and getting straight A grades. Mothers' experiences were portrayed from three perspectives: mothers as family members trying to realize academic success and experiencing tensions; mothers as individuals adjusting by trying to find new goals and standards; and mothers as members of a Korean-American social system. The mothers unknowingly provided a cross-national perspective of family resource management in everyday feelings, thoughts, and actions. *[Article copies available for a fee from The Haworth Document Delivery Service: 1-800-HAWORTH. E-mail address: <docdelivery@haworthpress.com> Website: <http://www.HaworthPress.com> © 2004 by The Haworth Press, Inc. All rights reserved.]*

Sungeun Yang is affiliated with Chosun University, College of Social Science, Department of Public Administration and Social Welfare, 70 Seosuk-dong, Dong-gu, Gwangju, South Korea (E-mail: yangx096@yahoo.com). Kathryn D. Rettig is affiliated with the University of Minnesota, Department of Family Social Science.

http://www.haworthpress.com/web/MFR
© 2004 by The Haworth Press, Inc. All rights reserved.
Digital Object Identifier: 10.1300/J002v36n03_04

KEYWORDS. Adolescents, academic success, Korean-Americans, phenomenological analysis

Academic success is one of the most important values in Korean-immigrant families. The children are encouraged to be high achievers, and parents are strongly committed to supporting their children's education (Tuan, 1995). However, there are few scholarly examinations of Korean-American mothers' unique perspectives on American schooling (Cheon, 1996), their meanings of academic success, or their emotions related to the processes of realizing children's academic success (Yang, 2001). There are few descriptions of interactions between children and parents (Pyke, 2000; Yang & Rettig, 2003), or between mothers and Korean-American social systems, while in the pursuit of academic success (Yang, 2001).

Previous studies have focused on correlations between demographic variables and children's grade point averages, SAT scores, or entrance rates into prestigious colleges in the United States (Fuligni, 1997; Hurh & Kim, 1984), but have been silent about whether or not parents have encountered difficulties as they assisted children in realizing academic success. Little is known about the consequences if children cannot reach parental expectations. Existing studies on Korean-Americans' academic success have not focused on the hidden, ambiguous, or contradictory aspects of family processes, and it is important to reflect on the empirical realities (Strauss & Corbin, 1990) of immigrant mothers' actual experiences.

The purpose of the current study was to gain a deeper understanding of the academic success phenomenon, from the perspectives of Korean-American mothers, by analyzing transcripts of personal interviews, using a phenomenological analysis method. The two central research questions were: What does academic success mean to the Korean-born mothers of adolescent children raised in the United States? What do mothers experience in facilitating academic success of their adolescents? The responses to these questions may be helpful for researchers studying immigrant families, educators of Korean-American students, and family life educators who work with Korean immigrant parents.

RELATED LITERATURE

The importance of academic success in Korean-American families originated from the Confucian tradition of placing high priority on the values of wisdom and competence acquired through education (Hyon, 1949; Park,

1997). Confucian philosophy has emphasized patriarchal authority and hierarchical relations between generations and genders (Hurh, 1998; Yang, 2001). Mothers, instead of fathers, were selected as participants for the current study for cultural reasons. There is a Confucian emphasis on the role of the mother in rearing children, and mothers are traditionally regarded as primary caregivers in Korean culture. Korean-American children have identified their mothers as primary caretakers (Park, 1995), and McCord (1991) noted that mothers, compared to fathers, were more influential in affecting children's behaviors.

Family researchers have acknowledged the importance of academic success in Korean-American families (Kwon, 1994; Lee & Cynn, 1991; Park, 1995), and reported that over one-third of Korean-American parents had bachelor's degrees from Korean Universities (U.S. Bureau of the Census, 1993). Korean parents have said they came to the United States because of a wish to provide their children with a good education (Schneider & Lee, 1990). They believed a good education was a way to (a) escape poverty, (b) gain financial security, (c) achieve upward mobility, (d) increase personal competence, (e) realize self-improvement, (f) acquire greater social prestige, and (g) improve perceptions of family status (Schneider & Lee, 1990).

It is estimated the Korean-American population in the United States is above 1.3 million. More than 72.7% of these individuals were Korean-born, 56.4% of them came to the United States after 1980 (U.S. Bureau of the Census, 1994), and 75.3% were married and had families with children under 18 years of age (Ishii-Kuntz, 1997). Thus, the majority of Korean-Americans in the United States lived in families consisting of first-generation immigrant parents and American-born or raised children. The children have been socialized in a different culture from their parents, who have lower levels of acculturation and assimilation. These cross national influences within families may affect the interpersonal interactions associated with realizing academic success, resulting in unique family experiences for Korean-Americans.

Strong ethnic attachment has been one of the most visible characteristics of Korean immigrants, compared to other ethnic groups (Min, 1995). Ethnic attachment refers to the extent to which members of an ethnic group maintain their native, cultural traditions, and participate in ethnic social networks (Hurh & Kim, 1984). One indicator of high levels of ethnic attachment is that more than 75% of Korean-Americans have been involved in Korean churches (Hurh & Kim, 1984; 1990; Min, 1995) where they have maintained their cultural traditions and language. Most Koreans living in the United States are Christians (Min, 1995), as they were when living in their country of origin. However, Koreans have also continued to be influenced simultaneously by Confucian ideology that has permeated Korean cultures across time (Cha, 1983).

There is speculation that an ethnic social system might provide immigrant parents with material, emotional, and informational resources to raise children in the United States (Cohen & Syme, 1985). However, social support needs to be investigated because of the Korean ideology that has emphasized familial interests over ethnic, nation, or race relations (Kim, 1980). It is important to bring forward the voices of mothers, regarding their own experiences in families and Korean-American social systems, in order to provide in-depth understanding of the realities of facilitating academic success for children. An exploratory investigation is needed to discover what difficulties Korean-American mothers encounter in the pursuit of academic success, how these difficulties affect parents and children, and what they do about these challenges in everyday life. Mothers' lived experiences can provide a process-oriented perspective, instead of focusing only on results or outcomes.

METHOD

A phenomenological analysis method was used (Giorgi, 1997) to reach a deeper understanding of the academic success phenomenon by systematically searching for meanings, perceptions, interpretations, feelings, and values (van Manen, 1990). The method was effective for revealing the ways mothers subjectively experienced their world (van Manen, 1990), and for exploring their experiences while trying to facilitate academic success for their children, within the contexts of their families and their Korean-American social systems.

Participants in the Study

The sampling method was criteria based and guided by the purposeful selection of participants who had experienced the phenomenon of interest (McClelland & Kao, 2000). The criteria required first-generation Korean immigrant mothers, who were educated in Korea, married to a first-generation Korean immigrant, and had at least one American-raised adolescent child. It was expected that first-generation mothers might have a different experience from their American-raised children in terms of the school curricula, peer influences, and teacher-student relationships (Feldman & Glen, 1990), all of which would be related to academic success.

Sample

When discussing appropriate sample size, ten subjects represents a reasonable size for a phenomenological study with interviews lasting as long as two hours (Creswell, 1998). Patton (1990) concluded, "The validity, meaningfulness, and insights generated from qualitative inquiry have more to do with the information richness of the cases selected, and the observational/analytical capabilities of the researcher, than with the sample size" (p. 185).

The first author recruited participants, during September 2000, at a "Parent-Child Rally" at a Korean Catholic Church in a city in the Midwest. Seven mothers volunteered, and ten mothers were obtained after hearing about the study (Patton, 1990), resulting in a total of 17 participants. The intension of the interviews was to generate rich descriptions of the participants' experiences (Girden, 2001) with academic success.

The 17 mothers in the study were middle aged (M = 44.2 years) and had arrived in the United States between 1979 and 1986. All of them had graduated from high school in Korea and some had additional years of schooling (M = 13.8 years). There were three housewives, two part-time, and 12 full-time working mothers. Eight mothers worked at the post office, three owned small businesses, two worked for non-profit organizations, and one was employed in a private company. Fifteen mothers had adolescent children born in the United States. The other two children were born in Korea and moved to the United States at age 11 years. All of the children started junior high school in the United States. The mean age of target children was 15.2 years and the eight males and nine females were in grades eight through twelve.

Interviews

Mothers were contacted by personal phone calls to schedule times and places for interviews. They were first invited to participate, informed of their rights, and the procedures of the interview were then explained. They had opportunities to ask questions, and if they agreed to participate, then a personal in-depth interview of one to two hours was conducted with each participant. The average amount of time for the interviews was about 90 minutes. The interviews were scheduled from September through November 2000, and held in the homes of participants, or the university office of the first author.

Prior to interviewing, five Korean doctoral students checked the interview questions in both Korean and in English languages. Changes were made in the wording of questions and were again verified by these consultants. The first author, a bilingual researcher, conducted all of the interviews, one with each mother. Each participant was given the option of having the interview conducted in English, Korean, or both languages, so that questions were understood, and answers explained. All mothers chose to speak Korean.

Mothers were then asked the following open-ended questions: (a) What does it mean for a Korean-American child to do well in the American school?

(b) How would you know if your child does well in school? (c) Are there any standards that you expect your child to meet? (d) How important is it for your child to do well in school? And why? (e) How do you help your child to do well in school? (f) What difficulties do you have with your child in terms of doing well in school? (g) What do you do about these difficulties? (h) What kind of person do you hope your child will be in terms of future competencies and work? (i) What kind of relationships do you have with other Korean-Americans regarding a child's doing well in school?

Analysis

Transcriptions were made verbatim in Korean, and the data were first analyzed in the original language. The quotations were translated at later stages of the analysis, and back translation methods were followed to establish validity from Korean to English. A bilingual translator checked the accuracy of the translations selected for reporting results.

Giorgi's (1997) phenomenological analysis approach was used to analyze the transcribed interviews. The analysis contains the following five stages: (a) Gaining a sense of the whole text to highlight the most important ideas; (b) Identifying the meaning units that emerge as spontaneous discriminations within the participants' statements during the line-by-line approach; (c) Transforming the participants' expressions into abstract language of the discipline to elucidate psychological and social aspects of the phenomenon; (d) Watching the modes of appearing, or the way in which the participants present the phenomenon for a meta communication analysis; and (e) Synthesizing the meaning units into a coherent description of the structure and/or processes of the phenomenon.

RESULTS

The results of the phenomenological analysis are presented in a linear manner that corresponds to the steps of the method authored by Giorgi (1997), although the processes of qualitative analyses tend to be more circular and overlapping than sequential and discrete. The participants are identified by numbers that are placed in parentheses at the end of the quotations.

Gaining a Sense of the Whole

The sense of the whole text describes the mothers' meanings of academic success and their justifications for their perspectives. All 17 Korean-American mothers in the study gave the same answer when asked about the meaning of academic success: "studying well and going to a good college." This goal-oriented meaning of the value of academic success was specified by the standards of "getting straight A's" and "going to an Ivy League University."

> To Korean mothers, it [doing well in school] means to study well and to go to a good college . . . to study well? Of course, it is to get straight A's. A good college means one of the Ivy League Universities. I mean Harvard. (# 08)

Mothers justified the high importance of academic success by their belief about the relationship between academic success and a better life.

> I want our son to go to college . . . If he studies more, he can get a high-class job . . . I also wish him to have a job, with a good salary, and with using his brain instead of body. Because we [parents] were neither raised here, nor educated well, we have a blue-collar job in the United States. We wish our children to have a better job than we have. (# 14)

IDENTIFYING THE MEANING UNITS

The second analysis stage of identifying meaning units, and the third stage of transforming them into abstract language, sometimes merged together because of the unique characteristics of language translation. The researcher separated the whole Korean text into manageable units, and translated repeated meaning units into English. The meaning units outlined in the following paragraphs are demonstrated by a summary, followed by at least one quotation that provides evidence for the meaning unit, as well as trustworthiness (Lincoln & Guba, 1985). The quotations were chosen to represent the voices of as many participants as possible, and also to describe accurately the meaning units that were found in so many of the transcripts. These processes encourage readers to participate in the verification of the results and conclusions of the study (Creswell, 1998).

Mothers' experiences of facilitating academic success were portrayed from three perspectives: (a) mothers as family members, trying to assist adolescents in realizing academic success in ways that created family tensions; (b) mothers as individuals, whose tensions led to adjusting personal goals and standards; and (c) mothers as members of a Korean-American social system, who made continuous comparisons of their adolescents with those of other families, that led to feelings of envy and loneliness.

Mothers, as Family Members, Trying to Realize Academic Success, and Experiencing Tensions

Korean-American mothers used many strategies to assist their adolescent in realizing academic success, and some of the strategies resulted in relationship tensions. These strategies required mobilizing human, economic, and community resources, and included several behavioral actions. They moved to good school districts and/or provided transportation to a distant good school. Mothers structured learning environments at home by establishing specific periods of time for study, and giving extra homework problems from workbooks purchased outside of school. They took adolescents to public libraries as often as possible. They strictly monitored television watching. They paid for private tutors and learning schools, and provided unconditional financial support for school expenses.

> Korean parents are different from American parents. We fully support the children's financial needs for schools. We make money and use it for children. All the Korean parents I know are supporting children's college expenses. (# 05)

Pressuring for higher goals and standards. Korean-American mothers held on to the high priority value of academic success, and continued to push their children to realize it. They agreed, "Education fever of Korean parents here [in the United States] is the same as it is in Korea" (# 11). Mothers knew, however, that their American-raised adolescents did not have the same standards, and the adolescents complained that their parents pressured them.

> Our son complains that we [parents] have too high expectations. He says we have too high standards that he cannot reach. He says it is our problem [laugh]. We know he has talent . . . We want him to do better. When I nag him, or tell him to study, it creates a big fight. He shouts at me to let him alone. There is a conflict coming from the difference. Our son strongly claims that Korean parents push children too much. (# 13)

Raising adolescents in a Korean way. Mothers in the study realized that Korean-American parents insisted on a traditional Korean parenting style that emphasized the values of obedience, conformity, and discipline, with minimal efforts to listen.

> When our daughter disagrees with my husband, he doesn't make her understand by logical language . . . When she talks back to him, she is

spanked by him. He has too much Korean style. It is his attitude. "I command, you obey." (# 06)

The mothers acknowledged that the Korean parenting style did not work well for their American-raised adolescents, and that changes were needed but difficult.

Children in American schools are taught to insist on their opinions when they think parents are wrong. At first, we [parents] didn't like it. We thought our daughter was against parents. I was upset and mad. Later, I realized that she acted, not for her rebellious mind, but for her own opinions. Her opinions were right. I think we [Korean-American parents] need to listen to them. However, we were not raised in that way. We just obeyed parents . . . The environments are so different here . . . I should change myself. . . . However, it is difficult. I know it is right but difficult. (# 15)

Mothers, as Individuals, Adjusting by Trying to Find New Goals and Standards

Each mother admitted that her child might not reach academic success, based on standards of the Korean-American social system. They tried to adjust their standards for particular children, as they explained by using the terms "accepting," "giving up," "changing," or "adjusting." Mothers' adjustments were not results that were accomplished, but were continual thinking processes, accompanied by feelings of sadness, anger, frustration, and disappointment. One mother said: "If I have small expectation, I have small disappointment" (# 07).

Mothers felt relieved and comforted, at the same time, because they no longer had to fight with their adolescent, pressure them, or feel anxious about failures to reach the standard.

I try to accept it [her real abilities and limitations]. While I am raising my children, I can say I have adjusted . . . I should be changed, depending on situations. Here is different from Korea . . . I expected her to do everything very well. Now I am just hoping she doesn't make any trouble . . . she is mentally and physically healthy . . . does what she wants [and] . . . is satisfied by her life. I try to think about it positively . . . Isn't it her life? I should give her a choice. We [parents] have nothing to do except stand by her. (# 10)

Mothers' hopes about adolescents' futures followed an adjustment process. One mother explained her adjustment saying, "I wish him to live an ordinary life, just like his mom and dad. Just a normal life" (# 04). The adjusting process came from mothers' conclusions that using the Korean parenting style of pressuring for higher standards in facilitating academic success, caused conflicts with their adolescents. In addition, mothers were seeing the challenges their adolescents faced, and were feeling guilty about failing to be helpful.

Seeing the challenges for adolescents of English and racism. Korean-American mothers knew their adolescents faced every day a cultural gap between home and school environments. The daily living of these families was highly similar to Koreans' living in Korea. There were few differences in eating habits, contacts with Korean media, or social contacts with other Koreans. Parents tried to teach children the same familial values and rules as if they were in Korea. However, their adolescents were supposed to "switch the cultural channel" (# 01) right after they stepped outside the house. The most visible challenge for Korean-American adolescents was learning English because they first learned Korean from their immigrant parents.

> Korean children have difficulty with language. We, Korean parents, don't speak English at home. Our child can learn English only from books, TV, friends, or school. Even though he was born here, he has a limitation for speaking English, compared to other American kids . . . Our child doesn't belong to American society. He lives in the United States, but he belongs to a Korean family. He has to be adapted to two cultures. Compared to American kids, he is slow to pick up the flow of [American] society. (# 04)

Korean-American adolescents often faced racism outside of home, but mothers did not take action, such as talking to teachers about experiences of racism. They tended to regard racial discrimination as a natural part of their living in the United States.

> I think my son was teased a lot on the school bus when he was in the middle school. Kids told him to go home or to go back to his country. He didn't talk to me about that. I thought he might be more bullied if I complained to teachers about that matter. As a mom, I thought it was better to let it be. Why? He had to overcome, and he had to learn something. He needed to know he was different . . . was not an American kid, and would often face that kind of situation in this society . . . I have let him handle the emotions since childhood. . . . He has done well until now. (# 04)

Failing to be helpful. Korean-American mothers felt they were unable to help their adolescents in terms of participating in school activities, or helping with studying. Mothers claimed their inability to help was mainly due to language, and their feelings of discomfort when they met with American teachers and parents.

> When I went to see an American teacher for the first time, I was too scared. I looked at the English dictionary and prepared sentences. But, I didn't say a word when I faced the teacher [laugh] . . . When our child was in an elementary school, I really tried to participate in school activities. There was nothing more difficult than that. English was so difficult. I gave it up when he went to middle school. I just couldn't do it anymore. (# 01)

Mothers' inabilities to help adolescents were also due to lack of knowledge about American schools and student activities.

> My husband and I don't like to go to the school meetings or activities. Sometimes I make an excuse for skipping meetings. I tell children I am uncomfortable with the meetings. I know children are disappointed. There are some school activities that I don't understand, such as Homecoming. We don't know school activities like that. . . . It would be great if we [parents] could participate in school activities. (# 10)

Mothers felt guilty about not being as helpful with homework as American parents. They also felt sorry their adolescents had to complete school-related work by themselves.

> Our child cannot catch up with American kids in those areas. He doesn't express anything, but I know he might have difficulties at school. A Korean child struggles by himself because we [Korean-American parents] don't know anything about American school systems. Many Korean parents say they are really sorry for their children. It is hard for a child to deal with all those school things by himself! (# 01)

Mothers, in a Social System, Comparing Adolescents, and Feeling Envy and Loneliness

Mothers went through the process of understanding their adolescents' realistic abilities, and adjusting their goals and standards, but they could not stop comparing their children with those in other Korean-American families.

Feeling envy, jealousy, and anxiety. The pursuit of academic success involved comparisons and competitions among Korean-American parents in the social system, instead of cooperation and support. Mothers revealed the rivalry.

There are some Koreans where my husband works. They have excellent children. My husband feels stressed by that. When he hears how good their children are in schools, he gets angry at our daughter's report card. He scolds her, "How did you get these damn grades?" He also blames me. He tells me to make her study, or send her to a learning center or a private school. He wants straight A's. (# 17)

Mothers expressed envy and jealousy that resulted from the comparison. One mother said, "Korean people cannot stand that other people do better than they do. In front of me, people say how wonderful my child is. However, people imply they don't like it. People are extremely jealous" (# 15). Another mother expressed her envy toward other parents whose adolescent reached the goals and standards of the Korean-American system, saying, "I envy other parents whose children go to Yale or MIT. I envy them to death" (# 02).

Most adolescents rarely achieved the level of academic success prescribed by the Korean-American social system because the standards were too high for them. Therefore, mothers felt anxious because other Korean-Americans might notice their child did not achieve academic success, and would gossip about it. The anxiety about gossiping caused mothers to remain silent, or to talk only of good things about their child's actual performance at school.

Most [Korean-American] parents don't open up to their child's problem. Although parents fight with the child seriously, they tell other people that the child does everything well . . . It doesn't matter how close you are to them. They don't tell you about the child's problem . . . Korean parents always say their child gets straight A's. How could it be possible? I don't understand it. Are all of them genius? Korean parents never open up their child's issues. (# 01)

Living with loneliness. Korean-American mothers hardly talked with anybody about difficulties with their adolescents in the pursuit of academic success. Their strategies to deal with envy, jealousy, and anxiety about gossiping in the Korean-American social system isolated them from each other. The expression, "I don't have a friend here," was repeated by most of the mothers in the study. Mothers experienced loneliness from isolation, and they were sad about the absence of close friendships.

I cannot open my heart. I was a very open person. However, I realize when I talk about my private thing, the rumor gets started right away. When I talk about a bad thing in the morning, someone calls me at night. When I tell people I feel bad for something that my child does, they talk about it with others. It is no good to talk to people. I never talk. I shut down the door. When Korean people get together, they talk about other families. I cannot open 100% of my heart to other Koreans . . . I cannot have a friend in the United States. I don't have a real close friend . . . It makes me stressed. That is the most difficult thing here. I have to solve problems by myself. Or just pray. All of us [Korean-Americans] are being hurt in the United States. We just live with it. We say that all the Korean-Americans are half psycho [laugh]. (# 15)

WATCHING THE MODES OF APPEARING

The fourth step of Giorgi's (1997) phenomenological analysis approach involved watching the modes of appearing, or the way in which the participants presented the phenomenon, for a meta communication analysis. The above quotation (#15) demonstrated mothers' feelings of inclusion and exclusion or detachment from their social system, that was also the way they talked throughout the interviews. The most visible mode of communication was mothers' use of the terms "we," "they," "I" and "my," indicating experiences of inclusion and detachment in their family and social group.

Mothers as Family Members and Individuals

The collective term "we" inside a family system implied "we, parents" in contrast to "they, children." Parental role identity seemed more like a joint experience to them. Mothers differentiated "we, parents" from "they, children" when talking about family tensions, although they emphasized strong bonds between mothers and children. The terms "I" and "my" had important meanings in the interviews, because Korean people rarely use them. Koreans use the word "uri" which means "we." Most things are referred to as "our" thing, instead of "my" something. Korean-American mothers used almost the same words, in the same order, when they described the meaning of academic success: "studying well and going to a good college." Their identical meanings were built in a Korean-American social system. Mothers seemed to automatically accept these cultural meanings of academic success that resulted from their strong ethnic attachment. "Our [Korean-Americans']" goals and standards were changed to "my" goals and standards when they explained their adjusted goals and standards of academic success for a particular child. The mothers' use of "I" or "my" represented their detachment from the Korean-American social system, their questioning about the absolute standards of the social system, their reassessment of the child's abilities, and their independent construction of personal reality.

Mothers in a Korean-American Social System

The word "we" inside a social system implied "we, Korean-Americans," compared to "they" non-Korean-Americans," mostly implying European Americans. Mothers used "we, Korean-Americans" when they compared and contrasted Korean traditional ideologies, values, norms, and parenting styles with American mainstream parents. None of the mothers in the study identified themselves as "American" or "Korean-American." They simply used the term "Korean" which was not distinguished from Koreans in Korea.

> When a child gets an A minus instead of an A, Korean parents yell at him. What is this A minus? How can you go to a good college? You will go to a damn shit college with this grade! I think it is Korean parents' greed. We [Korean-American parents] just push children in a Korean way . . . We [parents] had a lot of expectations for our son before. We wanted him to go to a good college. We had a lot of wishes for him. We did the same thing as other Korean parents do. "No! Obey parents' words. Follow mother's words. Do it in mother's way." However, it didn't work at all. While he grew up, I realized he didn't do well. What can I do? I should accept my son as he is. I should stand back instead of pushing him. The only thing I can do is to support him when he asks me to help. I often check him, "Are you studying [for the] SAT?" That's all I can do. (# 05)

SYNTHESIZING MEANING UNITS INTO A STATEMENT OF THE PHENOMENON

The relationships among the meaning units, as interpreted by the researchers, are integrated in Figure 1. This Korean symbol, without the words included, is called "Taeguk," which is a symbol of the "Supreme Ultimate," or the fundamental basis of all things. The three-parts of the "Taeguk" symbolize heaven, earth, and humanity. Each separate part exists in a dynamic movement of equal values that are ever changing and merging to make a perfect circle, and to create the universe. The "Taeguk" represents infinity and linkage (Hwang, 1568).

The modified "Taeguk" for the present study combined all of the interdependent meaning units and shows how mothers facilitated academic success within their simultaneous perspectives of family, individual, and social systems. There were mothers within the family trying to realize academic success for their adolescent by pressuring for higher goals and standards for academic success. The pressuring resulted in experiencing relationship tensions within the family system in which they were raising their children in a Korean way.

FIGURE 1. Korean-American Mothers' Processes of Realizing Academic Success

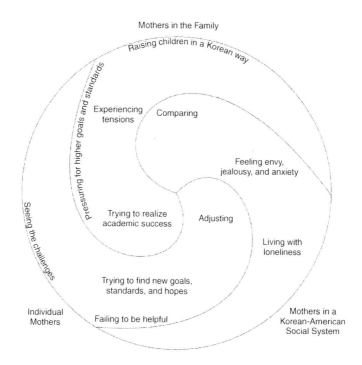

Mothers, at the same time, were individuals who were adjusting by trying to find new goals and standards, because their adolescents were resisting, and mothers were seeing challenges for children in learning English and facing racism. Mothers were feeling guilty about failing to be helpful to children. However, as they were adjusting from the Korean ideals, they were continuing to compare their adolescents to those in other Korean-American families. The comparisons led to feelings of envy, jealousy, and anxiety, which led to withdrawal from the Korean-American social system, and then to experience the resulting feelings of loneliness.

DISCUSSION AND IMPLICATIONS

The current study was an exploratory investigation, and one of the first to listen to Korean-American mothers' voices to reveal their meaning of academic success, and their experiences in facilitating academic success for their American-raised adolescents in American schools. The following paragraphs provide critique of the study with implications for research, implications for educators, contributions of the study, and conclusions.

Critique of the Study and Implications for Future Research

The unique contributions of the study must be accepted with the qualifications of inevitable limitations. The mothers provided very rich descriptions of their meanings, experiences, and feelings. These are strengths of qualitative research designs. However, the results from a small number of participants will not permit generalization beyond these mothers who live in a particular social system, and this would be a limitation as viewed by empirical social scientists. Second, the study intentionally included only the perspectives of mothers, without including fathers and adolescents. Fathers might experience academic success differently from mothers, although mothers regarded parental identity as a joint experience with fathers. The experiences of adolescents and fathers should be explored in future studies to give an integral family picture of meanings, values, and emotions when facilitating academic success.

The third limitation of the study is that the sample is limited to only one Korean-American social system in the Midwest. The mothers in this study may have had lower or higher levels of acculturation and assimilation than Korean-American immigrants in other locations. The social system represented in the study might have a smaller social network, with more frequent contacts, and may be more visible, due to the small percentage of ethnic minorities in this location, compared to larger cities. The experiences of mothers in other Korean-American social systems in various geographical areas should be examined in future studies.

A fourth limitation of the study may be that some qualitative researchers prefer methods of analysis that go beyond the descriptive emphasis of phenomenological analysis (Giorgi, 1997), and provide more depth in interpretation, or a more literary style of presenting research results (Espiritu, 2000; Pyke, 2000). There could also be criticism from phenomenology proponents who object to using a "scientific phenomenological analysis method that seeks reduction and meaning units influenced by a particular discipline" (Giorgi, 1997, p. 244). These researchers would criticize the absence of a phenomenological study design, believe there are too many interpretations, and find too much conceptualization from theories. We realize there are multiple meanings of good qualitative research (Brown, 1989).

Implications for Educators

The present study provides educators with insights about how realizing the value of academic success affects interpersonal relationships within Korean-American families, and in a Korean-American social system. Korean-American mothers might suffer from mental health problems caused by family tensions, isolation from other Korean-Americans, and distance from the mainstream American society. Korean-American adolescents might need support because they are struggling with parental pressures and with integrating Korean and American cultures.

There is a strong need to provide Korean parents with more opportunities to participate in the education of their adolescents in American schools (Esler, Godber, & Christenson, 2001). Mothers in the study expressed their inability to help their adolescents and their own strong feelings of guilt. They believed their inability to help adolescents came from their language barriers and ignorance about American school systems, and they were afraid of meeting teachers and other American parents. These same fears may make mothers hesitant to enroll in parenting workshops held by family life educators. Mothers may want to learn how they can interact with their child more effectively without giving up the value of academic success, but they might be less willing to share this information with other people. These fears would inhibit group discussion as an educational technique. The use of case studies might work more effectively, since the case studies place a 'theoretical problem' more distant from the people in the room, while retaining the advantages of portraying frustrations, failed solutions, and possible options.

Educators could use the experiences reported in the current study to encourage Korean-American mothers. The mothers provided excellent examples of the human ecological perspectives of family resource management in action (Bubolz & Sontag, 1993: Rettig, 1993). These managerial dynamics provided a cross-national perspective of one of the ten content areas of family life education (Arcus, Schvaneveldt, & Moss, 1993) required by the National Council on Family Relations for certifying family life educators (CFLE). The central concepts of family resource management include: problems, values, goals, standards, resources, decisions, and plans. Some of the processes of family resource management include: problem solving, decision-making and implementing; valuing, standard setting, and standard maintaining (Rettig, 1993; Rettig, Rossmann, & Hogan, 1993).

The mothers illustrated family resource management by their conscious and specific values, goals, and standards that were motivations for management. They clearly articulated that academic success (perceiving the challenge) could be obtained by establishing the explicit goal for their adolescent of admission to a good college, based on the specific standard of an Ivy League university. This long-term goal was facilitated by the short-term goal and behavioral actions of studying well with the standard of straight A grades. In addition, the mothers had alternative strategies for reaching their intentions (deciding what to do) and they mobilized resources in order to reach these important outcomes (actuating the decisions).

Mothers used their human resources of time and energy to drive their children to distant schools of higher quality. They used money resources and cognitive and psychomotor human resources in making decisions to buy a house in a better school district, to hire tutors to work with children, and to provide financial resources for school expenses. They utilized community resources, such as libraries, in order to provide better study environments and access a wider range of information resources. The social network was a potential source of social capital wealth that could not be accessed in this particular situation, and therefore, was not a resource for helping Korean-American children to do well in school.

Mothers planned the use of time at home that was designated for study, and they controlled the distractions from "studying well" by limiting television watching and taking the adolescents to libraries. They evaluated their own goals and standards for academic success, and made decisions about adjustments, because their Korean standards were unrealistic in their current American environment. They decided they needed to personally change, so they initiated alternative strategies of facilitating academic success, in order to realize an even higher priority goal of a good relationship with their adolescent.

The achievement of a good relationship with their adolescent was challenging for these mothers. However, several of the difficulties they described are also experienced by other parents of adolescents in the United States, regardless of their nationality, country of origin, or level of assimilation and acculturation. It is a time when parents learn to realistically accept the person their child is becoming, and along with that acceptance, are both strengths and limitations, as well as relationship tensions that are inherent in close relationships within the family context.

CONCLUSIONS

The in-depth interviews with Korean-American mothers in this study provided a process perspective that revealed some of the previously hidden, ambivalent, and contradictory ways of thinking and relating to others in the family and social systems, particularly the difficulties that were encountered and the tensions that resulted. The mothers were working continuously harder and longer for cognitive, academic achievement by asserting their power as parents. This Korean way of reaching a Korean ideal came in conflict with the American definitions of academic success, and the more democratic strategies of accomplishing this ideal. European-American parents have more often had an integrative definition of academic success that involved a balance of cognitive achievement and participation in school activities. The latter definition has often been accomplished by acceptance of the child's performance and accompanying encouragement and praise. These strategies have been viewed by Korean-American mothers as ineffective for reaching high levels of cognitive competence (Yang & Rettig, 2003).

The tensions in families resulted when adolescents resisted the parental strategies, and in doing so, violated the high priority Korean values of obedience and respect toward parents. The adolescents insisted on having freedom of speech and freedom to make their own decisions about time use, saying that "studying all the time" didn't work for them. Fathers blamed mothers for their failures to make the adolescents achieve in school. After long periods of family conflict, mothers realized their strategies were not working, and they began listening carefully to the perspectives of their adolescents. Mothers decided that cognitive academic achievement was not always worth the high cost of compromising a good relationship with their adolescents.

Adolescents had an important influence on their mothers, who began to change their expectations, and to think more in terms of long-term happiness for their adolescents. The results were a transformation in parenting behaviors to a style that was more accepting and encouraging. The outcomes of their personal changes indicated revised value priorities of love, respect, and harmony, along with academic success. The changes may have reduced personal anxieties, but increased conflicts with spouses, and furthered emotional distance from other mothers in their social system. Future studies will need to examine these interpersonal dynamics in greater depth.

ACKNOWLEDGMENTS

The research is a revision of part of a doctoral dissertation. The authors wish to acknowledge funding assistance from the Minnesota Experiment Station, Projects: "Decision making integral to relationship transitions," Kathryn D. Rettig, P.I.; and "Family systems and family realities," Paul C. Rosenblatt, P.I. Additional funding support was received from the American Association of Family and Consumer Sciences, International Fellowship 2000. The authors wish to thank Donghoh Kim for research assistance and Paul Rosenblatt, Harold Grotevant and Marilyn Rossmann for helpful comments on an earlier draft of the manuscript.

REFERENCES

Arcus, M. E., Schvaneveldt, J. D., & Moss, J. J. (Eds.). (1993). *Handbook of family life education: The practice of family life education* (Vol. 2, pp. 1-32). Newbury Park, CA: Sage Publications.

Brown, M. M. (1989). What are the qualities of good research? In F. H. Hultgren & D. L. Coomer (Eds.), *Alternative modes of inquiry* (pp. 267-297). Washington, DC: American Home Economics Association, Teacher Education Section.

Bubolz, M. M., & Sontag, M. J. (1993). Human ecology theory. In P. G. Boss, W. J. Doherty, R. LaRossa, W. R. Schumm, & S. K. Steinmetz (Eds.), *Sourcebook of family theories and methods: A contextual approach* (pp. 419-448). New York: Plenum.

Cha, C. H. (1983). *The ethical conceptions of the Korean people*. Seoul, Korea: The Academy of Korean Studies.

Cheon, H. (1996). *Korean immigrant mothers and American teachers: Mothers' experiences with their children's schooling and teachers' experiences with the mothers*. Doctoral Dissertation. Minneapolis, MN: University of Minnesota.

Cohen, S., & Syme, S. L. (1985). Issues in the study and application of social support. In S. Cohen & S. L. Syme (Eds.), *Social support and health* (pp. 3-22). New York: Academic Press.

Creswell, J. W. (1998). *Qualitative inquiry and research design*. Thousand Oaks, CA: Sage.

Esler, A., Godber, Y., & Christenson, S. L. (2001). Voices from home: How diverse families support children's learning similar ways. *CURA Reporter, 2001* (February), 9-15.

Espiritu, Y. L. (2000). "We don't sleep around like white girls do": Family, culture, and gender in Fillipina American lives. *Signs, 26,* 415-440.

Feldman, S. S., & Glen, R. E. (Eds.) (1990). *At the threshold: The developing adolescent*. Cambridge, MA: Harvard University Press.

Fuligni, A. J. (1997). The academic achievement of adolescents from immigrant families: The roles of family background, attitudes, and behavior. *Child Development, 68,* 351-363.

Giorgi, A. (1997). The theory, practice, and evaluation of the phenomenological method as a qualitative research procedure. *Journal of Phenomenological Psychology, 28,* 235-260.

Girden, E. R. (2001). *Evaluating research articles* (2nd ed.). Thousand Oaks, CA: Sage.

Hurh, W. M. (1998). *The Korean Americans*. Westport, CT: Greenwood Press.

Hurh, W. M., & Kim, K. C. (1984). *Korean immigrants in America: A structural analysis of ethnic confinement and adhesive adoption*. London: Fairleigh Dickinson University Press.

Hurh, W. M., & Kim, K. C. (1990). Correlates of Korean immigrants' mental health. *The Journal of Nervous and Mental Disease, 178,* 703-711.

Hwang, Y. (1568). *Songhakshipto* [Ten diagrams of the learning of the sage]. Seoul, Korea.

Hyon, S. Y. (1949). *A history of Korean Confucianism*. Seoul, Korea: Miuunsogwan.

Ishii-Kuntz, M. (1997). Intergenerational relationships among Chinese, Japanese, and Korean Americans. *Family Relations, 46,* 23-32.

Kim, K. D. (1980). *The future of Korean culture viewed in the historical context.* Seoul, Korea: The Academy of Korean Studies.

Kwon, H. Y. (Ed.). (1994). *Korean Americans: Conflict and harmony.* Chicago, IL: Covenant Publications.

Lee, J., & Cynn, V. (1991). Issues in counseling 1.5 generation Korean Americans. In C. Lee & B. Richardson (Eds.), *Multicultural issues in counseling: New approaches to diversity.* Alexandria, VA: American Association for Counseling and Development.

Lincoln, E.G., & Guba, Y. S. (1985). *Naturalistic Inquiry.* Beverly Hills, CA: Sage Publications.

McClellan, J. A., & Kao, S. C. (2000). *Parents' experience helping their children get into college.* Paper presented at the meeting of the National Conference on Family Relations, Minneapolis, MN.

McCord, J. (1991). Family relationships, juvenile delinquency, and adult criminality. *Criminology, 29*(3), 397-417.

Min, P. G. (1995). Korean Americans. In P. G. Min (Ed.), *Asian Americans: Contemporary trends and issues* (pp. 199-231). Thousand Oak, CA: Sage.

Park, E-J, K. (1995). Voices of Korean-American student. *Adolescence, 30,* 945-953.

Park, K. (1997). *The Korean-American dream.* Ithaca, New York: Cornell University.

Patton, M. Q. (1990). *Qualitative evaluation and research methods.* Newbury Park, CA: Sage.

Pyke, K. (2000). "The normal American family" as an interpretive structure of family life among grown children of Korean and Vietnamese immigrants. *Journal of Marriage and the Family, 62,* 240-255.

Rettig, K. D. (1993). Problem-solving and decision-making as central processes of family life: An ecological framework for family relations and family resource management. *Marriage & Family Review, 18,* 187-222.

Rettig, K. D., Rossmann, M. M., & Hogan, M. J. (1993). Educating for family resource management. In M. Arcus, J. D. Schevaneveldt, & J. J. Moss (Eds.), *Handbook of family life education: The practice of family life education* (Vol. 2, pp. 115-154). Newbury Park, CA: Sage Publications.

Schneider, B., & Lee, Y. (1990). A model for academic success: The school and home environment of East Asian students. *Anthropology and Education Quarterly, 21,* 358-377.

Strauss, A., & Corbin, J. (1990). *Basics of qualitative research: Grounded theory procedures and techniques.* Newbury Park, CA: Sage.

Tuan, M. (1995). Korean and Russian students in a Los Angeles high school: Exploring the alternative strategies of two high-achieving groups. In R. G. Rumbaut & W. A. Cornelius (Eds.), *California's immigrant children* (pp. 107-130). San Diego, CA: University of California.

U. S. Bureau of the Census. (1993). *1990 Census of population: Asians and Pacific Islanders in the United States.* Washington, DC: US Government Printing Office.

U. S. Bureau of the Census. (1994). *1990 Census of population, general social and economic characteristics, the United States.* Washington, DC: US Government Printing Office.

van Manen, M. (1990). *Researching lived experiences: Human science of an action sensitive pedagogy.* New York: State University of New York Press.

Yang, S. (2001). *Korean-American mothers' meanings of academic success and their experiences with children in American schools.* Doctoral Dissertation. Minneapolis, MN: University of Minnesota.

Yang, S., & Rettig, K. D. (2003). The value tensions in Korean-American mother-child relationships while facilitating academic success. *Personal Relationships, 10,* 351-371.

Sex Differences and Conjugal Interdependence on Parenthood Stress and Adjustment: A Dyadic Longitudinal Chinese Study

Luo Lu

ABSTRACT. This study explored sex differences and conjugal interdependence in stress and adjustment of young Chinese fathers and mothers in the half-year period following the birth of their children. Ninety pairs of married couples took part in this panel study conducted twice at six weeks and six months after the birth of their children. Results showed that (a) Wives reported heightened stress, worse health and lower marital satisfaction than husbands, (b) a substantial degree of conjugal interdependence was revealed in significant correlations of health and marital satisfaction between partners, and (c) conjugal discrepancy in stress had an adverse impact on personal well-being and marital satisfaction of wives. These results were discussed in relation to existing theories and research, as well as the distinct characteristics of contemporary Chinese society. *[Article copies available for a fee from The Haworth Document Delivery Service: 1-800-HAWORTH. E-mail address: <docdelivery@haworthpress.com> Website: <http://www.HaworthPress.com> © 2004 by The Haworth Press, Inc. All rights reserved.]*

Luo Lu is affiliated with the Department of Psychology, Fu-Jen Catholic University, Taiwan.

Address correspondence to: Dr. Luo Lu, Department of Psychology, Fu-Jen Catholic University, 510 Chong-Cheng Road, Hsing-Chuang 242, Taipei Hsien, Taiwan, ROC (E-mail: luolu@mails.fju.edu.tw).

This research was supported by a grant from the National Science Council, Taiwan, ROC, NSC89-2413-H-037-008.

http://www.haworthpress.com/web/MFR
© 2004 by The Haworth Press, Inc. All rights reserved.
Digital Object Identifier: 10.1300/J002v36n03_05

KEYWORDS. Chinese parents, conjugal interdependence, parenthood transition, sex differences

At the turn of the century, the traditionally conservative East Asia is undergoing profound economic and societal modernizations. As a consequence, the divorce rate has skyrocketed in this region. Even though Taiwan is a prototypical Chinese society with a strong Confucius family tradition, the latest official estimate indicates that for every three new marriages one ends up in divorce (Executive Yuan, 2001). Research has suggested that problems that lead to marital dissolution begin early in relationships (Thornes & Collard, 1979). Transition to parenthood has been described as a "crisis" for both men and woman (Cowan, Cowan, Heming, Garret, Coysh, & Curtis-Boles, 1985). However, extant research on parenthood adjustment has been heavily influenced by the dominant societal ethos of parenting being a "women's issue," and consequently little attention has been paid to sex differences, especially men's adjustment when they become fathers. The present study thus focused on these possible sex differences. Specifically, our dyadic design is a more rigorous method to examine conjugal similarities and discrepancies. Our two-wave panel design also allowed considerations of both the earlier (six weeks) and later (six months) transition stages to parenting. As it is not a foregone conclusion that western research findings can be generalized to a vastly different culture such as the Chinese one, our study with Chinese parents represents a pioneering study with important implications.

Although this paper focuses on the parenthood transition immediately following the birth of a child, what we explored has important implications for the entire duration of the parent-child relationship. First, the quality of parenthood adjustment and quality of the martial relationship may directly impact on the parent-child relationship. For example, Osofsky (1979) suggested that postnatal distress may hinder the crucial bonding between mother and child. Owen, Lewis, and Henderson (1989) also found that men and women who have close and confiding marriages are more likely as parents to be warm, sensitive, and to hold positive attitudes about their babies and their parenting roles. The stress of the transition to parenthood and changes in the quality of the marital relationship during this period may have crucial effects on the parent-child relationship.

Second, a more subtle kind of influence may involve family climate and social learning. Research has suggested that problems that lead to marital dissolution begin early in relationships (Thornes & Collard, 1979) and difficulties in parenthood transition may be just one such "crisis" (Cowan et al., 1985). Parental divorce adversely affected children in the areas of academic achievement, behavior/conduct, psychological adjustment, and social relations (see Amato & Keith, 1991a & b for reviews). The so-called "intergenerational transmission of instability in relationships" (MacAllister, 1998) is the saddest aspect of the long-term adverse effects of marital problems on children. Overall, the quality of parenthood adjustment can have important implications for the parent-child relationship, directly and indirectly, immediately and over a long period of time.

SEX DIFFERENCES IN MENTAL HEALTH AND MARITAL SATISFACTION AS PARENTHOOD ADJUSTMENT

In most societies, parenthood is generally regarded as a normative life change and has various positive associations such as love and affection (Burnell & Norfleet, 1986; Soloway & Smith, 1987). For both Chinese men and women, the "parental role" ranked the highest in importance among various critical adult roles (Lu & Lin, 1998). However, becoming parents also creates striking transformations of self, identity, and roles (Fiese, Hooker, Kotary, & Schwagler, 1993; Smith, 1995). This has a great impact on the individual's physical and mental well-being (Abbott & Brody, 1985). Furthermore, due to disparate social constructions of fatherhood and motherhood (Phoenix & Woollett, 1991), men and women may undergo very different psychological processes in becoming parents. "Parenting" has been generally constructed as a "women's business," coupled with demands of the role of a primary caregiver. Although becoming a mother greatly changes a woman's life, becoming a father has not been recognized historically as a major event in a man's life. Some researchers now argue that the transition into fatherhood is more abrupt, traumatic, and life altering for men than is their transition into marriage (Davidson & Moore, 1996). Men have recently become more attached to their family roles than ever before, including the nurturing aspects of fatherhood. However, academic interests in the implications of fatherhood on men's well-being and marital satisfaction are just beginning to be recognized.

In contrast to the extensive study on women's postpartum depression, there has been little examination of postnatal mental health problems in fathers. Rees and Lutkins (1971) found that up to 4% of postnatal fathers were identified as depressed by their family doctors. Ballard, Davis, Cullen, Mohan, and Dean (1994) found a similar figure of 5% among fathers six months after their children were born. However, both of these figures may still be underestimates.

Men's physical health, on the other hand, received somewhat more attention in scientific research. Ferketich and Mercer (1989) found that men's perception of their health was significantly poorer at eight months postnatal than during their partners' pregnancy. Quill, Lipkin, and Lamb (1984) found that men visited doctors more in the year after their children were born than during their partner's pregnancy. The strong relationship between physical and mental health (Lu & Hsieh, 1997; Lu, Shiau, & Cooper, 1997; Lu, Tseng, & Cooper, 1999) suggests that men experiencing a high level of physical symptoms may actually be having difficulties adjusting to their new role as a father. However, with the prevailing social pressure on women, we expected that parenting would exert a stronger impact on women than on men. Specifically, we hypothesized that women would report higher levels of stress and mental health problems than men (*Hypothesis 1*).

Transition to parenthood is also associated with a dip in marital satisfaction (Argyle, 1987). This adverse effect is probably caused by the competition for limited resources between parenthood and marriage (Belsky, 1990). Again, previous work has focused almost exclusively on mothers' reports of marital satisfaction; consequently, we know very little about men's perception of their marriage following the transition to fatherhood.

One study did examine reports of both men and women, and found that while women's marital satisfaction declined six months after childbirth, men's marital satisfaction declined between 6 and 18 months after their children were born (Cowan et al., 1985). This pattern of sex difference implies that both men and women feel the impact of parenthood on their marriage, but women feel it more quickly and strongly than do men. It is possible that the unique biological changes antenatal and postnatal coupled with the burden of childcare lead to more profound impact on women's lives than men's during early parenthood (Pfost, Stevens, & Matijcak, 1990). Consequently women are more sensitive to the impact of parenthood on their marital relationship and are more likely to detect early signs of warning. Men traditionally assume their roles of father as a provider rather than a nurturer (Atkinson & Blackwelder, 1993); thus, fathers may be more concerned with financial pressures at the early stage, and only eventually recognize the impact on their marital relationship. As our study focused on the relatively early stage of parenting (between six weeks and six months postpartum), we expected that women would report lower levels of marital satisfaction than men (*Hypothesis 2*).

CONJUGAL SIMILARITIES AND DISCREPANCIES IN PARENTHOOD ADJUSTMENT

Despite possible sex differences in the transition to parenthood, marriage is an intimate relationship within which husbands and wives continuously influence each other in every aspect of life (Cook, 1998). The marital relationship is a prototypical communal relationship in which strong interdependence is a defining characteristic (Argyle & Henderson, 1985). On the positive side, the "common fate" mentality facilitates the formation of marital alliance, which promotes marital adjustment (Cordova, 2001; Lu, 2000). For instance, Lu (2000) found that Chinese married couples reported strikingly high levels of conjugal congruence on their perceptions of three major family roles: spousal, parental, and filial roles. More importantly, the conjugal congruence on mental health and happiness was also high, whereas dyadic discrepancies on family role experiences were predictive of the individual's well-being. On the negative side, though, living with a psychologically distressed person is a considerable emotional burden and can even cause depressive symptoms in the non-depressed marital partner (Coyne, Kessler, Tal, Turnbull, Wortman & Greden, 1987; Krantz & Moos, 1987). Such emotional contagion results from the high level of interdependence between conjugal partners.

Accumulating evidence now suggests both the "common fate" mentality and "co-morbidity" of distress in couples, but no study has yet focused on this phenomenon during the crucial family stage of parenthood transition. We thus hypothesized that the interdependence of marital partners would manifest in conjugal similarities in stress, health, and marital satisfaction (*Hypothesis 3-1*). We also hypothesized that conjugal discrepancy in stress would impact on personal well-being and marital satisfaction (*Hypothesis 3-2*).

PARENTING IN A CHINESE CULTURAL CONTEXT

As noted by Phoenix and Woollett (1991), motherhood and fatherhood are socially and culturally constructed. Becoming a parent in a Chinese society may entail some distinct experiences. The aforementioned "common fate" thesis may be more applicable to Chinese couples than American marriages. As the most influential Confucian philosophy asserts, the life of each individual is only a link in that person's family lineage and that each individual is a continuation of his/her ancestors, and family is at the center of a Chinese person's existence (Lu, Gilmour, & Kao, 2001). Traditionally, becoming a parent is the ultimate purpose of a marriage. In so doing, a Chinese person not only acquires a socially desirable status and accomplishes the integrity of his/her personality, but also realizes the ultimate life goal of continuation, preservation, and prosperity of the family lineage and its collective well-being (Lu, 2001a). The Chinese family as a commune binds its members, especially marital partners, in health and sickness, in happiness and distress. Such family values are still central in modern Chinese life (Yang, 1988), although having a son and a daughter is increasingly perceived as equally desirable at least in Taiwan. The close-knit Chinese social institutions also help to nurture and maintain such a strong "common-fate" mentality among family members (Lu, 1997), especially married couples (Lu, 2000). On the other hand, because the Chinese culture places more emphasis on the father-son axis than the husband-wife axis (Hsu, 1953), the impact of the birth of a child on the marital relationship may be even greater than in a Western society.

Empirical studies of Chinese societies have indeed found that married couples view the parent-child relationship as more important than the conjugal relationship (Chen, 1978) and parental stress is detrimental for both sexes (Lu & Lin, 1998). The issue of sex differences is especially relevant in the Chinese context of parenthood transition. The Chinese paternalistic culture has gravely magnified the gender difference of agency vs. communion (Baken, 1966), which is prevalent in most societies. Specifically Chinese men are responsible for dealing with the "outside" world, whereas Chinese women are responsible for dealing with the "inside" world, with family borders as the dividing line. Using a dyadic design, Lu (2000) found that husbands were more committed to the worker role, whereas wives were more committed to the parental role. However, whether and/or how husbands and wives experience their parenthood transition differently has never been explored among the Chinese. The general expectation was that the aforementioned sex differences and conjugal interdependence would be magnified in a Chinese cultural context.

THE PRESENT STUDY

Thus far, we have argued that men and women may have different experiences and influence each other in their adjustment to parenthood. It is imperative, therefore, that the impact of parenthood be systematically examined for both men and women. However, most of the existing studies have either focused on men or women separately, or treated sex differences as aggregated group differences–namely, all married men contrasted with all married women, but not as married couples. There are two inherent methodological problems when study samples of men and women who are not married to each other are used. First, when men and women report their marital satisfaction, we cannot be sure that they are making judgments of the marital relationship as husbands and wives do. Second, the issue of "common fate" or "co-morbidity" in couples cannot be explored. To overcome these methodological shortcomings, a dyadic "within-subject" design must be adopted to examine the sex differences more rigorously. In other words, when men and women are married to each other in a study, a "purer" sex-related pattern (i.e., a conjugal pattern) should emerge.

The present analyses are based on data gathered as part of the Parenthood Transition Project (Lu, 2001b). These data have been used for testing a generic model of parenthood resources and adjustment (Lu & Kao, in press), delineation of trajectories of post-parenthood adjustment (Lu & Kao, 2002), and contrasting prenatal-postnatal adjustment against continuing adjustment after the parenthood transition (Lu, 2002). This represents the first attempt to explore sex/conjugal differences within this data.

The target population for the Parenthood Transition Project was parents who had a child born in two randomly drawn months and resided in the metropolitan city of Kaohsiung, Taiwan. Using the random sampling procedure, parents listed in the Kaohsiung Municipal Birth Registration were invited by phone to participate in the study. As a longitudinal (two-wave panel) study, each consenting participant answered a structured questionnaire twice, once when his/her child was six weeks old (Time 1), and another when the child was six months old (Time 2). Participation was anonymous and the survey was conducted by mail. A total of 483 parents (253F and 230M) with newly born children returned completed questionnaires at least once (response rate = 63%). This response rate is comparable to the reported average of mail surveys using general population (60% ± 20) (Baruch, 1999). Among our 483 participants, 204 had data for both Time 1 and Time 2, and 90 pairs were married to each other. Respondents were paid for their participation.

METHODS

Participants

The present dyadic sample was composed of the 90 pairs of married couples from the Parenthood Transition Project who have complete data for all relevant measures. The original sample in the project is a representative one compared against the national census data (Executive Yuan, 2001), and the present dyadic sample is not different from it in terms of demographics. To re-iterate, as a longitudinal study, each participant answered a structured questionnaire twice, six weeks and six months postpartum.

Measurements

Data for the present analyses came from three parts of the structured questionnaire.

Stress of parenthood. The Perceived Stress Scale was originally developed by Cohen, Kamarck, and Mermelstein (1983), translated and revised into Chinese by Kao and Lu (2001). This 14-item Chinese version has demonstrated good reliability and validity with both Chinese students (Kao & Lu, 2001) and community young adults (Tsai & Chen, 2002). The scale was used in the present study to measure stress of the parenthood transition. Five-point scales were used for rating the frequency of a particular stress feeling (0 = never, 4 = very often), and high score indicates a higher level of perceived stress. Sample items are "In the last month, how often have you been upset because of something that happened unexpectedly?" and "In the last month, how often have you felt confident about your ability to handle your personal problems?" (reverse scored). The average (across two times) Cronbach's α was .81 in the present study.

Mental health. Three subscales, depression (7 items), anxiety (7 items), and somatic symptoms (5 items) from the SCL-90-R (Derogatis, Rickels, & Rock, 1976) were used to assess mental health. The Chinese version was revised and applied to many and various independent samples, including students (Lu, 1994a & b), a community representative sample of adults (Lu & Shih, 1997), employees (Lu, 1999), and community elderly (Lu & Hsieh, 1997). Three-point scales were used for rating the severity of a particular symptom (0 = not at all, 2 = very severe), and high score indicates more mental symptoms, hence worse health. The average (across two times) Cronbach's α was .91 in the present study.

Marital satisfaction. This was rated by participants in reference to the marriage as-a-whole. A 7-point scale was used (1 = very dissatisfied, 7 = very satisfied), high score means greater satisfaction with marriage. Previous research has demonstrated that single-item global measures of satisfaction are acceptable, and may even be more indicative than the summation of facets (Wanous, Reichers, & Hudy, 1997).

In addition, sex, age, education attainment, and employment status were recorded.

RESULTS

Sample Characteristics

In our dyadic sample, husbands were between 22-47 years old and wives were between 21-44 years old. Husbands were significantly older than wives (see Table 1). The age distribution was comparable to the larger project sample (mean = 30.02, SD = 4.86). The distribution for educational attainment in this dyadic sample was also comparable to the larger pool (mean = 13.29, SD = 1.85). Husbands were better educated than wives as shown in years of formal education (see Table 1). Almost all fathers were working (95.5%), but only half of the mothers (53.3%) had paid jobs. Overall, our participants were young, well educated and half of these young mothers were combining career with motherhood. As some participants had missing data on some question-naire items, the actual sample size varied for each analysis. The pairwise dele-tion method was adopted to treat missing data against alternative methods (e.g., mean substitution or imputation or listwise deletion) in order to maxi-mize the utility of raw data without serious artificial distortion.

Sex Differences

Sex differences in stress and adjustment were examined by conducting paired t-tests. In this series of analyses, husbands and wives were treated as two "dependent samples." Results are incorporated in Table 1. Overall, wives reported greater stress, worse mental health, and lower marital satisfaction across both times. Therefore, our *Hypotheses 1 & 2* were supported.

We conducted more detailed analyses looking at conjugal discrepancies in specific aspects of mental health, namely, depression, anxiety, and somatic symptoms. Similar paired t-tests procedures were carried out. Results revealed that wives consistently reported significantly more depressive symptoms than husbands at both Time 1 and Time 2 (paired t = -2.74, df = 88, p < .01 and

TABLE 1. Sample Characteristics and Scores on the Research Variables

	Husbands (N = 90)		Wives (N = 90)		Paired t (df)		$r_{H \cdot W}$
	Mean	SD	Mean	SD			
Demographics							
Age	31.84	4.78	29.14	4.56	7.05***	(83)	.74***
Education	13.60	1.98	13.07	1.41	3.24**	(88)	.12
Research variables							
Stress 1	22.51	6.06	24.30	6.56	-1.96*	(79)	.16
Stress 2	23.19	5.74	25.12	6.45	-2.17*	(80)	.12
Mental health 1	25.02	6.11	27.07	6.08	-2.42*	(84)	.18
Mental health 2	25.17	5.14	26.60	5.58	-1.99*	(86)	.22*
Marital satisfaction 1	5.21	1.30	4.76	1.51	2.96**	(88)	.49***
Marital satisfaction 2	5.46	1.26	4.70	1.47	5.47***	(89)	.55***

*p < .05 **p < .01 ***p < .001

paired $t = -3.29$, df $= 87$, $p < .001$ respectively). However, husbands and wives were not at all different regarding anxiety and somatic symptoms at six weeks and six months postpartum.

We further examined the potential effects of spousal age differences on perceived stress, mental health, and marital satisfaction, to see if couples with larger age differences were any different compared to couples with smaller age differences. The spousal age difference (DIF) was represented by the absolute value of a wife's age subtracting her husband's age. First, Pearson correlations were computed between spousal age differences and personal (husbands' and wives') scores on perceived stress, mental health and marital satisfaction at both Time 1 and Time 2. No significant correlations were found between spousal age differences and any of the research variables. Second, Pearson correlations were computed between spousal age differences and conjugal discrepancies in perceived stress, mental health and marital satisfaction at both Time 1 and Time 2. Conjugal discrepancy (DIF) was represented by the absolute value of a wife's score of a particular construct subtracting her husband's. Only two significant correlations (out of 12) were found: between spousal age differences and (1) conjugal discrepancies in depressive symptoms (Time 1) ($r = .22$, $p < .05$), and (2) conjugal discrepancies in marital satisfaction (Time 2) ($r = .38$, $p < .001$). It seems that couples with larger age differences tended to have larger discrepancies in postpartum depressive symptoms and marital satisfaction compared to couples with smaller age differences.

Conjugal Interdependence and Its Impact on Personal Adjustment

Conjugal interdependence on stress and adjustment was examined by correlating scores of a husband and wife for a particular construct. The last column in Table 1 presents results of this correlation analysis. There were significant conjugal correlations in marital satisfaction across both times. There was also a significant conjugal correlation in health at Time 2. However, husbands and wives did not correlate in their stress scores. Overall conjugal interdependence was consistently observed for the evaluation of marital quality, less strongly for personal health, but not for perceived stress. Therefore, our *Hypothesis 3-1* was partially supported.

To examine whether conjugal discrepancy in stress was predictive of the individual's adjustment, four series of hierarchical regression analyses were carried out, with the husband's and the wife's health/marital satisfaction at Time 2 as dependent variables. As our sample had relatively large age and education ranges, these two variables were controlled in multiple regression analyses for their potential contributions to mental health and marital satisfaction. Thus, for all four sets of regression, age and education years were entered for statistical control at

Step 1. At Step 2, health/marital satisfaction at Time 1 was entered as a "baseline" control to take advantage of our longitudinal data. Conjugal discrepancy in stress at Time 2 was then entered. To statistically represent "conjugal discrepancy," a wife's score of a particular construct was subtracted from her husband's, and the absolute value of this result (DIF) was then used in the analysis. Full regression equations are presented in Table 2. Standardized β, standardized error, and F value were taken from the final equations.

Neither age nor education showed significant effects on any of the dependent variables. Nonetheless, all the subsequently identified significant predictors of mental health and marital satisfaction had been free of "contamination" by age and education. As shown in Table 2, husband's health at Time 1 was the only significant predictor of his health at Time 2. For wife's health at Time 2, however, her health at Time 1 and conjugal discrepancy in stress were both significant predictors. For husband's marital satisfaction at Time 2, again his marital satisfaction at Time 1 was the only significant predictor. For wife's marital satisfaction at Time 2, however, her marital satisfaction at Time 1, as well as conjugal discrepancy in stress were significant predictors. Overall, conjugal discrepancy in stress exerted adverse effects on wives' well-being and marital satisfaction, but not on husbands'. Therefore, our *Hypothesis 3-2* was partially supported.

DISCUSSION

The present study was set against the Chinese cultural background. Adopting a dyadic panel study design, longitudinal data were collected at two times

TABLE 2. Hierarchical Regression Analyses Predicting Personal Adjustment

Dependent variable	step	Entered variable	β	R^2	F (df)	
(H) Health 2	1	(H) Health 1	.65***	.39		
	2	(DIF) Stress 2	.02	.40	12.65***	(4, 79)
(W) Health 2	1	(W) Health 1	.41***	.18		
	2	(DIF) Stress 2	.20*	.37	10.61***	(4, 78)
(H) Satisfaction 2	1	(H) Satisfaction 1	.47***	.21		
	2	(DIF) Stress 2	.11	.23	5.61***	(4, 79)
(W) Satisfaction 2	1	(W) Satisfaction 1	.34***	.16		
	2	(DIF) Stress 2	−.21*	.27	6.97***	(4, 78)

*p < .05   ***p < .001

postpartum, from a paired sample of husbands and wives. With these method-ological strengths, hypotheses regarding sex differences and implications of conjugal interdependence were tested. Sex differences were pronounced for both stress and adjustment, as women reported heightened stress, worse health, and lower marital satisfaction. Conjugal similarities were generally high except for stress, indicating a fair extent of conjugal interdependence. Conjugal discrepancy in stress was predictive of wives' adjustment but not husbands'. It seems that conjugal interdependence is present in some aspects of parenthood transition and indeed has important implications for women's adjustment. Thus far, our four hypotheses have been fully or partially sup-ported. The following discussion elaborates on implications of these findings.

Before doing so, however, one sampling condition must be qualified. Our current dyadic sample was composed solely of people in their first marriages. In other words, none of the parents had children from previous relationships or marriages. Our sample was thus rather homogenous regarding marriage his-tory and family developmental stage to warrant the subsequent general discus-sions.

Sex Differences as Conjugal Discrepancies in Parenthood Transition

Most extant research relating to the transition of parenthood has focused on maternal distress and adjustment. Consequently we know very little about men's experiences of fatherhood. However, the present study used a commu-nity paired representative sample with men and women equally represented. We examined a "purer" form of sex differences in terms of conjugal discrep-ancies. Our results have revealed a stable pattern over a half-year period after the child was born. Wives consistently reported higher stress, worse psycho-logical health, and lower marital satisfaction than did husbands. More detailed analyses revealed that wives' poorer mental health was attributable to their in-flated depression levels at both testing times, but not anxiety and somatic symptoms.

Our finding of women's heightened stress and poorer health, especially de-pression, is consistent with existing research on maternal distress and adjust-ment (Brody, 1985; Cowan et al., 1985). In particular, Chinese culture places great emphasis on the continuation of the family line, and places the responsi-bility of childrearing squarely on the shoulders of women (Kao & Lu, 2001; Lu, Gilmour & Kao, 2001; Yang, 1988). Becoming a mother is not only the most salient role for women (Chen, 1978; Lu & Lin, 1998) but also culturally sanctioned as a women's legitimate occupation.

Social institutions, customs, and practices in daily life often support cul-tural ideas. In the Chinese culture there is the custom of a "honeymoon for the mother" immediately following the childbirth. There is a full set of rituals and practices to be observed, many originating from traditional Chinese medicine. The grandmother usually moves in to live with the young family and take on all household chores and baby-care activities. This custom of "honeymoon for the mother after the birth of a child" is still intact in modern Chinese societies, and it helps to strengthen the cultural discourse that parenting is "a women's business." Chinese women have largely internalized these cultural values and even high-achieving professional women are prepared to sacrifice their own career pursuits in order to be "a good mother" (Lin & Liu, 1996). It is thus understandable that becoming a mother may be far more salient and stressful than becoming a father. Worse still, in a modern society when women have to juggle jobs and family responsibilities, as did half the mothers in this sample, motherhood becomes even more taxing.

However, men's experiences of fatherhood are also experiencing rapid change in a modern society. Traditionally, Chinese fathers were sole bread earners and had little to do with child caring. Contemporary fathers though are expected to share household duties including childcare responsibilities, especially when mothers also are working. Although women still assume a greater share of homemaking activities, the pressure of being "a new good man" is increasing. As we found elsewhere, parenthood stress also was detrimental to men's health and marital happiness (Lu & Kao, in press). Previous research has even found that husbands report the greater degree of unhappiness (Cowan et al., 1985). Although husbands in the present sample were better off than their wives in overall mental health, they nonetheless reported comparable levels of postpartum anxiety and somatic symptoms. It is clear that both men and women feel the negative effects of having a child on their health and marital relationship. Although wives are generally more committed and carry more burdens of parenting, husbands' contributions are increasing. Hence scientific research and intervention should better address the needs and concerns of both genders.

Conjugal Interdependence in Parenthood Transition

Despite the acknowledgement that spousal support is important during the parenthood transition, few studies have focused directly on the interdependence of marital partners during this crucial period of family life. However, the present study did test the effects of conjugal interdependence on personal adjustment for both husbands and wives. Overall, the conjugal interdependence was substantial in both aspects of parenthood adjustment: health and marital satisfaction. Our results were thus consistent with the "co-morbidity" proposition and had further extended the research on conjugal interdependence beyond emotional contagion already documented in the literature (Coyne et al., 1987; Krantz & Moos, 1987; Noh & Avison, 1988).

However, the finding that the wives' but not husbands' health and marital satisfaction were related to conjugal discrepancy in stress seems to suggest that women were more vulnerable than men. This is somewhat consistent with results from research by Cordova (2001) who found that variance in husbands' teamwork (marital alliance) better accounted for marital and parental functioning than did wives' teamwork. Teamwork was also the best predictor of depression, especially for wives. Furthermore, wives' evaluation of supportive co-parenting was predicted by husbands' teamwork. Taken together, Cordova's findings and ours suggest that men may still assume more relative power in the intimate conducts of a marital relationship, and women are more sensitive to the fine grain tone of a relationship. The proposition that women are more sensitive to the impact of parenthood on their marital relationship, and detect early signs of warning, seems to have been supported by the empirical evidence.

Our findings should also be read in the cultural milieu of a modern Chinese society. In all contemporary Chinese societies, traditional and modern values coexist as a result of societal modernization and Western cultural influences (Lu & Kao, 2002b). The once rigid gender division of men as providers and women as homemakers is increasingly transgressed. More and more men are "returning to the family" to take on a caring and involvement in the father role (i.e., the so-called "new good man") while more and more women are stepping out of home to combine career with motherhood. The young, educated urban residents exhibit the strongest trend of synthesizing the traditional and modern values as well as the old and new ways of life (Lu & Kao, 2002b). Our sample evidently belongs to this section of the population, as additional information revealed that 65.7% of the couples jointly cared for their newborn baby (i.e., co-parenting). It is ironic that when husbands are getting more involved in parenting and other aspects of family life, wives' expectations raise and perceived disappointments may be even more distressing. On a positive side, husbands are learning to be more sensitive to their wives' burden and stress (Tsai & Chen, 2002).

Marriage is "a holy mystery in which man and woman become one flesh . . . that husband and wife may comfort and help each other . . . that they may have children . . . and begin a new life together in the community" (Alternative Service Book, 1980). These are some of the central features of marriage—sharing bed, food and property, producing children, and caring for one another; it is a commitment to a biological partnership and a social alliance. To realize the promise of marriage, the husband and the wife need to work together in close coordination, including co-parenting at the early stage of family life. Scientific research can help couples to better achieve this goal by appreciating and understanding their idiosyncratic needs and developing more effective intervention programs.

Limitations and Conclusions

It should be kept in mind that these data came from a cross-sectional self-report design. One cannot draw causal conclusions, and there is the concern about possible percept-percept bias. Arguing against this possibility are the findings that over half of the correlation and regression coefficients were non-significant (see Tables 1 and 2). This suggests that there was no pervasive underlying bias inflating these relationships. Nonetheless, one should still be cautious in interpreting the data, as well as data from other studies using similar designs.

The other limitation of the present study pertains to the generalizability of our findings. We adopted random sampling methods in our Parenthood Transition Project to minimize sampling bias, and the current dyadic sample is not different from the larger project sample in terms of demographics. Still, Taiwan is a heterogeneous and vibrant society with rich albeit subtle regional differences, especially between the fast developing industrial urban areas and the more traditional agricultural rural areas. Hence, a sample drawn from a booming metropolitan southern city (the second largest in Taiwan) could not be regarded as representative of the entire country. The potential differences between Taiwan and other major Chinese societies such as the People's Republic of China (PRC) may be even more profound due to their unique political, economic, and social characteristics (Lu, Cooper, Kao, & Zhou, in press). Further research needs to target other distinctive groups in these Chinese societies, such as rural populations and young parents in the PRC in search of convergence or divergence of evidence.

What do our findings inform family scholars of parent-child relationship? Previous research has suggested that postnatal distress may hinder the crucial bonding between the parent and the child (Osofsky, 1979). As we found that wives generally suffered higher postnatal distress than their husbands, this pattern of sex difference may imply that the mother-child relationship is more at risk than the father-child one. This implication is especially grave as in most societies the mother is still the primary caregiver for the child, and the psychic costs of a less than satisfactory mother-child relationship on both the mother and the child is not to be overlooked. On the other hand, we found a substantial degree of conjugal interdependence between partners during the parenthood transition. This is encouraging as marital alliance or co-parenting is beneficial for both postnatal distress alleviation (Cordova, 2001) and the establishment of a warm parent-child relationship (Owen, Lewis, & Henderson, 1989). It seems reasonable to suggest that efforts made to foster and nurture marital alliance or co-parenting would most likely yield beneficial effects on the developing parent-child relationship, especially the mother-child relationship.

Of what do our findings inform family policy makers and practitioners then? Since previous work has suggested that the problems that lead to marital breakdown start early within relationships (Thornes & Collard, 1979), early preventive measures are most likely to be effective as they would address problems before conflicts have become serious. As we have found that the birth of a child does entail substantial stress and costs on personal well-being as well as marital satisfaction for both men and women, preventive interventions aimed at supporting couples at this family stage are likely to have long term beneficial effects on the functioning of their developing family, including, of course, the evolvement of a healthy parent-child relationship. Although we found that women seemed to bear the brunt of parenthood transition more than men, and interventions to support family have traditionally been directed towards women, men's needs should not be ignored. As we have demonstrated that men were not better off than women in terms of postnatal anxiety and somatic symptoms, support offered to fathers should be increased. Perhaps even at the national policy level, fathers should be encouraged to get more involved in the co-parenting teamwork amongst other aspects of the family life. One foreseeable consequence of the greater paternal involvement is a warm and constructive father-child relationship, which is often absent in traditional family life.

REFERENCES

Abbott, D. A., & Brody, G. H. (1985). The relation of child age, gender, and number of children to the marital adjustment of wives. *Journal of Marriage and the Family*, *47*, 77-84.

The Alternative Service Book. (1980). Oxford: Oxford University Press.

Amato, P. R., & Keith, B. (1991a). Parental divorce and adult well-being: A meta-analysis. *Journal of Marriage and the Family*, *53*, 43-59.

Amato, P. R., & Keith, B. (1991b). Separation from a parent during childhood and adult socio-economic attainment. *Social Forces*, *70*, 187-206.

Argyle, M. (1987). *The psychology of happiness*. London: Methuen.

Argyle, M., & Henderson, M. (1985). *The anatomy of relationships*. London: Heinemann and Harmondsworth: Penguin.

Atkinson, M. P., & Blackwelder, S. P. (1993). Fathering in the 20th century. *Journal of Marriage and the Family*, *55*, 975-986.

Baken, D. (1966). *The duality of human existence*. Chicago: Rand McNally Press.

Ballard, C. G., Davis, R., Cullen, P. C., Mohan, R. N., & Dean, C. (1994). Prevalence of postnatal psychiatric morbidity in mothers and fathers. *British Journal of Psychiatry, 164,* 782-788.

Baruch, Y. (1999). Response rate in academic studies: A comparative analysis. *Human Relations, 52,* 421-438.

Belsky, J. (1990). Children and marriage. In F. D. Fincham & T. N. Bradbury (eds.) *The psychology of marriage: Basic issues and applications* (pp. 63-72). New York: The Guildford Press.

Brody, E. M. (1985). Parent care as a normative family stress. *Gerontologist, 25,* 19-29.

Burnell, G. M., & Norfleet, M. A. (1986). Psychosocial factors influencing American men and women in their decision for sterilization. *The Journal of Psychology, 120,* 113-119.

Chen, J. F. (1978). *Marital role behavior and marital satisfaction.* Master dissertation, National Taiwan University.

Cohen, S., Kamarck, T., & Mermelstein, R. (1983). A global measure of perceived stress. *Journal of Health and Social Behavior, 24,* 385-396.

Cook, W. L. (1998). Integrating models of interdependence with treatment evaluations in marital therapy research. *Journal of Family Psychology, 12,* 529-542.

Cordova, A. D. (2001). Teamwork and the transition to parenthood. Dissertation Abstracts International: The Sciences & Engineering, 61(9-B), 5052.

Coyne, J. C., Kessler, R. C., Tal, M., Turnbull, J., Wortman, C.B., & Greden, J. F. (1987). Living with a depressed person. *Journal of Consulting and Clinical Psychology, 55,* 347-352.

Cowan, C., Cowan, P., Heming, G., Garrett, E., Coysh, W., & Curtis-Boles, H. (1985). Transitions to parenthood: His, hers and theirs. *Journal of Family Issues, 6,* 451-482.

Davidson, J. K., & Moore, N. B. (1996). *Marriage and the family: Change and continuity.* Boston: Allyn and Bacon.

Derogatis, L. R., Rickels, K., & Rock, A. F. (1976). The SCL-90MMPI: A step in the validation of a new self-report scale. *British Journal of Psychiatry, 128,* 280-289.

Executive Yuan. (2001). *Report on the nation's family life.* Taipei: Executive Yuan.

Ferketich, S. L., & Mercer, R. T. (1989). Men's health status during pregnancy and early fatherhood. *Research in Nursing and Health, 12,* 137-148.

Fiese, B. H., Hooker, K. A., Kotary, L., & Schwagler, J. (1993). Family rituals in the early stages of parenthood. *Journal of Marriage and the Family, 55,* 633-642.

Hsu, L. G. (1953). The Chinese and the Americans: Two ways of life. New York: Henry Schuman.

Kao, S. F., & Lu, L. (2001). The relationship between parental rearing attitudes and the perceived stress of JHSEE among junior high school students. *Research in Applied Psychology, 10,* 221-250.

Krantz, S. E., & Moos, R. H. (1987). Functional and life context among spouses of remitted and non-emitted depressed patients. *Journal of Consulting and Clinical Psychology, 55,* 353-360.

Lin, D. M., & Liu, S. M. (1996, December). The psychological adjustment of female managers. Paper presented at the Taipei Conference of Mental Health. Taiwan: Taipei.

Lu, L. (1994a). University transition: Major and minor life stressors, personality characteristics and mental health. *Psychological Medicine, 24*, 81-87.

Lu, L. (1994b). Stressors, personality and mental health: A follow-up study. *Kaohsiung Journal of Medical Sciences, 10*, 492-496.

Lu, L. (1997). Social support, reciprocity, and well-being. *The Journal of Social Psychology, 137*, 18-628.

Lu, L. (1999). Work motivation, job stress and employees' well-being. *Journal of Applied Management Studies, 8*, 61-72.

Lu, L. (2000). Gender and conjugal differences in happiness. *Journal of Social Psychology, 140*, 132-141.

Lu, L. (2001a). Understanding happiness: A look into the Chinese folk psychology. *Journal of Happiness Studies, 2*, 407-432.

Lu, L. (2001b). *Adjusting to be first-time parents: A panel study*. Taipei, Taiwan: National Science Council.

Lu, L. (2002). Adjustment of parenthood transition: A follow-up study from prenatal to postnatal. Taipei, Taiwan: National Science Council.

Lu, L., Cooper, C. L., Kao, S. F., & Zhou, Y. (In press). Work stress, control beliefs and well-being in Greater China: An exploration of sub-cultural differences between the PRC and Taiwan. *Journal of Managerial Psychology, 18*, 479-510.

Lu, L., Gilmour, R., & Kao, S. F. (2001). Culture values and happiness: An East-West dialogue. *Journal of Social Psychology, 141*, 477-493.

Lu, L., & Hsieh, Y. H. (1997). Demographic variables, control, stress, support and health among the elderly. *Journal of Health Psychology, 2*, 97-106.

Lu, L., & Kao, S. F. (2002a). *Internal and external resources for coping with parental stress*. Paper presented at XXV International Congress of Applied Psychology. Singapore.

Lu, L., & Kao, S. F. (2002b). Traditional and modern characteristics across the generations: Similarities and discrepancies. *Journal of Social Psychology, 142*, 45-60.

Lu, L., & Kao, S. F. (In press). Impact of parenthood: A two-wave panel study in Taiwan. In A. D. Nor Ba'yah (Ed.) *Women, children, and subjective well-being*. Sarawak, Malaysia: University Malaysia Sarawak.

Lu, L., & Lin, Y. Y. (1998). Family roles and happiness in adulthood. *Personality and Individual Differences, 25*, 195-207.

Lu, L., Shiau, C., & Cooper, C. L. (1997). Occupational stress in clinical nurses. *Counseling Psychology Quarterly, 10*, 39-50.

Lu, L., & Shih, J. B. (1997). Personality and happiness: Is mental health a mediator? *Personality and Individual Differences, 22*, 249-256.

Lu, L., Tseng, H. J., & Cooper, C. L. (1999). Managerial stress, job satisfaction and health in Taiwan. *Stress Medicine, 15*, 53-64.

MacAllister, F. (1998). *Marital breakdown and the health of the nation (2nd ed.)* London: One Plus One.

Noh, S., & Avison, W. R. (1988). Spouses of discharged psychiatric patients: Factors associated with their experience of burden. *Journal of Marriage and the Family, 50*, 377-389.

Osofsky, J. D. (1979). *Handbook of infant development*. New York Chichester: Wiley.

Owen, M. T., Lewis, J. M., & Henderson, V. K. (1989). Marriage, adult adjustment, and early parenting. *Child Development, 60*, 1015-1024.

Pfost, K. S., Stevens, M. J., & Matijack, A. J. (1990). A counselor's primer on post-partum depression. *Journal of Counseling & Development, 69*, 149-151.

Phoenix, A., & Woollett, A. (1991). Motherhood, social construction and psychology. In A. Phoenix, A. Woollett & E. Lloyd (Eds.) *Motherhood: Meanings, practices and ideologies* (pp. 13-27). London: Sage.

Quill, T E., Lipkin, M., & Lamb, G. S. (1984). Health seeking by men in their spouse's pregnancy. *Psychosomatic Medicine, 46*, 277-283.

Rees, W. D., & Lutkins, S. G. (1971). Parental depression before and after childbirth. *Journal of the Royal College of General Practitioners, 21*, 26-31.

Smith, J. (1995). Qualitative methods, identity and transition to motherhood. *The Psychologist, 8*, 122-125.

Soloway, N. M., & Smith, E. M. (1987). Antecedents of late birthtiming decision of men and women in dual-career marriages. *Family Relations, 36*, 258-262.

Thornes, B., & Collard, J. (1979). *Who divorces?* London: Routledge and Kegan Paul.

Tsai, S. M., & Chen, C. H. (2002). The Covet syndrome, stress and social support of expecting fathers. *Nursing Research, 2*, 153-165.

Wanous, J. P., Reichers, A. E., & Hudy, M. J. (1997). Overall job satisfaction: How good are single-item measures. *Journal of Applied Psychology, 82*, 247-252.

Yang, K. S. (1988). A conceptual analysis of filial piety among the Chinese people. In K. S. Yang (Ed.) *Psychology of the Chinese people* (pp. 39-73). Taipei: Laurent.

Parent-Child Relationships in Childhood and Adulthood and Their Effect on Marital Quality: A Comparison of Children Who Remained in Close Proximity to Their Parents and Those Who Moved Away

Yoav Lavee
Ruth Katz
Tali Ben-Dror

ABSTRACT. This study examines the links between parent-child relationships in childhood and adulthood and the marital quality of adult children. Additionally, the study tests the hypothesis that this association is moderated by residential proximity and frequency of contact between the two generations. In order to test these hypotheses, 54 kibbutz children who have remained in close proximity and daily contact with their parents ("Remainers") were compared with a matched group of 55 kibbutz-born respondents who moved away ("Leavers"). Findings indicated a strong association between family experiences during childhood (family cohesion, parental marital happiness, and parent-child relationships) and emotional and contact solidarity with parents in

Yoav Lavee, Ruth Katz, and Tali Ben-Dror are affiliated with the Center for Research and Study of the Family, Faculty of Social Welfare & Health Studies, University of Haifa, Israel.

Address correspondence to: Yoav Lavee, PhD, School of Social Work, Faculty of Social Welfare & Health Studies, University of Haifa, Haifa 31905, Israel (E-mail: lavee@research.haifa.ac.il).

http://www.haworthpress.com/web/MFR
© 2004 by The Haworth Press, Inc. All rights reserved.
Digital Object Identifier: 10.1300/J002v36n03_06

adulthood. Adult children's marital quality was explained by parent-child relations in childhood and by the interaction between parent-child relationships in adulthood and living proximity. Marital quality was found to be associated with parent-child relations only for the Remainers but not for the Leavers. The findings have implications for parent-child relationships and marital quality among broader populations experiencing geographical mobility. *[Article copies available for a fee from The Haworth Document Delivery Service: 1-800-HAWORTH. E-mail address: <docdelivery@haworthpress.com> Website: <http://www.HaworthPress.com> © 2004 by The Haworth Press, Inc. All rights reserved.]*

KEYWORDS. Parent-child relations, marital quality, kibbutz children, adult children

Interest in the relations between adult children and their parents has grown dramatically over the past three decades (Lye, 1996; Suitor, Pillemer, Bohanon, & Robison, 1995). The most popular organizing framework for understanding intergenerational relationships within the family is that of *intergenerational solidarity* (Bengtson & Roberts, 1991), in which parent-child relations are characterized by reciprocity of exchange and solidarity along multiple dimensions. Research in this tradition has emphasized shared values across generations, enduring ties between parents and children, and normative obligations to provide help and mutual support. Along this line, researchers have found that parents and adult children maintain regular relations of exchange and support–both instrumental and emotional–and that this exchange has positive as well as negative implications for adult children's well-being (Antonucci, 1990; Bengtson, Rosenthal, & Burton, 1990; Mancini & Blieszner, 1989).

Whereas the research conducted on intergenerational relationships has yielded valuable knowledge about the implications of these relations for adult children's *individual* well-being, relatively little attention has been given to their effect on adult children's families, in general, and their marital relationships in particular (Ward & Spitze, 1998). Additionally, this research has been narrowly focused on their contemporary relations and has largely ignored the influence of their earlier relationships (Rossi & Rossi, 1990).

The purpose of the present study is to examine the association of parent-child relationships in childhood and adulthood with the marital quality of adult children. The underlying assumption is that this association is moderated by residential proximity and frequency of contact between the two generations. More specifically, the study tests the hypothesis that adult children's marital quality is influenced by parent-child emotional solidarity for those who live in close proximity and maintain daily contact, but not for those who are geographically distant from their elderly parents and who maintain less frequent contact. In order to test these hypotheses, children who have remained in close proximity and daily contact with their parents are compared with those who have chosen to move away, using the kibbutz setting as a "natural laboratory" for examining close vs. distant living arrangements.

Following is a review of both theory and research on the association between parent-child relationships in childhood and in adulthood; the effect of these relationships on adult children's marital quality; and the moderating effect of parent-child living proximity on adult children's marital quality.

PARENT-CHILD RELATIONSHIPS IN CHILDHOOD AND ADULTHOOD

Research on parent-child relationships has typically focused on either the beginning of the life course, during childhood and adolescence, or on its end, dealing with adult children's relationships with their elderly parents. This trend, characterized as the alpha-omega tendency in parent-child research (Hagestad, 1987), has brought about a paucity of knowledge regarding the association between early and later parent-child relationships.

In one of a few studies on parent-child relationships in childhood and adulthood, Rossi and Rossi (1990) examined the extent to which early family experiences contribute to variation in social interaction, affective closeness, and the exchange of help between parents and children. They found that greater intimacy and a tighter bond in relations between parents and adult children were related to a higher level of affection and acceptance during childhood, a stronger sense of family cohesion, and closer parent-child relations during adolescence. They concluded that intergenerational relations are primarily the result of a "snow-ball" effect, with the qualities of early parent-child relationships continuing to typify relations into the children's adulthood. We therefore expect that parent-child relationships in adulthood will be related to the parent-child and other family relationships of childhood.

PARENT-CHILD RELATIONSHIPS AND ADULT CHILDREN'S MARITAL QUALITY

Adult children's marital quality may be shaped both by early family experiences and parent-child relationships and by existing intergenerational relationships. The link between parent-child relationships in childhood and intimate relationships in adulthood has been the focus of a number of theoretical frameworks, including psychoanalytic theory (Freud, 1949); life-span developmental approach (Baltes & Reese, 1984); attribution theory (Kelly, 1972); attachment theory (Bowlby, 1969, 1988); and Bowen's (1978) intergenerational theory. Psychoanalytic and object relations theorists have long argued that the parent-child relationship is the prototype for later love relationships. Similarly, attachment theory posits that working models of childhood attachment relationships are strongly related to the quality of couple relationships in adulthood (Bowlby, 1969, 1988; Shaver, Hazan, & Bradshaw, 1988).

A number of studies have documented the link between the quality of parent-child relationships in childhood and later intimate adult relationships (Belsky & Pensky, 1988; Caspi & Elder, 1988; Rossi & Rossi, 1990). There is evidence to suggest that patterns of infant-parent attachment can be translated into patterns of adult attachment relationships (Hazan & Shaver, 1987). Furthermore, adult attachment is linked to relationship satisfaction (Collins & Read, 1990), self-disclosure (Feeney & Noller, 1990) and improved functioning (Cohn, Silver, Cowan, Cowan, & Pearson, 1992) between partners.

In addition to parent-child relationships, patterns of intimate relationships may be shaped by other experiences in one's family of origin. For example, positive associations were found between family cohesion and functioning during childhood and marital satisfaction in adulthood (Fisiloglu & Lorenzetti, 1994; Rossi & Rossi, 1990). Adult children's marital quality may also be related to their parents' marital relationships (Amato & Booth, 2001; Booth & Edwards, 1990; Lewis & Spanier, 1979; Feng, Giarruso, Bengtson, & Frye, 1999). Rossi and Rossi (1990) found that adult children whose parents had greater marital happiness tended to show more affection and cooperation in their own intimate relationships.

During adulthood, parent-child relations are likely to have both negative and positive implications for adult children and their families. The literature on adult children's caregiving of elderly parents tends to emphasize burden and stress (e.g., Mancini & Blieszner, 1989; Pearlin, Mullan, Semple, & Skaff, 1990; Pearlin, Aneshensel, Mullan, & Whitlatch, 1996), problems and conflicts (Suitor & Pillemer, 1988) as well as ambivalence in intergenerational relations (Luescher & Pillemer, 1998). Caregiving for parents is a potential source of strain and conflict in marital relations. It may interfere with marital roles by reducing the time and energy available for interaction with a spouse (Suitor & Pillemer, 1992, 1994).

However, other research on the relationships of adult children with their parents points to positive outcomes. Studies indicate that for the adult child, good relations with and support from parents alleviate psychological strain and enhance one's sense of satisfaction with life (Barnett, Marshall, & Peck, 1992; Wan, Jaccard, & Ramey, 1996).

All in all, there is inconsistent evidence regarding the effects of parent-child relations on the marital quality of the adult child. A number of researchers found only scattered evidence, if any, for the effect of intergenerational exchanges on the marital quality of adult children (Suitor & Pillemer, 1992, 1994; Ward & Spitze, 1998). Thus, it appears that the quality of the marital relationship has little association with intergenerational exchange per se, but rather is more consistently associated with the quality of parent-child relations. In particular, problematic parent-child relations are associated with distress and lower reported marital quality (Krause, 1995; Ward & Spitze, 1998; Umberson, 1992) as well as with increased marital conflict (Suitor & Pillemer, 1988).

THE MODERATING EFFECT OF GEOGRAPHICAL PROXIMITY

A missing link in understanding the association between intergenerational relationships and adult children's marital quality is the geographical proximity of adult children and their elderly parents. Geographical proximity enables the continuity of parent-child relations, face-to-face interactions, and exchanges of support between generations, whereas geographical mobility increases the physical distance between generations, thereby impeding the exchange of social and instrumental support (Dewit, Wister, & Burch, 1988). In his theoretical framework of intergenerational solidarity, Bengtson and his colleagues (Bengtson & Roberts, 1991; Bengtson, Giarrusso, Mabry, & Silverstein, 2002) conceptualized the opportunity for contact between parents and adult children in terms of structural solidarity, and the frequency of contact in terms of associational solidarity.

Geographical proximity, social contact, and affection also may have a reciprocal effect on each other. Lawton, Silverstein and Bengtson (1994) found that greater contact is associated with greater affection and, in turn, greater affection is associated with greater contact, especially among mother-child dyads. Thus, residential proximity encourages emotional intimacy insofar as it facilitates opportunities for shared experiences. Lin and Lewis (1996) further suggest that families with a stronger sense of cohesion in earlier periods of family life tend to maintain more frequent contact. The greater the physical proximity, the greater the accessibility and opportunity to notice and respond to family members' needs.

We hypothesized that current intergenerational relations would be associated with early parent-child relationships. Specifically, this meant that one's early experiences in the family, especially parent-child relations, would influence the adult child's choice of whether or not to stay in close geographical proximity to the parents. This intergenerational residential proximity, in turn, would moderate the association between current parent-child relationships and the adult child's marital relationship. More specifically, we hypothesized that adult children's marital quality would be negatively associated with a conflicted intergenerational relationship and positively associated with a supportive intergenerational relationship only for those who live in close proximity to, and have daily contact with, their parents.

THE SOCIAL CONTEXT:
ADULT CHILDREN WHO STAY OR LEAVE THE KIBBUTZ

The kibbutz is a type of collective unique to Israel, with an average of about 100 families in residence in each community. In the past, child socialization and economic functions were accorded to the collective. However, the privatization process in recent years has "normalized" the kibbutz family, turning it into a "regular" household that is responsible for most of its own functions and services (Palgi, 1997).

Over the years, the extended family has become an important component of the kibbutz community, with several generations and several separate household units within the community maintaining daily contact. For the older generation, living in such proximity and daily contact with their offspring provides a major contribution to their psychological well-being. For the younger generation, however, this arrangement represents an added psychological and emotional burden, despite its instrumental benefits.

One of the focal issues addressed by kibbutz researchers involves the decision-making process of kibbutz-born children about whether to leave or to stay on the kibbutz. Researchers have found that family environment is an important factor in this decision, with those who choose to remain on the kibbutz having a greater need to stay near their parents and a stronger sense of commitment to the kibbutz (Mitleberg & Lev-Ari, 1991).

Within this context, we examine parent-child relationships in childhood and adulthood as predictors of marital quality among kibbutz children who have remained in close and daily contact with their parents and among those who have chosen to move away.

METHOD

Sample

The sample was composed of 109 couples in which at least one member was born and raised on a kibbutz. Fifty-four of the kibbutz-born respondents currently live on the kibbutz (the "Remainers"), together with at least one parent, whereas the other 55 kibbutz-born respondents have moved to other locations in Israel (the "Leavers").

Procedure

The respondents were recruited from 30 kibbutzim across the country. In order to recruit the sample, contact was first made with a liaison person in each kibbutz, who was informed about the study and was asked to provide the names and addresses of appropriate subjects. The information requested included current kibbutz members as well as former members, matched by age and marital status, who had moved away. A self-report questionnaire was then sent to each potential subject, together with a letter inviting them to take part in the study, a brief explanation of the study, and a stamped return envelope. The packet included a questionnaire booklet for the focal respondent–the kibbutz-born person–and a one-page questionnaire for the spouse (see Measures section below for a more detailed description). Four weeks later, potential subjects who had not responded were contacted by phone to encourage participation. In all, 116 questionnaires were returned (representing a return rate of 49%), of which seven questionnaires were discarded due to incomplete data. Analyses were therefore conducted with data from 109 focal respondents and their spouses, of whom 54 are kibbutz members (the "Remainers") and 55 ex-kibbutz members (the "Leavers").

Table 1 provides demographic data of the two groups. As the data show, there were no significant group differences in any of the background variables. In each group, there was an equal gender distribution (27 males and 27 females in the Remainers group; 27 males and 28 females in the Leavers group). The mean age of the respondents was about 39, and on average they had a little more than 14 years of education. Respondents were married for 13-15 years and had, on average, between two and three children.

Group differences also were examined with respect to the respondents' parents, such as marital status, age, and health, but no differences were found on these variables either. The only significant difference between groups was in the distance between the respondents' and their parents' residence. While all Remainers live within walking distance from their parents, the distance be-

TABLE 1. Personal and Family Characteristics: Comparison of the Two Research Groups

			Remainers	Leavers	Difference
Gender	Male	N	27	27	x^2 = .009
		%	(50)	(49)	
	Female	N	27	28	
		%	(50)	(51)	
Age	Mean		38.6	39.35	t (103) = 1.44
	S.d.		6.8	6.09	
Education	Mean		14.6	14.5	t (107) = .408
	S.d.		2.07	2.3	
Years of marriage	Mean		12.9	15.0	t (107) = .87
	S.d.		7.8	6.5	
Number of children	Mean		2.6	2.8	t (107) = .86
	S.d.		1.3	1.0	

tween the Leavers' place of residence and that of their parents ranged between 20 miles and more than 100 miles ($z = 5.22$, $p < .001$).

Measures

A set of standardized measures was used to collect data on the respondents' current relationship with their parents, family relationships during childhood, and perceived marital quality. The parent-child and family relationship measures, both current and in childhood, were adopted from Rossi and Rossi's (1990) study on intergenerational relations in American families.

Current parent-child relationship. Relationship between the respondents and their parents was measured by two solidarity dimensions: associational and affectional.

Associational solidarity was measured by the frequency of face-to-face interaction (visiting) with each parent, ranging from 1 (1-2 times a year) to 8 (every day) and the frequency of phoning (measured on the same eight-point range). A value of zero was assigned if no contact at all was made during the last year. The Cronbach alpha reliability of this measure was .82. As expected, a significant difference was found between the Remainers and the Leavers in their frequency of contact with their parents ($F_{(4,66)} = 33.85$, $p < .001$). The analysis indicated that the Remainers are in closer contact with their parents than are the Leavers, both in terms of visiting ($F_{(2,68)} = 69.74$, $p < .001$) and phone contacts ($F_{(2,68)} = 11.32$, $p < .001$).

Affectional solidarity was measured in terms of closeness and intimacy versus distance and strain in the relationship with each parent. Respondents were asked to rate the relationship with each parent on a scale ranging from 1 (very strained relationship) to 7 (very close relationship).

Two other solidarity dimensions used in Rossi and Rossi's (1990) study were also measured: functional (amount of help given and received) and consensual (value consensus). However, their internal consistency reliabilities were too low (alpha = .57 and .58, respectively) to be included in the data analysis. All variables concerning current relations with parents were computed so that, if both parents were alive, the variable was a sum of responses regarding both parents, whereas, if one parent was deceased, the variable referred to the relationship with the surviving parent.

Family-of-origin relationships. Family relations in the respondents' childhood were examined by four variables: emotional bond, parental affection, family cohesion, and parents' marital happiness.

Emotional bond in childhood was measured in terms of closeness and intimacy versus distance and strain in the relationship with each parent in childhood (around age 10), in adolescence (around age 15), and during young adulthood (around age 25). Respondents were asked to rate the relationship with each parent, at each age, on a scale ranging from 1 (very strained relationship) to 7 (very close relationship). The Cronbach alpha reliabilities of emotional bond with mother and father were .74 and .71, respectively.

Parental affection was measured by a four-item scale rating the extent to which each parent was available when needed, was easy to talk to, showed love and affection, and encouraged sharing of troubles. The reliabilities of these scales for mothers and fathers were .75 and .81, respectively.

Family cohesion was measured by a four-item scale tapping family relationships (e.g., "the family had lots of fun together") and activities (e.g., "the family did interesting things together on weekends") during childhood and adolescence. The Cronbach alpha reliability of this scale was .80.

Parental marital happiness was measured by a single item, "How would you describe the relationship between your parents when you were growing up?" Response categories ranged from 1 (very unhappy) to 5 (very happy).

Marital quality. Marital quality was measured by the Hebrew adaptation of the short version of *ENRICH* (Fowers & Olson, 1992). The original scale is a 10-item Likert-type scale that assesses the respondent's perceived quality of his/her marriage across 10 dimensions of the relationship (spouse's personal traits, communication, conflict resolution, financial management, leisure activities, sexuality, parenting, relationship with the extended family, division of household labor, and religious practices). Fowers and Olson (1992) reported good reliability estimates of the short ENRICH scale, as well as high concurrent and predictive validity.

Similar estimates were found in the modified Hebrew version (Lavee, 1995). In this version, items and response categories were modified in order to decrease the response set. Instead of the original Likert scale in which items are ranked between "fully agree" and "disagree," each item is given two extreme response categories and the respondent is asked to check a number on a scale ranging between these responses (for example: "When we have conflicts or disagreements–[1] We always come to an agreement . . . [7] We seldom are able to bridge our differences"). A scale of this type (see, for example, Antonovsky, 1987) was found to be less affected by social desirability than the typical Likert scale. Indeed, the modified version was found to correlate only modestly (r = .16) with a social desirability scale (Lavee, 1995). The scale has been extensively used in studies in Israel. Evidence for its validity has been shown by high correlation estimates (.86 to .91) between scores of the short and the long scales, as well as its ability to discriminate clinical from non-clinical samples.

In the present sample, the internal consistency reliability (Cronbach alpha) of the marital quality scale was .78. This instrument was completed by both spouses. Initial analyses indicated no significant difference between spouses (t = .13) and a high correlation between spouses in their evaluation of marital quality (r = .79, p < .01). Based on Larsen and Olson's (1990) suggestion, the spouses' evaluations were averaged.

RESULTS

The data were analyzed in three steps. First, differences between groups were examined regarding their past family relations. Second, we examined the association between past family relations and current relationships with parents. Finally, the effect of past family relations and current relationships with parents on marital quality was examined.

In order to examine the differences between the Leavers and the Remainers in past family relations, a multivariate analysis of variance (MANOVA) was conducted, testing for group and gender differences. The analysis indicated a significant difference between groups across the six family-of-origin variables (F = 3.95, p < .05), but no gender differences were found (F = 1.45, p = .23) nor was there a significant interaction between group and gender (F = 1.07, p = .30). The findings of the univariate analyses for differences between groups in the family-of-origin variables are presented in Table 2.

The data in Table 2 show that the Remainers report closer family relationships in their childhood than do the Leavers. As compared with the Leavers, they report a stronger emotional bond with their mothers in childhood, a higher level of mother's affection, a more cohesive family, and a higher level of marital happiness between their parents. However, no differences were found between groups in their past relationships (i.e., emotional bond and affection) with their fathers.

Next, we examined the association between current relationships with parents, in terms of emotional bond and contact solidarity, and past family relations.

As Table 3 shows, relationships with parents in adulthood, especially in regard to emotional bond, are highly related to the relationships in childhood. The emotional bond with the parents is associated with all past family relations, with the exception of father's functioning. A regression analysis of current

TABLE 2. Means, Standard Deviations, and Differences Between Groups in Past Family Relationships

Family Relationship	Leavers		Remainers		Difference
	M	SD	M	SD	$F_{(1,102)}$
Mother's emotional bond	4.66	1.09	5.27	.87	13.01**
Father's emotional bond	4.79	1.03	4.81	.89	.02
Mother's affection	2.07	.56	2.33	.53	5.99*
Father's affection	1.97	.59	2.05	.55	.76
Family cohesion	2.00	.57	2.87	.47	5.28*
Parents' marital happiness	3.05	.83	3.65	.87	12.47**

$F_{(5, 98)} = 3.95, p < .05$
Note: * $p < .05$ ** $p < .01$

TABLE 3. Correlations (Person r) Between Past Family Relationships and Current Adult-Child–Parent Relationships

	Current Family Relations	
	Emotional Bond	Contact Solidarity
Past Family Relationships		
Emotional bond with mother	.369**	.354**
Emotional bond with father	.243*	.157
Mother's affection	.337**	.240*
Father's affection	.138	.179
Family cohesion	.454**	.323**
Parents' marital relations	.311**	.325**

* $p < .05$ ** $p < .01$

emotional bond on past family relations indicated that these variables to-gether explain 32% of the variance in emotional bond ($F_{(6,82)} = 6.52$, $p <$ .001). A stepwise regression indicated that family cohesion and emotional bond with the mother in childhood best explain current emotional bond ($R^2 =$ .28, $F_{(2,86)} = 16.97$, $p < .001$).

Contact solidarity is associated with childhood relationships with the mother, with family cohesion, and with the parents' marital relations. A re-gression analysis of contact solidarity on past family relations indicated that these variables together explain 16% of the variance in frequency of contact with the parents ($F_{(6,82)} = 2.59$, $p < .05$). A stepwise regression indicated that parents' marital relationship and emotional bond with the mother in childhood best explain current contact solidarity ($R^2 = .15$, $F_{(2,86)} = 7.41$, $p < .001$).

Marital Quality of Leavers and Remainers

In the final phase of the analysis, we examined how past and current rela-tionships with parents are related to the respondents' marital quality among the Leavers and the Remainers. First, group and gender differences in percep-tions of their marital relations was examined by a two-way analysis of vari-ance. The analysis showed a significant group difference, with the Leavers reporting a higher level of marital quality than the Remainers ($F(1,104) = 5.18$, $p < .05$). However, no gender differences were found nor was there a signifi-cant group x gender interaction effect.

Second, the contribution of past and current family relationships to the adult children's marital quality was analyzed utilizing a hierarchical regression analy-sis (see Table 4). In the first step of this analysis, group, past parent-child rela-tions and current parent-child relations were entered. The results of the first step indicated that marital quality is explained by group affiliation and by past family

TABLE 4. Hierarchical Regression Analysis for Variables Explaining Marital Quality

Step		B	Se.B	β
1	Group	−0.36	0.13	−0.26**
	Past parent-child relations	0.19	0.08	0.24*
	Current parent-child relations	0.15	0.14	0.11
2	Group	−1.31	0.47	−0.96**
	Past parent-child relations	0.20	0.08	0.26**
	Current parent-child relations	−0.14	0.19	−0.10
	Group x current p-c relations	0.56	0.27	0.74*

Note: $R^2 = .12$ for Step 1 ($F_{(3,102)} = 4.45**$); $\Delta R^2 = .04$ for Step 2 ($F_{(1,101)} = 4.45*$); Total model $R^2 = .15$, $F_{(4,101)} = 4.57**$
* $p < .05$. ** $p < .01$.

relations, but not by current relationships with parents. In the second step of the analysis, an interaction term of group and past family relations was entered, followed by an interaction term of group and current parent-child relations. The group X past family relations interaction did not yield a significant F change, and the interaction term was not found to be statistically significant. In contrast, the group X current parent-child relations interaction added significantly to the explained variance of marital quality (F_{change} = 4.45, p < .05), with a significant effect of this interaction term on marital quality (beta = .74, p < .05).

In order to examine the interaction effect of group and current relationships with parents, respondents were divided into two categories of their relationship with parents, based on the median statistic of this variable: *strained* and *close* relationships. A plot of marital quality by each relationship category for the Leavers and the Remainers is presented in Figure 1. Figure 1 shows that among the Leavers, marital quality is nearly equal for both levels of the relationship with parents. Among the Remainers, in contrast, marital quality depends on the current parent-child relationship insofar as close relationships are associated with high marital quality, whereas strained relationships are associated with a significantly lower level of marital quality. These results are further confirmed by the finding that marital quality and current relationships with parents are highly correlated among the Remainers (r = .35, p < .01), but not among the Leavers (r = .12, p = .37).

FIGURE 1. Marital Quality as a Function of Parent-Child Relationship Among "Leavers" and "Remainers"

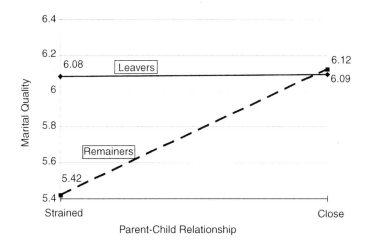

DISCUSSION

Family scholars have long emphasized the correspondence between parent-child relationships and the capacity of adult children to form intimate relationships. One research tradition emphasizes early parent-child and family relationships as predictors of intimate relationships in adulthood (Bowen, 1978; Bowlby, 1969, 1988; Cohn et al., 1992; Shaver et al., 1988). Another line of research is more focused on the intergenerational relationships between elderly parents and their adult children as they relate to the latter's psychological well-being and marital quality (Bengtson et al., 1990; Mancini & Blieszner, 1989; Suitor & Pillemer, 1988; Ward & Spitze, 1998).

The present study attempts to add to the accumulating knowledge about the links between parent-child relationships and adult children's marital quality in two respects. First, we consider parent-child relationships both in childhood and adulthood, thus bridging the gap characterized as the alpha-omega tendency in parent-child research (Hagestad, 1987). Second, we examine the moderating role of residential proximity on the association between intergenerational relationships and the quality of adult children's marital relationships.

Before we discuss the findings, several caveats should be noted. First, parent-child relationships during childhood were retrospectively reported. Since this memory is not necessarily compartmentalized into distinct domains and periods of life, it loses its acuity as time passes. Furthermore, this memory may be biased by current life situations. Second, given that this is a cross-sectional research, causal relations between parent-child relationships and children's marital quality cannot be ascertained. Bearing these limitations in mind, our findings do provide some new perspectives on the links between parent-child relationships and the quality of adult children's marital relationships. Furthermore, our confidence in the validity of the findings is based on previous research on parent-child relationships in childhood and adulthood (Rossi & Rossi, 1990) and the association between intergenerational relationships and marital quality (Ward & Spitze, 1998).

The findings indicate several associations that may attest to the developmental nature of parent-child relations and their correspondence with adult children's marital quality. The closer the relations with parents were in childhood, the stronger they were in adulthood. In particular, parent-child emotional relations and contact solidarity are strongly related to emotional relations with the mother, parents' marital happiness, and the level of family cohesion during childhood. This finding provides further evidence for the continuity of contact throughout life and corroborates Rossi and Rossi's (1990) finding that greater intimacy and a stronger emotional bond between adult children and their parents are associated with better parent-child relations in childhood. Such families tend to manifest more expressions of affection and a stronger sense of family cohesion.

Our findings also indicate that offspring who had more positive family experiences and closer relations with parents in childhood tend to remain in close proximity and to have more intensive contact with them. In contrast, those whose childhood relations with parents were experienced as less affectionate tend to move away. In particular, the decision to remain in close residential proximity was related to emotional relations with the mother, family cohesion, and parents' marital happiness. These findings provide support for other studies indicating that the parent-child assistance relationship is weaker when parental marital quality is poor and when offspring do not regard their parents as sources of help (Amato, Rezac, & Booth, 1995; Lin & Lewis, 1996). Presumably, families in which parents' marital relations are stronger also have a stronger sense of family cohesion and a closer emotional bond between offspring and parents.

However, positive family experiences during childhood are not the sole explanatory factor in the decision to stay in close proximity to parents or to move away. Some children remained close to parents even though they reported unfavorable family experiences. According to intergenerational theories (Bowen, 1978), when unresolved parental tensions exist, a child may fulfill an emotional role in the parental relationship–usually within the matrix of a rigid triangle–making separation more difficult. Unsatisfactory relationships with parents also may invoke a low self-image and a lack of self-reliance among children, making it more difficult for them to cope with the "outside world." Thus, we find adult children who choose to live in close proximity and to maintain frequent contact with their parents despite having strained relationships.

Upon examining the factors that explain the marital quality of children–those who remained close to or moved away from their parents–the findings show that their marital quality is related to the past emotional bond with their parents. The association between marital quality and current parent-child relationships, however, depends upon residential proximity. More specifically, the marital quality of children who moved away remained the same, regardless of whether they had close or strained relationships with their parents. In contrast, the marital quality of those who remained in close proximity to their parents was affected by their current parent-child relationship. Those with strained relationships experienced poorer marital quality than did those whose relations with parents were defined as close. This finding should be evaluated in light of previous research (e.g., Ward & Spitze, 1998) indicating that there is little association between marital quality and intergenerational exchange per se, but rather a more consistent association with the quality of parent-child relationships. In the same vein, Suitor and Pillemer (1994) found that in the context of intergenerational relationships, adult children's marital satisfaction declined for some but increased for others.

The present study further suggests that offspring who physically distance themselves from their parents are less affected in their marriages by relations with their parents. For those who live near their parents and encounter them on a daily basis, close emotional relationships with parents may enhance marital relationships, whereas strained parent-child relationships may have an unfavorable effect on adult children's marital quality.

This study is based on a unique sample of kibbutz families, which serves as a natural setting for assessing the moderating effect of residential proximity and contact solidarity between adult children and their parents. Although additional research is needed, we believe that the findings have implications for broader populations. Given the highly mobile nature of modern society, a norm of "remote intimacy" has emerged, with many offspring choosing their place of residence on the basis of such criteria as school, work, and proximity to leisure centers, rather than staying in close proximity to their parents' home. The findings presented here shed light on this phenomenon and point to the importance of the state of the relationship between parents and their offspring in the formation of adult children's marital relationships.

REFERENCES

Amato, P. R., & Booth, A. (2001). The legacy of parents' marital discord: Consequences for children's marital quality. *Journal of Personality and Social Psychology, 81,* 627-638.

Amato, P. R., Rezak, S. J., & Booth, A. (1995). Helping between parents and young adult offspring: The role of parental marital quality, divorce, and remarriage. *Journal of marriage and the Family, 57,* 363-374.

Antonovsky, A. (1987). *Unraveling the mystery of health: How people manage with stress and stay well.* San Francisco, CA: Jossey-Bass.

Antonucci, T. (1990). Social supports and social relationships. In R. Binstock & L. George (Eds.), *Handbook of aging and the social sciences* (pp. 205-226). New York: Academic Press.

Baltes, P. B., & Reese, H. W. (1984). The life-span perpective in developmental psychology. In M. Borenstein & M. Lamb (Eds.), *Developmental psychology: An advanced textbook* (pp. 499-532). Hillsdale, NJ: Lawrence Erlbaum.

Barnett, R. C., Marshall, N. L., & Pleck, J. H. (1992). Adult son-parent relationships and their associations with sons' psychological distress. *Journal of Family Issues, 13,* 505-525.

Belsky, J., & Pensky, E. (1988). Developmental history, personality and family relationships: Toward an emergent family system. In R. Hinde & J. Stevenson-Hinde

(Eds.), *Relationships within families: Mutual influences* (pp. 193-217). Oxford: Oxford University Press.

Bengtson, V. L., & Giarrusso, R., Mabry, J. B., & Silverstein, M. (2002). Solidarity, conflict, and ambivalence: Complementary or competing perspectives on intergenerational relationships? *Journal of Marriage and Family, 64*, 568-576.

Bengtson, V. L., & Roberts, R. E. L. (1991). Intergenerational solidarity in aging families: An example of formal theory construction. *Journal of Marriage and the Family, 53*, 856-870.

Bengtson, V. L., Rosenthal, C., & Burton, L. (1990). Families and aging: Diversity and Heterogeneity. In R. Binstock & L. George (Eds.), *Handbook of aging and the social sciences* (pp. 263-287). New York: Academic Press.

Booth, A., & Edwards, J. N. (1990). Transmission of marital and family quality over the generations: The effects of parental divorce and unhappiness. *Journal of Divorce, 13*, 41-58.

Bowen, M. (1978). *Family therapy in clinical practice.* New York: Jason Aronson.

Bowlby, J. (1969). *Attachment and loss, Vol. I: Attachment.* New York: Basic Books.

Bowlby, J. (1988). *A secure base: Parent-child attachment and healthy human development.* New York: Basic Books.

Caspi, A., & Elder, G. H. (1988). Emergent family patterns: The intergenerational construction of problem behavior and relationships. In R. Hinde & J. Stevenson-Hinde (Eds.), *Relationships within families: Mutual influences* (pp. 218-240). Oxford: Oxford University Press.

Cohn, D. A., Silver, D. H., Cowan, C. P., Cowan, P. A., & Pearson, J. (1992). Working models of childhood attachment and couple relationships. *Journal of Family Issues, 13*, 432-449.

Collins, N. L., & Read, S. J. (1990). Adult attachment, working models and relationship quality in dating couples. *Journal of Personality and Social Psychology, 58*, 644-663.

Dewit, D., Wister, A., & Burch, T. (1988). Physical distance and social contact between elders and their adult children. *Research on Aging, 10*, 56-80.

Feeney, J. A., & Noller, P. (1990). Attachment style as a predictor of adult romantic relationships. *Journal Personality and Social Psychology, 58*, 281-291.

Feng, D., Giarruso, R., Bengtson, V. L., & Frye, N. (1999). Intergenerational transmission of marital quality and marital instability. *Journal of Marriage and the Family, 61*, 451-463.

Fisiloglu, H., & Lorenzetti, A. F. (1994). The relation of family cohesion to marital adjustment. *Contemporary Family Therapy, 16*, 539-552.

Fowers, B. J., & Olson, D. H. (1992). ENRICH marital satisfaction scale: A brief research and clinical tool. *Journal of Family Psychology, 7*, 176-185.

Freud, S. (1949). *An outline of psychoanalysis.* New York: Norton.

Hagestad, G. O. (1987). Parent-child relations in later life: Trends and gaps in past research. In J. B. Lancaster, J. Altmann, A. S. Rossi, & L. R. Sherrod (Eds.), *Parenting across the life span: Biosocial dimensions* (pp. 405-433). Hawthorne, NY: Aldine Publishing.

Hazan, C., & Shaver, P. (1987). Romantic love conceptualized as an attachment process. *Journal Personality and Social Psychology, 52*, 511-524.

Kelley, H. H. (1972). Causal schemata and the attribution process. In E. E. Jones, D. E. Kanouse, H. H. Kelley, R. E. Nisbett, S. Valins, & B. Weiner (Eds.), *Attribution: Perceiving the causes of behavior* (pp. 151-174). Morristown, NJ: General Learning Press.

Krause, N. (1995). Negative interaction and satisfaction with social support among older adults. *Journal of Gerontology: Psychological Sciences and Social Sciences, 50B(2):* P59-P73.

Larsen, A. S., & Olson, D. H. (1990). Capturing the complexity of family systems: Integrating family theory, family scores, and family analysis. In T. W. Draper & A. C. Marcos (Eds.), *Family variables: Conceptualization, measurement, and use* (pp. 19-47). Beverly Hills, CA: Sage.

Lavee, Y. (1995, October). *The Israeli Marital Quality Scale (I-MQS): Clinical and research applications.* Paper presented at the annual conference of the Israeli Psychological Association, Beer Sheva, Israel.

Lawton, L., Silverstein, M., & Bengtson, V. (1994). Affection, social contact, and geographic distance between adult children and their parents. *Journal of Marriage and the Family, 56,* 57-68.

Lewis, R. A., & Spanier, G. B. (1979). Theorizing about the quality and stability of marriage. In W. R. Burr, R. Hill, F. I. Nye & I. L. Reiss (Eds.), *Contemporary theorizing about the family, Vol. I.* (pp. 268-294). New York: Free Press.

Lin, L. W., & Lewis, R. A. (1996). Intergenerational interdependence: Models of help-exchange among three generations. *Family Science Review, 9,* 207-229.

Luescher, K., & Pillemer, K. (1998). Intergenerational ambivalence: A new approach to the study of parent-child relations in later life. *Journal of Marriage and the Family, 60,* 413-425.

Lye, D. N. (1996). Adult child-parent relationships. *Annual Review of Sociology, 22,* 79-102.

Mancini, J., & Blieszner, R. (1989). Aging parents and adult children: Research themes in intergenerational relations. *Journal of Marriage and the Family, 51,* 275-290.

Mitleberg, D., & Lev-Ari, L. (1991). *Kibbutz-born children living overseas: Reasons for immigration and return possibilities.* Unpublished manuscript, Institute for the Study of the Kibbutz, University of Haifa.

Palgi, M. (1997). Women in the changing world of the kibbutz. *Women in Judaism: A Multidisciplinary Journal, 1,* 1-9.

Pearlin, L., Mullan, J., Semple, S., & Skaff, M. (1990). Caregiving and the stress process: An overview of concepts and their measures. *Gerontologist, 30,* 583-594.

Pearlin, L., Aneshensel, C., Mullan, J., & Whitlatch, C. (1996). Caregiving and its social support. In R. Binstock & L. George (Eds.), *Handbook of aging and the social sciences* (pp. 283-302). New York: Academic Press.

Rossi, A. S., & Rossi, P. H. (1990). *Of human bonding: Parent-child relations across the life course.* New York: Aldine de Gruyter.

Shaver, P., Hazan, C., & Bradshaw, D. (1988). Love as attachment: The integration of three behavioral systems. In R. Sternberg & M. Barnes (Eds.), *The psychology of love* (pp. 68-99). New Haven, CT: Yale University Press.

Suitor, J. J., & Pillemer, K. (1988). Explaining intergenerational conflict when adult children and elderly parents live together. *Journal of Marriage and the Family, 50,* 1037-1047.

Suitor, J. J., & Pillemer, K. (1992). Status transitions and marital satisfaction: The case of adult children caring for elderly parents sugffering from dementia. *Journal of Social and Personal Relationships, 9,* 549-562.

Suitor, J. J., & Pillemer, K. (1994). Family caregiving and marital satisfaction: Findings from one-year panel study of women caring for parents with dementia. *Journal of Marriage and the Family, 56,* 681-690.

Suitor, J. J., Pillemer, K., Bohanon, K. S., & Robison, J. (1995). Aged parents and aging children: Determinants of relationship quality. In V. Bedford & R. Blieszner (Eds.), *Handbook of aging and the family* (pp. 223-242). Westport, CT: Greenwood Press.

Umberson, D. (1992). Relationships between adult children and their parents: Psychological consequences for both generations. *Journal of Marriage and the Family, 54,* 664-685.

Wan, C. K., Jaccard, J., & Ramey, S. L. (1996). The relationship between social support and life satisfaction as a function of family structure. *Journal of Marriage and the Family, 58,* 502-513.

Ward, R.A., & Spitze, G. (1998). Sandwiched marriages: The implications of child and parent relations for marital quality in midlife. *Social Forces, 77(2),* 647-666.

Parental Separation and Adolescents' Felt Insecurity with Mothers: Effects of Financial Hardship, Interparental Conflict, and Maternal Parenting in East and West Germany

Sabine Walper
Joachim Kruse
Peter Noack
Beate Schwarz

ABSTRACT. This study investigates effects of living in nuclear, separated single mother, or stepfather families on adolescents' relationship to their mothers. Focusing on adolescents' felt insecurity toward mother, effects of family type are expected to be mediated by economic pressure and impaired family dynamics. Subsamples from East ($n = 220$) and West Germany ($n = 273$) allow a comparison of relevant

---

Sabine Walper and Joachim Kruse are affiliated with the University of Munich. Peter Noack is affiliated with the University of Jena. Beate Schwarz is affiliated with the University of Konstanz.

Address correspondence to: Sabine Walper, University of Munich, Department of Education, Leopoldstr. 13, D-80802 Munich, Germany (E-mail: walper@du.uni-muenchen.de).

This research was supported by a grant of the German Research Council to the first author (Wa 949/3-1 to 3-5). The authors would like to thank Mechtild Goedde and Anna Katharina Gerhard for their support in conducting this research, and are grateful to the families for their cooperation.

http://www.haworthpress.com/web/MFR
© 2004 by The Haworth Press, Inc. All rights reserved.
Digital Object Identifier: 10.1300/J002v36n03_07

processes according to contextual conditions. Although no simple as-sociation between family type and adolescents' felt insecurity is ob-served, tests of path models confirm that interparental conflict, impaired parenting, mothers' pressure to side against the father, and adoles-cents' feelings of being caught in the middle link family type to adoles-cents' relationship to their mothers. Similarities between the regional subsamples outweigh differences. *[Article copies available for a fee from The Haworth Document Delivery Service: 1-800-HAWORTH. E-mail address: <docdelivery@haworthpress.com> Website: <http://www.HaworthPress.com> © 2004 by The Haworth Press, Inc. All rights reserved.]*

KEYWORDS. Adolescents, financial hardship, insecurity, parental conflict, parental separation

As in many other Western countries, divorce rates have more or less steadily increased in Germany since the turn to the 20th century (Statistisches Bundesamt Deuschland, 1998; Walper & Schwarz, 1999). In 2001, almost 10 out of 1,000 existing marriages experienced divorce, and more than one-third of all marriages in Germany are estimated to end in court (Statistisches Bundesamt, 2002). Despite substantial divorce rates, the consequences of pa-rental divorce and remarriage have only recently become the target of more sys-tematic investigation among German researchers (Walper & Schwarz, 1999). Moreover, the majority of studies address aspects of children's psychosocial ad-aptation as outcomes of concern (Amato & Keith, 1991). Less is known con-cerning the development of parent-child relations as they are affected by parental separation. While research analyzing patterns of parental child-rearing in nuclear families, single-parent families, and stepfamilies is informative in this respect (Demo & Acock, 1996; Hetherington & Clingempeel, 1992), it does not address likely variations in the normative, age graded transformation of par-ent-child relationships directly.

The present study examines mother-adolescent relationships in different family structures. As suggested by individuation theory (Grotevant & Cooper, 1986; Youniss & Smollar, 1985), the development of more mutuality and indi-viduality in the family during adolescence depends on parents' and adoles-cents' success in remaining connected and maintaining supportive relationships. Our central hypothesis is that concurrent problems in the family system interfere with the normative transformation of parent-child relation-ships (Ullrich, 1999; Walper & Schwarz, 2001). More specifically, we expect parental separation to affect social-emotional bonds between adolescents and their mothers by fostering feelings of ambivalence and insecurity. In line with earlier research (cf. Amato, 1993), we assume that family structure differences during adolescents' development are related to interparental conflict as well as by financial pressures typically resulting from divorce. Drawing on data collected in West and East Germany allows us to examine to what extent the assumed processes vary in different macro-contextual conditions in both parts of the country. For example, the prevalence of divorced and single parent families is clearly higher in East Germany and the institutional support system such as day-care facilities or after-school care is more extensive than in the West. In this article,we will first discuss the development of parent-child relationships during adolescence and possible effects of parental separation on this process. Next, we introduce variables which we expect to mediate the postulated linkage between parental separation and impaired socio-emotional bonds between adolescents and their parents. Before summarizing our conceptual framework, we will provide more detailed information on the societal background of family life in East and West Germany.

PARENT-CHILD RELATIONS DURING ADOLESCENCE AND PARENTAL SEPARATION

Although little evidence exists that supports traditional notions of adolescence as a volatile period of 'storm and stress' in individual development and interpersonal relations, most scholars agree that parent-child relations are subject to considerable change during the second decade of life (Steinberg, 2001). In particular, relationships have to adjust to adolescents' increasing need for autonomy and self-direction. While earlier theoretical accounts (e.g., Blos, 1962) posited a growing detachment from parents as the process accommodating adolescents' changing needs, more recent proponents of individuation theory (e.g., Grotevant & Cooper, 1986; Youniss & Smollar, 1985) have voiced doubt concerning this notion. They claim that changes toward a more peer-like relationship and toward mutual perceptions as autonomous individuals do not require weakening the socio-emotional bonds that link parents and their children. Instead, it is suggested that warm and supportive emotional bonds form a basis that greatly facilitates the normative transformation of parent-child relations.

Findings from studies examining parent-child relations during adolescence mostly confirm claims of individuation theory. For example, there is little evidence for a severe impairment of socio-emotional bonds in the family (e.g., Buhrmester & Furman, 1987) and using meta-analysis, Laursen, Coy, and Collins (1998) found no dramatic peak of conflict between parents and youth adolescence. Only a small minority of families go through strong and extended conflicts during this period of family development (Montemayor, 1983). By the same token, a structural transformation of parent-child relations accompanied by emotional detachment is predictive of adolescents' poor psychosocial adjustment (Noack & Puschner, 1999). In particular, not only the denial of attachment needs, but also anxieties in relation to parents during the individuation process pose a risk for a variety of personality problems (Holmbeck & Leake, 1999).

Typically, the modal family manages to successfully maneuver through the relationship transformation during adolescence (Steinberg, 2001). However, the individuation process is characterized by a lag between adolescents' striving for autonomy, and parental hesitation to grant leeway and give up control which requires constant negotiations (e.g., Smetana, 1988). Additional strain on the family or conflict between parents could hamper the individuation process by preventing parents from supporting this process and by creating general insecurity about the reliability of relationships. Due to the many stressors faced by single mothers (Simons, Johnson, & Lorenz, 1996), divorced mothers are more likely to be depressed and to exhibit impaired parenting, even beyond detrimental effects of these risk factors (Simons & Johnson, 1996; cf. Amato, 2000 for an overview). Furthermore, parent-adolescent relationships have been shown to be more conflicted in divorced families (Smetana, 1996), threatening a problematic trajectory between middle adolescence to parental separation during early adulthood (Amato & Booth, 1996). This suggests that parental problems coinciding with the normative relationship changes during adolescence may affect the socio-emotional basis of the process (Ullrich, 1999). While detachment from parents may be a long-term outcome, subtle uncertainty concerning the relationship, feelings of being drawn back and forth between closeness and distance, and insecurity concerning positive parental regard and support are likely to emerge from conflict-ridden homes (Davies & Cummings, 1994; Davies, Harold, Goeke-Morey, & Cummings, 2002).

So far, little research has addressed the question of how parental conflict may interfere with the individuation process during adolescence. Findings from studies of divorce suggest that separated families are more likely to foster early—perhaps premature–development of autonomy (e.g., Smetana, 1993), which can be explained by increased risk for family discord, lack of parental support, and higher demands on children's self-reliance (Sessa & Steinberg, 1991). While remarriage provides an additional adult as a resource in family management and child support, parental monitoring proves to be lower in single-parent as well as stepfamilies when compared to nuclear families (Kerns, Aspelmeier, Gentzler, & Grabill, 2001). Most research shows that children in stepfamilies are not better off than their age-mates in single mother families (Amato, 1994; Hetherington & Clingempeel, 1992), and that parent-child relationships are predictive of early detachment from the family (Hetherington & Jodl, 1994).

Mediators Linking Parental Separation and Psychosocial Outcomes

Findings that moderate negative effects of parental separation (cf. Amato & Keith, 1991) suggest a need for more differentiated approaches that consider conditions and processes before and during parental separation in order to explain problematic outcomes (e.g., Amato, 1993; Hetherington, Bridges, & Insabella, 1998). Particular attention has been paid to economic pressure experienced by families after divorce and to interparental conflict as mediators of separation effects.

A typical consequence of parental separation is financial hardship particularly among single-mother families (Burkhauser, Duncan, Hauser, & Berntsen, 1991; McLanahan & Sandefur, 1994). Starting with Elder's seminal research on the children of the Great Depression (Elder, 1974), the evidence points to the detrimental effects of poverty and economic pressure on family dynamics and children's development (Duncan & Brooks-Gunn, 1997). Indeed, financial hardship has been identified as a factor strongly contributing to disadvantages faced by children from single-mother families (McLanahan & Sandefur, 1994). Following findings from research on nuclear families (Elder, Conger, Foster, & Ardelt, 1992; Walper, 1999), it can be assumed that effects of financial deprivation in families after parental separation operate largely indirectly through their negative effects on the parental relationship and parents' child-rearing practices.

Interparental conflict often is a concomitant of parental divorce and sometimes an ongoing stressor. Emery (1982) pointed out that it is not parental divorce but interparental conflict that explains children's adjustment problems after divorce. Since then, a large number of studies have supported this hypothesis (cf. Amato, 1993, 2000). Moreover, children from nuclear families characterized by considerable spousal conflict show adjustment problems similar to those of age-mates from divorced parents (Jenkins & Smith, 1993; Peterson & Zill, 1986; Reis & Meyer-Probst, 1999). It seems to be children's perceptions of their parents' conflicts which are important in determining the stressfulness of parental disagreements (Grych & Fincham, 1993). Conflict has been shown to be particularly problematic if perceived as being frequent, intense, and focused on sons or daughters themselves as the topic of arguments (e.g., Harold, Osborne, & Conger, 1997). While parental conflict may directly affect children (e.g., Emery, Fincham, & Cummings, 1992), there is considerable evidence for a spill-over of interparental conflict into parent-child inter-actions, contributing to increased negativity and lower levels of support by parents (Erel & Burman, 1995; Fauber & Long, 1991).

Comparably less attention has been paid to more subtle modes of impairment of parent-child relationships as a consequence of interparental problems. Weak or antagonistic marital relationships may result in parents' attempts to form an intergenerational coalition with their sons or daughters against the spouse (Christensen & Margolin, 1988; Minuchin, 1974). As many children may want to remain loyal to both parents, they could easily find themselves caught between their parents. While little research has addressed such loyalty conflicts and their consequences, available evidence is suggestive of negative effects on the child (Buchanan, Macoby, & Dornbush, 1991; Lopez, 1991).

To summarize, sons and daughters who experienced the separation of their biological parents can be assumed to show more insecurity in the relationship with their parents than their age-mates. However, we expect a moderate effect which is mediated by economic pressure and interparental conflict. Previous findings suggest that negative consequences of economic problems and of conflict between parents operate through dysfunctional parenting. Besides decreased parental support and more restrictive child-rearing strategies, it may be that parents' attempt to press their children to side with them in the spousal conflict, leaving children caught in the middle between their fathers and mothers. While economic pressure may also affect parenting directly, it can be expected that the effect is partly mediated by interparental conflicts which are likely to emerge from economic hardship (Conger, Elder, Lorenz, Conger, Simons, & Whitbeck, 1990).

Parental Separation in East and West Germany

Before German unification, divorce rates in East Germany were consistently higher than in the West (Walper & Schwarz, 1999). It would be premature, however, to conclude that marriage and family had a lower significance during the socialist regime. It is suggested that lower economic risks associated with separation contributed to the high divorce rates in the former German Democratic Republic (GDR) (Schneider, 1994). Moreover, an extensive childcare system facilitated mothers' lives after separation. GDR policies supported of full-time employment of all adults below age 65. As a consequence, about 85% of all women between the ages of 15 and 65 were employed, and women with children were no less likely to be in the labor force than women without children, which sharply contrasted with the West German situation (Maier, 1993). State-subsidized public provisions of child care up to adolescence greatly fostered maternal employment (Walper & Galambos, 1997).

After unification, divorce rates in East Germany dropped dramatically and fell well below West German figures, and even now they have not reached the West German level. At the same time, the economic risks associated with divorce and single parenting in East Germany increased resulting in a pattern of poverty similar to that prevalent in West Germany (Joos, 1997). Although the situation in both parts of the country has become more similar in this respect, other differences may continue to matter. It seems plausible to assume that the higher readiness in the former GDR to end a problematic marriage may have prevented an escalation of interspousal conflict prior to divorce which, in turn, could have resulted in a less conflictual post-separation phase (cf. Maccoby, Depner, & Mnookin, 1990). Moreover, contact with the non-custodial parent was less promoted and sought-after than in the West. Consequently, in the East conflictual ex-spouse relationships were not as common as in the West. Such patterns may have persisted beyond the rapid social and material changes after reunification. Thus, parental separation in East German families may still be less predictive of spousal conflict and pressures on the child to side with one parent than in the West German context.

Although the extensive system of institutional child care in the East may have weakened parent-child relationships in East Germany, currently parent-child relationships seem to show remarkable similarities to those in West Germany (Behnken, Gunther, Kabat vel Job, Kaiser, Karig, & Kruger, 1991; Walper, 1995). Some scholars suggest that, in East Germany, the family partly played the role of a private "counter-structure" in the light of considerable public control exerted by the socio-political system (Schneider, 1994). Moreover, child-rearing goals seem to be quite similar in both parts of Germany except for some greater emphasis placed on autonomy and self-reliance by West German parents as well as a lesser emphasis on conformity (Feldkircher, 1994).

Aims and Hypotheses of the Present Study

The major objective of the present study is to analyze effects of parental separation on adolescents' felt insecurity in the relationship. All adolescents, regardless of the present family structure (nuclear, single mother, and stepfather families) live with their biological mother. The analyses focuses on adolescents' felt insecurity in the relationship to their mother, testing for possible differences by family type. Drawing on earlier research, we expect such effects to be mediated by economic pressure and interparental conflict thought to result in dysfunctional patterns of child-rearing. At the same time, we consider the subtle, albeit powerful problem of adolescents' loyalty conflicts in the wake of parental separation as an additional mediating variable. Parental separation, particularly if resulting in extensive interparental conflict, is hypothesized to increase the likelihood of maternal pressure on adolescents to side with them against fathers and to lead to adolescents' feelings of being caught in the middle. This, in turn, may foster feelings of insecurity in the mother-child relationship.

Despite the sharp contrast in the conditions characterizing the socio-economic systems ruling the two parts of the country up until a decade ago, the previous literature sources suggest similarities between family relationships in both parts of the country outweigh differences. The associations between parental separation, family dynamics, and adolescents' felt insecurity is the focus of this study rather than socioeconomic differences. Even though some studies suggest somewhat stronger effects of divorce and parenting on adolescent outcomes in the West than in the East (Forkel & Silbereisen, 2001; Silbereisen, Meschke, & Schwarz, 1996), most of the findings address outcomes such as competence and problem behavior among adolescents. Against this backdrop, our study is largely exploratory with respect to regional variations in effects on adolescents' relationship to their mothers. The postulated model is tested separately for the East and West German subsamples in order to reveal possible differences.

METHOD

Sample

The present analyses are based on a sample of 493 children who participated in the first wave of a longitudinal study of families in the former East and West Germany. The overall sample of this study is larger ($N = 743$), but the present analyses required several restrictions concerning the target group. All families had a target child in grade 5 to 11. These children were recruited through a school-based screening involving over 6,000 children and adolescents in five large cities in Germany. Selection for the longitudinal study followed a design which asked for similar proportions of nuclear, single mother, and stepfather families. The latter two groups comprise families in which both biological parents were separated, divorced, or never married to each other. Stepfather families include remarried as well as coresiding couples. All three family types are stratified by the target children's age and gender.

Since our research questions address the interparental relationship, not all separated families could be included in the present analyses. Only those who reported at least some contact of the noncustodial father to their children as well as the child's mother were considered. This restriction yielded a higher loss in the East than the West German subsample, since 53.3% of the East German children from separated families had lost contact with their fathers, as compared to 33.8% of the West German children from separated families. This difference is most pronounced among single mother families, where 50% of East German, but only 28.5% of the West German children were no longer in contact with their biological fathers. In those families who qualified for the target group in the present analyses, missing data were accounted for by using full information maximum likelihood (FIML) estimation for the computation of the path models.

Children's mean age is 14.1 years ($SD = 1.8$) with a range of 9.5 to 19.2 years. Half of the subjects are male (51.3%), half female. The sample is biased toward more highly educated parents with 62.9% attending the highest school track ("Gymnasium"). Due to the selection criteria used here, family types are not equally presented. Of those youth who could be included, 50.9% ($n = 251$) live in a nuclear family with both biological parents, 29.4% ($n = 145$) are raised by their single mother, and 19.7% ($n = 97$) live with their biological mother and a stepfather. There are no significant differences between the three family types concerning children's age, gender, or school track, but their distribution clearly differs by region as explained above ($Chi^2 = 53.51$, $df = 2$, $p < .001$). While in the East German sample 69.1% of the adolescents ($n = 152$) come from nuclear families, in the West German sample the proportion is only 36.3% ($n = 99$). Furthermore, in the West German sample 39.6% ($n = 108$) live with a single mother and 24.2% ($n = 66$) in stepfather families, but in the East German sample the respective percentages are only 16.8% ($n = 31$) and 14.1% ($n = 37$).

Variables

Most indicators for the present analyses are based on children's questionnaire data which were assessed during extensive individual interviews in children's home. Maternal reports which are available for 81% of the children and adolescents were used to indicate economic conditions. Overall, the analyses presented here highlight adolescents' perspective on family dynamics. Although this approach may increase shared measurement variance, it seems nonetheless most appropriate for addressing the subjective representation of parent-child-relationship qualities such as ambivalences and anxieties which may easily be masked in social interaction and may not be validly perceived by other family members. Furthermore, even effects of family stressors like interparental conflict have been shown to be mediated by children's and adolescents' perceptions (Harold & Conger, 1997), thus pointing to the importance of adolescents' perspective on family dynamics in predicting adolescent outcomes. All scales have at least satisfactory, in most cases rather high internal consistency given the low number of items for some of the indicators.

Information on *family structure*, obtained from the interview data, is based on household composition rather than legal family status and distinguishes nuclear families from single mother families (without a new partner of the mother in the household) and stepfather families (comprising remarried as well as coresiding couples). *Economic pressure* in the family household was reported by mothers using two scales which were adapted from Elder et al. (1992). The first scale ("material needs") comprises seven items asking whether the family has sufficient money for different kinds of expenditure (i.e., housing, clothing, household, food, car, traveling, leisure time) using 5-point-ratings (from "not at all true" = 1 to "very true" = 5). Ratings for single items were inverted and averaged (α = .92). The second scale ("financial adjustments") consists of nine items concerning the use of savings for regular payments, the reliance on governmental transfer payments, borrowing money from friends or relatives, delayed payments of bills, and reduced expenditures in various domains (each answered in a yes/no format). The number of "yes" answers was summed (α = .75). Both scales are used to estimate economic pressure as a latent construct. *Frequency of Interparental Conflict* was assessed using a three-item scale with a 4-point rating which is part of a German short version of the Children's Perception of Interparental Conflict Scales (CPIC) developed by Grych, Seid, and Fincham (1992; German translation by Goedde & Walper, 2001; e.g., "My parents have arguments"). Cronbach's Alpha is high with .80.

With respect to maternal parenting, two aspects were considered as predictors of adolescents' felt insecurity in relation to mother. The first was estimated as a latent construct from two scales measuring the degree of *Maternal Supportive Parenting* and *Maternal Sensitivity* to the child's well-being and needs. The Supportive Parenting Scale (translated from Simons, Lorenz, Conger, & Wu, 1992) consists of nine items (e.g., "How often does your mother talk to you about things that bother you?") to be answered with a 4-point frequency rating (ranging from "never/rarely" = 1 to "very frequently" = 4). Items were averaged (α = .84). The scale on Maternal Sensitivity consists of four items which address maternal empathy as experienced by the child and was derived from other measures (cf. Schwarz, Walper, Goedde, & Jurasic, 1997; e.g., "My mother realizes immediately if I am afraid of something."). The 4-point ratings (from "not true" = 1 to "very true" = 4) were averaged (α = .69). The second indicator of maternal parenting assesses *Maternal Restrictiveness* toward the child. It consists of nine items concerning strict control (e.g., "My mother always thinks that she is right and I should not oppose.") and restrictions experienced due to parental overprotectiveness (e.g., "My mother does not credit me with anything and always wants to do everything for me."), which were developed from other scales (cf. Schwarz et al., 1997). The items were to be answered with 4-point ratings (from "not true" = 1 to "very true" = 4) and were averaged ($\alpha = .75$).

As a third aspect of maternal behavior toward the adolescent child, *Mother's Pressure to Side* was indicated by three items (to be answered with a 5-point frequency rating) which were developed for this study. This scale focuses on maternal strategies to get the child involved in a coalition against the father (e.g., "My mother wants me to love her more than I love my dad.") and has a moderate internal consistency ($\alpha = .67$). As a separate indicator, the scale concerning adolescents' *Feelings of Being Caught in the Middle* measures the experience of loyalty conflicts which may result from such maternal behavior, other aspects of parenting, or interparental conflict per se. It consists of six items, each to be rated on a 4-point scale (e.g., "I feel torn back and forth between my parents.") and has high internal consistency ($\alpha = .80$).

Finally, a scale assessing adolescents' *Feelings of Insecurity* in relation to mother was used. It was derived from the Munich Individuation Test of Adolescence (MITA) (Walper, 1998), a revised version of the Separation-Individuation Test of Adolescence (SITA) as developed by Levine and colleagues (Levine, Green & Millon, 1986; Levine & Saintonge, 1993). The MITA allows assessment of individuation in relation to the mother, father, and friends separately, with comparable scales for each of these relationships. Using a combination of two subscales, Feelings of Insecurity are indicated by 10 items. One of these subscales assesses Fear of Losing Parents' Love which emerged as a distinct aspect of the heterogeneous SITA scale "Separation Anxiety" (e.g., "When I disappoint my mother, I am afraid that she does not love me anymore."); the other was newly developed to assess Ambivalence as a feature of insecure relationships which was not included in the SITA (e.g., "I would like to do more things with my mother, but I am afraid to get on her nerves.") This combination of subscales into larger scales, based on theoretical consideration, was confirmed by findings from second order factor analyses (Walper, 1998). Cronbach's Alpha of the combined scale is $\alpha = .77$.

Analyses

In a first step, main and interaction effects of family structure, region, adolescents' age and gender on the dependent variable (Feeling Insecure in Relation to Mother) were tested by analysis of variance in order to explore differential effects of family structure as related to region as well as adolescents' age and gender. Age and gender were considered as possible moderating variables since other studies suggest different reactions to single parenting or living in a stepfamily as dependent on age and gender (Hetherington, 1993), but findings are not consistent (Amato, 2001; Amato & Keith, 1991). Hence, we first tested whether combining boys and girls and all age groups for the subsequent analyses would be legitimate. Three age groups were distinguished: children up to age 12 (preadolescence), youth age 13 and 14 (puberty/early adolescence), and those age 15 and older (middle adolescence). Only main effects, two-way and three-way interactions were considered. In a second step, regional differences concerning the mediating variables were explored employing t-tests. Thirdly, given the considerable age range of our sample, age- and gender-related differences concerning all mediating factors were explored conducting separate correlation analyses for both regions. These three kinds of analyses were conducted for cases with full information. For testing the path model, however, missing information (including missing data due to mothers' lower participation rate) was accounted for by using the FIML approach. This estimation method uses all information of the observed data. The likelihood is computed for the observed portion of each case's data and then accumulated and maximized (Arbuckle, 1996). It usually yields results equivalent to Schafer's multiple imputation approach (Schafer & Graham, 2002; Schafer & Olsen, 1998).

Finally, the hypothesized structure of the path model was tested using AMOS 4.0.1 which allows researchers to estimate path models with latent as well as observed variables (Arbuckle, 1997). Since effects of gender were largely insignificant and the two significant correlations found for the total sample proved to be restricted to the East, gender was not included in the path analyses. Age, however, was significantly and substantially related to perceived interparental conflict and mothers' pressure to side in both subsamples. Hence, we controlled for effects of age by including age as additional predictor, assuming that it affects adolescents' exposure and sensitivity to interparental conflict directly, while effects on maternal pressure to side should be indirect, being mediated by frequency of interparental conflict.

Using family type as a predictor (exogenous) variable in the path model, the three comparison groups were contrasted using two effect coded variables (cf. Cohen & Cohen, 1975; for the use of categorical predictors in path models see Kline, 1998, p. 17). The first effect coded variable compares nuclear families (coded "1") to both groups of separated families (single mother families coded as "0" and stepfather families coded "−1"), while the second effect coded variable tests differences between single-mother families (coded "1") and both groups of two-parent families (nuclear families being coded as "0" and stepfather families being coded as "1").[1] *Direct effects of family structure* were assumed on economic pressure, interparental conflict, and parents' pressure to side. Although the latter pertains to mothers' behavior toward their children and might be assumed to be only contingent on interparental conflict, we tested for direct effects of family structure assuming that more covert forms of interparental antagonism may be particularly prevalent in separated families. These are not captured by overt conflict between parents but may as well contribute to maternal pressure to side. *No direct, but only indirect effects of family structure* were assumed for maternal parenting, which was hypothesized to be linked to family structure by economic pressure and interparental conflict. Both economic pressure as well as interparental conflict were expected to be higher in separated families and should, in turn, undermine sensitive support as well as contribute to more restrictive parenting. Furthermore, indirect effects of family structure were assumed for adolescents' feelings of being caught in the middle. Such effects of family structure should be mediated by interparental conflict and mothers' behavior toward adolescents.

We assumed that increased conflict among parents in separated families would explain higher feelings of being caught in the middle among youth in separated families. In addition to conflict, maternal behavior and particularly maternal pressure to side might contribute to adolescents' feelings of being caught in the middle and could also mediate between family structure and adolescents' feelings of being caught in the middle. Finally, effects of family structure on adolescents' feelings of insecurity in relation to the mother should also be indirect, being mediated by maternal behavior (parenting and pressure to side) and adolescents' feelings of being caught in the middle.

As to *relations between the mediating variables*, economic pressure was expected to contribute to interparental conflict, and the latter was assumed to promote maternal pressure to side. Since the three indicators of perceived maternal behavior toward the child were assumed to be interrelated, their error terms were allowed to covary. As can be seen in Table 1, the correlations vary between $r = .14$ (mothers' pressure to side and restrictive parenting in the East) and $r = -.35$ (mothers' sensitivity/support and restrictiveness in the West). Figures 1 and 2 (see results) show the specification of the path model, but disregard the covariation of error terms and do not show the indicators of the latent variable for the sake of greater clarity. Also, as stated above, interparental conflict, maternal pressure to side, and both indicators of parenting are tested for their effects on children's feelings of being caught

With respect to *regional variations*, multi-group comparisons were employed testing first whether the model accommodated the data of both samples, when no restrictions as to size of coefficients was assumed. Thereafter, differences between single path coefficients were tested by constraining the path to an equal size in both subsamples where a path was found to be significant in only one regional group. This procedure follows suggestions by Jøreskog and Sørbom (1996) and Kline (1998, p. 181f).

TABLE 1. Means, Standard Deviations, and Intercorrelations Between Variables for the West and East German Sample

	M (East)	M (West)	S (E)	SD (W)	1	2	3	4	5	6	7	8	9	10	11
1 Nuclear vs. Separated Families	0.55	0.12	0.73	0.77	/	0.37	-0.02	-0.29	0.00	-0.14	-0.12	-0.05	0.06	0.04	0.09
2 Single-Mother vs. 2-Parent Families	0.03	0.15	0.56	0.78	0.31	/	-0.02	0.11	0.17	0.31	0.20	0.07	-0.01	0.03	0.09
3 Age	13.90	14.26	1.82	1.77	-0.04	-0.04	/	0.18	0.19	-0.05	-0.06	0.00	0.04	-0.07	-0.17
4 Mother's Pressure to Side	1.75	1.96	0.62	0.74	-0.37	0.08	0.11	/	0.56	0.05	0.02	0.37	-0.32	0.23	0.04
5 Parental Conflict	1.90	2.06	0.77	0.89	0.09	-0.02	0.21	0.25	/	0.16	0.10	0.42	-0.20	0.29	0.09
6 Material Needs	2.16	2.03	0.80	0.92	-0.08	0.23	-0.11	0.12	-0.06	/	0.75	0.16	-0.08	0.00	0.12
7 Financial Adjustments	1.24	1.23	0.22	0.22	-0.15	0.20	-0.09	0.15	0.02	0.68	/	0.14	-0.07	0.00	0.07
8 Feeling Caught in the Middle	1.37	1.36	0.48	0.45	0.08	0.12	-0.04	0.21	0.48	0.11	0.11	/	-0.24	0.20	0.35
9 Maternal Support and Sensitivity	3.02	3.11	0.51	0.48	-0.01	0.06	-0.01	-0.18	-0.09	-0.10	-0.08	-0.20	/	-0.35	-0.33
10 Maternal Restrictiveness	2.00	1.92	0.44	0.49	0.05	0.05	-0.09	0.14	0.14	0.06	-0.01	0.42	-0.24	/	0.49
11 Feeling Insecure in Relation to Mother	1.79	1.59	0.48	0.42	0.20	0.06	-0.10	0.01	0.22	0.08	0.07	0.38	-0.30	0.46	/

Note. Coefficients for the West German sample ($n = 273$) are shown above the diagonal and for the East German sample ($n = 220$) below the diagonal. Significant correlations (p at least < .05, two-tailed significance) are underlined.

FIGURE 1. Path Model Linking Family Structure to Adolescents' Attachment to Mother. Findings for the West German Sample (*n* = 273); Standardized Solution; Fit Indexes Are Based on the Joint Analysis of East and West via a Multiple Group Approach; Bold Paths and Path Coefficients = *p* < .05

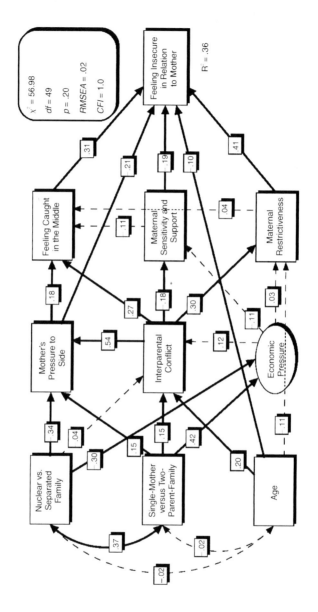

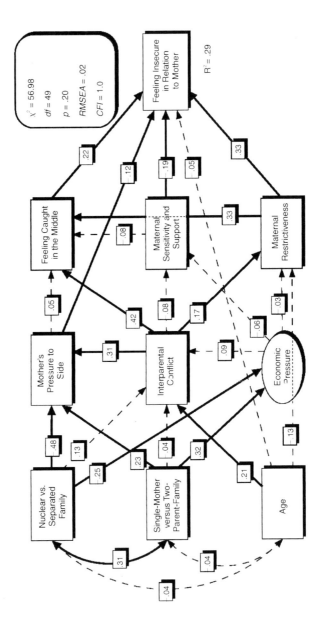

FIGURE 2. Path Model Linking Family Structure to Adolescents' Attachment to Mother. Findings for the East German Sample ($n = 220$); Standardized Solution; Fit Indexes Are Based on the Joint Analysis of East and West via a Multiple Group Approach; Bold Paths and Path Coefficients = $p < .05$

RESULTS

Family Type, Region, Age, and Gender Effects on Feeling Insecure Relative to Mother

The analysis of variance concerning adolescents' feelings of insecurity yielded marginally to highly significant main effects for three of the four factors. As to *region*, East German youth report significantly higher feelings of insecurity in relation to their mothers than their West German age mates: $M = 1.72$ vs. 1.57; $F(1, 452) = 9.12, p < .01$. A closer inspection of subscales reveals that this is restricted to adolescents' fear of losing mother's love and approval which is higher in East Germany ($M = 1.91$ vs. 1.70), while no significant differences are found for children's ambivalence. The effect of *family structure* is also highly significant, $F(2, 452) = 4.77, p < .01$, but not in the expected direction: children from nuclear families report the highest feelings of insecurity while youth from stepfather families feel least insecure ($M = 1.73$ vs. 1.66 vs. 1.55 for nuclear, single mother, and stepfather families). *Gender* differences are not significant, $F(2, 452) = 2.60, p = .11$. Finally, *age* differences indicate a marginal drop of insecurity in relation to mother between the second and third age group: $M = 1.66$ vs. 1.71 vs. 1.57; $F(2, 452) = 2.95, p = .05$.

None of the interaction effects were significant (all $p > .20$). Hence, effects of family structure are fairly homogenous across region, age, and gender. Contrary to our expectations, living apart from one's biological father, be it with a single mother or with the mother and her new partner, does not seem to contribute to adolescents' feelings of insecurity in relation to their mother. Rather, we find that children from separated and particularly stepfather families feel less insecure toward the mother.

Comparing East and West Germany

T-tests were used to test for differences in age and the six indicators, which are considered to link family structure to adolescents' felt insecurity in relation to mother. Adolescents' mean age was higher in the Western than in the Eastern sample, $M = 14.26$ vs. 13.90, $t(491) = 2.20, p < .05$, but does not differ in variance. Economic pressure had significantly higher variance in the East than in the West ($SD = .93$ versus $.81$; $F = 4.73, p = .03$), but there were not significant regional differences, $t(379.17) = -1.50$, n.s. for material needs or $t(390) = -.21$, n.s. for financial adjustments. Interparental conflict as perceived by youth differed marginally in variance with higher variation in the West than in the East ($SD = .90$ versus $.77$, $F = 3.66, p = .06$), but mean values did not differ by region, $t(394) = 1.41$, n.s. Both indicators of maternal parenting show marginal mean differences but not differences in variance between both regions. Mothers' sensitivity and support is reported as being somewhat higher in the West ($M = 3.11$) than in the East ($M = 3.02$), $t(484) = 1.95$, $p = .05$, and East German youth indicate slightly more restrictive parenting ($M = 2.00$) than their West German age-mates ($M = 1.92$), $t(484) = -1.82$, $p = .07$. Substantially stronger differences emerge for maternal pressure to side which is higher in the West ($M = 1.95$) than in the East ($M = 1.75$), $t(481.1) = 3.18$, $p = .00$, and also shows more variation in the West when variances are compared ($SD = .74$ versus .63, $F = 6.30$, $p = .01$). However, children's and adolescents' feelings of being caught between parents do not differ by region, $t(480) = -.47$, n.s. (variance: $F = 1.11$, n.s.).

Effects of Age and Gender

As shown by correlational analyses for all mediating variables, effects of gender were largely insignificant and the two significant correlations found for the total sample were to be restricted to the East, where gender was related to perceived interparental conflict (with higher values for girls: $r = .17$, $p = .02$, $n = 180$) and restrictive parenting (with lower values for girls: $r = -.15$, $p = .02$, $n = 217$). In the West German sample, these correlations were not or only marginally significant (interparental conflict: $r = .06$, n.s., $n = 216$; restrictive parenting: $r = -.11$, $p = .08$, $n = 269$). Hence, gender was not included in the path analyses. Age, however, was significantly and substantially related to perceived interparental conflict in the entire sample ($r = .22$, $p < .001$) as well as in both subsamples ($r = .21$ and .23, each $p = .00$). Furthermore, mothers' pressure to side was higher among older youth ($r = .16$, $p < .001$) in the entire sample. Accordingly, age was controlled in the following path analyses.

Testing the Path Model

In the general path model, adolescents' feelings of insecurity in relation to the mother were found to support the assumptions of this study (comparison of both regional subgroups with the same model structure but without restrictions as to path size: $Chi^2 = 56.98$, $df = 49$, $p = .20$, $CFI = 1.00$, $RMSEA = .02$). Figure 1 shows the findings for West Germany, while Figure 2 presents the path coefficients for East Germany.

Linking family structure to economic pressure, interparental conflict, and mothers' pressure to side. As expected, in the West German sample economic pressure was lower in nuclear than in separated families ($\beta = -.30$, $p < .05$) and there was additional disadvantage for single mother families as compared to two-parent families (β = .42, p < .05). However, in the Eastern sample, both coefficients were comparable (β = $-$.25 and .32, p < .05). Contrary to our expectations, parental separation did not seem to affect family finances more strongly in the West. Hence, the hypothesis concerning regional differences in the vulnerability to economic hardship among separated families was not supported by the data.

As expected, family structure was also linked to interparental conflict, but it was not to both types of separated families, which reported increased conflict between biological parents (dummy contrasting nuclear and separated families: β = $-$.04 and .13 for West and East Germany, both n.s.). Only single mothers in the West seemed to have a more conflicted relationship to their child's father (β = .15, p < .05 vs. β = $-$.04, n.s. for the East). The difference between the Western and Eastern sample was not significant (Δ Chi^2 = 2.12, df = 1, p = .14). Furthermore, there was no indirect effect of family structure on interparental conflict, which was expected to be mediated by economic pressure. Contrary to our expectations, economic pressure did not contribute to interparental conflict, in either the West (β = .12, n.s.) or in the East (β = .09, n.s.). Taken together, the effect of family structure on interparental conflict was weaker than might have been expected, suggesting that many separated parents, if keeping in contact with each other, managed to resolve their conflicts or at least keep their children unaware of still existing tensions.

Much stronger effects of family structure were found for mothers' pressure to side, which was consistently lower in nuclear than separated families (β = $-$.34 and $-$.48 for West and East Germany, both p < .05) and in addition was even higher in single mother than two-parent families (β = .15 and .23 for West and East Germany, both p < .05). Hence, antagonisms between parents still seemed to prevail after separation spilling over into maternal behavior toward their children in both regions. As expected, there were no further direct effects of family structure on maternal parenting or adolescents' feelings of being caught in the middle (i.e., as suggested by the good fit of the model to the data).

Effects of economic pressure and interparental conflict. Findings for both regions were highly similar and contrary to our expectations for these two variables. Mothers' sensitive support was not affected by economic hardship in either region (West vs. East: β = $-$.11 vs. $-$.06, both n.s.), and no independent impact on restrictiveness was found (West vs. East: β = .03 vs. $-$.03, both n.s.). There was not even an indirect connection between economic strain and restrictive parenting, as might have been mediated by increased conflict between parents, since economic pressure as reported by mothers did not contribute to increased interparental conflict in the eyes of children.

Interparental conflict, however, emerged as a significant predictor for all aspects of maternal behavior as well as for children's feelings of being caught between parents. In addition to the direct effects of family structure, maternal pressure to side increased substantially with the frequency of conflict between both (ex-) partners (West vs. East: β = .54 vs. .31, both $p < .05$). This effect was stronger in the West than in the East as indicated by a significantly worse fit to the data if this effect is assumed to be of the same size in both regions (Δ *Chi*^{2} = 8.92, *df* = 1, $p < .01$). It seems that although mothers in both regional samples were more likely to seek an alliance with their child against the father if their relation to the father was conflicted, this risk was lower in the East than in the West.

More frequent conflict contributed to higher maternal restrictiveness (West vs. East: β = .30 vs. .17, both $p < .05$). The path linking interparental conflict to lower maternal sensitivity and support was somewhat weaker. While it reached significance only in the West (β = $-.18$, $p < .05$ vs. $-.08$, n.s. in the East), this variation in the size of coefficients was not statistically reliable (Δ *Chi*^{2} = 0.62, *df* = 1, n.s.). Hence, interparental conflict undermined the quality of mothers' parenting quite similarly in both regions. Furthermore, interparental conflict was directly linked to children's feelings of being caught, regardless of maternal behavior. This path was significant in both regions (West vs. East: β = .27 vs. .42, both $p < .05$) and in the expected direction: the more conflicted the interparental relationship, the higher adolescents' feelings of being caught in the middle.

Effects of perceived maternal behavior. Mothers' pressure to side did not emerge as a significant predictor in the East German sample (β = .05, n.s.). Despite significant bivariate correlations in both regions (see Table 1), a significant path was found only in the West (β = .18, $p < .05$). While this might suggest that West German adolescents were more vulnerable to maternal pressure, this difference between coefficients is not statistically reliable (Δ *Chi*^{2} = 1.22, *df* = 1, n.s.). Hence, contrary to our expectations, adolescents' loyalty conflicts did not seem to be consistently dependent on mothers' efforts to pull them into an alliance against their father, but rather seem to have been provoked directly by interparental conflict. In addition, other aspects of maternal behavior were important, though quite different in each region. In the Eastern sample, maternal restrictiveness emerged as a significant predictor of feeling caught in the middle (β = .32, $p < .05$), while no such effect was found in the Western sample (β = .04, n.s.). The difference was statistically significant (i.e., the model fit suffers) if the path coefficient is restricted to being equal in both regions (Δ *Chi*^{2} = 13.62, *df* = 1, $p < .001$).

Predictors of adolescents' felt insecurity in relation to the mother. As noted above, links between family structure and adolescents' feelings towards mother cannot be interpreted as mediators, since both variables were unrelated in the Western subsample, and the correlation which was observed in the East is not in the expected direction. However, the finding supports a mediation hypothesis for the East German sample: interparental conflict is significantly related to higher feelings of insecurity in the East ($r = .20$ vs. $.09$ in West Germany), but the test of the path models did not suggest any additional direct effect.

All paths which were specified as leading to felt insecurity in relation to mother were significant in at least one subsample and explained a substantial share of the variance in adolescents' insecure relationship to their mother (West: $R^2 = .36$; East: $R^2 = .29$). In fact, age was the only factor which was not consistently significant in both samples, but this regional variation was at the chance level ($\Delta\ Chi^2 = 0.32$, $df = 1$, n.s.). The strongest effect was found for maternal restrictiveness (West vs. East: $\beta = .41$ vs. $.33$, both $p < .05$) with higher restrictiveness contributing to stronger feelings of insecurity in relation to the mother. Mothers' sensitive support had a weaker but also significant independent effect ($\beta = -.19$ in East and West Germany, both $p < .05$), with high support preventing adolescents' felt insecurity. In addition to parenting variables, adolescents' feelings of being caught between parents contributed to increased insecurity (West vs. East: $\beta = .31$ vs. $.22$, both $p < .05$). Hence, impaired maternal parenting and particularly their increased restrictiveness as well as adolescents' loyalty conflicts emerged as important mediators between interparental conflict and adolescents' insecure attachment to the mother.

While the findings from this study generally support our hypotheses, the remaining path suggests effects contrary to our expectations. Maternal pressure to side shows a surprising negative effect (West vs. East: $\beta = -.21$ vs. $-.12$, both $p < .05$), which seemed to indicate that higher pressure to side reduces insecurity in relation to mother. Since the correlation between pressure to side and insecure attachment is about zero (West: $r = .01$ and East: $r = .04$, both n.s.), there seemed to be a suppressor effect in both subsamples. Only if the impact of parenting and loyalty conflicts are controlled does this "opposite" effect of maternal pressure to side emerge. This may be seen as evidence for two different types of adolescents' reactions to maternal pressure to side.

DISCUSSION

This study addresses a variety of family factors related to specific problems in adolescents' individuation process: their felt insecurity about the mother's affection and approval. Our aim was to link a lack of adolescents' security in the family context to family structure and dynamics, taking possible moderating influences of the larger social context into account. Given the complexity of the model investigated here, the organization of the summary and discussion of the results follows the sequence of factors as they are assumed to be interrelated in affecting adolescents' felt insecurity.

Effects of Family Structure on Adolescents' Felt Insecurity in Relation to the Mother

Our initial expectation was that adolescents' felt security in relation to the mother would suffer from parental separation and the entry of a new partner in the family system, perhaps somewhat more in the West than in the East. However, neither any disadvantage of separated families in general, nor the hypothesized difference between East and West Germany was supported by our findings. To the contrary, the data presented here point to somewhat higher insecurity among East German youngsters living in a nuclear family. Upon closer inspection, this effect turned out to be restricted to children's increased fear of losing mother's approval if misbehaving or failing at school. Hence, it might reflect differences in parenting practices not captured here. More conventional and achievement-oriented child rearing in nuclear families could be relevant, particularly in the East, where mothers' parenting is in general somewhat stricter than in the West.

Given that the large majority of youth studied here experienced parental separation or divorce many years prior to our interviews, it seems that possible disruptions in children's and adolescents' security in relation to mother have been overcome in the meantime. However, even if we compare youth with recently separated parents to their age-mates whose parents separated earlier, we do not find differences in children's relationship to their mother (Walper, 1998). In line with other research (Coiro & Emery, 1998), this would suggest that adolescents' relationship to their mother is rather immune to the stresses associated with parental separation and living in a single mother or stepfather family.

Economic Pressures as Mediator

Exploring differential links between family structure and adolescent outcomes in East and West Germany, financial hardship was of particular interest here, since we expected to find more pronounced economic disadvantage of separated and particularly single mother families in the West. However, economic differences between family types proved to be quite similar in both regions, evidencing the expected disadvantage of separated and particularly single mother families not only in the West, but as well in the East. Moreover, no links between economic pressure and family relations could be observed in either region. Given that economic insecurity and unemployment are rather "new" experiences for East German families, one might have expected these families to be somewhat more stressed by financial hardship. However, economic stress does not seem to spill over into the interparental relationship and maternal parenting. Given that the larger share of our sample consists of separated families, the lack of any effect of economic pressure on the interparental relation may largely be due to the reduced contact between biological parents in most families. As to maternal parenting, our findings are in line with other research on economic deprivation which suggests that mothers may suffer less from financial hardship than fathers for whom the provider role may be more crucial than for mothers (McLoyd, 1989). Although there is also considerable evidence that mothers' psychological well-being and their interaction with adolescent children may be impaired by financial problems (Conger, Ge, Elder, Lorenz, & Simons, 1994; Simons & Johnson, 1996), the findings reported here indicate mothers' considerable resilience in coping with economic stress.

Parenting and Alliances as Mediators to Attachment

Turning to the significance of a conflicted relationship between parents for adolescents' development, it was claimed that not only maternal parenting, but also unhealthy triadic alliances and children's loyalty conflicts mediate the negative effects of interparental conflict on adolescents' relationship to their mother. This expectation is confirmed by the data presented here. Although interparental conflict seemed to promote more restrictive parenting among mothers which, in turn, increased the risk for adolescents' felt insecurity regarding maternal affection, parenting did not provide the only mediating link. Irrespective of mothers' behavior toward their children, interparental conflict has been shown to increase the risk for loyalty conflict among youth from conflict-ridden families, and such feelings of being caught between parents seem to account for much of the negative impact of interparental tensions on children's and adolescents' felt security in relation to the mother. Hence, our findings do not support the position held by Fauber and Long (1991), who reported that impaired parenting is the single most important factor explaining negative effects of interparental conflict on children. Rather, our findings are in line with Emery et al. (1992) who stress that impaired parenting does not explain all detrimental effects of interparental conflict. As suggested by family systems theory (Minuchin, 1974), a weak alliance between parents increases the risk for unhealthy triadic patterns which, in turn, contribute to children's less optimal development. In both regional samples, loyalty conflicts are significantly linked to adolescents' increased feelings of insecurity in relation to the mother. In particular, this finding may be best understood in light of the emotional security hypotheses (Davies & Cummings, 1994; Davies et al., 2002). Interparental conflict seems to increase the risk that children are forced to monitor their behavior toward parents since positive affection for one parent may cause the other to feel rejected and answer with disappointment, disapproval, and even negative sanctions. This lack of an independent position in relation to both parents, in turn, directly undermines children's felt security in relation to the mother–and most likely to the father, too.

Some of our findings require additional considerations, and these relate particularly to mothers' pressure on their children to enter an alliance against the father. While we assumed that maternal pressure to side provides an important link between interparental conflict and children's feelings of being caught between parents, this could only be shown for the West Germany sample. Obvious tensions between parents seem to promote such maternal strategies more strongly than in the East, and where maternal pressure to side was indeed found to contribute to children's loyalty conflicts, even though not strongly. Hence, at least in West German families, mothers' pressure to side seems to provide a mediating link which accounts for some of the negative impact of parental discord on adolescents' feelings towards their mother.

It is not easy to explain why this should be more likely to happen in West German families than in the East. Interestingly, it is only interparental conflict which predicts maternal pressure to side more strongly in the West than in the East, whereas effects of family structure are similarly strong in both regions. Hence, factors related to the mothers' coping with separation and divorce or single parenthood do not seem to play a role in these regional differences. In considering why a conflict-ridden relationship with one's (former) partner might increase mothers' striving for exclusive loyalty and affection from their children particularly in the West, the notion of a "compensation effect" may be helpful, which has been put forward in research on the effects of marital conflict on the parent-child relationship (Erel & Burman, 1995). Given that the role of mother is particularly salient for West German women, whereas East German mothers have more strongly been socialized to value their employment role (cf. Walper & Galambos, 1997), West German women may be more inclined to make up for the lack of support and consideration experienced in relation to their (former) spouse by turning to their children. East German mothers may have other options to compensate for problems in the relationship to their child's father. Another interpretation refers to mothers' position in the family, particularly their significance in children's lives. As shown by Behnken et al. (1991), East German mothers' advice is more valued by youth than West German mothers' competence in providing advice about school, political questions, and life goals. This may increase mothers' security in their relationship to children and thus pressure them less to strive for an alliance with the child. However, both interpretations are speculative and await further evidence from other studies pointing to similar differences as found here.

The Role of Mothers' Pressure to Side

Of further interest is that mothers' pressure to side lacks more substantial effects on children's and adolescents' feelings of being caught between parents. One might have expected this to be the most important predictor, but it proved to be much less relevant than conflict between parents. Based on the limitations of this research, multi-source information, and particularly observational evidence would seem helpful. Children's awareness of such maternal strategies may at least partly caution them against the pitfalls of becoming triangulated. Parents' demands for an alliance against the other parent may function as an intended push-factor leading to adolescents' detachment instead of coalition formation (Walper & Schwarz, 2001). Furthermore, it should be kept in mind that we focus on mothers' behavior only.

Finally, the effect of maternal pressure to side on insecure attachment was unexpected: the more the mother was perceived as pressing the child into a coalition against the father, the *lower* adolescents' insecurity in relation to their mother in both regions. Interestingly, this effect was not evident in simple correlations but only emerged in the path model where parenting and effects of interparental conflict via children's feelings of being caught in the middle were controlled. Interrelations between mothers' parenting and their pressure to side were not depicted in the path model. It seems that the lower support and higher restrictiveness which were reported for mothers who seek to draw their child in an alliance against the father obscure this relationship. According to adolescents, mothers' pressure to side was accompanied by impaired parenting, and the latter contributed to increased feelings of insecurity among youth in relation to the mother. However, once these indirect negative effects are taken into account, mothers' efforts to gain their children's exclusive love may actually make youth feel quite secure about their mothers' affection. This is not to say that adolescents join a coalition with their mother. Children who become aware of their mother's pressure to side are more likely to detach themselves emotionally from her, which may allow them to escape feelings of insecurity. This interpretation would be in line with attachment theory and recent research on emotional autonomy, which suggests that detachment from an emotionally stressful relationship is a major way to avoid the stress of feeling caught, insecure, and vulnerable in this relationship thus allowing for healthy development (Bartholomew, 1990; Fuhrman & Holmbeck, 1995; Walper & Schwarz, 2001).

Some caveats should be mentioned. First, our study is based on cross-sectional data. The causal interpretation of relationships specified in the path model is theory driven and needs to be empirically substantiated by longitudinal data. Second, while maternal reports on the families' financial situation were included, the main part of the analyses highlights children's and adolescents' perspective. Although focusing on information provided by children and adolescents might inflate the interrelation of indicators we chose to do so. Several indicators would seem to be less valid if assessed from an outsider perspective (e.g., adolescents' feelings of being caught between parents and their felt insecurity in relation to mother). The children's report (e.g., on maternal behavior like her pressure to side) might be less biased by social desirability than maternal self-report. Finally, although children may have only limited insight into conflict between their parents, the validity of their report on interparental conflict has been demonstrated by substantial correlations with both parents' report on marital conflict (Goedde & Walper, 2001).

Our study suggests that interparental conflict is an important risk factor for adolescents' individuation process by undermining their felt security in relation to the mother. Whether this holds similarly or even more so for the father-adolescent relationship will be addressed in future analyses. Furthermore, our study has shown that it is valuable to focus not only on parenting when trying to explain negative effects of interparental conflict, but to consider the increased risk for children's involvement in intergenerational alliances, too. Despite the regional variations in maternal strategies to draw their children into an alliance against the father, adolescents' feelings of being caught in loyalty conflicts between parents emerges as a similarly important link to their lack of security in relation to the mother in West and East Germany.

NOTE

1. Different from dummy coding, effect codings assign the value -1 to that group which is not the target of either contrast. Entering both effect coded predictors simultaneously allows estimation of independent effects of each target group in comparison to the respective remaining groups. Both effect coded family type variables as well as age were included as predictors (exogenous variables), while economic pressure, parental conflict, mothers' pressure to side, maternal parenting, and adolescents' feelings of being caught were mediating variables.

REFERENCES

Amato, P. R. (1993). Children's adjustment to divorce: Theories, hypotheses, and empirical support. *Journal of Marriage and the Family, 55,* 23-38.

Amato, P. R. (1994). The implications of research findings on children in stepfamilies. In A. Booth & J. Dunn (Eds.), *Stepfamilies. Who benefits? Who does not?* (pp. 81-87). Hillsdale, NJ: Erlbaum.

Amato, P. R. (2000). The consequences of divorce for adults and children. *Journal of Marriage and the Family, 62,* 1269-1287.

Amato, P. R. (2001). Children of divorce in the 1990s: An update of the Amato and Keith (1991) meta-analysis. *Journal of Family Psychology, 15,* 355-370.

Amato, P. R., & Booth, A. (1996). A prospective study of divorce and parent-child relationships. *Journal of Marriage and the Family, 58,* 356-365.

Amato, P. R., & Keith, B. (1991). Parental divorce and the well-being of children: A meta-analysis. *Psychological Bulletin, 110,* 26-46.

Arbuckle, J. L. (1996). Full information estimation in the presence of incomplete data. In G. A. Marcoulides & R. E. Schumacker (Eds.), *Advanced structural equation modeling: Issues and techniques* (pp. 243-277). Hillsdale, NJ: Lawrence Erlbaum.

Arbuckle, J. L. (1997). *AMOS user's guide. Version 3.6*. Chicago, IL: Small Waters Corporation.

Bartholomew, K. (1990). Avoidance of intimacy: An attachment perspective. *Journal of Social and Personal Relationships, 7*, 147-178.

Behnken, I., Günther, C., Kabat vel Job, O., Kaiser, S., Karig, U., Krgüer, H.-H. (1991). *Schlüerstudie '90* (Study on students '90). Weinheim: Juventa.

Blos, P. (1962). *On adolescence: A psychoanalytic interpretation*. New York: Free Press.

Buchanan, C. M., Maccoby, E. E., & Dornbusch, S. M. (1991). Caught between parents: Adolescents' experience in divorced homes. *Child Development, 62*, 1008-1029.

Buhrmester, D., & Furman, W. (1987). The development of companionship and intimacy. *Child Development, 58*, 1101-1113.

Burkhauser, R. V., Duncan, G. J., Hauser, R., & Berntsen, R. (1991). Wife or frau, women do worse: A comparison of men and women in the United States and Germany after marital dissolution. *Demography, 28*, 353-360.

Christensen, A., & Margolin, G. (1988). Conflict and alliance in distressed and non-distressed families. In R. A. Hinde & J. Stevenson-Hinde (Eds.), *Relationships within families: Mutual influences* (pp. 263-282). Oxford: Clarendon Press.

Cohen, J., & Cohen, P. (1975). *Applied multiple regression/correlation analysis for the behavioral sciences*. New York: Wiley.

Coiro, M. J., & Emery, R. E. (1998). Do marriage problems affect fathering more than mothering? A quantitative and qualitative review. *Clinical Child and Family Psychology Review, 1*, 23-40.

Conger, R. D., Elder, G. H., Jr., Lorenz, F. O., Conger, K. J., Simons, R. L., Whitbeck, L. B., Huck, S. M., & Melby, J. N. (1990). Linking economic hardship to marital quality and instability. *Journal of Marriage and the Family, 52*, 643-656.

Conger, R. D., Ge, X., Elder, G. H., Jr., Lorenz, F. O., & Simons, R. L. (1994). Economic stress, coercive family process, and developmental problems of adolescents. *Child Development, 65*, 541-561.

Davies, P. T., & Cummings, E. M. (1994). Marital conflict and child adjustment: An emotional security hypothesis. *Psychological Bulletin, 116*, 387-411.

Davies, P. T., Harold, G. T., Goeke-Morey, M. C., & Cummings, E. M. (2002). Child emotional security and interparental conflict. *Monographs of the Society for Research in Child Development, 67* (Serial No. 270). Boston, MA: Blackwell.

Demo, D. H., & Acock, A. C. (1996). Family structure, family process, and adolescent well-being. *Journal of Research on Adolescence, 6*, 457-488.

Duncan, G. J., & Brooks-Gunn, J. (Eds.) (1997). *Consequences of growing up poor*. New York: Russell Sage Foundation.

Elder, G. H., Jr. (1974). *Children of the great depression*. Chicago: University of Chicago Press.

Elder, G. H., Jr., Conger, R. D., Foster, E. M., & Ardelt, M. (1992). Families under economic pressure. *Journal of Family Issues, 13*, 5-37.

Emery. R. E. (1982). Interparental conflict and the children of discord and divorce. *Psychological Bulletin, 92,* 310-330.

Emery, R. E., Fincham, F. D., & Cummings, E. M. (1992). Parenting in context: Systemic thinking about parental conflict and its influence on children. *Journal of Consulting and Clinical Psychology, 60,* 909-912.

Erel, O., & Burman, B. (1995). Interrelatedness of marital relations and parent-child-relations: A meta-analytic review. *Psychological Bulletin, 118,* 108-132.

Fauber, R. L., & Long, N. (1991). Children in context: The role of the family in child psychotherapy. *Journal of Consulting and Clinical Psychology, 59,* 813-820.

Feldkircher, M. (1994). Erziehungsziele in West- und Ostdeutschland. In M. Braun & P. P. Mohler (Hrsg.), *Blickpunkt Gesellschaft 3. Einstellungen und Verhalten der Bundesbürger* (S. 175-208). Opladen: Westdeutscher Verlag.

Forkel, I., & Silbereisen, R. K. (2001). Family economic hardship and depressed mood among young adolescents from former East and West Germany. *American Behavioral Scientist, 44,* 1955-1971.

Fuhrman, T., & Holmbeck, G. N. (1995). A contextual-moderator analysis of emotional autonomy and adjustment in adolescence. *Child Development, 66,* 793-811.

Gödde, M., & Walper, S. (2001). Elterliche konflikte aus der sicht von kindern und jugendlichen: Die deutsche kurzfassung der Children's Perception of Interparental Conflict Scale (CPIC) [Interparental conflict from children's and adolescents' point of view: The German short version of the Children's Perception of Interparental Conflict Scale (CPIC)]. *Diagnostica, 47,* 18-26.

Grotevant, H. D., & Cooper, C. R. (1986). Individuation in family relationships: A perspective on individual differences in the development of identity and role-taking skills in adolescence. *Human Development, 29,* 82-100.

Grych, J. H., & Fincham, F. D. (1993). Children's appraisals of marital conflict: Initial investigations of the cognitive-contextual framework. *Child Development, 64,* 215-230.

Grych, J. H., Seid, M., & Fincham, F. D. (1992). Assessing marital conflict from the child's perspective: The children's perception of interparental conflict scale. *Child Development, 63,* 558-572.

Harold, G. T., & Conger, R. D. (1997). Marital conflict and adolescent distress: The role of adolescent awareness. *Child Development, 68,* 333-350.

Harold, G. T., Osborne, L. N., & Conger, R. D. (1997). Mom and Dad are at it again: Adolescent perceptions of marital conflict and adolescent psychological distress. *Developmental Psychology, 33,* 333-350.

Hetherington. E. M. (1993). An overview of the Virginia longitudinal study of divorce and remarriage with a focus an early adolescence. *Journal of Family Psychology, 7,* 39-56.

Hetherington, E. M., Bridges, M., & Insabella, G. M. (1998). What matters? What does not? Five perspectives on the association between marital transitions and children's adjustment. *American Psychologist, 53,* 167-184.

Hetherington, E. M., & Clingempeel, W. G. (1992). Coping with marital transitions. *Monographs of the Society for Research in Child Development, No. 227, 57* (2-3).

Hetherington, E. M., & Jodl, K. M. (1994). Stepfamilies as settings for child develop-ment. In A. Booth & J. Dunn (Eds.), *Stepfamilies: Who benefits? Who does not?* (pp. 55-79). Hillsdale, NJ: Lawrence Erlbaum.

Holmbeck, G. N., & Leake, C. (1999). Separation-individuation and psychological adjustment in late adolescence. *Journal of Youth and Adolescence, 28,* 563-581.

Jenkins, J. M., & Smith, M. A. (1993). A prospective study of behavioral disturbance in children who subsequently experience parental divorce: A research note. *Journal of Divorce and Remarriage, 19(1/2),* 143-160.

Joos, M. (1997). Armutsentwicklung und familiale Armutsrisiken von Kindern in den neuen und alten Bundesländern. In U. Otto (Hg.), *Aufwachsen in Armut. Erfahrungswelten und soziale Lage von Kindern armer Familien* (S.47-78). Opladen: Leske & Budrich.

Jøreskog, K. G., & Sørbom, D. (1996). *LISREL 8: User's reference guide (2nd ed.).* Chicago, IL: Scientific Software International.

Kerns, K. A., Aspelmeier, J. E., Gentzler, A. L., & Grabill, C. M. (2001). Parent-child attachment and monitoring in middle childhood. *Journal of Family Psychology, 15(1),* 69-81.

Kline, R. B. (1998). *Principles and practice of structural equation modeling.* New York: Guilford.

Laursen, B., Coy, K. C., & Collins, W. A. (1998). Reconsidering changes in parent-child conflict across adolescence: A meta-analysis. *Child Development, 69,* 817-832.

Levine, J. B., Green, C. J., & Millon, T. (1986). The Separation-Individuation Test of Adolescence. *Journal of Personality Assessment, 50,* 123-137.

Levine, J. B., & Saintonge, S. (1993). Psychometric properties of the Separation-Indi-viduation Test of Adolescence within a clinical population. *Journal of Clinical Psy-chology, 49,* 492-507.

Lopez, F. G. (1991). Patterns of family conflict and their relation to college student ad-justment. *Journal of Counseling & Development, 69,* 257-260.

Maccoby, E. E., Depner, C. E., & Mnookin, R. H. (1990). Coparenting in the second year after divorce. *Journal of Marriage and the Family, 52,* 141-155.

Maier, F. (1993). The labour market for women and employment perspectives in the af-termath of German unification. *Cambridge Journal of Economics, 17,* 267-280.

McLanahan, S., & Sandefur, G. (1994). *Growing up with a single parent.* Cambridge, MA: Harvard University Press.

McLoyd, V. C. (1989). Socialization and development in a changing economy. *American Psychologist, 44,* 293-302.

Minuchin, S. (1974). *Families and family therapy.* Cambridge, MA: Harvard Univer-sity Press.

Montemayor, R. (1983). Parents and adolescents in conflict: All families some of the time and some families most of the time. *Journal of Early Adolescence, 3,* 83-103.

Noack, P., & Puschner, B. (1999). Differential trajectories of parent-child relationships and psychosocial adjustment in adolescents. *Journal of Adolescence, 22,* 795-804.

Peterson, J. L., & Zill, N. (1986). Marital disruption, parent-child relationships, and be-havior problems in children. *Journal of Marriage and the Family, 48,* 295-307.

Reis, O., & Meyer-Probst, B. (1999). Scheidung der eltern und entwicklung der kinder: Befunde der Rostocker Längsschnittstudie [Parental divorce and children's development: Findings from the Rostock Longitudinal Study]. In S. Walper & B. Schwarz (Eds.), *Was wird aus den Kindern? Chancen und Risiken frü die Entwicklung von Kindern aus Trennungs- und Stieffamilien* (pp. 49-72). Weinheim: Juventa.

Schafer, J. L., & Graham, J. W. (2002). Missing data: Our view of the state of the art. *Psychological Methods, 7,* 147-177.

Schafer, J. L., & Olsen, M. K. (1998). Multiple imputations for multivariate missing-data problems: A data analyst's perspective. *Multivariate Behavioral Research, 33,* 545-571.

Schneider, N. (1994). *Familie und private Lebensfhürung in West- und Ostdeutschland [Family and private life in West and East Germany].* Stuttgart: Enke.

Schwarz, B., Walper, S., Goedde, M., & Jurasic, S. (1997). Dokumentation der Erhebungsinstrumente der 1. Haupterhebung (überarb. Version). *Berichte aus der Arbeitsgruppe "Familienentwicklung nach der Trennung" # 14/1997.* München: Ludwig-Maximilians-Universittä München.

Sessa, F. M., & Steinberg, L. (1991). Family structure and the development of autonomy during adolescence. *Journal of Early Adolescence, 11,* 38-55.

Silbereisen, R. K., Meschke, L. L., & Schwarz, B. (1996). Leaving the parental home: Predictors for young adults raised in former East and West Germany. In J.A. Graber & J.S. Dubas (Eds.), *Leaving home: Understanding the transition to adulthood* (New Directions for Child Development No.71, pp. 71-86). San Francisco.CA: Jossey-Bass.

Simons, R. L., & Johnson, C. (1996). Mothers' parenting. In R. L. Simons (Ed.), *Understanding differences between divorced and intact families* (pp. 81-93). Thousand Oaks, CA: Sage

Simons, R. L., Johnson, C., & Lorenz, F. O. (1996). Family structure differences in stress and behavioral predispositions. In R. L. Simons (Ed.), *Understanding differences between divorced and intact families* (pp. 45-64). Thousand Oaks, CA: Sage.

Simons, R. L., Lorenz, F. O., Conger, R. D., & Wu, C. I. (1992). Support from spouse as mediator and moderator of the disruptive influence of economic strain on parenting. *Child Development, 63,* 1282-1301.

Smetana, J. (1988). Adolescents' and parents' conceptions of parental authority. *Child Development, 59,* 321-335.

Smetana, J. G. (1993). Conceptions of parental authority in divorced and married mothers and their adolescents. *Journal of Research on Adolescence, 3,* 19-39.

Smetana, J. (1996). Adolescent-parent conflict: implications for adaptive and maladaptive development. In D. Cichetti & S. L. Toth (Eds.), *Rochester Symposium on Developmental Psychopathology. Volume 7. Adolescence: opportunity and challenges* (pp. 1-46). Rochester, NY: University of Rochester Press.

Statistisches Bundesamt Deutschland (1998). *Statistisches jahrbuch frü die Bundesrepublik Deutschland [Statistical yearbook for the Federal Republic of Germany].* Stuttgart: Metzler-Poeschel.

Statistisches Bundesamt (2002). Weitere Zunahme der Scheidungen im Jahr 2001 [Further increase in divorces in the year 2001]. Press Release from August 27, 2002. *http://www.destatis.de/presse/deutsch/pm2002/p3000023.htm.*

Steinberg, L. (2001). We know some things: Parent-adolescent relationships in retrospect and prospect. *Journal of Research on Adolescence, 11,* 1-19.

Ullrich, M. (1999). *Wenn kinder jugendliche werden. Die bedeutung der familienkommunikation im übergang zum jugendalter [When children become adolescents. The importance of family communication for the transition into adolescence]* Weinheim: Juventa.

Walper, S. (1995). Youth in a changing context: The role of the family in East and West Germany. In J. Youniss (Ed.), *After the wall: Family adaptation in East and West Germany* (pp. 3-21). New Directions for Child Development (No. 70). San Francisco, CA: Jossey-Bass.

Walper, S. (1998). *Individuation Jugendlicher in Konflikt-, Trennungs- und Stieffamilien. Theorie, Diagnostik und Befunde* [Adolescents' individuation in conflicted, separated, and stepfamilies]. Unpublished thesis for habilitation. Munich: University of Munich.

Walper, S. (1999). Auswirkungen von Armut auf die Entwicklung von Kindern [Effects of poverty on children's development]. In Deutsches Jugendinstitut (Eds.), *Normalität, Abweichung und ihre Ursachen* (Materialien frü den 10. Kinder- und Jugendbericht, Band 1, S. 291-359). München: DJI Verlag.

Walper, S. & Galambos, N. L. (1997). Employed mothers in Germany. In J. Frankel (Ed.) *Families of employed mothers. An international perspective* (pp. 35-65). New York: Garland.

Walper, S. & Schwarz, B. (1999). Risiken und Chancen frü die Entwicklung von Kindern aus Trennungs- und Stieffamilien: Eine Einfhürung [Risks and chances for children's development in separated and stepfamilies: an introduction]. In S. Walper & B. Schwarz (Hrsg.) *Was wird aus den Kindern? Chancen und Risiken frü die Entwicklung von Kindern aus Trennungs- und Stieffamilien* (S. 7-22). Weinheim: Juventa.

Walper, S., & Schwarz, B. (2001). Adolescents' individuation in East and West Germany: Effects of family structure, financial hardship, and family processes. *American Behavioral Scientist, 44,* 1937-1954.

Youniss, J., & Smollar, J. (1985). *Adolescent relations with mothers, fathers, and friends.* Chicago: The University of Chicago Press.

From Patriarchy to Egalitarianism: Parenting Roles in Democratizing Poland and Kyrgyzstan

Barbara Wejnert
Almagul Djumabaeva

ABSTRACT. This paper offers an analysis of how parenting can be understood as an artifact that articulates and portrays the cultural, economic and political reality of transitional democratic vs. communist societies. In this framework, we specifically compare forms of family life and parental roles in the democratizing former Soviet countries: Poland and Kyrgyzstan. In these countries traditional culture, stemming in part from Moslem or Catholic traditions, operates as a noteworthy segment of societal structure that plays a significant role in holding societies together. Accordingly, two tendencies can be observed in these countries: (a) a move towards Western democratic values, including the idea of egalitarianism and small nuclear families, and (b) a revival of cultural traditions relating to family life and marital relation-

---

Barbara Wejnert is affiliated with Cornell University. Almagul Djumabaeva is affiliated with Kyrgyz State National University.

Address correspondence to: Barbara Wejnert, Department of Human Development, 21 G Martha Van Rensselaer Hall, Cornell University, Ithaca, NY 14853 (E-mail: bw15@cornell.edu).

The research reported below was supported by an International Research and Exchange Board Grant (2001) and with funds provided by the US Department of State (Title VIII program) and the National Endowment for Humanities (granted to Wejnert), the Soros Open Society Foundation (awarded to Djumabaeva and Wejnert), and also by a fellowship from the Soros Open Society Program (granted to Djumabaeva). None of these organizations is responsible for the views expressed here.

http://www.haworthpress.com/web/MFR
© 2004 by The Haworth Press, Inc. All rights reserved.
Digital Object Identifier: 10.1300/J002v36n03_08

511

ships. Although families have become solely responsible for how they choose to organize themselves, whether in the spirit of Western values and egalitarian roles, or in the spirit of traditional patriarchy, this paper posits that recent democratization and diffusion of Western, egalitarian models of family relationships have a stronger effect on parenting roles than religious traditionalism. *[Article copies available for a fee from The Haworth Document Delivery Service: 1-800-HAWORTH. E-mail address: <docdelivery@haworthpress.com> Website: <http://www.HaworthPress.com> © 2004 by The Haworth Press, Inc. All rights reserved.]*

KEYWORDS. Democratic transitions, gender roles, post-communist states, parenting, parent-child relationships

This paper explores the cultural and ideological understanding of parental roles that reflects and defines the social reality of the communist and post-communist (transitional democracy) periods. The current democratic transformation taking place in the former communist states, accompanied by the transition toward a capitalistic market economy, have brought substantial changes in the lives of residents of countries from the former Soviet bloc (Czapiński, 1994; Reboud & Hoaquan, 1997; Stephenson, 1998). Among these changes are the establishment of political freedom, free elections, the transition to a market economy, and the opening of opportunities for private entrepreneurship. Moreover, the ongoing political and economic openness, and contact with the Western world, have exposed former Soviet-bloc societies to the lifestyle of Western countries, and to their liberal, egalitarian culture (Dąbrowski & Antczak, 1996; Wejnert, 2002; Wejnert & Spencer, 1996).

These changes have generated trends of rising expectations and yearning for material comforts at the same time as a tendencies to adopt Western models of social behavior. Such Western practices include modern parental roles characterized by marital relations that are egalitarian as well as the active involvement of fathers in child care and child-rearing duties. Consequently, this paper offers an analysis of how parenting can be understood as a social mechanism that articulates and portrays the cultural, economic and political reality of communist and post-communist societies.

In this framework, we specifically compare family relationships and parental roles in the communist and post-communist periods of two former Soviet countries: Poland and Kyrgyzstan. In these countries, traditional culture operates as an articulated segment of societal structures, and thus, plays a significant role in holding societies together.

AN OVERVIEW OF PARENTING ROLES DURING COMMUNISM

> It is true that in the Soviet bloc women keep the wheels of industry turning. Virtually no factory could keep going without female labor, no hospitals could function in a country where women constitute about 70 percent of all doctors, and service industries would collapse without women hairdressers and waitresses, ticket-sellers, and shop assistants . . . But women also do *all* the shopping, cooking and cleaning. (Binyon, 1983, p.36)

Every year on March 8th, the men of Eastern European and former Soviet societies used to officially honor their wives with a holiday that was a celebration of women's liberation during the communist revolution–a recognition of their achievement of equality. The celebration of this *International Women's Day* was acknowledged by tributes in the press, speeches in the Politburo, and flowers and gifts for female coworkers, wives and mothers. Women, however, recognizing that their equality under communism was, at the least, equivocal, often used these celebrations as an occasion to send letters to newspaper editors describing their bitter lives.

Since the establishment of the communist system in the early 1920s, women were proclaimed to be equal to men across communist states. Potential problems with the equality of women were solved through the establishment of laws prohibiting gender discrimination. For the next fifty years, the problem of gender inequality was considered to be nonexistent (Gontarczyk, 2001, p.213). To some extent, the equality of women and men was achieved in education, labor force participation, and representation in political organs was more extensive than in Western democracies. Women also received many social benefits that were rarely seen in Western countries, such as maternity leaves lasting as much as 3 years, long-term maternity benefits, low-cost day-care centers, and state funds for child support provided to married couples (Wejnert, 1996a).

Nonetheless, the view of social equality promoted by communist states failed to acknowledge that women were also expected to be the sole care-provides for family members, and practically the sole care-givers of children. The lack of state interest in the domestic sphere led to women being overburdened and to the submissive position of wives-mothers, a circumstance that contrasted with what appeared to be their equal position in the public sphere. The neglect of domestic issues was reflected by a lack of studies on the overburdened condition of women. In fact, such studies were considered Western political propaganda and any initiative with the goal of raising public awareness of women's inequality at home was categorized as dissident political activity

(Binyon, 1983, p.36). In addition, the communist government exerted control over media coverage of feminist issues and the media was remarkably timid about the issue of domestic inequality. Patriarchal authority prospered under such a climate. Fathers' involvement in child rearing was limited and there was a lack of emphasis placed on modern paternal roles. Similar to other Soviet bloc countries, patriarchal culture dominated family life in Poland and Kyrgyzstan.

Poland. Throughout nineteenth and twentieth century Polish history (e.g., the time of partition in the nineteenth century, World War I and II), Polish men were killed, imprisoned, or sent to Siberia, while women were left to raise children, support families, and maintain cultural traditions (Titkov, 1992). These historical circumstances eventually led to the emergence of a model of "Matka Polka" (the Polish Mother). The image of *Matka Polka* envisioned a woman who was strong and selfless, "a figure of courage and great strength." At the same time, this ideal woman was to have "no meaningful life of her own" but was supposed to be fully devoted to her family (Reading, 1992).

Thus, across the last two centuries, women's self-sacrifice for the family was glorified in literature, movies, songs, paintings and monuments. This cultural tradition, deeply embedded in Polish society, was an important element in the prevailing "models of womanhood" within communist systems. In particular, during a brief period from the mid-1940s to the mid-1950s, the "socialist hero-worker" model of women came to predominate, presenting women as brick layers, tractor drivers, miners and factory workers. This model rested entirely on women's occupational involvement. In the years 1945 54, when all hands were needed for labor, the streets were full of posters with women tractor drivers and women streetcar drivers who were joyfully smiling. By the end of the 1950s, when no more laborers were needed, the traditional domestic view of women replaced previous propaganda and the previous posters vanished from streets (Reading 1992, p.39). From the 1960s until the end of the 1980s, the hero-worker model for women was being abandoned and replaced by a more traditional and difficult, "working mother" model.

Thus, within the communist past, contrasting cultural models of motherhood, ranging from total engagement in occupational activities to the more traditional worker-mother, were propagated. Nonetheless, the prevailing model of mother-homemaker was never completely revived and working, career-oriented involvements are still expected of mothers, though perhaps only implicitly. Such expectations have been supported by the Catholic tradition of promoting sexual abstinence before marriage and forbidding the use of birth-control methods by married couples, a practice that indirectly encourages larger families. The promotion of larger families was accompanied by several ideas rooted in the traditional culture. These traditional ideas included patriarchal authority of husbands/fathers, combined with the absence of ex-pectations conveyed by religious, state-run, or non-governmental institutions, that fathers should be actively involved in parental duties. Consequently, child-parent relationships, lasting until adulthood, were expected to be domi-nated by strong emotional ties developed between children and mothers, but were extremely limited if not absent in relationships between fathers and chil-dren.

This mother-centered parenting was generally free of substantial conflicts between parents and children. For example, in Skorupska-Sobańska's 1967 study, 73% of children age 11-18 reported having a strongly positive relation-ship with their parents and 91% of children reported feeling loved by their par-ents. However, the relationships between mothers and children were much stronger than relationships between fathers and children. The great majority of children reported having a close affiliation with mothers (97% of children) but only 3% of girls and no boys reported having close relationship with fathers (Skorupska-Sobańska, 1967). In another study by Skorupska-Sobańska (1971), close to one-fifth of youth were reported to believe that parents do not understand their problems and hence wanted to expand relationships with them. However, while almost all of those children (over 90%) were certain that mothers would support them during times of difficulty, only 3% believed that they could always count on the support of fathers. Middle and high school students perceived mothers as caring, patient, dedicated to children, seeking contact with children, and having interest in their problems, while fathers were perceived as controlling, interested in discipline, unwilling to spend time with children, and not having any interest in children's lives. Fathers also were crit-icized for not helping mothers with housework and/or child-care (Rachalska, 1968).

Only 3% of youth felt alienated at home, attesting to very positive relation-ships between children and parents and almost nonexistent conflicts (Skorupska-Sobańska, 1967). If conflicts were noticed, they tended to be short-term in nature, with over one-fifth (22%) of youth reporting frequent, short-term disagreements with parents (Skorupska-Sobańska, 1971). More frequent but also short-term disagreements were observed in families of farm-ers where, according to one study (Grzybek, 1977), as many as 75% of high school students reported having minor conflicts with parents. Youth described most disagreements as relating to parental requirements to help with house-care duties or about children's behavior. Conflicts occurred more fre-quently with mothers than with fathers (Kowalski, 1980). It is not surprising, however, that fathers rarely disagreed with children because child-father contacts were extremely limited and children were emotionally distant from fathers (Kowalski, 1980).

Overall, in communist Poland, parent-child relationships were dominated almost solely by the care that mothers provided. Not surprisingly, society's and children's perceptions of the role of Polish mothers versus fathers reflected the prevailing cultural image of "*Matka Polka*" (the Polish Mother).

Kyrgyzstan. In order to understand the changes in roles of mothers and fathers introduced during communism, it is necessary to summarize briefly the traditions that prevailed in pre-Soviet times. Kyrgyz people used to lead a nomadic life with a patriarchal culture strongly consolidated by a hierarchy of social status based on sex and age. Polygamy and extended families were among the most common family forms, with families consisting of parents (the core of the family), grandparents, children, and unmarried siblings. Father was the breadwinner and had the unquestionable authority in his family over children and his one or more wives.

To establish a family, an adult son needed to pay the bride's family *kalym*, a bride-price, which led to the treatment of the acquired wife and her children as the property of the husband and his family (Olcott, 1991). Mothers, who often had 10 or more children, were solely responsible for childcare and all domestic tasks. At the same time, they had no authority in the family, and were fully subordinated to their husband, older male children, the husband's parents and his family. If a husband died, a mother did not gain authority in her family nor control over her children. Often, a widow could not keep her children because they were taken in by the husband's family members. In order to keep the widow and her children as property of her husband's family, her husband's brother would marry her (the practice of *levirate*) or a widower would marry the sister of his wife (the practice of *sororate*).

The Soviet experience was crucial to women's emancipation in Central Asia and to changes in parental roles. By two decades after the establishment of communism, free education was implemented and, for children under the age of 25, mandatory schooling leading to the full literacy of boys and girls was achieved. The communist government banned polygamy, introduced abortion policies, taught about birth control methods, included women into the labor force, and opened networks of preschools and after school programs. Parental duties, child-parent relationships, and the relationship between the nuclear and the extended families drastically changed. Following recommendations of the Communist Party and communist ideology, the communist government in Kyrgyzstan designed regulations and laws regarding parenting, marriage, and egalitarian family relationships. Parents were taught that education, including moral guidance, as well as the upbringing of children should be left to preschools, schools, and after school activities in social organizations, like the Pioneer Organization, and the Young Communist Union. Mothers as well as fathers were not involved in child-care and child-rearing with the exception of mothers' responsibility to feed and clothe children. Parenting by mothers and fathers was fully replaced by state institutions. Children were taught to respect parents, but they spent most of their time at preschool, school, and at after school activities.

Consequently, by the end of 1990s, women's involvement in the labor force reached 49% of the total labor force (Semya v SSSR, 1991). High levels of women's employment, together with an increase in urbanization, strengthened the position of wives and mothers. However, families were far from egalitarian in terms of the roles of women compared to men. Working mothers were obligated to perform all the domestic duties, to care for husbands, provide food and clothing for children and, in most traditional families, care for the husband's parents and other members of the husband's extended family. Husbands were considered the heads of families while wives and children had subordinated positions. The role of a father was reduced to being an authority in the family and an economic provider with no expectations in the area of child rearing, childcare, or household duties.

AN OVERVIEW OF PARENTING ROLES IN POST-COMMUNISM

In the early 1990s, together with new economic and political transitions, increased unemployment and privatization of industry brought an end to women's participation in the labor force and maternity-type benefits (day care centers in company facilities, maternity leave, and sick child leave), that were common during the communist period (Wejnert, 2002). Moreover, in the new political, economic, and social climate, the model of "working mother" was changed to that of "mother-homemaker," as religious institutions joined governments in encouraging women to be mothers above all else, rather than professional achievers. This newly propagated role for women was used, in part, as a mechanism to free up jobs in a downsizing job market (Lissyutkina, 1993).

The new perspective on the role of *Mother* was mirrored by the acceptance of legislative changes encouraging higher fertility and in some countries making abortion illegal. Famous at that time was a slogan: *Women Returned to a Family*. Despite going back to traditional roles of mothers, the parental role of fathers did not change much and husbands continued to be viewed as the sole breadwinners (even in cases where mothers were working and fathers were unemployed). However, in some of the former Soviet bloc countries, fathers' involvement in childcare and domestic duties started to increase.

Despite models to promote larger families, a rapid transition to a market economy generated economic hardship, which influenced the decision of many couples to reduce planned procreation. The fertility rate dropped from an average of 2.1 to 2.3 children at the end of the 1980s, to 1.4 to 2.0 children per woman a decade later (United Nations, 2002). Except for a small percent of families that grew in affluence, many families could not afford to fulfill children's needs and "wishes" especially since new consumer goods were introduced to the market causing increases in both basic needs and more luxurious wishes.

The new ideology promoting women as homemakers, combined with the difficult economic situation of many families were reflected in child-parent relationships and in parental roles. In the two countries presented in this article, changes observed in these relationships were as follows.

Poland. During the period of rising unemployment and the rule of conservative political groups in the early 1990s, an ideological concept was widely propagated that the survival of the Polish nation required the strengthening of traditional family values, including putting women back into home to take care of the house and children. This early 1990s trend found expression in the new restrictive abortion policy and in the closing of the Office for Women and Family Matters in the Polish Government (i.e., Pełnomocnictwo Rządu do Spraw Kobiet i Rodziny) in 1993, which used to represent women's rights in the public and domestic spheres. Released as a Director of this latter office, Minister Anna Popowicz stated: "as soon as the right wing politicians win the election to the Polish government, women's role will be limited to that of mother, care giver, and homemaker . . . and nobody will invest in the education of women whose only role will be to bear children" (Paradowska, 1992, p.5).

Economic difficulties, however, led to the reduction of family size and a decrease in fertility rates, but did not disturb parent-child relationships. The great majority of children increasingly felt loved by parents (an increase from 81% in 1992 to 83% by 1999) and more children felt understood by their parents (an increase from 39% in 1992 to 43% in 1999). At the same time the percentage of children that felt unloved by parents decreased from 6% to 3% (Kwak, 2001) (see also Table 1).

To some degree, children-parent relationships were a function of the family's economic well-being. Children from more wealthy families, more often reported having strong, positive relationships with parents than children from poorer families (Kwak, 2001). Moreover, children of wealthy families, when compared to children from poor families, almost twice as often reported feeling loved by parents (59% vs. 39%, respectively) and less frequently felt alienated from parents (10% vs. 16%, respectively) (Filipiak, 1999). At the same

TABLE 1. Relationship of Polish Youth with Their Parents (in Percent)

Describe your relationships with your parents	Data collected in April 1994*	Data collected in April 1996	Data collected in December 1998
With mothers			
Very good	35	36	47
Rather good	43	39	37
Sometimes good sometimes bad	17	20	13
Rather not good	3	3	2
Not good	2	2	2
With fathers			
Very good	17	21	31
Rather good	31	29	29
Sometimes good sometimes bad	31	33	23
Rather not good	14	11	9
Not good	7	6	8

Source: Data from Central Office of Public Opinion Research. 1999. Polish Census Data on the representative sample of middle and high schools youth in Poland. See also Kwak, Anna (2001, p. 237). * For 1994 N = 1260, for 1996 N = 1275, and for 1998 N = 1316. The percentage depicts percent of the respondents in each sample in the particular year.

time, however, children who reported that parents do not understand them came mainly from families with college-educated parents who tended to be more economically affluent. According to Wrzesień (2001, 2002) higher educated parents believed that education is the key to success in the post-communist society and hence had high educational expectations for their children. Having high expectations for their children, in turn, led to many conflicts between parents and youth. However, as Marzec (2001) showed, 15% of children from very wealthy families, who lived in luxurious conditions and whose parents fulfilled all of their material desires and needs, reported that their home was a stressful place. These youth preferred to spend time with their friends' families because their own parents had no time for them.

Observed differences in child-parent relationships also were a function of family residence and parental religiosity. Throughout the 1990s, compared to rural families, children of urban families reported feeling loved and understood by parents almost twice as often (55% vs. 37%, respectively) and felt alienated at home less than half as often (9% versus 21%). Similarly, significant differences were found between religious and non-religious families. Children who had religious parents felt loved by parents twice as often as those who had non-religious parents (56% vs. 27%, respectively) and were over six times less likely to report feeling alienated at home (4% vs. 26%, respectfully) (Filipiak, 1999).

The most visible change was demonstrated in the roles of fathers. Partially as a result of the diffusion of Western models of fatherhood (e.g., the popular Scandinavian model), fathers became more involved in child rearing. Interestingly, the change in parental roles of fathers was supported and promoted by the Polish Catholic church, which may have been influenced by increasing contacts with more liberal Catholic churches of Western countries. By the end of the 1990s, therefore, though mothers still performed most household and childcare duties, fathers were increasingly viewed by children not only as the breadwinners but also as the caregivers.

As reported by middle and high school students, children had closer relationships with mothers than fathers but 30% of them, as compared to 3% in communist times, believed that fathers would help them at times of difficulty (63% of children believed that mothers would always help them) (Kwak, 2001). Children reported being able to discuss their problems with parents, but most discussion was still with mothers. For example, 67% of girls and 40% of boys reported being able to talk with mothers about a broad range of problems from sex and personal friendships to professional careers and educational plans. However, college-educated fathers were considered discussion partners as well (Kwak, 2001). Under communism, none of the boys ever discussed their problems with fathers, and only 3% of girls reported talking about their problems with fathers. By contrast, in post-communist Poland, 1% of the boys and 13% of the girls reported discussing problems with their fathers. This small but visible change was significant for parent-youth relationships, especially since it occurred in just one decade. By 1999, children still predominantly had relationships with mothers, who were the main persons in their lives–children talked to mothers about intimate problems, engaged with them in discussion about various issues, could count on them when in trouble, and cared the most about their opinions and approval (Zielińska, 2001). Nonetheless, the strong attachment of children to mothers was becoming slowly supplemented by the development of relationships between children and fathers.

Kyrgyzstan. The Communist ideology was displaced by the transition to democracy, and thus, children's social organizations disappeared and issues of educating children, teaching morality and ethics, along with the responsibility for children's upbringing returned to families. The traditional division of labor at home, with the mother being fully responsible for domestic duties and child care, returned with the abolishment of communism. The democratic transition, with its introduction of personal freedom, also stimulated a rebirth of an old, banned custom of wife-kidnapping and women wearing *parandjas*[1] that were still formally banned, but, being considered religious practice, were tolerated. To clarify and document changes in the roles of mothers and fathers that emerged in the post-communist system, we conducted field research in Poland and Kyrgyzstan (presented below) and compare the results with the parental roles described in the literature mentioned above.

FIELD RESEARCH IN POLAND AND KYRGYZSTAN

Methodology

Two consecutive questionnaire interview studies were conducted in Poland in 1995 and 1999. The first research, conducted under the direction of Wejnert and Joseph Stycos, took place in the regions of Konin and Poznan (West-central Poland), which, compared to the whole country, are characterized by an average level of socioeconomic development, an average mean income per resident, and an average unemployment rate, including women's unemployment. The later (1999) study was conducted under the direction of Anna Wachowiak in one of the poorest rural areas in Poland, the region of Zielona Gora (South-Western Poland). The first study consisted of 50 interviews, and was intended to test the questionnaire developed by Stycos, Wejnert and Tyszka (Stycos, Wejnert & Tyszka, 2001, Stycos, Wejnert, & Zbigniew, 2002) for its application to Polish and Kyrgyzstan studies; the later (1999) project consisted of 306 interviews (Wachowiak, 1999).

Data were collected in Kyrgyzstan during 2001 using the Polish questionnaire interview translated into Russian. Kyrgyz data were collected from 100 female and 100 male respondents who resided in two villages located to the North and to the West of the capital city Bishkek. These villages consisted of multinational populations having largely an average standard of living for Kyrgyzstan. Included in this multinational population were the larger Kyrgyz and Russian (settled during communism) ethnic groups as well as the smaller German and Kazakh ethnic groups.

In the 1995 study the respondents were 35-60 years of age with about four-fifths being married and two-thirds being employed outside the home. In 1999-2001, almost all the respondents were married (97% in Poland and 91% in Kyrgyzstan), with 92.5 % in Poland and 84% in Kyrgyzstan being married to their first partner. The general tendency in Kyrgyzstan was to marry early, with female respondents being married between 16 and 23 and males between 20 and 26 years old. In comparison, the majority of Polish female respondents married between the ages of 21 and 25 and males between 21 and 29 years old indicating that Polish couples tended to marry later. Most Polish couples formed nuclear families, which consisted of parents, children, and sometimes older grandparents. The family composition in Kyrgyzstan, in turn, varied depending upon parents' ethnic background. Following tradition, Kyrgyz and Kazakh couples lived in multigenerational, extended families with parents, children, grandparents and unmarried siblings of parents (usually the husband), whereas Russian and German families were mainly nuclear in their structure.

Results

In both countries, women were the sole childcare providers, being almost fully responsible and involved in bringing up children prior to communism. Moreover, in Poland, women remained fully responsible for these roles during the communist period. Consequently, to demonstrate the effect of democratization and economic transition on parental roles, we tested whether the roles of fathers changed and whether fathers became more involved in parental duties.

Indicators of husbands' help with childcare and the upbringing of children and of husbands' help in domestic duties were selected for our study. The selected indicators represent active (involved) vs. passive (uninvolved) parenting functions of fathers. They also indicated the general models for paternal and maternal roles that the younger generation was socialized into within families. The initial analyses provide a presentation of different types of childcare tasks performed by fathers, which describe the participation of fathers in child rearing in each country. In the next step, we examined several potential predictors of fathers' parental involvement, a procedure that assessed parental roles as a function of a set of variables depicting family structure and parental cultural tradition. Specifically, the variables for this study were:

Structure of Families

- family size (measured as the number of children in each family)
- current husband's employment status
- current wife's employment status

Parents' Cultural Tradition

- parents' traditionalism
- religiosity
- liking/disliking housework

The traditionalism of the father/mother was measured by agreement/disagreement with the statement "the man is the decision maker and the woman is the subordinated follower." Religiosity was assessed by statements indicating frequency of religious practice, whereas liking/disliking housework (a domestic activity) was self-assessed by respondents indicating agreement/disagreement.

Types of Parenting Roles. In both countries, a slow increase in fathers' involvement in childcare indicated a change towards modern paternal roles. Although the specific tasks related to childcare differed, unlike circumstances in prior history, nearly 45.4% of Polish fathers and 42% of Kyrgyz fathers helped with childcare duties either a lot or somewhat. Kyrgyzstan fathers helped mainly with homework and played with children, while Polish fathers most frequently played with children, took children for walks, or cooked meals for them (see Figure 1).

Parenting Roles and Family Size. In Kyrgyzstan as well as in Poland, children were strongly desired by families, as demonstrated by the first baby being born in these families during the first 1-2 years of marriage. However, significant differences between countries and ethnic groups were observed in reference to family size. Polish families were small, with an average of 1.5 children per family (the national average was 1.37 as of 2/2001) (GUS, 2002), while the number of children in families in Kyrgyzstan varied depending on parents' ethnicity. Kyrgyz and Kazakh couples had significantly more children than Russian or German families. On average, Kyrgyz families had 3-4 children, which despite being large, was a smaller number of children than during Soviet times, when the average Kyrgyz family size was 4.6 children. Moreover, also during Soviet times, 20.3% of all families and 35.4% of Kyrgyz families had 7 or more children (Lubin, 1991). In addition, couples in Kyrgyzstan frequently adopted children when they could not have their own children. The practice of adoption was very rare in Poland, and there were no cases of adoption in our sample.

Family planning had been commonly practiced in both countries during the communist period. This trend continued into post-communism, when economic difficulties and increasing expectations for higher material standards of living became prevalent. Other developments that encouraged family planning were reductions in the number of many state-run, inexpensive preschool institutions (daycares and kindergartens) that influenced parents to have only as many children as they could afford (Falkingham, 1997).

As our studies show, Polish and Kyrgyz couples controlled childbearing, particularly using conventional methods of contraception, with twice as many husbands in Poland (60%) as in Kyrgyzstan (30%) using some form of birth control (see Table 2). The conventional methods were complemented by abortion and in Poland also by contraception pills and less often by IUD. Despite recently

FIGURE 1. Forms of Active Paternal Roles of Fathers Measured by the Type of Childcare Involvement*

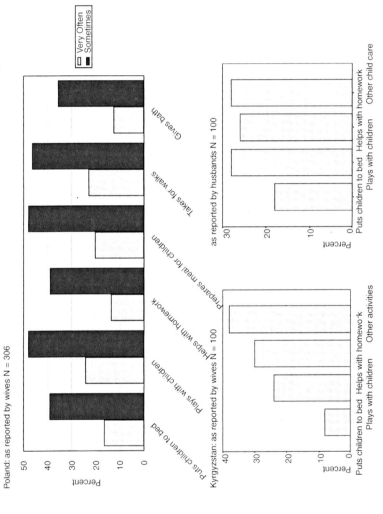

Note: *Overall, as respondents indicated, 45.4% of Polish fathers and 35.4% of Kyrgyz fathers were involved in parental duties

TABLE 2. The Use of Birth Control by Husbands in Relation to Family Size in Number of Respondents

Kyrgyzstan*: Husband's birth control N = 100						Total
		yes	no	sometimes	N/A	
How many children	1	1				1
	2	2	3			5
	3	12	28			40
	4	6	18		1	25
	5	6	9			15
	6	1	6			7
	7	1	1			2
	8	1	3	1		5
Total		30	68	1	1	100
Poland: Husband's birth control N = 306						Total
How many children	0	4	2			6
	1	42	27			69
	2	90	33			123
	3	29	23			52
	4	8	4			12
	more than 4	5	9			14
Missing data						30
Total		178	98			276

Note: * The recorded data were derived from interviews with Kyrgyz men. The interviews with Kyrgyz women closely resembled data obtained during interviews with husbands.

growing religiosity among the mainly Moslem population of Kyrgyzstan (near 90% of the population is considered Moslem), and the large Catholic population in Poland (over 90% of Poles declare themselves as Catholics), only 10% of Polish and 11% of Kyrgyz female respondents believed that abortion should be banned, while 38% of Kyrgyz men believed that it should be (see Figure 2). Abortion is more commonly practiced in Kyrgyzstan, where women on average have 4 to 10 abortions in their lifetime (United Nations, 1999).

Women tried to increase their incomes, especially at times of economic hardship (as our study shows, 65% of female respondents preferred working to increase income and to achieve relative financial stability) even if it implied reducing family size. Nonetheless, the pro-family traditions influenced parents to prefer to have larger families than they actually had, if they could afford to do so. As our data demonstrates, 37% of mothers and 100% of fathers in Kyrgyzstan would have liked to have more children. Many Kyrgyzstan women (30% of women) with three children expressed a preference to have more children and many men (38% of men) with 4 children would like to have more children. In

FIGURE 2. Attitudes Towards Abortion in Poland and Kyrgyzstan

Percent of Respondents

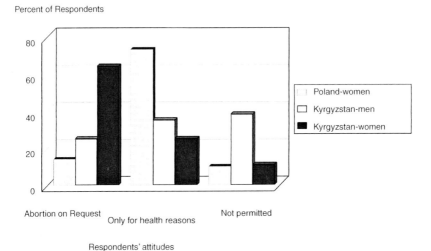

Note: In Poland N = 306 (women), in Kyrgyzstan N = 100 (women) and N = 100 (men).

contrast, Polish families preferred to have two children. In Kyrgyzstan, the desire to have more children was not determined by the family size; but, on the contrary, in larger families parents (mothers and fathers alike) continued to prefer having more children than they had currently (see Table 3). For example, most working mothers indicated that poor economic conditions had caused them to stop procreation but, regardless whether they currently had two or more than five children, they continued to want one more child than their present number.

The size of a family has also a non-linear effect on parenting roles or shared domestic duties in Poland and in Kyrgyzstan. Specifically, in Kyrgyzstan, husbands helped the most with childcare when families had 3-4 children (twice as many fathers helped than not helped–43% vs. 22%, respectively); for families with five and more children, the figures were 16% helped vs. 13% did not help while for families with two children only 3% helped. When there was only one child, the husband did not help at all. It seems that husbands do not feel the need to help when there are 1-2 children or when there are five or more children. Since the most common are families with 3-4 children and the families that are larger follow the traditional Muslim norms, the most traditional

TABLE 3. Respondents' Attitude for Having More Children as Corresponding with Family Size

		no more	one more	two more	three more	seven and more	Total
			**Wants more children**				
			Women-Kyrgyzstan N = 100				
How many children in the family	1	1					1
	2	1	4				5
	3	10	29			1	40
	4	7	15		1	2	25
	5	7	8				15
	6	3	3			1	7
	7	1	1				2
	8	3	1			1	5
Total		33	61		1	5	100
			Men-Kyrgyzstan N = 100				
How many children in the family	1		1				1
	2			4			4
	3		5	10	5		20
	4		16	14	8		38
	5		8	8	2		18
	6		4	5			9
	7			2			2
	8		3	5			8
Total			37	48	15		100
			Poland N = 306				
How many children in the family	No children	8	.3				9
	1	56	17				73
	2	123	4				127
	3	49	.3				50
	4	11	.3				13
	5						12
Missing							22
Total		259	25				306

Note: Data are presented in number of respondents.

husbands are least likely to help women. When there was only one or two children, help may not have been seen as needed.

Polish fathers' help also did not have a linear relationship based on the number of children. Fathers were actively engaged in childrearing in families with one or two children (51.7% of fathers were involved vs. 9.5% were not). In families with three or more children, nearly one quarter of fathers (22.8%) were helping with childcare and only 0.1% did not help. Thus, the pattern observed in Poland is similar to Kyrgyzstan. In families with 1-2 children that are considered more modern, husbands were more likely to help, but in more traditional, larger families, closely following the Catholic norms, husbands were less likely to help.

Polish fathers with 1-2 children were 10 times more likely to help with household chores than were Kyrgyz fathers with the same number of children (51.7% and 5.0% respectively). See Table 4.

Parenting Roles and Employment Status. Interestingly, the strongest indicator of a husband's help with housework and childcare was his employment status. *Working fathers helped much more* in housework *than unemployed fathers.* In Poland, the percentage of working fathers who helped was higher and the percentage of unemployed fathers who were not helping was lower than in Kyrgyzstan. In Kyrgyzstan, husbands who help at home were much more likely to be working (59%) than unemployed (32%). Among those husbands who did not help at home 3% were working and 5% were unemployed. In Poland, 74.6% of those husbands who help at home were working compared to 11% who were unemployed (see Table 4).

It seems that in Kyrgyzstan, the prevailing traditional culture affected the non-working fathers' involvement in domestic duties. Only the employed father, who fit the image of a successful man and breadwinner, had a sufficiently high self-esteem to break the gender role boundaries of what was often considered not a masculine activity, and to engage in help with house chores and childcare. We assume that in a society with a traditional culture, fathers who have lost their jobs and cannot fulfill the expected breadwinner role are reluctant to engage in the "non-masculine" activity of parenting. This trend was not so strongly visible in Poland where, historically, women had held strong positions in the family, making the implementation of a new tradition of husbands helping with domestic chores much easier.

Not surprisingly, in Kyrgyzstan the employment status of mothers did not predict greater involvement of fathers in parental duties. As discussed earlier, it was common during communism for mothers to be employed full time in addition to being full time mothers which led to an expectation for women to do both tasks simultaneously. As demonstrated, husbands more likely helped non-working than working wives (22% of Kyrgyz mothers who had full time jobs were helped by their spouses with child upbringing in comparison to 40% who were not helped; and 35% of working mothers were helped vs. 53% were not helped with domestic duties).

In contrast, Polish husbands helped their working wives. Of those wives who were helped with childcare, 64% were employed and only 19.7% of

TABLE 4. Variables that Influenced Kyrgyz and Polish Husbands' Help with Childcare and Domestic Duties (in percent)*

Variables	Kyrgyzstan				Poland			
	Help with childcare		Help in domestic duties		Help with childcare		Help in domestic duties	
	yes	no	yes	no	yes	no	yes	no
1. Wife: has a job	22 (22%)	19 (19%)	35 (35%)	6 (6%)	184 (64%)	11 (3.8%)	168 (59.2%)	25 (8.8%)
does not have a job	40 (40%)	19 (19%)	53 (53%)	6 (6%)	56 (19.7%)	6 (2.1%)	57 (20%)	14 (4.9%)
2. Husband: has a job	26 (26%)	17 (17%)	59 (59%)	3 (3%)	202 (71%)	14 (4.9%)	212 (74.6%)	27 (9.5%)
does not have a job	20 (20%)	9 (9%)	32 (32%)	5 (5%)	37 (13%)	1 (.03%)	34 (11.1%)	10 (3.5%)
3. Family size:								
0 child	0	0	0	0	0	0	6 (2.1%)	0
1-2 children	3 (3%)	3 (3%)	5 (5%)	0	144 (50.7%)	12 (4.2%)	147 (51.7%)	27 (9.5%)
3-4 children	43 (43%)	22 (22%)	59 (59%)	6 (6%)	65 (22.8%)	3 (.1%)	61 (21%)	10 (3.5%)
5 or more children	16 (16%)	13 (13%)	19 (19%)	5 (5%)	5 (1.7%)	0	6 (2.1%)	0
4. Father's traditionalism**								
traditional	19 (19%)	10 (10%)	36 (36%)	4 (4%)	14 (4.9%)	1 (.03%)	14 (4.9%)	1 (.03%)
not sure	22 (22%)	8 (8%)	37 (37%)	3 (3%)	12 (4.2%)	4 (1.4%)	15 (5.2%)	3 (1%)
not traditional	8 (8%)	5 (5%)	19 (19%)	1 (1%)	214 (75.3%)	11 (3.8%)	215 (75.7%)	34 (11.9%)
5. Father's religiosity								
religious	29 (29%)	16 (16%)	57 (57%)	6 (6%)	191 (67.2%)	9 (3.1%)	194 (68.3%)	23 (8.1%)
not religious	17 (17%)	10 (10%)	34 (34%)	2 (2%)	48 (16.9%)	6 (2.1%)	51 (17.9%)	14 (4.9%)

Note: *The percent indicates % of husbands and numbers the Ns of husbands who were helping or not with childcare and helping/not helping in domestic duties as a function of each variable. **Percent agreeing that man is a decision maker, the woman is a submissive follower.

529

non-employed mothers, while 59.2% of working and only 20% of not working mothers were helped in domestic tasks (see Table 4).

Parenting Roles and Religiosity. Interestingly, in Kyrgyzstan the religious husbands were less involved in paternal roles than were religious husbands in Poland (29% of religious fathers were involved in childcare in Kyrgyzstan while 67.2% of fathers in Poland) while the percent of nonreligious fathers who were involved in childcare was about the same in both countries. This finding reflects that Kyrgyz cultural tradition is strongly rooted in religion (Islam), whereas, while Polish tradition also stems from traditional religion (Catholic), it became modified most likely due to contacts with modern Western European and North American Catholic churches and the diffusion of cultural models of paternal roles. The diffusion of paternal roles, we believe, is to some degree reflected by recent changes in the Polish Catholic church's perspective on families and its broad emphasis on fathers' and husbands' involvement in childcare (see Table 4).

Parenting Roles and Traditionalism. Similarly, the increased involvement of fathers in child and house care positively correlated with egalitarian marital relationships in Poland but opposite trend was found in Kyrgyzstan. Accordingly, Polish wives, in general, had more authority in the family and a greater ability to make decisions regarding family matters than Kyrgyz women. Polish wives who did not hold traditional beliefs were able to persuade husbands to be egalitarian spouses and involved fathers, and to share parenting and house duties (75.3% of non-traditional vs. 4.9% of traditional husbands helped). An unanticipated finding for Kyrgyzstan was that, unlike Poland, husbands with traditional beliefs were two and a half times more likely to help with childcare than were husbands with non-traditional beliefs (19% vs. 8%).

A similar pattern was observed for help with domestic duties. In Poland, 75.7% of husbands with non-traditional beliefs provided help as compared with 4.9% of husbands with traditional beliefs. However, in Kyrgyzstan, 36% of husbands with traditional beliefs provided help with domestic duties as compared with 19% of those holding nontraditional beliefs (see Table 4). In additional analysis it was found that Kyrgyz women who were liberated (and hence fully disagree with the statement that "a man is a decision maker and a woman is a submissive follower" were much less likely to be helped by their spouses–14.3% traditional vs. 4.8% of non-traditional, liberated wives were helped by their spouses. It seemed that it paid off to be submissive and subordinated women in Kyrgyzstan. Perhaps traditional Kyrgyz husbands felt threatened by their wives' independence and tried to preserve their position in the family by refusing to be involved in perceived as not masculine activities of child and house care.

CONCLUSION

In both countries, despite differences in family composition, parenting roles were a function of: (a) family size, (b) fathers' employment status, (c) religiosity, and (d) traditionalism. At the same time, wives' working status and the degree to which wives liked domestic duties had no effect on performed parental roles. Based on this study, two tendencies can be observed in Poland and Kyrgyzstan today. First, there is movement toward Western democratic values, including the ideas of egalitarianism and greater emphasis on small nuclear families. Second, tendencies exist in the direction of reviving traditional cultural patterns relating to family life, marital, and parent-child relationships. These opposite tendencies can lead to conflict, particularly when the state does not interfere and does not support any ideology through its policies. Under these circumstances, families become solely responsible for decisions pertaining to family patterns, socialization practices, and the education of children in terms of either Western values and egalitarian relations versus the traditional relationships of patriarchy within families. Given such contradictory viewpoints, families must resolve questions related to morality and the role of religion, particularly in reference to such issues as family planning, abortion, and the family roles of women and men. The first years of this major transition may be the turning point, which will determine which model prevails in the future.

Our 1995 Polish study depicted that marriage and family are the strongest determinants of life satisfaction (Stycos, Wejenrt & Tyszka, 2001), a finding supported by several American studies (Andrews & Whithey, 1976; Andrews & Robinson, 1991; Campbell, 1981). However, a corresponding finding is that women have lower marital and life satisfaction than men.

Why should women consistently report lower levels of satisfaction in these studies? One possibility is their increasing dissatisfaction with male contributions to household tasks. As Elina Haavio-Mannila (1992, p.105) has concluded, "women were happier . . . the more the spouse participated in domestic work." For example, only half of our respondents in 1995 reported that their husbands often help with household chores and this data was consistent with earlier World Bank studies conducted in five European countries, including Poland (World Bank, 1994).

As demonstrated five years later in Poland and in Kyrgyzstan (see Tables 2-4), while domestic work still was not equally shared, our respondents were crossing parental role boundaries as fathers were helping with childcare and domestic duties more extensively. This contrasts with the periods prior to and during communism, when mothers performed almost all of the childcare duties and were responsible for children's well-being. Fathers were the authorities within families but were uninvolved parents and the emphasis on equalizing men and women did not generate egalitarian parental roles. In contrast, recent trends toward democratization, assisted by the diffusion of the Western European and American egalitarian models of family relationships (both marital and parent-child relationships), have started to influence parenting roles by overcoming cultural traditionalism.

Changes are already being observed, some of which are responses to economic conditions and preferences for improved material well-being. An example of change is that our respondents have established smaller families despite expressed preferences for larger families. Moreover, active fatherhood (i.e., fathers involved in childcare) in Poland is actually promoted by the Catholic Church, most likely because of the diffusion of more modern religious attitudes. The formation of Women's Studies programs and majors in Poland, which are also starting to be established in Kyrgyzstan, have generated numerous studies on men's and women's social positions, including their parental roles. This trend also might bring the awareness and recognition that mothers are overburdened and might help to encourage egalitarian parental models.

At the same time, however, the more traditional behavioral norms, such as traditional attitudes regarding abortion, birth control and the desired family size, are reemerging. The rebirth of traditionalism in part results from the growth of religious freedom and increasing religiosity, but also from the newfound freedom to regain parenting roles that had been performed by state-run childcare facilities under communism. Therefore, following Mukherjee's (1998, p.4) argument that "culture does not change on its own because 'by definition,' culture is not capable of self-revision or self-production: it registers the worldview which may or may not change over time" we may expect intertwined modern and traditional parenting styles during the post-communist transition. On one hand, the encouragement of Western examples of parenting should progressively encourage greater egalitarianism for men's and women's domestic and childcare duties, and improve father-child relationships. On the other hand, an important role in shaping parenting styles may also be traditionalism.

At time of contradicting parenting models, active fatherhood could serve as a source of help for somewhat confused youth, as well as a source of guidance and a constructive role model. Active fathering could help manage a new youth subculture inundated with pathological behaviors that were extremely rare, if not nonexistent, within strictly controlled communist societies (Pielkowa, 2001). Hence, the models of involved, active parenting are especially important within liberal democratic systems where the parent-child relationships are challenged by increases in youthful drug use, teen prostitution, as well as teen and out-of-wedlock pregnancy.

NOTE

1. *Parandja* is a burqa-type cover for face and body which is worn by women and girls. Under the Soviet regime, this tradition was forbidden and local authorities, fulfilling the Party's instructions, organized public burnings of *parandjas*.

REFERENCES

Andrews, F. & Robinson J. (1991). Measures of well-being. In J. Robinson, P. Shaver & L. Wrightsman (Eds.) *Measures of personality and social psychological attitudes.* San Diego, CA: Academic Press: pp. 1-115.

Andrews, F. & S. Withey (1976). *Social indicators of well-being: Americans' perceptions of life quality.* New York: Plenum Press.

Campbell, A. (1981). *The sense of well-being in America. Recent patterns and trends.* New York: McGraw Hill.

Czapiński, J. (1994). Uziemnienie duszy Polskiej. *Kultura i spoleczenstwo [culture and society], 1,* 19-37.

Dąbrowski, M. & Antczak R. (Eds.) (1996). *UkrainskadDroga do gospodarki rynkowej 1991-1995.* Warszawa: Wydawnictwo Naukowe, PWN.

Falkingham, J. (Ed.) (1997). *Household welfare in Central Asia.* Macmillan Press; New York: St. Martin's Press, pp. 183-200.

Filipiak, G. (1999). Funkcja wsparcia społecznego w rodzinie (The role of social support in the family). *Annals of Sociology of Family, 11,* pp. 131-145.

Gontarczyk, E. (2001). Kobiety i zmieniajace sie relacje plci. (Women and change in gender relations) In: A. Wachowiak (Ed.) Jak zyc? (How to live?) (pp. 205-224). Poznan: Wydawnictwo fundacji Humanitora.

GUS (Glowny Urzad Statystyczny). (2002). *Rocznik statystyczny.* Warszawa, Poland: Zaklad Wydawnictw Statystyczych.

Grzybek, H. (1977). Konflikty dorastajacej młodziezy z rodzicami. (Conflicts between youth and parents). *Family Problems, 3,* 20-23.

Haavio-Mannila, E. (1992). *Work, family and well-being in five North and East European capitals.* Helsinki: Suomalainen Tiedeakatemia.

Kowalski, W. (1980). Percepcja postaw rodzicielskich przez młodzież w zależności od płci rodziców i płci dziecka. (Children's perception of parental roles as a function of parents' and children's sex). *Problemy Rodziny, 4,* 35-42.

Kwak A. (2001). Relacje mołdziezy z perspektywy przemian społecznych: Stałość czy modyfikacja? (Adolescents-parents relationships from the perspective of social transformation: Constancy or modification?). In Z. Tyszka (Ed.) *Wspocłzesne rodziny polskie-ich stan i kierunk przemian* (pp. 231-243). Poznań: Wydawnictwo Naukowe UAM.

Lissyutkina, L. (1993). Soviet women at the crossroad of perestroika. In N. Funk & M. Mueller, *Gender politics and post-communism* (pp. 274-287). New York: Routledge.

Lubin, N. (1991). *Implications of ethnic and demographic trends.* In W. Fierman (Ed.) the *Soviet Central Asia: The failed transformation* (pp. 36-59). Boulder: Westview Press.

Marzec, H. (2001). Sytuacja dziecka w rodzinie o wysokim standarcie economicznym (A child in a family of high economic status). In: Z. Tyszka (Ed.) *Wspocłzesne rodziny polskie-ich stan i kierunk przemian* (pp. 323-333). Poznań, Wydawnictwo Naukowe UAM.

Mukherjee, R. (1998). Social reality and culture. *Current Sociology*, *46*, 39-50.

Olcott, M. B. (1991). Women in Central Asia. In W. Fierman (Ed.) *Soviet Central Asia: The failed transformation* (pp. 241-246). Boulder: Westview Press.

Paradowska, J. (1992). Kobieta do domu. *Polityka*, March, 21:5.

Pielkowa, J. A. (2001). Zmiany w pelnieniu funckji socjalizacyjnej w rodzinie. (Change in families' socialization function). In: Z. Tyszka (Ed.) *Wspocłzesne rodziny polskie-ich stan i kierunk przemian* (pp. 255-261). Poznań, Wydawnictwo Naukowe.

Rachalska, W. (1968). Ojciec w oczach dziewcząt. (Father as perceived by girls). *Family and School*, 7/8, 4-5.

Reading, A. (1992). *Polish women, solidarity and feminism.* Macmillan Academic and Professional Press.

Reboud, M. & Hoaquan C. (1997). *Pension reforms and growth in Ukraine: An analysis focusing on labor market constraints.* Washington, D.C.: World Bank.

Semya v SSSR. (1991). (Dannye perepisi 1989) (*Family in the USSR* (census data 1989). Moscow: Finances and Statistics.

Skorupska-Sobańska, J. (1967). *Młodzież i dorośli.* (*Youth and adults*). Warsaw, Poland: PZWS.

Skorupska-Sobańska, J. (1971). *Potrzeby nastolatków a wychowanie w rodzinie. (Needs of teenagers and family socialization).* Warsaw: Nasza Księgarnia.

Stephenson, P. (Ed.). (1998). *Improving women's health services in the Russian Federation: Results of a pilot project.* Washington, D.C.: World Bank.

Stycos, M. J., Wejnert, B.& Tyszka, Z. (2001). Polish women and quality of life: A preliminary research report. *Roczniki Socjologii Rodziny (Annals of Sociology of Family)*, 9: 17-29.

Stycos, M. J., Wejnert, B., & Zbigniew T. (2002). Polish women during transition to democracy: A preliminary research report. In Wejnert, B. (Ed.) *Transition to democracy in Eastern Europe and Russia: Impact on politics, economy and culture* (pp. 259-279). NJ: Praeger Press.

Titkov, A. (1992). Political change in Poland: Cause, modifier, or barrier to gender equality?, In Funk, N. and Magda M. (Eds.) *Gender politics and post-communism* (pp. 253-256). New York: Routledge.

United Nations (1999). *From Beijing to New York. (1995-2000): Report on the status of women in the Kyrgyz Republic* (pp. 8-14). Bishkek, Kyrgyzstan.

United Nations, Department of International and Social Affairs. (2002). *The world's women 1970-2000. Trends and statistics.* New York: United Nations.

Wejnert, B. (1996a). Political transition and gender transformation in the communist and post-communist periods. In: Wejnert, B. & M. Spencer (Eds.) *Women in post-communism* (pp. 3-19). Connecticut: JAI Press.

Wejnert, B. (Ed.). (2002). *Transition to democracy in Eastern Europe and Russia. Impact on politics, economy and culture.* NJ: Praeger Press.

Wejnert, B. & Spencer, M. (Eds.), (1996). *Women in post-communism,* Connecticut: JAI Press.

World Bank. (1994). *World development report 1994.* Oxford University Press.

Wrzesień, W. (2001). Napięcia pomiedzy pokoleniami w rodzinie bliskiej generacji pokolenia końca wieku. (Tensions between generations in the end of the century generations families). In Z. Tyszka (Ed.) *Wspołczesne rodziny polskie-ich stan i kierunk przemian* (pp. 243-255). Poznań, Wydawnictwo Naukowe UAM.

Wrzesień, W. (2002). Rodzina jako sposób bycia dwcóh pokoleń w świecie życia codzinnego. Family–the two generations in the world of everyday life). In Z. Tyszka (Ed.) *Rodzina w czasach szybkich przemian* (pp. 71-81). Poznań, Wydawnictwo Naukowe UAM.

Zielińska, M. (2001). Ochronna funkcja wspólnot. Przyczynek do badań nad jakościa zycia młodziezy. Family function of social support. In A. Wachowiak (Ed.) *Jak zyć? (How to live?)* (pp. 95-113). Poznan, Poland: Wydawnictwo Humanitora.

Parent-Youth Relationships and the Self-Esteem of Chinese Adolescents: Collectivism versus Individualism

Gary W. Peterson
Jose A. Cobas
Kevin R. Bush
Andrew Supple
Stephan M. Wilson

ABSTRACT. This study sought to determine how several child-rearing behaviors within the Chinese parent-adolescent relationship were predictive of youthful self-esteem through either collectivistic or individualistic socialization approaches. Theoretically based relationships were tested with structural equation modeling to examine whether dimensions of parental behavior (i.e., support, reasoning, monitoring, and punitiveness) influenced the self-esteem of Chinese adolescents through the mediating influences of either conformity (i.e., collectivism) or autonomy (i.e., indi-

Gary W. Peterson is affiliated with the Department of Family Studies and Social Work, Miami University, McGuffey Hall, Room 451, Oxford, OH 45056-3493 (E-mail: petersgw@muohio.edu). Jose A. Cobas is affiliated with the Department of Sociology, Arizona State University, Arizona State University, Tempe, AZ 85287. Kevin R. Bush is affiliated with the Department of Child and Family Development, University of Georgia, 112a Dawson Hall, Athens, GA 30602-3622. Andrew Supple is affiliated with the Department of Human Development & Family Studies, The University of North Carolina at Greensboro, PO Box 27160, Greensboro, NC 27402-6170. Stephan M. Wilson is affiliated with the Department of Human Development and Family Studies, University of Nevada, Reno, Mail Stop # 140, Reno, NV 89557-0131.

http://www.haworthpress.com/web/MFR
© 2004 by The Haworth Press, Inc. All rights reserved.
Digital Object Identifier: 10.1300/J002v36n03_09

vidualism) in reference to parents. The sample for this study consisted of 497 adolescents from Beijing, China, ranging in age from 12-19 years of age. Data were acquired with self-report questionnaires administered in school classrooms. Results provided support for parental behaviors as predictors of self-esteem development through individualistic patterns of socialization. Although collectivistic parent-adolescent patterns did not predict the self-esteem of Chinese adolescents, several results supported a collectivistic conception of socialization through significant relationships involving parental behaviors as predictors of adolescent conformity to parents. Some results of this study highlight the significance of parental support and dimensions of moderate parental control (e.g., reasoning and monitoring) within the Chinese parent-adolescent relationship, while identifying only a minimal role for punitive behavior.   *[Article copies available for a fee from The Haworth Document Delivery Service: 1-800-HAWORTH. E-mail address: <docdelivery@haworthpress.com> Website: <http://www.HaworthPress.com> © 2004 by The Haworth Press, Inc. All rights reserved.]*

KEYWORDS. Chinese parent-adolescent relations, Chinese self-esteem, Chinese parental behavior, collectivism, individualism

INTRODUCTION

A person's sense of self, a focus of western social science for more than a century, is both a constantly changing social process and a product of development (Cooley, 1902; Gecas & Burke, 1995; Harter, 1999; James, 1890; Mead, 1934; Rosenberg, 1965, 1979). Adolescence, in particular, is a time when the self becomes more complex, resulting partly from emerging cognitive abilities, but also from dynamic interaction within diverse social-cultural contexts (Gecas & Burke, 1995; Harter, 1999).

The most frequently researched aspect of the self is a person's self-esteem, the criterion variable for this study, designating the positive or negative feelings adolescents have about themselves (Gecas & Burke, 1995; Harter, 1999; Rosenberg, 1965, 1979). A positive self-esteem is commonly viewed as a psychological resource for competent psychosocial development and a protective mechanism that shelters the young from involvement in problem behavior (Covington, 1992; Gecas & Burke, 1995; Lui, Kaplan, & Risser, 1992; Owens, 1992; Rosenberg, 1965, 1979).

Parent-Adolescent Socialization and Self-Esteem in China: Mediated Effects Model

Belief in the importance of youthful self-esteem has led to substantial cross-cultural interest in how parents either foster or inhibit this attribute in children and adolescents (Bush, Peterson, Cobas, & Supple, 2002; Gecas & Burke, 1995; Kagitcibasi, 1996). Extensive Western research demonstrates that youthful self-esteem is encouraged by parents who use support and firm control, whereas negative self-evaluations are fostered by being punitive and non-supportive (Barber, Chadwick & Oerter, 1992; Demo, Small, & Savin-Williams, 1987; Gecas & Schwalbe, 1986; Peterson & Hann, 1999).

The purpose of this study, in turn, was to examine these issues with data provided by adolescents from Mainland China. The intent was to examine how several child-rearing behaviors were predictive of youthful self-esteem within a society often viewed as fostering the "self" through more collectivistic (i.e., group-oriented) socialization approaches compared to Western patterns. A collectivistic pattern of socialization is often thought to be more characteristic of Asian cultures, whereas an individualistic pattern is proposed to be more common in Western societies (Triandis, 1989, 1995; Kagitcibasi, 1996). Consequently, a theoretical model was tested with structural equation modeling *to determine whether the influences of parental behaviors on the self-esteem of Chinese adolescents are conveyed through mediating variables that are indicators either of a collectivistic or an individualistic pattern of socialization* (see Figure 1). A collectivistic pattern of socialization would be evident if dimensions of parental behavior (i.e., reasoning, monitoring, punitiveness, and support) predict the self-esteem of Chinese youth through the mediating influence (or indirect influence) of conformity to their parents' expectations (see Figure 1). The variable conformity to parents is an indicator (at the family relationship level) of a collectivistic socialization pattern to the extent that youthful self-development is rooted in extensive orientation toward one's family, and particularly by being responsive (or conforming) to parents' expectations.

In contrast, a more individualistic pattern of socializing adolescent self-esteem occurs if the influences of parental behaviors are conveyed indirectly through the process of gaining autonomy from parents, a specific indicator (at the family relationship level) of individualistic socialization patterns within families (see Figure 1). *Results consistent with an individualistic pattern would be evident if dimensions of parental behavior (i.e., reasoning, monitoring, and support) predict the self-esteem of Chinese adolescents through the mediating influence of increased autonomy from parents* (see Figure 1). According to Western conceptions, youthful self-esteem develops in association

FIGURE 1. Theoretical Model

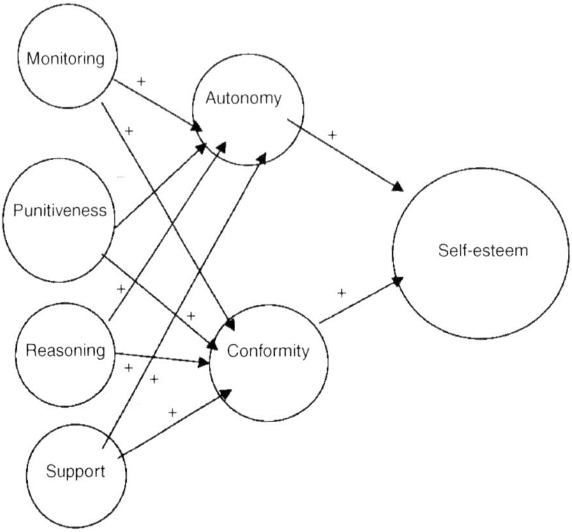

Note--The following predictions for the direct effects of parental behaviors on self-esteem are not shown: Parental educ +, Monitoring +, Punitiveness −, Reasoning +, Support +

with the process of gaining autonomy from family and parents (Fuligni, 1998; Peterson, 1995; Sessa & Steinberg, 1991).

GENERAL CULTURAL ORIENTATIONS AND THE SELF: INDIVIDUALISM AND COLLECTIVISM

Investigators of socialization issues in Chinese cultures often utilize the general cultural orientations *collectivism* and *individualism* to conceptualize how socialization patterns differ across societies. Scholars who view Asian socialization as differing substantially from Western patterns have frequently attributed many of these variances to collectivistic patterns that appear to characterize Chinese culture (Lam, 1997; Meredith, Abbott, & Shu, 1989; Triandis, 1989, 1995; Yang, 1981, 1986). China is commonly viewed as emphasizing familistic or group-focused values, whereas Western societies, such as the United States, are thought to focus on individualistic values, including personal agency and autonomy (Lam, 1997; Triandis, McCusker, Hui, 1990;

Yang, 1981, 1986). Frequent contrasts are made between the differing cultural patterns used in eastern and western societies to foster the "self" (Tafarodi & Swann, 1996).

Collectivistic societies, such as China, are commonly thought to encourage interdependence and connectedness, or relationship patterns in which self-concept development is associated with family loyalty, responsiveness to group expectations, interpersonal togetherness, and conformity (obedience) to authority figures (Ho, 1994). Compared to *individualistic values* of Western parents, Chinese parents are expected to place less emphasis on independence and to discourage such things as the expression of hostility, aggression, and impulsive behavior by the young (Ho, 1986; Meredith et al., 1989). Chinese youth are socialized to think of themselves as being prepared more extensively to serve societal rather than individual goals (Ho, 1994; Lam, 1997; Meredith et al., 1989). Consequently, self-esteem in Chinese society is supposed to be rooted in relational aspects of collectivism such as the Confucian doctrine of filial piety and the economic-political ideology of socialism (Ho, 1994; Lam, 1997; Wang & Hsueh, 2000). Perhaps to a greater degree than Western youth, Chinese adolescents may base their self-esteem on how effectively they view themselves as connected to parents by conforming to their elders' expectations (Gecas & Burke, 1995; Tafarodi & Swann, 1996).

In contrast, individualistic societies are described as emphasizing independence, freedom, and personal assertiveness as socializing climates in which a person's self-esteem develops (Kagitcibasi, 1996; Triandis, 1989; 1995). A Western view of self-awareness is based on the idea that one's "private self" resides within each person consistent with such cultural themes as the separateness and distinctiveness of each person (Gecas & Burke, 1995). Central goals of Western parenting include encouraging freedom of action, refraining from severe restrictiveness, and encouraging self-confidence for exploratory behavior.

Although such theoretical distinctions exist, current scholarship on the *individualistic* versus *collectivistic* basis of self-esteem in Chinese and Asian youth is characterized by much contradiction. Most of the theory and some of the research indicates that Asian, Chinese, and Asian-American socialization patterns are collectivistic in the sense that a "connected" self is fostered (Berndt, Cheung, Hau, & Lew, 1993; Chun & McDermid, 1997; Fuligni, 1998; Ho, 1986; Lam, 1997; Stevenson, Chen, & Lee, 1992). In contrast, other research conducted with Chinese samples, focusing on parental behavior as predictors of self-esteem, has revealed patterns quite similar to the individualistic approaches found in Western cultures. Specifically, socialization behavior such as independence-granting, warmth, and parental organization (i.e., a non-authoritarian form of firm control) were found to encourage adolescent self-esteem (Cheung & Lau, 1985; Lau & Cheung, 1987). Contrary to collectivistic conceptions, such findings suggest that the self-esteem of Chinese youth may be anchored in psychological autonomy and moderate, but firm types of parental control.

An important qualification is that most existing studies have significant methodological limitations that may explain some of the current inconsistency. Studies on the self-esteem of Chinese adolescents, for example, have been conducted quite frequently either with samples of Chinese-American adolescents or samples of youth from Hong Kong. A problem with these studies is that, given Hong Kong's unique Western history, Chinese populations from this location are more likely to be exposed to Western values than are populations located elsewhere in Mainland China (Cheung & Lau, 1985). More precise examination of these issues has been hampered because, until recently, little data was gathered on parent-youth relationships within The People's Republic of China. Moreover, Chinese-American populations are likely to be more attuned to Western values associated with the dominant culture in the U.S. through acculturation processes (Cheung & Lau, 1985; Yau & Smetana, 1996).

Chinese Parent-Adolescent Relations and Adolescent Self-Esteem

Further theoretical understanding is needed (see below) about the specific predictions proposed in Figure 1 involving parental support, punitiveness, reasoning, and monitoring as either direct or indirect influences on adolescent self-esteem.

Parental support as a predictor of adolescent self-esteem. Some of the previous scholarship on Chinese and Chinese American parents has portrayed their socialization strategies as being less warm (i.e., less supportive) (Bond & Wang, 1983; Wu, 1986) and more restrictive, coercive, and authoritarian than European-American parents (Chao, 1994; Chiu, 1987; Dornbusch, Ritter, Leiderman, Roberts, & Fraleigh, 1987; Steinberg, Lamborn, Dornbusch, & Darling, 1992; Yang, 1981; 1986). Current work includes a debate about the efficacy of parental nurturance as a means of socializing Chinese youth (Wang & Hsueh, 2000). Compared to European-American parents, for example, some observers have reported that Chinese, Chinese American, and other Asian parents are less warm (supportive) or less emotionally demonstrative toward adolescents (Bond & Wang, 1983; Bush et al., 2002; Chao, 2001; Chiu, 1987; Dornbusch et al., 1987; Stevenson et al., 1992; Wu, 1996). One possibility is that Chinese parents convey supportiveness differently, not as emotional demonstrativeness, but as care and concern that becomes evident through their efforts to control and provide governance (Chao, 2000). Such conceptions suggest that clear distinctions may not exist between supportive and controlling dimensions in the Chinese socialization process. However, contradictory results, similar to scholarship on Western samples, indicate that supportive behavior from parents is a prominent positive predictor of self-esteem in Chinese adolescents (Cheung & Lau, 1985; Ho, 1989; Lau & Cheung, 1987; Lin & Fu, 1990). Consequently, this study addresses this issue by *examining the extent to which parental support, as a separate variable, is either a direct or indirect influence on adolescent self-esteem* (see Figure 1).

If it were found that parental support predicts adolescent self-esteem in China, in turn, a question remains about the precise mechanism through which this influence is conveyed (see Figure 1). Current scholarship in the West suggests that support contributes both to the autonomy of adolescents from parents as well as continued conformity to their expectations (Peterson & Hann, 1999; Peterson, Bush, & Supple, 1999; Peterson, Rollins, & Thomas, 1985), though comparable conceptualizations for China do not exist. Western parents appear to use supportive behavior as a means of encouraging adolescents to balance their progress toward self-direction (i.e., autonomy) with the need for continued receptiveness (i.e., conformity) to parental influences (Peterson & Leigh, 1990). Another objective of this study, therefore, is to examine *whether parental support influences the self-esteem of Chinese adolescents primarily through one of the following means: (1) autonomous processes (i.e., an individualistic pattern), (2) conforming processes (i.e., a collectivistic pattern), or (3) some combination of these paths (see Figure 1).* Moreover, besides the indirect tests specified in Figure 1, additional analyses were conducted to determine if parental support was a direct positive predictor of self-esteem.

Punitive Behavior versus Organized Control as Predictors of Adolescent Self-Esteem

Another controversy in the Chinese parent-youth scholarship concerns the role of authoritarian, restrictive, or punitive child-rearing behavior. A conclusion in some of the research and theoretical scholarship is that, beyond the early years of childhood, Asian parent-youth relationships are characterized by restrictive or authoritarian discipline, perhaps often more so than in Western socialization processes (Chao, 1994; Chiu, 1987; Kelley & Tseng, 1992; Ho, 1989; Wolf, 1970). Compared to Western patterns, this strict or authoritarian parenting style is viewed by some as having fewer problematic or even possibly positive consequences for Asian youth. Authoritarian parenting, for example, has been shown to be less strongly linked to poor academic achievement by Asian American youth as occurs within European American samples

(Steinberg et al., 1992; Steinberg, Lamborn, Darling, Mounts, & Dornbush, 1994).

Such a benign conception of punitive or restrictive parenting might have important implications for additional outcomes in Chinese youth such as self-esteem. Authoritarian parenting by Chinese parents might foster a variety of psychosocial outcomes that are consistent with traditional Chinese cultural values but differ from consequences commonly found in the West. Examples of such outcomes might be strong connections to others (e.g., conforming to parent's expectations) and subordinating one's concept of self to the interests of the group. Compared to Western parenting, therefore, higher self-esteem in Chinese youth might result from more restrictive (even autocratic) forms of parental control that encourage feelings of intergenerational solidarity with others and greater receptivity to parental influences (i.e., conformity to parents' expectations).

Such conceptions of restrictive child-rearing practices are a source of much controversy in the study of Chinese parent-child relations. Chinese scholars, in particular, have criticized Western researchers by for failing to articulate the cultural meaning of the proposed "restrictive" character of Chinese parenting (Chao, 1994; Gorman, 1998). According to this perspective, Western researchers tend to use rather global conceptions of parenting that fail to capture essential elements of Chinese child-rearing. Western parenting concepts, such as the "authoritarian style," are composed of several parental behaviors, expectations, and emotional qualities (Darling & Steinberg, 1993; Peterson & Hann, 1999), some of which may be expressions of values specific to a particular culture. Such multi-dimensional parental styles (e.g., authoritarian parenting) may fail to generalize effectively from one cultural setting to another and, at worst, may simply be reflections of cultural bias that mask subtle differences in meaning. Of particular concern is the tendency for cultural meanings of Chinese parenting to be inadequately captured by such ethnocentric Western constructs as authoritarian parenting (Berndt et al., 1993; Chao, 1994, 2000, 2001). A multifaceted conception of child-rearing, *authoritarian parenting*, is prevalent when parents have uncompromising expectations associated with hostile and mistrustful feelings toward the young. Strict behavior codes are expected as parents seek to dominate the young through excessively forceful and arbitrary behaviors. A frequent intention of authoritarian parenting (without much scientific evidence of effectiveness) is to prevent children from drifting into problematic or deviant involvements. These purposes of punitive/authoritarian parenting are deeply rooted in Judeo-Christian and Puritan traditions of Western and American thought (Day, Peterson, & McCracken, 1998; Peterson & Hann, 1999).

A contrasting viewpoint of Chinese parental guidance is provided by current scholarship on *dysfunctional control* within Chinese and Chinese-American families. Specifically, dysfunctional control, a construct used in studies of Chinese parenting, seems similar to Western versions of restrictive or authoritarian parenting, and has been reported by some scholars to *inhibit,* not foster, self-esteem in Chinese youth (Cheung & Lau, 1985; Lau & Cheung, 1987). Adding to the complexity of this debate are the proposals by some observers that Chinese parenting is rooted in distinctive traditions of strict control having their origins in traditional Chinese culture. Thus, in contrast to Western thought, traditional parenting themes, based in Confucian thought, emphasize responsibility to others, the importance of group interests, filial piety, parental authority, and the provision of guidance as goals of restrictive control (Berndt et al., 1993; Chao, 1994; Gorman, 1998). Rather than harshly punitive strategies, these parenting approaches are consistent with the traditional Chinese principles of *chiao shun* and *guan,* which refer to processes of *training* or *teaching.* Although emphasizing firm restrictiveness and obedience, *chiao shun* and *guan* differ from Western punitive approaches by being expressions of care and concern, not simple demonstrations of arbitrariness and hostility aimed at dominating the young. As such, Chinese parenting may be more accurately characterized as firm and demanding, with the goals being harmony, guidance, teaching, monitoring, and supportiveness (Berndt et al., 1993; Chao, 1994, 2000, 2001; Gorman, 1998).

Scholarship on parent-adolescent relationships within Chinese or Chinese American families often deals with such concepts of firm and non-punitive behavior in terms of the concepts *parental organization* or *functional control* (Cheung & Lau, 1985; Lau & Cheung, 1987). Instead of authoritarian or punitive behavior (i.e., dysfunctional control), Chinese parental control appears more comparable to such Western conceptions of non-authoritarian control as reasoning and monitoring. Such forms of functional control are used to foster an atmosphere of structure, order, and clear rules, combined with expressions of parental support. Contrary to punitive strategies, current conceptions of Western research indicate that monitoring and reasoning are aspects of firm control that contribute both to growing autonomy from parents and to continued conformity to parental expectations (Baumrind, 1991; Peterson et al., 1999; Peterson & Hann, 1999; Peterson & Leigh, 1990; Peterson et al., 1985). Based on these ideas, therefore, this study sought to determine which form of control, *punitiveness (i.e., dysfunctional/authoritarian control) or reasoning/ monitoring (i.e., functional or firm control) fosters positive self-esteem in Chinese adolescents through either direct or indirect paths* (see Figure 1). Specifically, the theoretical model tested whether these forms of control influenced the self-esteem of Chinese adolescents through one of the following pathways: (1) autonomous socialization processes (i.e., an individualistic pattern), (2) conforming socialization processes (i.e., a collectivistic pattern), or (3) some combination of these paths (see Figure 1). Additional tests were conducted to test for the direct effects of both forms of parental control (i.e., punitiveness versus reasoning and monitoring) on adolescents' self-esteem.

A particular contribution of this study was the effort to avoid some of the cultural bias involved in using global parental styles (e.g., authoritarian or authoritative styles) to predict adolescent self-esteem. Criticisms of parental styles have prompted the present investigators to use adolescent reports of specific dimensions of parental behavior instead of global parental styles (e.g., authoritarian or authoritative) composed of diverse but often culturally specific (or culturally biased) attributes. Well-defined dimensions of perceived socialization behavior, such as punitiveness, reasoning, monitoring, and support, are less constrained by cultural limitations than are multidimensional styles–or complex collections of expectations, motivations, values and behavior that are encompassed by parental styles (Darling & Steinberg, 1993; Peterson & Hann, 1999).

METHODOLOGY

Sample

Participants consisted of 497 adolescents selected from six state-funded high schools in Beijing, China, who volunteered to complete the questionnaire. Contacting adolescents through the schools was a convenient and cost-effective means of sampling a diverse population of sufficient size so that statistical models with multiple predictors could be examined. The selected high schools were classified in terms of test score standards required for enrollment. Although probability sampling was not possible, the socio-demographic characteristics (age, gender, and family characteristics) of the participants varies sufficiently to be a reasonable representation of a larger population of adolescents from Beijing, the economic, social, and political capital of the People's Republic of China.

Adolescent respondents were drawn from schools classified in terms of four different test score classifications in proportionate numbers (i.e., high to below average test scores). In Beijing, a particular school's academic level may reflect, in part, the socio-economic status of an adolescents' family, though class definitions are difficult to determine in a society that remains influenced by Marxist thought.

The final sample consisted of adolescents who ranged in age from 12 to 19 years having a mean age of 15.42 years. The gender of these participants was fairly evenly distributed, with 242 of the youthful respondents being female, and 238 being male. Average scores on the parental education variable were "some high school" for fathers, and "completion of middle school" for mothers. For their fathers' education, adolescents reported that 1.6% completed grade school, 28.8% completed middle school or technical school, 18.5% completed high school, 41.9% had attended or completed undergraduate college, and 1.2% attended or completed graduate school. For their mothers' education, adolescents reported that 1.6% completed grade school, 41.6% completed middle school or technical school, 19.9% completed high school, 26% had attended or completed their undergraduate years in college, and 0.2% attended or completed graduate school.

Procedure

Six hundred questionnaires were distributed in classrooms of the participating secondary schools, 497 (or 83%) of which were completed and/or provided useful data for this study. Teachers were trained to administer a standard protocol for the survey to the participating students. Respondents were instructed to complete the questionnaire independently in their classrooms and answer each item in a way that best corresponded with their experience. During administration, teachers provided assistance to participants by remaining in the classroom to answer questions of clarification about the items.

Measurement

The questionnaire for the larger project consisted of survey items that assess adolescents' self-reports of their own self-esteem, dimensions of social competence, several aspects of the parent-adolescent relationship, family relationship dimensions, and sociodemographic variables. Questionnaire translation was conducted using the technique of back translation in which the survey first was translated from English to Chinese and then from Chinese back to English. This procedure sought to ensure that both versions of the questionnaire conveyed item meanings that were as comparable as possible.

Specific measures used for this study assessed parental support, monitoring, reasoning, punitiveness, conformity to parents' expectations, behavioral autonomy from parents, and adolescent self-esteem. Research on the dependent variable, adolescent self-esteem, has demonstrated that youthful perceptions of parental behavior are more strongly predictive of the their own self-perceptions than are parents' reports of their own child-rearing behavior

(Buri, 1989; Gecas & Schwalbe, 1986). Moreover, assessing parental behaviors directly from parents' perceptions is subject to possible response bias from parents who may attempt to conceal certain behaviors (e.g., harsh or punitive behaviors) that are socially sanctioned (Gecas & Schwalbe, 1986; Peterson & Hann, 1999). A methodological (and theoretical) assumption of this study, therefore, is that adolescents' self-perceptions (e.g., self-esteem) are more likely to be influenced by their own constructions of reality (i.e., their own perceptions of parental behavior) than would their parents' conceptions of the same phenomenon.

Self-Esteem. Adolescents' global self-esteem was measured with 4 items taken from the Rosenberg Self-Esteem Scale (Rosenberg, 1965, 1979). The participants responded to the items in terms of a four-point Likert scale which varies from "Strongly Agree" (SA) to "Strongly Disagree" (SD). The items were phrased as positive assessments (e.g., "I feel I have a number of good qualities") involving evaluations of (1) one's personal worth, (2) good qualities, (3) ability to do things, and (4) satisfaction with self. Moderate internal consistency was demonstrated for these items with a Cronbach's alpha reliability coefficient of .71.

Parental Behaviors. The parental behaviors examined in this study were assessed by items from the Parent Behavior Measure (PBM). The PBM is a self-report instrument that measures adolescents' perceptions of several supportive and controlling dimensions of behavior that parents direct at adolescents (Henry & Peterson, 1995; Peterson et al., 1985; Peterson et al., 1999). The PBM assesses several parental behaviors, including support, reasoning, monitoring, punitiveness, and love withdrawal and is indebted, in part, to other investigators for its conceptualizations (Barber et al., 1992; Devereaux, Bronfenbrenner, & Rodgers, 1969; Heilbrun, 1964; Hoffman, 1980; Schaefer, 1965; Small, 1990). Most items composing the scales of the PBM are from previously existing instruments and were selected based on having the highest loadings on identified factors in previous factor analytic studies (Peterson et al., 1985). Many of the PBM items were taken from the 80 item Rollins and Thomas Parent Behavior Inventory that was, in turn, a distillation of the best items from the 192 item Schaeffer's Parent Behavior Inventory (Schaefer, 1965). Items that measured parental support originated from a scale developed through a factor analytic study that examined the Heilbrun (1964) and Cornell measures (Devereaux et al., 1969) of parental support. The items measuring reasoning were developed from Hoffman's (1980) conception of induction, whereas monitoring items were based on the work of several previous researchers (Small, 1990; Barber et al., 1992). Participants responded to the items composing the PBM in terms of a four-point Likert scale varying from "Strongly Agree" (SA) to "Strongly Disagree" (SD).

Perceptions of parental support were measured by three items assessing the degree to which adolescents viewed mothers and fathers as being accepting, warm, and nurturant. Specifically, the items assessed adolescents' perceptions of their parents' tendencies (1) to be there if needed, (2) give love, and (3) give approval to him/her. The 4 items that measured parental reasoning assessed the extent to which mothers and fathers are perceived as explaining to (or use reasoning with) adolescents concerning how they should feel about disciplinary circumstances and how their behavior affects the internal feelings of others. Specifically, the items provided teenagers' perceptions of their parents' tendencies to explain (1) how good adolescents should feel when something was shared with other family members, (2) how good adolescents should feel when they have done what is right, (3) how good other family members feel when something was shared with them by the adolescent, and (4) how good others feel when adolescents had done what is right. Parental punitiveness was assessed by 6 items measuring adolescents' perceptions of their mothers' and fathers' use of verbal coerciveness, physical punishment, and the imposition of arbitrary control (i.e., dysfunctional control). Specifically, the items provided adolescents' perceptions of their parents' tendencies to (1) yell at them, (2) hit them, (3) hit them when they are wrong, (4) not give them any peace, (5) not let them do what they really enjoy, and (6) not let them do things with other teenagers. Parental monitoring was measured by 4 items that assessed how much mothers and fathers are perceived as supervising adolescents' activities. The items assessed the adolescents' perceptions of the degree to which (1) parents are told where adolescents are going when the young go out, (2) parents know where the adolescents are when they are away from home, (3) parents know the adolescents' friends, (4) parents know how adolescents spend their money. When combined into scales, these observed measures of parental behavior demonstrated moderate to good internal consistency reliability, with Cronbach's alphas ranging from .71 to .84.

Conformity and Autonomy. Adolescents' reports of their conformity to mothers' and fathers' expectations were assessed by three self-report items from the Rollins and Thomas Adolescent Conformity Scale (Peterson et al., 1999; Peterson et al., 1985; Thomas, Gecas, Weigert, & Rooney, 1974). The participants responded to these items separately for mothers and fathers in terms of a four-point Likert-type items ranging from "Strongly Agree" to "Strongly Disagree." The constituent items assessed the extent to which adolescents conformed to parents' expectations about their choices of friends, decisions about education, as well as their parents' general expectations for their behavior. Specific content of these items dealt with whether the adolescent would (1) choose friends their parent preferred, (2) go to a different school that their parent wanted, and (3) would do, in general, what the parent wanted.

Moderate internal consistency was demonstrated with Cronbach's alpha reliability coefficients of .73 for adolescents' conformity to fathers' and .70 for youthful conformity to mothers' expectations.

Autonomy from parents was measured by 6 items from a scale dealing with the growth of self-direction (behavioral autonomy) by the young (Peterson et al., 1999; Sessa & Steinberg, 1991). These items measure the extent to which mothers and fathers were perceived as allowing adolescents to make their own decisions and engage in activities without excessive parental intrusion. Specific content of these items dealt with whether adolescents viewed their parents as allowing them (1) to choose their own friends, (2), enough freedom, (3) to make their own decisions, (4) to help make decisions about family matters, and (5) to make their own decisions about educational goals. Good internal consistency was demonstrated for the scale composed of these observed measures, with Cronbach's alpha reliability coefficients of .85, both for autonomy from mothers and fathers.

ANALYSIS AND RESULTS

The theoretical relationships represented by Figure 1 were tested with structural equations models consisting of five exogenous and three endogenous latent variables. Structural equation models combine the features of confirmatory factor analysis with simultaneous equation models to test theoretically based predictions in a system of variables (Bollen, 1989; Hayduk, 1987). The central idea is that sets of observed variables (e.g., quantitative measures on questionnaire items) are dependent on latent or unobserved variables that are defined through confirmatory factor analysis. The results of structural equation modeling (SEM) commonly include (1) a measurement model of latent constructs based on measured data, (2) a derived structural model that includes latent variables, (3) estimates of observed variables that are dependent on latent constructs, (4) linear structural equations reflecting theoretically based predictions. Advantages of SEM over OLS multiple regression approaches include the capacity to correct for the biasing effect of measurement error and the prevention of multicollinearity. Two empirical models, one dealing with adolescents' relationships with fathers and the other concerning adolescents' relationships with mothers, were fitted with the LISREL 8 statistical package. Results for the father's model are shown in Figure 2, while the mother's model is shown in Figure 3. Estimates were obtained through maximum likelihood, the appropriate method when the observed variables approximate a continuous level of measurement.

FIGURE 2. Model for Fathers

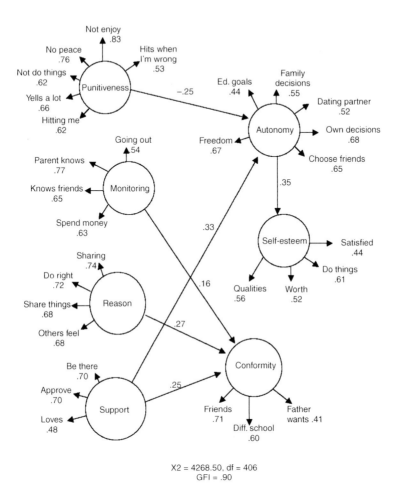

X2 = 4268.50, df = 406
GFI = .90

Tables 1 and 2 present the descriptive statistics and bivariate correlations for the data consisting of the means, standard deviations, and ranges for each variable. Results for the structural equations models are shown in Figures 2 (fathers) and 3 (mothers), with particular focus on the significant paths for the theoretical model and their associated coefficients. Both models demonstrate an adequate fit to the data, as manifested by the diagnostic values Critical N and Goodness of Fit Indices (see Figures 2 and 3), which in both cases fall within acceptable ranges. This is further supported by the RMSEA values of .05 for both the mothers' and fathers' models. Moreover, the lambda coefficients, which are akin to factor loadings, are fairly strong for all the variables, indicating that the constructs in this model have merit.

Perhaps the most central set of findings indicate that conformity to parents' expectations does not function as a mediating variable for the influence of either mothers' or fathers' parental behavior on self-esteem (see Figures 2 and 3). Although parental behaviors are moderate predictors of conformity to parents, the subsequent linkage between conformity to parents and adolescent self-esteem was not significant. Consequently, the expectation was not supported that self-esteem for Chinese adolescents would result from a collectivistic socialization pattern. Instead, both the mothers' and fathers' models sustained individualistic conceptions of self-esteem, with significant indirect paths leading from both parental punitiveness and support to self-esteem as conveyed through the mediating variable, autonomy from parents (see Figures 2 and 3). Specifically, both maternal and paternal punitiveness were negative predictors, whereas both maternal and paternal support were positive predictors of adolescent autonomy from parents. This was followed in sequence by strong predictive relationships for adolescent autonomy from both mothers and fathers on the self-esteem of Chinese youth (see Figures 2 and 3).

Although not a mediating construct, the findings were notable that conformity to parents' expectations was moderately predicted by all of the mothers' and fathers' parental behaviors, except for punitiveness (see Figures 2 and 3). Specifically, three of the exogenous parental behaviors (i.e., parental monitoring, reasoning, and support) have significant positive effects in reference to conformity to parents' expectations. Of considerable importance, therefore, is the finding that parental punitiveness failed to predict adolescent conformity to parents' expectations, whereas more moderate forms of firm control and parental support were positive predictors of responsiveness by the young to their parents' expectations. Consequently, these Chinese adolescents were more responsive to parents who use forms of parental behavior based on supervision (i.e., monitoring), rationality (i.e., reasoning), and supportiveness, rather than more dysfunctional (punitive) kinds of control. These results also indicate that maternal monitoring is the only exogenous variable to *directly* predict the self-esteem of Chinese adolescents.

An important general result of this study, therefore, was the empirical support provided for the latent constructs in the proposed model, both in terms of the confirmatory factor results (i.e., the latent variables) and some of the relationships among these constructs that were consistent with theory. Consequently, the constructs self-esteem, autonomy from parents, conformity to parents' expectations, support, monitoring, reasoning, and punitiveness were

TABLE 1. Descriptive Statistics

Latent	*Maternal Model* Observed	M SD	*Paternal Model* Observed	M SD
Punitiveness		**5.70 (5.15)**		**6.12 (5.37)**
	Hitf	1.13 (1.11)	Hitm	1.03 (1.10)
	peacef	1.22 (1.28)	peacem	1.50 (1.35)
	enjoyf	1.07 (1.24)	enjoym	1.14 (1.26)
	yellf	.81 (1.10)	yellm	.95 (1.20)
	punishf	.63 (1.05)	punishm	.72 (1.13)
	hittingf	.87 (1.07)	hittingm	.83 (1.07)
Monitoring		**7.37 (3.95)**		**8.04 (3.90)**
	wheref	1.75 (1.38)	wherem	1.91 (1.39)
	withf	2.22 (1.35)	withm	2.38 (1.27)
	whof	1.57 (1.22)	whom	1.74 (1.24)
	moneyf	1.85 (1.37)	moneym	2.01 (1.33)
Reasoning		**7.64 (3.76)**		**7.86 (3.94)**
	sharef	1.84 (1.20)	sharem	1.89 (1.22)
	dorightf	2.45 (1.10)	dorightm	2.48 (1.14)
	thingsf	1.50 (1.21)	thingsm	1.58 (1.29)
	rightf	1.89 (1.24)	rightm	1.94 (1.24)
Support		**5.67 (2.79)**		**6.36 (2.80)**
	needf	2.00 (1.23)	needm	2.27 (1.22)
	appovef	2.26 (1.10)	appovem	2.37 (1.05)
	lovemef	1.44 (1.34)	lovemem	1.74 (1.37)
Autonomy Grnt.		**17.2 (3.20)**		**17.1 (3.20)**
	freedomf	3.00 (.73)	freedomm	3.00 (.69)
	friendsf	3.01 (.70)	friendsm	2.94 (.72)
	datingf	2.60 (.85)	datingm	2.60 (.85)
	confidnf	2.84 (.76)	confidnm	2.80 (.76)
	encourgf	2.90 (.81)	encourgm	2.92 (.80)
	educf	3.05 (.71)	educm	3.05 (.69)
Conformity		**7.14 (1.61)**		**7.10 (1.67)**
	schoolf	2.34 (.74)	schoolm	2.34 (.75)
	groupf	2.20 (.71)	groupm	2.19 (.71)
	wantsf	2.64 (.71)	wantsm	2.62 (.75)
Self-Esteem		**11.7 (2.04)**		
	satisfy	2.52 (.75)		
	dothing	2.90 (.77)		
	worth	3.30 (.70)		
	quality	3.10 (.75)		

TABLE 2. Pearson's Correlation Coefficients for Paternal and Maternal Model

Variables	1	2	3	4	5	6	7
1. Self-Esteem	1.00	-.035	.185**	.175**	.156**	.259**	.144*
2. Punitiveness	-.094	1	-.037	.015	-.161**	-.179**	-.024
3. Monitoring	.127**	.016	1	.241**	.261**	.095*	.191**
4. Reasoning	.150**	-.024	.209**	1	.491**	.223**	.170**
5. Support	.120**	-.176**	.273**	.438**	1	.234**	.200**
6. Autonomy granting	.264**	-.273**	.063	.178**	.255**	1	.050
7. Conformity	.090*	-.019	.182**	.120*	.193**	.039	1

Note. Maternal correlations are in the upper diagonal and paterna correlations are in the lower diagonal. *p < .05; **p < .01

FIGURE 3. Model for Mothers

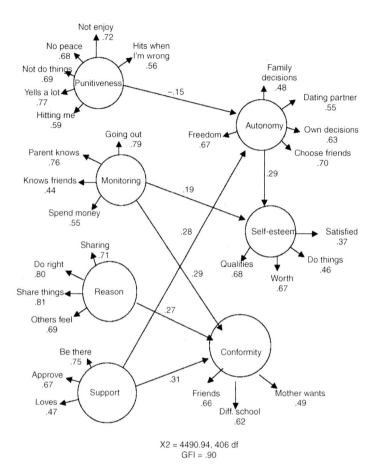

X2 = 4490.94, 406 df
GFI = .90

provided empirical support as meaningful constructs within the Chinese parent-adolescent relationship.

DISCUSSION AND CONCLUSIONS

The primary purpose of this study was to determine whether parental behaviors provided either an individualistic or collectivistic socialization climate for the development of self-esteem in Chinese adolescents (see Figure 1). Tests of a mediated effects model indicated that parental behavior influences the self-esteem of Chinese adolescents by way of indirect paths emphasizing an individualistic rather than either a collectivistic theme or one conveyed by direct effects. That is, the development of self-esteem in Chinese adolescents is the mediated consequence of two types of socialization behaviors, parental support and punitiveness, the effects of which are conveyed as adolescents either acquire or are denied autonomy (or individuality) from their parents. Rather than a collectivistic climate, adolescent self-esteem is fostered through a pattern of socialization that conveys such "individualistic" themes as the need for self-direction and personal separateness (indicated by autonomy as the mediating variable) (Cheung & Lau, 1985; Lau & Cheung, 1987).

Besides the identification of autonomy as a mediator, the fact that conformity to parents' expectations failed to predict adolescent self-esteem provided further evidence that a collectivistic conception of the self was not supported. That is, conformity to parents' expectations, an indicator of collectivism at the relationship level, failed to function as a mediator for the influences of child-rearing behaviors (i.e., reasoning, monitoring, punitiveness, support) on the self-esteem of Chinese adolescents (Gecas & Burke, 1995; Taforadi & Swann, 1996). Consequently, these results, for the particular type of self-esteem measured, did not sustain traditional Chinese conceptions of self development, but seemed more akin to Western patterns rooted in the affirmation of one's individuality. Adolescent self-esteem was encouraged by Chinese parents who fostered individualism by granting a form of autonomy facilitated by supportiveness and by avoiding punitive behavior. These findings do not preclude, of course, the possibility that other dimensions of self-esteem may exist that are based more extensively in collectivistic or relational sources (Kagitcibasi, 1996; Taforadi & Swann, 1996).

Prominent was the present finding that Chinese parents who use supportive behavior often encourage the young to become more autonomous, which, in turn, creates a relationship climate that fosters the development of adolescent self-esteem. In contrast, punitive parenting contributes to a highly restrictive climate, diminishes the ability of Chinese adolescents to assert their autonomy, and inhibits self-esteem development. In general, therefore, adolescent self-esteem is fostered when Chinese parents are supportive, refrain from dysfunctional control, and encourage autonomous behavior by the young.

Despite this evidence for individualism as the basis for self-esteem development, some findings provide moderate support for the view that Chinese parents use child-rearing strategies to foster a collectivistic relationship climate by encouraging adolescent conformity to their expectations. Specifically, several parental behaviors (i.e., reasoning, monitoring, and support) were direct positive predictors of youthful conformity to parents, suggesting that an important goal of Chinese parenting efforts is to retain influence over adolescents (though conformity is not linked, in turn, to self-esteem). Thus, while youthful self-esteem is not rooted in collectivism, other objectives of Chinese parents, such as maintaining influence over adolescents, may be moderately evident in the findings of this study.

These complicated and seemingly contradictory findings raise the possibility that general efforts to classify the socialization patterns of particular cultures as either collectivistic or individualistic may be too simplistic for the complex realities of social life. A more complicated conception is necessary, in part, due to rapid value changes occurring both across and within societies through the process of globalization. Instead, both individualistic and collectivistic orientations may coexist in varying degrees within cultures, depending upon how they are relevant to particular outcomes of socialization and are compatible with other aspects of the culture (Kagitcibasi, 1996; Peterson, 1995). Urban Chinese parents may use complementary socialization strategies to foster an individualistic form of adolescent self-esteem, while simultaneously encouraging conformity through more traditional, collectivistic approaches.

This "duality" in socialization approaches avoids the view that individualism and collectivism are contradictory forces in favor of the idea that autonomy and interdependence, at the relationship level, can potentially coexist and complement each other (Kagitcibasi, 1996). Conceptualizing the coexistence of these cultural orientations also avoids such value-laden pitfalls as equating individualism with progressive "modernity" in "advanced" societies and collectivism with "traditional" and "less advanced" cultural circumstances (Kagitcibasi, 1996; Stevenson et al., 1992; Wang & Hsueh, 2000). Instead, both individualism and collectivism are potentially complementary themes that may function together, especially when expressed in degrees appropriate to unique cultural and familial circumstances.

Results for specific parental behaviors provide additional insights into current controversies about Chinese parent-youth relations. First, these results for the supportiveness of Chinese parents stand in sharp contrast with traditional themes suggesting that warmth, compared to Western parenting, may be either emphasized or conveyed, not as a separate dimension, but more subtlely as part of the control dimension (Chao, 1994; 2000; 2001). Instead, the present data indicate that support is a distinct dimension of parental behavior that operates independently of parental control and is a positive predictor of both autonomy from and conformity to parents (Bond & Wang, 1983; Chiu, 1987; Dornbusch et al., 1987; Stevenson et al., 1992; Wu, 1996). These findings are consistent with earlier studies on Chinese parent-youth relations indicating that parental support is an important predictor of positive socialization outcomes for adolescents (Cheung & Lau, 1985; Lau & Cheung, 1987; Lin & Fu, 1990).

An interesting paradox that occurs is the way that both autonomy and conformity are jointly encouraged by supportive behavior from Chinese parents. Parental support, on the one hand, may communicate how much the young are valued and accepted and is used to foster the conformity of adolescents to their parents' expectations by fostering trust, internalized commitment, and receptivity to parental influence (Peterson et al., 1985; Rohner, 1986). Paradoxically, parental support provides the basis for a seemingly opposite development, that of the progress of adolescents toward autonomy. Specifically, supportiveness by parents provides the emotional context or a secure base, rooted partially in the acceptance of parental standards (i.e., internalized conformity to parents), from which the young safely explore beyond family boundaries (Peterson et al., 1999; Peterson & Hann, 1999). Chinese adolescents appear to use supportive parent-youth relationships as a secure base from which to engage with confidence the world outside the family and face both the risks and benefits of self-directed activities (Kobak & Sceery, 1988). Consequently, adolescents who receive sufficient parental supportiveness are more likely to balance the seemingly contradictory attributes of individuality with responsiveness to others, or prosocial attributes central to social competence (Peterson & Leigh, 1990).

Results for parental punitiveness also address a controversy on the type of parental control that is characteristic of parent-adolescent relations in China. Specifically, punitiveness failed to foster self-esteem, both by not predicting conformity to parents' expectations through the collectivistic path and by inhibiting adolescent autonomy (i.e., as a negative predictor) through the individualistic path. Such findings contradict the view that Chinese parents commonly use restrictive, autocratic, or punitive approaches to foster self-esteem or related prosocial outcomes (Chao, 1994; Chiu, 1987; Dornbusch et al., 1987; Steinberg et al., 1992; Yang, 1981, 1986). Instead, similar to Western research (Peterson & Hann, 1999), punitiveness either inhibits self-esteem by restricting the autonomy of adolescents or fails to predict self-esteem through socializing approaches emphasizing conformity to parents.

In contrast to results for punitiveness, parental reasoning and monitoring are consistent positive predictors of adolescent conformity to parents' expectations. Moreover, monitoring was the only behavior to directly predict adolescent self-esteem, demonstrating a positive relationship in the mothers' model. According to Western scholarship (Baumrind, 1991), firm control is a central feature of the authoritative parenting style and includes such practices as clearly defining rules, consistently enforcing discipline, using reason, and supervising the activities of youth (Peterson & Hann, 1999). Although disagreements exist about the comparability of Western and Chinese parenting concepts (Chao, 1994), firm control seems similar to a culturally specific form of influence defined by Chinese and Chinese-American scholars as "functional or organizational control." Specifically, functional control involves providing guidance, a clear definition of rules, firm and demanding influence, high parental involvement, and a quest for harmony (Lau & Cheung, 1987; Chao & Sue, 1996). A central feature of the similarity between "firm" and "functional" control is their shared rejection of coercive or arbitrary control, without surrendering the parents' abilities to be in charge. The results of the present findings, in turn, support the view that adolescent self-esteem and conformity to Chinese parents are fostered primarily by functional control that is neither punitive or arbitrarily restrictive (Chao, 1994).

The first dimension of functional control that fosters conformity to mothers and fathers, parental reasoning, refers to rational explanations that provide guidance and convince children to voluntarily accept their parents' viewpoints and modify their behavior (Baumrind, 1991). Adolescents use these internalized expectations as guides or standards in reference to which their behavior is governed (Peterson & Leigh, 1990). Parents often use reason to explain why role expectations and rules are important, why certain behaviors are forbidden, how the actions of adolescents will influence others, and how to take responsibility for one's own mistakes (Peterson & Hann, 1999). Such conceptions of reasoning are consistent with the Chinese emphasis on child training or teaching as embodied in the concept *chiao-yang*. This idea emphasizes that parents should actively teach and structure the child's environment, encourage character development, and mold the young to become functional members of society, all of which are compatible with fostering adolescent conformity to parents' expectations (Bernt et al., 1993; Chao, 1994, 2000, 2001; Ho, 1989; Lin & Fu, 1990).

A second dimension of functional control, parental monitoring, was a positive predictor of both conformity to parents (both mothers' and fathers' monitoring) and adolescent self-esteem (mothers' monitoring only). Monitoring refers to the extent that parents are aware of and seek to manage their adolescents' schedules, free time activities, peer associations, school work, and physical whereabouts (Barber et al., 1994; Peterson & Hann, 1999). Effective monitoring requires that parents maintain a clear set of rules about such things as the expected time to return home from school, when homework should be finished, what school grades are expected, when to return from peer activities, with whom to associate, and places to venture. Effective monitoring also requires that parents "verify" their youngster's compliance by "checking up" on them and by implementing consequences when rules are violated. Studies on children and adolescents in the U.S. have long supported the idea that self-esteem is fostered by firm (not arbitrary) parental control that provides structure and clear expectations to the young (Gecas & Seff, 1990). Chinese adolescents appear to assess their personal self-worth more favorably when the standards that parents set are clear and relatively easy to use for making self-evaluations.

Combined assessments of parental support, reasoning, and monitoring as predictors of adolescent self-esteem and conformity seem consistent with the principle of *guan*, or the Chinese belief that parents should create an atmosphere combining control and governance with care and concern (Chao, 2000; Ho, 1989). That is, common practices used by Chinese parents include supervising, governing, and controlling so that order, discipline, self-control and conformity are fostered firmly but not through punitiveness (Wu, 1996). Such aspects of firm control are complemented by parental care and concern that fosters both self-esteem and conformity, which apparently is neither a muted form of parental warmth nor one that is simply embedded in parental control. Instead, supportiveness by Chinese parents is a clearly expressed, distinctive behavior that fosters both individualistic (e.g., self-esteem) and collectivistic outcomes (e.g., conformity to parents' expectations) in the young. This finding contrasts with previous research indicating that traditional Chinese parents, especially fathers, are less warm and emotionally expressive than Western parents (Bond & Wang, 1983; Wu, 1996). Another possibility is that parental support may be an expanding dimension of Chinese parenting that fosters both newer individualistic themes as well as maintaining the traditional focus on respect for parents and filial piety (Wang & Hsueh, 2000).

Despite the logic of these results, certain methodological and sampling issues may limit the interpretation of these findings. One shortcoming was the restricted geographic area (Beijing, China) from which the sample was drawn and the resulting limitations for generalization. Moreover, the use of cross-sectional and predictive approaches means that the proposed directions of influence in the theoretical model (i.e., parental behavior as an *influence* on adolescent outcomes) were offered for heuristic value only. Other limitations involve validity issues when all the variables in the model (i.e., predictor and criterion variables) are measured from one person's (or the adolescent's) perception.

A general way of interpreting these findings, however, is that a pattern of parent-youth relationships may be emerging in China, with the result being a mixture of individualistic and collectivistic patterns, referred to as *psychological interdependence* (Ho, 1989; Wang & Hsueh, 2000). Depending upon the particular outcome addressed, parental behaviors such as support and dimensions of functional control (i.e., reasoning and monitoring) may prepare the young to pursue both personal goals that encourage their individuality and collectivistic values that sustain the more traditional focus of Chinese culture on interpersonal relatedness.

REFERENCES

Baumrind, D. (1991). Effective parenting during the early adolescent transition. In P.A. Cowan & M. Hetherington (Eds.). *Family transitions* (pp. 111-163). Hillsdale, NJ: Lawrence Erlbaum.

Barber, B.K., Chadwick, B.A., & Oerter, R. (1992). Parental behaviors and adolescent self-esteem in the United States and Germany. *Journal of Marriage and the Family, 54*, 128-141.

Berndt, T.J., Cheung, P.C., Hau, K. Lew, W. J.F. (1993). Perceptions of parenting in Mainland China, Taiwan, and Hong Kong. *Developmental Psychology, 29*, 156-164.

Bollen, K.A. (1989). Structural equations with latent variables. New York: Wiley.

Bond, M.H. & Wang, S. (1983). China: Aggressive behavior and the problems of maintaining order and harmony. In A.P. Goldstein & M.H. Segall (Eds.), Aggression in global perspective (pp. 58-74). New York: Pergamon.

Buri, J.R. (1989). Self-esteem and appraisals of parental behavior. *Journal of Adolescent Research, 4*, 33-39.

Bush, K.R., Peterson, G. W., Cobas, J.A., Supple, A. J. (2002). Adolescents' perceptions of parental behaviors as predictors of adolescent self-esteem in Mainland China. *Sociological Inquiry, 72*, 503-526.

Chao, R. K. (1994). Beyond parental control and authoritarian parenting style: Understanding Chinese parenting through the cultural notion of training. *Child Development, 65*, 1111-1119.

Chao, R.K. (2000). Cultural explanations for the role of parenting in the school success of Asian-American children. In R. Taylor & M.C. Wang (Ed.). *Resilience across contexts: Family, work, culture, and community* (pp. 333-363). Temple University: Center for Research in Human Development.

Chao, R.K. (2001). Extending research on the consequences of parenting style for Chinese Americans and European Americans. *Child Development, 72*, 1832-1843.

Chao, R. K. & Sue, S. (1996). Chinese parental influence and their children's school success: A paradox in the literature on parenting styles. In S. Lau (Ed.) *Growing up the Chinese way: Chinese children and adolescent development* (pp. 93-120). Sha Tin, N.T., Hong Kong: The Chinese University Press.

Cheung, P.C. & Lau, S. (1985). Self-esteem: Its relationship to the family and school social environments among Chinese adolescents. *Youth and Society, 16* 438-456.

Chiu, L.H. (1987). Child-rearing attitudes of Chinese, Chinese-American, and Anglo-American mothers. *International Journal of Psychology, 22*, 409-419.

Chun, Y.J. & MacDermid, S.M., (1997). Perceptions of family differentiation, individuation, and self-esteem among Korean adolescents. *Journal of Marriage and the Family, 59*, 451-462.

Cooley, C.H. (1902). *Human nature and the social order.* New York: Scribner's.

Covington, M.V. (1992). *Making the grade: A self-worth perspective on motivation and school reform.* Cambridge, England: Cambridge University.

Darling, N. & Steinberg, L. (1993). Parenting style as context: An integrative model. *Psychological Bulletin, 113*, 487-496.

Day, R., & Peterson, G., McCracken, C. (1998). Predictors of frequent spanking of younger and older children. *Journal of Marriage and the Family, 60,* 79-94.

Demo, D.H., Small, S.A., & Savin-Williams, R.C. (1987). Family relations and the self-esteem of adolescents and their parents. *Journal of Marriage and the Family, 49,* 705-715.

Devereaux, E., Bronfenbrenner, U., & Rodgers, R.R. (1969). Child-rearing in England and the United States: A cross-national comparison. *Journal of Marriage and the Family, 31,* 257-270.

Dornbusch, S.M., Ritter, P.L., Leiderman, P.H., Roberts, D.F., & Fraleigh, M.J. (1987). The relation of parenting style to adolescent school performance. *Child Development, 56,* 326-341.

Fuligni, A.J. (1998). Authority, autonomy, parent-adolescent conflict and cohesion: A study of adolescents from Mexican, Chinese, Filipino, and European Backgrounds. *Developmental Psychology, 34,* 782-792.

Gecas, V. & Burke, P.J. (1995). Self and identity. In K. S. Cook, G.A. Fine, & J.S. House (Eds.), *Sociological perspectives on social psychology* (pp. 41-67). Boston, MA: Allyn & Bacon.

Gecas, V. & Schwalbe, M. L. (1986). Parental behavior and adolescent self-esteem. *Journal of Marriage and the Family, 48,* 37-46.

Gecas, V. & Seff, M.A. (1990). Adolescents and families: A review of the 1980s. *Journal of Marriage and the Family, 52,* 941-958.

Gorman, J.C. (1998). Parenting attitudes and practices of immigrant Chinese mothers of adolescents. *Family Relations, 47,* 73-80.

Harter, S. (1999). *The construction of the self.* New York: Guilford.

Hayduk, L.A. (1987). Structural equation modeling with LISREL: Essentials and advances. Baltimore, MD: Johns Hopkins University Press.

Heilbrun, A.B. (1964). Parent model attributes, nurturant reinforcement, and consistency of behavior in adolescents. *Child Development, 35,* 151-167.

Henry, C. H., & Peterson, G. W. (1995). Adolescent social competence, parental behavior, and parental satisfaction. *American Journal of Orthopsychiatry, 65,* 249-262.

Ho, D.Y.F. (1986). Chinese patterns of socialization: A critical review. In H.M. Bond (Ed.), *The psychology of Chinese people* (pp.1-37). Hong Kong: Oxford University Press.

Ho, D. Y. F. (1989). Continuity and variation in Chinese patterns of socialization. *Journal of Marriage and the Family, 51,* 149-163.

Ho, D.Y.F. (1994). Filial piety, authoritarian moralism, and cognitive conservatism in Chinese societies. *Genetic, Social, and General Psychology Monographs, 120,* 347-365.

Hoffman, M.L. (1980). Moral development in adolescence. In J. Adelson (Ed.), *Handbook of adolescent psychology* (pp.295-343). New York: Wiley.

James, W. (1890). *Principles of psychology.* Chicago: Encyclopaedia Britannica, Inc.

Kagitcibasi, C. (1996). Family and human development across cultures: A view from the other side. Mahwah, NJ: Lawrence Erlbaum Associates.

Kelley, M.I., & Tseng, H-M. (1992). Cultural differences in child-rearing: A comparison of immigrant Chinese and Caucasian American mothers. *Journal of Cross-Cultural Psychology, 23,* 444-455.

Kobak, R. & Sceery, A. (1988). Attachment in late adolescence: Working models, affect regulation, and representation of self and others. *Child Development, 59,* 135-146.

Lam, C.M. (1997). A cultural perspective of the study of Chinese adolescent development. *Child and Adolescent Social Work Journal, 14,* 85-113.

Lau, S. & Cheung, P.C. (1987). Relations between Chinese adolescents' perception of parental control and organization and their perception of parental warmth. *Developmental Psychology, 18,* 215-221.

Lin, C.C., & Fu, V.R. (1990). A comparison of child-rearing practices among Chinese, immigrant Chinese, and Caucasian-American parents. *Child Development, 61,* 429-528.

Lui, X., Kaplan, H.B., & Risser, W. (1992). Decomposing the reciprocal relationships between academic achievement and general self-esteem. *Youth and Society, 24,* 123-148.

Mead, G.H. (1934). *Mind self & society* Chicago: The University of Chicago Press.

Meredith, W.H., Abbott, D.A., & Shu, L.T. (1989). A comparative study of only children and sibling children in the People's Republic of China. *School Psychology International, 10,* 251-256.

Owens, T. J. (1992). The effect of post high school social context on self-esteem. *Sociological Quarterly, 33,* 553-577.

Peterson, G.W. (1995). Autonomy and connectedness. In R.D. Day, K.R. Gilbert, B.H. Settles, W.R. Burr (Eds.) *Research and theory in family science.* Pacific Grove, CA: Brooks/Cole.

Peterson, G.W., Bush, K.R., & Supple, A. J. (1999). Predicting adolescent autonomy from parents: Relationship connectedness and restrictiveness. *Sociological Inquiry, 69,* 431-457.

Peterson, G. W., & Hann, D. (1999). Socializing parents and children in families. In M. B. Sussman, S. K. Steinmetz, & G. W. Peterson (Eds.). *Handbook of marriage and the family* (pp. 327-370). New York: Plenum Press.

Peterson, G.W., & Leigh, G.K. (1990). The family and social competence in adolescence. In T.P. Gullotta, G.R. Adams, & R. Montemayor (Eds.). *Developing social competency in adolescence: Advances in adolescent development. Vol. 3* (pp. 97-138). Newbury Park, CA: Sage.

Peterson, G.W., Rollins, B.C., & Thomas, D.L. (1985). Parental influence and adolescent conformity: Compliance and internalization. *Youth and Society, 16,* 297-420.

Rohner, R.P. (1986). *The warmth dimension. Foundation of parental acceptance-rejection theory.* Beverly Hills, CA: Sage Publications.

Rosenberg, M. (1965). *Society and the adolescent self-image.* Princeton, NJ: Princeton University Press.

Rosenberg, M. (1979). *Conceiving the self.* New York: Basic Books.

Sessa, F.M., Steinberg, L. (1991). Family structure and the development of autonomy during adolescence. *Journal of Early Adolescence, 11,* 38-55.

Schaefer, E.S. (1965). Children's reports of parental behavior. *Child Development, 36,* 552-557.

Small, S. (1990). Preventive programs that support families with adolescents. *Working paper: Carnegie Council on Adolescent Development.* Carnegie Corporation: Washington, DC.

Steinberg, L., Lamborn, S.D., Darling, N., Mounts, N.S., & Dornbusch, S.M. (1994). Over-time changes in adjustment and competence among adolescents from authoritative, authoritarian, indulgent, and neglectful families. *Child Development, 65,* 754-770.

Steinberg, L., Lamborn, S.D., Dornbusch, S.M., & Darling, N. (1992). Impact of parenting practices on adolescent achievement: Authoritative parenting, school involvement, and encouragement to succeed. *Developmental Psychology, 63,* 1266-1281.

Stevenson, H. W., Chen, C., & Lee, S. (1992). Chinese families. In J. L. Roopnarine & D. B. Carter (Eds.) *Parent-child socialization in diverse cultures* (pp. 17-33). Norwood, NJ: Ablex Publishing.

Tafarodi, R.W., & Swann, W.B. (1996). Individualism-collectivism and global self-esteem: Evidence for a cultural trade-off. *Journal of Cross-Cultural Psychology, 27,* 651-672.

Thomas, D.L., Gecas, V., Weigert, A., & Rooney, E. (1974). *Family socialization and the adolescent.* Lexington, MA: Lexington Books.

Triandis, H.C. (1989). The self and social behavior in differing cultural contexts. *Psychological Review, 96,* 506-520.

Triandis, H.C. (1995). *Individualism & collectivism.* Boulder, CO: Westview Press.

Triandis, H.C., McCusker, C., & Hui, C.H. (1990). Multimethod probes of individualism and collectivism. *Journal of Personality and Social Psychology, 59,* 1006-1020.

Wang, Q. & Hsueh, Y. (2000). Parent-child interdependence in Chinese families: Change and continuity. In C. Violato & E. Oddone-Paolucci (Eds.) *The changing family and child development* (pp. 60-69). Aldershot, England: Ashgate Publishing Ltd.

Wolf, M. (1970). Child training and the Chinese family. In M. Freedman (Ed.), *Family and kinship in Chinese society.*

Wu, D.Y.H. (1996). Chinese childhood socialization. In M. H. Bond (Ed.), *The handbook of Chinese psychology* (pp. 143-154). Hong Kong: Oxford University Press.

Yang, K.S. (1981). Social orientation and modernity among Chinese students in Taiwan. *Journal of Social Psychology, 113,* 159-170.

Yang, K.S. (1986). Chinese personality and its change. In M. Bond (Ed.), *The psychology of the Chinese people* (pp. 106-170). New York: Oxford University Press.

Yau, J. & Smetana, J.G. (1996). Adolescent-parent conflict among Chinese adolescents in Hong-Kong. *Child Development, 67,* 1263-1275.

Parental
versus Government Guided Policies:
A Comparison of Youth Outcomes
in Cuba and the United States

Suzanne K. Steinmetz

ABSTRACT. This paper examines the outcomes of youth who live in Cuban and United States societies characterized by two distinct political systems. Although both societies claim to be child-centered, the value placed on health care, especially for children, and education, as well as the percentage of the budget allocated to support children is greater in Cuba than the United States. It also appears that, though the United States is a major world power that leads in technology and medical advance, there are few differences between the two nations in health and educational outcomes. In fact, statistics from numerous sources demonstrate the greater success of Cuban youth in terms of educational attainment, health promotion activities, and avoidance of negative outcomes as a result of risky behaviors. *[Article copies available for a fee from The Haworth Document Delivery Service: 1-800-HAWORTH. E-mail address: <docdelivery@haworthpress.com> Website: <http://www.HaworthPress.com> © 2004 by The Haworth Press, Inc. All rights reserved.]*

Suzanne K. Steinmetz is affiliated with the Department of Sociology, Indiana University-Purdue University at Indianapolis.

Address correspondence to: Suzanne K. Steinmetz, 425 University Blvd., IUPUI, Indianapolis, IN 46202 (E-mail: sksteinm@iupui.edu).

The author thanks Yaima Gonzalez, a sociology student at the University of Havana, Cuba, for her valuable assistance in locating sources of data and providing the translation. The author also thanks Elizabeth Henderson, a sociology graduate student at Indiana University-Purdue University at Indianapolis, for locating sources of data and analyzing the data on parenting used in this paper.

http://www.haworthpress.com/web/MFR
© 2004 by The Haworth Press, Inc. All rights reserved.
Digital Object Identifier: 10.1300/J002v36n03_10

KEYWORDS. Adolescence, communism, Cuba, parenting, youth, political systems, United States

INTRODUCTION

In Cuba, the real parent is the Marxist state.

–Quoted by Jeff Jacoby after reviewing Cuba's Code of the Child

Cuba has been both a thorn in the United States' side and a major curiosity because of its Communist government and ability to adapt and modernize in spite of numerous challenges. Cuba's strong commitment to the highest quality of health and educational accomplishments far exceed what one might anticipate in a relatively poor Caribbean island. Cuba, which is about the size of Pennsylvania, has 11 million people of whom 70% live in urban areas. The racial composition is 37% white; 11% black; 1% Chinese, and 51% mulatto (Bureau of Western Hemisphere Affairs, 2002). The workforce of 4.5 million is composed of government and services (30%), industry (22%); agriculture (20%), commerce (11%), construction (11%), as well as transportation and communications (6%). About 70 percent of the population lives in urban areas, with Havana, the largest city, having a population of 2 million, which is six times larger than the next largest city (U.S. Department of State, 1998; Latin American Alliance, 1997). In rural areas there are one room schools as well as schools that serve only a few students.

A LIVING MARXIAN LABORATORY

A Different Paradigm

In many ways Cuba can be thought of as a living Marxian Laboratory. Although the material provided below might suggest an overwhelming positive appraisal of Cuba's political, educational, health and economic system, this is not the goal. However, in order to assess the effectiveness of Cuba's ruling regime in supporting the welfare of children and parents, one must do so under the values and operating principles of the system. Consequently, this goal will be evaluated within the context of Cuban efforts (1) to provide a classless society, (2) to provide equal access to health care, education, and cultural enrichment, and (3) to have all citizens buy into the same value system.

Children and youth are considered Cuba's most valuable resource and the programs provided to them reinforce this value at all levels. Families in rural areas may not have electricity for cooking but their children will have access to electricity for computers. In times of food or medical shortages, children, especially young children, are always the first priority. Thus, an examination of various youth outcomes that result from the different values, health care and educational systems of Cuba can provide some interesting insights into the issue of cultural variability.

The Communist Manifesto: 10 Goals

In many ways, the values and goals held by the government and citizens of Cuba mirror many of the goals described by Marx and Engels in their 1884 publication of *The Communist Manifesto*. Thus, a review the 10 goals as stated in *The Communist Manifesto* (Marx & Engels, 1948:30-31) provide a basis for the ideology that shapes many of the family and community decisions that make Cuba unique. The first three: (1) the abolition of property in land and the application of all rents of land to public purposes; (2) implementation of a heavy progressive or graduated income tax, and (3) the abolition of all right of inheritance, a policy intended to level the playing field for each succeeding generation. The fourth goal, (4) the confiscation of the property of all emigrants and rebels had the effect of redistributing property. Those who chose to stay in Cuba kept their homes, whereas those who left had their property confiscated and turned into museums, governmental buildings or multi-family housing. It is interesting to note that the tax structure in the United States also attempts to level the intergenerational playing field to a much lesser degree through graduated income taxes and inheritance taxes.

Nationalization and centralization of a national bank, factories, and the means of communication and transport in the hands of the state (goals 5-7) are mechanisms not only of control by the government, but of efficiency. For contemporary society, this enables the government to quickly establish the needed industries (e.g., the rapid development of their oil industry when the U.S.S.R. collapsed); finance those family-related programs it deems most important; as well as controlling the means of communication to assure that the politically endorsed message is delivered.

The next two goals revolve around work and education: (8) equal obligation of all to work and the establishment of industrial armies especially for agriculture; (9) the gradual abolition of the distinction between town and country by more equally distributing the population over the country. This philosophy was further elaborated by Jose Martí, a national hero of Cuba, who specifically condemned the separation of work from study in modern education as "a monstrous crime" and "an error of the utmost gravity." Martí suggested that in the future every school should operate an "agricultural station" in which the students would be able to not only describe but handle a plough (Cheng & Manning, 2003). Marx once commented positively on the implementation of the British Factory Reform Act of 1864, which proposed a half-day study, half-day labor project for working-class children (Marx, 1936 p. 526 as cited by Cheng & Manning, 2003). Marx also suggested that this integration of education with labor would "raise the working class far above the level of the higher and middle class" (Marx, 1973 p. 113 as cited by Cheng & Manning, 2003).

The 10th goal further elaborated on the importance of free education for all children in public school, the abolition of child factory labor in its present form, and the combination of education with industrial production. Karl Marx conceptualized the future of education in terms of emphasizing the integration of work and study. For Marx, the development of a "well-developed man" in communist society, as opposed to the alienated man under capitalism, required thorough educational reform. Although proposed by Marx and Engels in 1848, it was during the 20th century that free public education became widely available in most western and developing societies and child labor was abolished.

Applying These Principles

One's mindset shapes our view of various situations. If the goal is that all children should have equal access to resources needed to create circumstances of equality, then children from families with more challenges (e.g., such as a parent with a chronic mental or physical illness, or one who is hospitalized or in prison) must be provided with additional resources to compensate for his or her family situation. Likewise, children who reside in outlying geographic areas should have access to the same resources as do children living in tourist-rich, and therefore currency-rich, cities. This may mean that a family will be provided with solar panels so that their children, who live far from other residential areas, may have the same access to computers (even when they lack electricity) as youth who live in cities (Grogg, 2003). Having goals of "equality" also means that children from families who face challenges do not produce a subsequent generation of disadvantaged children. Thus, every attempt is made to avoid the "cycle of poverty" that is characteristic of the underclass in the U.S.

A personal experience, as a member of a humanitarian group that has taken medical, educational, and personal items to Cuba, illustrates how difference between the Cuban and American value system can effect decisions.

When viewed from the perspective that *all* children should have equal access to all resources, it make sense that those students who attended schools in tourist areas would receive many more gifts than students in outlying areas if care was not taken by the government to redistribute these goods. In the United States, we express support for the value of equality for all children. However, in reality this value is more in terms of providing a safety net for the disadvantaged than in providing a totally level playing field for all children. Thus, providing additional resources for our own children (or those selected for us to interact with) is not seen as a conflict with our value of equality.

As a result, many in our humanitarian group were disappointed when they learned that the gifts given to the children with whom we directly interacted would not remain in the specific school we visited, but were to be sent to a re-distribution center. Instead, members of our group viewed this as denying *these* children the extra gifts, rather than viewing it from the perspective of the Cuban value system in which the goal truly is to share resources among *all* children.

Another value that has been observed is use of scientific research as the foundation for decision making. Since policies are not party-bound, the goal of deciding the best way to prevent or intervene in a problem is approached as a scientific endeavor. When Attention Deficit Disorder (ADD) in children became a growing problem, the situation was investigated and remedial and pre-ventative programs were enacted in a manner that resulted in reducing the problem. Likewise, when teenage pregnancy became a growing problem, this was approached in a manner similar to that used in most European societies, with early, realistic education combined with the availability of contraception. This is in direct contrast to the approach in the U.S. of "Just say no" or to have youth take a pledge of virginity.

Health care and education is the primary focus of the Cuban government and results of this effort are reflected in comparisons with the U.S. on mea-sures of health status and educational attainment. For the larger Cuban society and the government, their children represent the human capital for the next generation. The government recognizes that the future of their society is intri-cately tied to the health and education of their youth. An inevitable conclu-sion, therefore, is that resources required to support these programs must be preserved at all costs.

Measuring Parenting Attitudes and Values

Measuring individual attitudes and beliefs on parenting in a society in which the State defines these matters is problematic. Jacoby (2000), in a sum-mary of some of the articles in Law 16: *Code of the Child,* notes some of the values as expressed in this code:

The communist formation of the younger generation is a valued aspiration of the state, the family, the teachers, the political organizations, and the mass organizations that act in order to foster in youth the ideological values of communism. (Article 3)

In article 5, the emphasis is on developing the youths' personality: "Society and the state watch to ascertain that all persons who come in contact with the child . . . constitute an example for the development of his communist personality." This is further reinforced in Article 8: "Society and the state work for the efficient protection of youth against all influences contrary to their communist formation" (Jacoby, 2000).

Thus, examining difference in expressed childrearing beliefs would not appear to be fruitful, or even possible. However, one can indirectly measure the efficacy of these beliefs by examining family circumstances and youth outcomes.

DEMOGRAPHICS, HEALTH CARE AND EDUCATION

Demographic Characteristics

Although Cuba is a relatively poor country with few resources when compared to the United States, many indicators of health, sociodemographics, and socioeconomic indicators in Cuba are comparable to those in the U.S. Many of these indicators provide substantial insight into the circumstances and general welfare of parents, children, and adolescents in Cuba. For example, the Cuban life expectancy at birth in 2003 was 74.7 years for males and 79.4 years for females. These life expectancy averages are similar to the comparable U.S. statistics for the same year of 74.4 and 80.0 years for males and females respectively (World Factbook, 2003). One difference observed was in the annual rate of population growth of 0.34% (one of the lowest in the Caribbean), was lower than the U.S. rate of 0.92%. Two factors contribute to the similarities in total median age of 35.8 years for U.S. and 34.5 years for Cuba: a low birth rate and increasing life expectancy (World Factbook, 2003).

Decreasing Infant Mortality and Low Birthweight. Infant mortality in Cuba by the end of 1997 had reached a low of 7.2 per 1000 live births, compared with 7.9 in 1996. Infant mortality rates for 2002 are similar for both countries: 7.15 deaths/1,000 live births in Cuba and 6.75 deaths/1,000 live births in the U.S. (World Factbook, 2003) However, the infant mortality rates in 2002 reported for Washington, DC, for minority and poor women was about twice the rate reported for the larger U.S. population (Chelala, 1998; De La Osa, 2004;

The State of the World's Children, 2004). Comparable differences in infant mortality rates based on geographic area, SES, or race do not exist in Cuba. In contrast, in the United States, African Americans and Hispanics have infant mortality rates that are two to three times higher than among Caucasian groups.

Mortality for children under 5 years of age were 9/1,000 for Cuba in 2002 and 8/1,000 for the U.S. (The State of the World's Children, 2004, Table 1). However, the tremendous improvement in both Cuba's and the United States' health care can be seen by examining the data for 1960 and 2002. Between 1960 and 2002, U.S. reduced infant mortality for youth under 5 from 30/1,000 to 8/1,000. Cuba experienced an even more dramatic reduction from 54/1,000 in 1960 to 9/1,000 in 2002 (The State of the World's Children, 2004, Table 1).

Cuba's prenatal health care and education has resulted in decreasing the percentage of low birthweight infants (less than 2,500 grams) to 6%; comparable percentage of low birthweight infants in the U.S. is 8% (The State of the World's Children, 2004, Table 2). Cuba now ranks among the 25 countries in the world with the lowest infant mortality. See data summarized in Table 1.

Standard of Living. The standard of living, specifically the discrepancy between those in the most privileged social classes and those lacking access to resources, had been identified as a major factor in a number of high risk behaviors by the young, such as lowered educational motivation that results in dropping out of school (Applebee, Langer, & Mullis, 1986). Youth from economically disadvantaged homes are twice as likely as middle-income youth and nearly 11 times more likely than high-income youth to drop out of school (Sherman, 1994). Minority youth and youth from lower SES are also more likely to engage in delinquent and risky behaviors such as substance

TABLE 1. General Indicators of Health*

	Cuba	U.S.
Infant mortality under 1/1,000 (2002)	7	7
Under 5 mortality	9	8
Rank of country** (2002)	152	158
Percent of infants with low birthweight***	6%	8%
Percent immunized 2002****	98-99%	88-94%
HIV/AIDS 2001 children 0-14	1<100	10,000
Contraceptive prevalence (1995-2002)	73%	76%

* Data adapted from The State of the World's Children (2004) Tables 1, 2, 3, 4, 8.
** Countries ranked with highest rank indicate a low number of infant mortality under 5 years. of age. Sweden received the highest rank, 193, with 3 death/1,000
*** The most recent year available between 1998-2002
**** TB, DPT3, Polio3, HebB3

TABLE 2. Comparison of Homicide and Suicide Victims per 100,000: Cuba and United States

	Age Groups			
Suicide*	**5-14**		**15-29**	
	Males	Females	Males	Females
Cuba	-----	-----	16.4	9.5
	(N = 5)	(N = 6)	(N = 235)	(N = 130)
U.S.	1.2	0.4	20.2	3.7
	(N = 241)	(N = 83)	(N = 5,718)	(N = 1,029)
Homicide**				
Cuba	-----	-----	35.7	15.7
	(N = 17)	(N = 14)	(N = 511)	(N = 208)
U. S.	3.0	2.2	44.2	8.3
	(N = 894)	(N = 613)	(N = 12,511)	(N = 2,297)

* Cuban data is for 1997, U.S. data for 1998. Data adapted from Dahlberg, Mercy, Zwi, & Lozano, R. (2002). World Report on Violence and Health. Geneva: World Health Organization. Table A.9: Mortality Caused by Suicide.
** Cuban data is for 1997, U.S. data for 1998. Data adapted from Dahlberg, Mercy, Zwi, & Lozano, R. (2002). World Report on Violence and Health. Geneva: World Health Organization. Table A.7: Mortality Caused by Intentional Injury.

abuse and risky sexual behavior (see Steinmetz, 1999 for a discussion of these findings).

Demographic data from international sources (World Health Organization, 2002; World Factbook, 2003; and World Bank, 2002) as well as published studies, report that gender, social class, and race do not operate as factors predicting school leaving, literacy rate, and youth-related problems in Cuba.

Homelessness and Home Ownership. In Cuba, 85% of people own their own homes and do not pay property taxes on those homes (Castro, 2003; Lippman, 2001). Home ownership is the universal goal for all citizens in Cuba. Although there are no homeless people, the housing shortage is extremely severe, especially in areas such as Havana, characterized by tourism.

By comparison, homelessness represents a growing problem in the U.S., with families constituting a growing proportion of this population. A study of the homeless in the U.S. estimates that 80% are temporarily homeless (one short spell), 10% are episodically homeless (intermittent frequency, usually for short periods), and 10% are chronically homeless (protracted and frequent homeless experience, often lasting a year or longer). Approximately 200,000 individuals will experience chronic homelessness each year (U.S. Department of Health and Human Services, 2003). A United States Cities Mayors' Survey (2002) found that requests for emergency shelter assistance grew an average of 19% in the 518 cities that reported an increase, the steepest rise in a decade.

A lack of secure housing has impact on youth in numerous ways. Homelessness and constant moving contributes to truancy and dropping out of school (Donahue & Tuber, 1995; Winborne & Murray, 1992; Horowitz, Springer & Kose, 1988). Although the national dropout rate is just above 28%, this rate ranges between 40 to 70% in some of larger urban school districts where homelessness is a greater problem, with percentages increasing annually (Sherman, 1994).

Family Wealth. Attempting to compare economic factors for the average income of individuals in the U.S. and Cuba is like comparing oranges and watermelons. In the UNICEF report, *The State of the Worlds Children, 2004* (Table 7), the Gross National Income/per capita (GNI) for Cuba in U.S. dollars in 2002 was $1,170 and for U.S. it was $35,060. The annual growth rate between 1990 and 2002 was 3.7% for Cuba and 2.1% for the United States.

Another measure is the Household Wealth Index (Prescott-Allen (2001) based on data collected during the mid-to-late 1990s and is the average of indicators of needs and income. A higher value indicates a greater level of household wealth. Based on this index, the U.S. has a score of 85.00 while Cuba has a score of 37.00. However, this does not take into account the high level of subsidies for housing and housing-related costs, food, transportation as well as the free education and health care provided by the Cuban government.

Although the average Cuban salary is only about 200-250 pesos/month (the Cuban peso is roughly exchanged at the rate of 20 to the U.S. dollar), this can provide a skewed comparison. Cubans do not pay taxes and rent (for the minority who do not yet own their home), utilities, food and clothing is heavily subsidized. Lippman (2001) provides the following comparisons between Havana and Los Angeles. In Havana, the monthly gas, electricity, water and phone bill is $0.11, $0.80, $0.06 and $0.40 respectively. For comparison purposes, in Los Angeles, the average monthly cost would be: $40.00 for gas, $70.00 for electricity, $25.00 for water, and $30.00 for the phone. Furthermore, there is virtually no cost associated with health care and education (from daycare and kindergarten to graduate and professional degrees) in Cuba.

Access to Communication. Most Cuban homes have television or access to TV, and some hotels and bars have cable TV, including ESPN, HBO, CNN, and Mexican stations. In a speech given in December 2002, Castro reported that in rural areas without electricity, the use of solar panels has enabled the establishment of 1,885 television and video clubs to serve one-half million citizens and made computers available in 2,300 country schools that lacked electricity. To emphasize the importance of education, Castro further noted that ". . . we have brought electricity to all of the country's rural schools. Not electricity for cooking, but electricity for televisions and computers in the schools" (Castro, 2003; Grogg, 2003). In a speech in 2004, Castro reported that all schools now have computers.

Cuban citizens also have access to a range of Western media and are quite aware of current cultural trends and technological innovations. Because a large number of citizens have relatives in the United States or other economically enriched countries, many citizens have access to the same range of technology "toys" as are found in the U.S. Many resources such as telephones and access to the Internet are in short supply, primarily because of the lack of infrastructure to support the demand. In 2001 there were 112 phones and 50 Internet users/100 population in the United States compared to 5 phones and 1 Internet user/100 population in Cuba (The State of the World's Children, 2004, Table 5). On a recent visit to Cuba, the tour guide remarked that we [Cubans] live in a third world country but we have a first world mindset and knowledge.

Divorce and Single Parent Families. The U.S. divorce rate of with 4.35 divorces/1000 inhabitants currently ranks third among all surveyed nations (Aneki.com, 2003). Divorce or single parenthood is much less of a problem in some countries such as Sweden or Cuba because child-related services are enriched for children from divorced or single-parent families. However, in the U.S. single parenthood is linked to lower SES and a range of parent-youth problems. In Cuba, no SES differences are observed between single and two-parent families. Not only are additional resources provided in day cares and schools for children from families facing challenges, SES differences are extremely small. Thus, the relationship between single-parent families, poverty and high rates of teen pregnancy, delinquency, school dropouts, and substance abuse prevalent in the U.S. (Lerner & Galambos, 1998; Jarjoura, Triplett, & Brinker, 2002; Steinmetz, 1999; White, 2002) do not appear to be prevalent in Cuba.

Gender Equity. The Gender Equity Index (Prescott-Allen, 2001) is based on the ratio of male to female income, the difference between male and female school enrollment rates, and the percentage of seats in the national parliament held by women. A higher value on this index indicates better gender equity. Based on data collected from the 180 countries during the mid-to-late 1990s, Sweden, a country that actively supports gender equity, received a high score of 82.0. Cuba and the U.S. had similar scores of 51 and 58 for Cuba and the U.S. respectively.

Health Care

In Cuba, with a population of about 11 million, there are 22 medical schools resulting in a physician per population ratio in Cuba of 1 per 255 as compared to a ratio in the U.S. of 1 per 430 (Waitzkin, Wald, Kee, Danielson, & Robinson, 1997). This small island has 222 Research centers (employing 34,000 people) and 1.8 scientists and engineers for every 1,000 inhabitants (Grogg, 1999). It is widely acknowledged that the efforts and material resources devoted to health care have been a good investment. Freid and Gaydos (2002) note that Cuba (along with Costa Rica and Jamaica) has much better health outcomes such as life expectancy at birth and child survival than might be predicted based on the relatively low GNPs per capita. The Cuban government contributes to 88% of the cost of health care and 8.2% of Cuba's GNP spent on health care compared to U.S. which spends about 6.5% of the GNP on health care (Fried & Gaydos, 2002).

Lippman (2001) reports that foreigners often travel to Cuba to take advantage of its advanced medical technologies that provide Cuba with a source of hard currency. As an example, he notes that Cuba has used lasers with acupuncture, a practice developed in China for some time. In contrast, enabling legislation for this technique has yet to be adopted in the U.S. Health care researchers have taken note of Cuba's innovative public health initiative, treatment in green medicine and thermalism, as well high-technology achievement in pharmacology, biotechnology, surgical procedures and HIV care (Waitzkin et al., 1997). Cuba has developed the only effective vaccines against meningitis meningococcus groups B and C, vaccines for hepatitis B and monoclonal antibodies used to prevent the rejection of transplanted organs (Grogg, 1999). Currently, the Cuban Neuroscience Center is part of a nine country project, mapping the brain using Cerebral Electrical Tomography (Riera, 2004).

In a *British Medical Journal* article, Veeken (1995) noted that, in spite of the "special period," the years following the 1989 Soviet collapse and the end of support to Cuba, as well as the 35+ year trade embargo by the U.S., Cuban health figures are on par with developed countries having 20 times the Cuban budget. Most noteworthy, however, is that the Cuban health system guarantees accessibility to the entire population, is free of charge, and emphasizes preventative medicine.

In 1997, several diseases, such as congenital syphilis, meningitis, tetanus, and typhoid fever, reached their lowest rates ever (Chelala, 1998). By early 1999, The National Vaccination Program protected the population against 13 preventable diseases. These significant advances happen at a time of continuing restrictions in food and medicines as a consequence of the embargo imposed by the United States. The State of the World's Children (2004) reports that Cuba's youth immunization rates are 98-99%; comparable rates for the U.S. were 88-94% (see Table 1).

Education

Education is a critical variable not only for defining the level of modernization and standard of living in a society, but also because education is so critically linked to social class, standard of living, and the ability to make informed decisions. For youth, fulfilling educational goals provides a mechanism for preparing for the workforce; dropping out of school has been linked to a variety of negative outcomes such as delinquency, early pregnancy, unemployment, and substance abuse (Steinmetz, 1999). Thus the value a society places on education, and the resources devoted to this enterprise, provides insights into current and future ability to meet societies' demands.

Education is held in very high esteem in Cuba, with literacy being one of Castro's first goals. As a UNESCO foreword for a Cuban education report in 1975 pointed out, it was "one of the extreme cases where everything in the education system constitutes a break, not only with the past, but also with what exists everywhere" (Figueroa, Prieto, & Gutierrez, 1974, p.3, as cited by Cheng & Manning, 2003).

In the Third World, educational innovations in Cuba were considered to be an efficient procedure making education and literacy universally available. As Castro stated, "In the future, practically every plant, agricultural zone, hospital, and school will become a university" and "One day we will all be intellectual workers!" (Castro, (n.d.) Revolutionary Offensive. p. 217; Castro, (n.d.) Fidel Castro on Chile, p. 134, As cited in Cheng & Manning, 2003).

Literacy. As a result of emphasis placed on education, Cuban citizens are extremely well educated with literacy rates of 97% using the criteria "15 or older can read or write." The U.S. literacy rate was also 97%, but this was based on a 1979 estimate (World Factbook, 2003). In "The State of the World's Children," a 2004 UNICEF publication, the Cuban literacy rate was 97%, whereas there was NO information on literacy rates for the U.S. In fact a fairly comprehensive search did not reveal a more recent national literacy rate that was easily accessible.

However, the National Institute for Literacy (2004:2) did report that 40%-60% of college freshmen need remedial courses, and international comparisons of 16-18-year-olds revealed that even the top 10% in the U.S. cannot compete with the top 10% of comparable students in other industrialized countries. This article also noted that many of the 25% of high school students who leave school without a diploma do so because serious reading problems do not enable them to do the required coursework. Furthermore, reading levels were found to decline between 4th and 8th grades and again between 8th and 12th grade (National Institute for Literacy, 2004). This is a curious finding given that those who experience less success in school are more likely to have dropped out between the 10th and 12th grades, leaving the better students in school.

Willms and Somers (2001:409), using UNESCO data from the third and fourth grades in 100 schools in 13 Latin American countries, found that "The most successful country, Cuba, has uniformly effective schools, and relatively small inequities along social class lines and between the sexes" (National Institute for Literacy (2004:2). This finding is also supported by the virtually identical percentage of males and females who are literate. Unlike the data reported from Cuba, race and socioeconomic status does influence literacy rates in the United States. When average non-white or more disadvantaged 8th graders were compared with white or more advantaged students, they read at three to four grade levels lower.

These data did not go unnoticed in Cuba. In a speech on May 26, 2003, Castro noted the statistics from a UNESCO study on education. He reported that Cuban students in

> fourth and fifth grades of grammar school have almost twice the knowledge in language skills and mathematics as children of the same age in the rest of Latin America, and not just Latin America but the United States as well. (Castro, 2003)

Recently Cuba was awarded the UNESCO sponsored Rey Sejong Honorary Mention for Literacy based on its development of a high quality system of education over the past 40 years that has provided literacy and education to many peoples in less developed areas of the world (Castañeda, 2003). By comparison, in the United States, television commercials suggest that many parents are purchasing products such as "Hooked on Phonics," and the nationwide system of Sylvan Learning Centers for reading and mathematics to overcome the shortfall in the U.S. educational system.

FAMILY-YOUTH PROBLEMS

The focus in this section is to compare a variety of family-related problems and their effect on U.S. and Cuban youth. Although it is not possible to directly connect the health and educational status with youth related problems, difference in outcomes between the countries cannot be overlooked. In this section we will examine youth with educational challenges, dropping out of school, homicide and fatal child abuse, suicide, pregnancy, abortion, STDs, and runaway teens.

Youth with Educational Challenges. The links between infant and toddler care and later cognitive abilities has also been explored in numerous studies. The effect that nutrition in infants and children has on cognitive development has been well-documented in numerous counties (Mendeza & Adair, 1999; Pollitt, Gorman, Engle, Rivera, & Martorell, 1995; Scrimshaw, 1998). These data were noted by Castro who stated that if children are not provided with all of the required nutrients up until two and a half years of age, they will reach the age of six and begin school with a diminished intelligence in comparison with children who receive adequate nutrition. He noted that ". . . one of the most essential things, if we advocate equality, is the right to reach the age of six with the mental capacity with which a child is born . . ." (Castro, 2003:9).

Later in this speech Castro emphasized the importance of every child being in school ". . . at this moment, we have every case recorded, and not only the children, but also the slightly more than 140,000 people with some form of mental incapacity. All children with some type of physical or mental disability, or who are blind, or deaf-mute, or something even more terrible, blind and deaf-mute at the same time, are all registered" (Castro, 2003:12). Data from Cuban scientists at a recent Cuba-U.S. Workshop on Biological Psychiatry noted that 45% of mental retardation is linked to pre-natal factors; only 15.9% is genetically based (Riera, 2004).

Research in the United States has documented increasing levels of depression, including clinical depression and dysphoric mood (Craighead, 1991; Rutter, 1995), both of which have been related to numerous problem behaviors in children and adolescents. In *The State of America's Children* (Children's Defense Fund, 1995), an estimated 7.7 million youth in the United States were reported to suffer from serious emotional disorders. Not only do 48% of these youth drop out of high school compared with 30% of youth with other disabilities, but 73% are arrested within five years of leaving school (Children's Defense Fund, 1995).

Cuba has 55,000 children enrolled in special education schools from 6th to 9th grade. Children without the cognitive ability to attend senior high school up to 12th grade or to attend a technological school for vocational training, remain in school to complete the work expected in 9th grade and are provided with skill training and a job based on that skill (Castro, 2003).

In 2002, 19% of 4th graders, 17% of 8th graders, and 11% of 12th graders in United States were identified as special needs students. Other NAEP assessments show a pattern of increasing numbers of special needs students (Plisko, 2002). Furthermore, in 1996, approximately 79% of public school teachers had mainstreamed students with disabilities. The experiences of the learning-disabled youth may be even more stressful and lead to a higher incidence of behavioral dysfunction. Zeitlin (1993) noted that learning-disabled students faced the additional tasks of trying to fit the norms of achievement exhibited by peers and siblings, while attempting to overcome their parents' over-protective behavior. The most recent remedy, "No Child Left Behind" (Bush, January 8, 2002), is an attempt to remedy identified shortcomings in our educational system. However, many school-related problems begin in the home.

Unfortunately, social service programs, especially those that provide access to health care and adequate diet for all children, are being cut. One cannot forget that that during the Reagan administration, the government unsuccessfully attempted to define ketchup as a vegetable in school lunches. However, in 1998 the Agriculture Department decreed that school lunch programs can use salsa as a component of a nutritionally balanced menu, enabling it to be a reimbursable item under the federal school lunch program (Associated Press, July 1, 1998).

Dropping Out of School. There are numerous obstacles to achieving independence today. Unlike earlier eras when youth dropped out of school in order to supplement the family income–an indication of a sense of responsibility and maturity–today's youth tend to drop out of school because they lack the ability or maturity to complete the tasks required in school or behave in an acceptable way.

The U.S. Department of Justice (1996) estimates that 80% of individuals currently incarcerated started out as truants and an even higher rate is observed among juvenile offenders. Truancy is clearly the gateway to crime; daytime burglary, vandalism, and violent juvenile crime have been linked to truancy (Steinmetz, 1999).

The graduation rate for 1995-96 was 71.5% suggesting that approximately 30% of our youth, attending both public and private schools, do not graduate from high school (Snyder, Hoffman, & Geddes, 1996, Table 98). Since the mid-1960s when rates of 75-76% for high school graduation were observed, there has been a continual decrease in the percentage of students graduating. Those graduating from high school not only have advantages in terms of occupational opportunities, but they are also extremely likely to continue their education. Furthermore, early warning signals exist that predict, with 75% accuracy, those students who are at risk for dropping by the 3rd grade (Finn, 1989) and with 90% accuracy by the 9th grade (Lloyd, 1978).

Data from the World Bank (2002) provides information on the Cuban secondary educational system, which has a large vocational component for the less academically inclined secondary students. The United States and Cuba share considerable similarities in terms of enrollment status. The net primary enrollment for 2000, i.e., the percent of relevant age group enrolled, was 97.3% for Cuba and 94.4% for the United States; net primary enrollment in secondary school was 82.2% for Cuba and 88.1% for the U.S.

Homicide and Fatal Child Abuse. Noting that the U.S. may more carefully investigate child deaths, a report from the United Nations Children's Fund reported that each week there were 27 abuse-related deaths in the U.S. and along with Mexico and Portugal the U.S. leads the world's 27 richest nations in deaths from child abuse (Dowdy, 2003). Although it is not possible to assume that child abuse cases were considered as homicide, there were clear differences in the rates of victims of homicide.

Homicide data was obtained from the World Report on Violence and Health Organization (Krug, Dahlberg, Mercy, Zwi, & Lozano, 2002, Table A9) and reports data from Cuba in 1997 and from the U.S. in 1998. Several patterns are observable. First, in general, males are more likely to be victims of homicide than females. Second, U.S. males in the 15-29 age group were somewhat more likely to be victims than Cuban males (16.4 versus 20.2 for Cuba and U.S. respectively). Third, in the older age group, Cuban females were about 2.5 times more likely to be victims of homicide than were U.S. females (see Table 2). One similarity between the countries was that the age group 15-29 years was the category most likely to be victims of homicide.

Suicide. The Suicide rate of adolescents and young adult provides insights into the general chemical imbalances that may have genetic links as well as the result of social and economic factors that may result in the individual no longer being able to cope. Data from the World Health Organization (2002, Table A.9) found only 5 suicides for males and 6 suicides for females in Cuba for youth 5 to 14 years of age. Rates for those 15-29 years old were 16.4 and 9.5.1/100,000 for males and females, respectively. Data for the U.S., collected during 1998, found rates of 1.2/100,000 for males and 0.4/100,000 in the 5-14 age group. For those youth in the 15-29 age group, the rates were 20.2/100,000 for males and 3.7/100,000 for females (World Health Organization, 2002, Table A.9).

Three patterns were found when examining the data on suicide. First, in general, males have higher rates of suicide than do females. Second, although females in the 1-14 age group in the U.S. were more likely to commit suicide than comparable females in Cuba, within the older 15-29 age group category, Cuban females were nearly 4 times more likely to commit suicide than U.S. females in this age group. Third, Cuban males in the 15-29 age group were somewhat less likely than their male counterparts in the U.S. to commit suicide (14.2 and 18.9 for Cuba and U.S. respectively).

A recent conference on mental health in Cuba reported that research into factors leading to identification of depression as well as treatment modalities had reduced the total suicide rate from 24.6/100,000 in 1984 to a current rate of 14.3/100,000 (Riera, 2004). The relatively high rate of suicide for Cuban youth, in contrast to their overall health status, may reflect a lack of medicine to treat depression and other mental illnesses. The American Association for World Health found that since the tightening of the embargo in 1992 (Helms-Burton, 1996), Cuban physicians now have access to only 889 medicines compared to 1,297 available in Cuba in 1991 (Nations Health, 1997; Robinson, 1999).

Pregnancy and Abortion. Despite declines in the past decade, U.S. teenage pregnancy rates and birthrates are among the highest in the industrialized world (Manlove, Ryan & Franzetta, 2003; Singh & Darroch, 2000), much of which is unintended (Henshaw, 1998). A large number of international studies on teens have found that they all begin sexual activity at the same age as teens in the U.S. and they change partners at about the same rate (see Steinmetz, 1999 for a discussion of this data). However, these western and third world countries have little or no unplanned pregnancy. The major difference between the United States and other countries is the availability of adequate sex-education programs and contraceptives.

The relationship between levels of contraceptive use and the incidence of induced abortion were examined in a number of countries (Marston & Cleland, 2003). In seven countries, Kazakhstan, Kyrgyz Republic, Uzbekistan, Bulgaria, Turkey, Tunisia and Switzerland, the incidence of abortion declined as prevalence of modern contraceptive use rose. However, both the U.S. and Cuba were among six countries in which an increase in both contraception use and abortion took place.

When a group of University of Wisconsin-Madison medical, nursing, and physician's assistant students visited Cuba's public health system, a second-year medical student reported: "This is a Third World country achieving standards we don't even have in the United States." "It was inspiring." This article also noted that condoms and sex education are widely available. Support groups combined with a social emphasis on community and early intervention had reduced problems such as teenage pregnancy and domestic violence (Wisconsin State Journal, 1999).

A study of 4651 Cuban women surveyed in their first trimester in 1994 found that 1,978 had an abortion (Public Health Ministry, n.d.). Approximately 57% of pregnant women in this study had their sexual debut between 15-17 years of age and were more likely to seek abortion than birth (63.4% versus 49.9%). However, only slight differences were observed for pregnant women whose sexual debut was 18-19 years of age (26.9 % chose abortion; 27.9% gave birth. For those under 18 years of age, 39.8% had an abortion and 31.2 gave birth, whereas for those 18 to 19 years of age, just over half (52.1%) had an abortion.

Women living with their partners were more likely to give birth, but living with other family members did not make a significant difference. Although women's educational levels did not reveal a consistent pattern, students were far more likely to have an abortion rather than give birth (22.2% and 6.4% respectively) than were employed women (33.9% versus 35.5%) and housewives (43.9 versus 58.1%). This may reflect the younger age of this group.

Data from the Alan Guttmacher Institute (McClam, 2004) indicated that between 1994 and 2000, a decrease of 40% occurred in abortion (from 24/1,000 to 15/1,000) for women 15-17 years of age in the United States. Differences were observed according to the degree of poverty and ethnic status. The abortion rate rose 25% among all women below the poverty line and among minority women (32% of abortions are among blacks; 20% among Hispanics). Finally, contraception use, for women who are currently in a relationship aged 15-49, was quite similar: 73% for Cuban women and 76% for U.S. women (The State of the World's Children, 2004, Table 8).

Risky Sexual Behavior and STDs. Sexually transmitted infections among adolescents are a concern in both the U.S. and Cuba. Nearly half of the 1,641 patients treated for STDs at the Ramón Gonz lez Coro obstetric-gynecological hospital in Havana from 1993 to 1996 were under 25. The STDs most frequently seen among young women were human papilloma virus (HPV), followed by genital herpes and trichomoniasis, which appeared as a secondary infection in 92.5 percent of the cases. A 1996 survey of 1,108 adolescents between the ages of 11 and 15 found that 26 percent of the respondents said they had become sexually active between the ages of nine and 11 (Acosta, 2000).

New programs are targeting teens and young adults 15-29 years of age because of rising rates of STDs. The Public Health Ministry reported 23,225 cases of gonorrhea and 12,285 cases of syphilis last year in Cuba, a country of 11.1 million during 2000 (Acosta, 2000). Consensus existed, however, among both female and male respondents on condom use: condoms were reportedly used in casual relationships or in early stages of a relationship, but not considered necessary in a committed relationship (defined as one lasting two or more months). Adolescents reported fears of poor quality condoms and condom breakage, rather than limited access, as obstacles to use.

STDs in the U.S. showed similar patterns. Among all racial groups, the number of high school students reporting that they had ever had sexual intercourse decreased between 1991 and 2001 (Centers for Disease Control, 2002). However, over one-third (34.4%) of 9th graders reported that they had engaged in sexual intercourse, a number that increased to 40.8 for 10th graders, 51.9 for students in the 11th grade, and 60.5 for students in their senior year of high school. Data collected in 2001 indicated that a greater percentage of students who were currently sexually active reported the use of condoms during the last sexual intercourse–a consistent increase from 1991 to 2001. However, younger students were more likely to report condom use during the last sexual intercourse than were older students: 67.5%, 60.1%, 58.9%, and 49.3% for 9th-12th grades respectively.

A study of 12,000 teens between the ages of 12 and 18 who pledge to remain virgins until marriage were questioned again six years later. The study found that these adolescents did delay having sex, had fewer sex partners, and married earlier, but they had the same rates of STDs as those who did not pledge abstinence. Apparently abstinence pledgers were less likely to use a condom, a practice suggesting that "just say no" may work in the short term, but the long-term findings were not promising (Bearman & Buckner, 2004).

The Centers for Disease Control (2002, Tables 11, 21, 34) reported the following data for 2001 for the age groups 10-14 and 15-19 respectively: gonorrhea rates per 100,000 were: 26.5 and 476.4; for primary and secondary syphilis were 0.1 and 1.7 per 100,000; and for chlamydia were 73.2 and 1,426.0 per 100,000. In the U.S., adolescents are particularly at risk for chlamydia and gonorrhea, whereas in Cuba the primary STDs reported were HPV, followed by genital herpes.

Runaway Teens. A Department of Justice survey (1990) reported that there were 446,700 "broad scope runaways" (i.e., children who left home without permission and stayed away overnight), and an estimated 127,100 "broad scope throwaways" (i.e., a child has been out of the home for at least one night because: (1) the child had been directly told to leave the household; (2) the child had been away from home and a caretaker refused to allow the child back; (3) the child had run away, but the caretaker made no effort to recover the child or did not care whether or not the child returned; or (4) the child had been abandoned or deserted). In the course of a year, an estimated 500,000 to 1.5 million young people run away from or are forced out of their homes, and an estimated 200,000 are homeless and living on the streets (U.S. Department of Justice, 1990). Although their ages range from younger than 11 to over 18, over half are between the ages of 15 to 16. Because of Cuba's approach to homelessness and care of children, there were no data on these phenomena from Cuba for comparisons. One might hypothesize that given Cuba's policies there would be few cases of homelessness among adolescents.

CHILDREARING TECHNIQUES

A recent survey of 1125 Cuban families with adolescent children examined the methods that parents used to control the conduct of their children (Suárez, Reyes, Casañ, and Marrero, n.d.) The authors reported the following results:

- Mothers use better methods to control their children's conduct, as they are considered more persuasive as parents.
- 33% of the sample showed physically and verbally aggressive patterns being employed by one parent, while the other parent is always persuasive. Thereby, a typical sanction pattern is for one parent to threaten the child that he/she will tell the other member of the couple about the child's misbehavior.
- Children are having greater difficulty communicating with their parents
- Boys are punished more than girls, and particularly with non-persuasive methods.

A study of 520 youths 6-12 years of age used three indirect methods for investigating physical abuse towards children. The Phrase Completion component requested student to complete sentences such as "When there is an argument in my family . . . ," "When my father gets angry . . . ," "If I misbehave . . ." and "When my mother gets upset . . ." The Graphic Stories technique consisted in elaborating stories from three comics in which children are asked to create the end to a story. The Family Drawing asked youth to *"Draw yourself and your family when you misbehave"* and write a story about what happened (Gondar, Tenorio, Jiménez, Córdova & Hernández, 2003).

Almost one-third of youth reported being beaten with a hand or object, and two in every three children who reported physical abuse did so in two or, in some cases, three of the indirect methods used, which suggested consistency. The authors note that, because these are indirect methods, it does not indicate that all of these children were actual victims of physical abuse.

Another study used a more direct method to explore youth reports of the methods used by parents to discipline adolescents and the techniques used to encourage respect for a parent (Medina, 2001). Two hundred youth, ages 11-19, were randomly selected from the municipality of Old Havana and, subsequently, completed a self-administered survey. The adolescents were asked to identify parenting techniques that could be used to encourage respect for a parent, though these were not necessarily used within the respondent's family. Results indicated that the mother figure is the most respected, with over 70% of the adolescents reporting that love was the greatest reason for respecting their parents. Setting an example and reasoning were the next highest reported responses given (57% and 51% respectively), whereas punishments (11.5%), yelling (18.5%), beating (.04%), and obligation (.01%) were not seen as fostering respect.

This study also asked students to report on the methods that their parents used when disciplining them. The data revealed that discussing the problem (47.5%) was the most consistent technique employed, while silence and yelling (29.0% and 27.5) were the next most frequent techniques employed by parents. Pushing, hair pulling and beating were reported by 12.5%, 4.0% and 8.5% respectively (Medina, 2001). These findings were similar to those found in the U.S. (see Table 3).

It was difficult to find a direct comparison for specific techniques in a recent sample of adolescents in the U.S. Therefore, data were adapted from two articles based on a 1995 Gallup Poll of 1000 parents of children from infancy to 19 years of age (Straus, Hamby, Finkelhor, Moore & Runyan, 1998; Straus & Field, 2003), and an analysis of a sample of 556 students from six high schools in a midwestern city was undertaken by the author.[1]

The Straus and Field (2003) study found that 89% of parents of youth 13-17 years of age reported shouting, yelling, and screaming; 33.5% reported swear-

TABLE 3. A Comparison of Parents' Disciplinary Techniques in Cuba and the United States

	Cuba	United States	
	Percent	Percent	Percent
Discussion/Explained	47.50	96.52[a]	------
Omissions/Avoids	11.50	------	30.35[b]
Grounded/No Privileges	-------	77.80[a]	44.10[c]
Silence	29.00	-----	31.50
Guilt	-----	-----	29.55
Disrespect/Swore at	10.50	33.50[d]	------
Harasses/Nag	-----	-----	35.50
Yells	27.50	85.50[d]	30.30
Humiliation/Name Calling	6.00	30.00[d]	------
Beating/Slapped/Hit	8.50[e]	60.00[af]	19.30[g]
Pushes	12.50	------	------
Hair Pulling	4.00	-------	------

* Adapted from survey of 200 Cuban youth ages 11-19 (Medina, 2001)
** Adapted from survey of 1000 parents of children aged infancy through 19, using the Conflict Tactics Scale Parent-Child (Straus et al., 1998, Table 1; Straus & Field, 2003, Table 3)
*** Analysis of Midwest sample of youth ages 13-18 years from six public high schools who "Strongly Agreed" or "Agreed" that their mother and father (combined) used these behavior to discipline them.
[a] Prevalence based on the "last year," and represents ages 1-19 years (Straus, 1998, Table 1)
[b] Average of "Send out of room" and "Avoid eye contact"
[c] Average of "No enjoyable activities" and "No activities with friends."
[d] Ages 13-17 (Straus & Field, 2003, Table 3)
[e] "Beating" is the wording in the Cuba sample
[f] "Slapped on hand, arm or leg" (Straus et al., 1999 Table 1)
[g] Average of "Parents hit me when they think I am doing something wrong" and "Parents punish me by hitting me" in Midwestern sample analyzed for this paper.

ing at the child, 30% engaged in name-calling. Data for discussion and hitting were not reported for each age group, but another study using this data set (Straus et al., 1998) found that during the "last year" 96.52% of parents of youth 1-19 used explanation, 77.80% grounded or removed privileges, and 60% slapped their child on the hand, arm, or leg.

Although there were different items used and the cultural context of the items may be problematic, in general, non-verbally or physically aggressive methods appear to be most common. Verbally aggressive methods such as yelling, nagging, swearing, are used less frequently than non-aggressive methods. Finally, although it is difficult to compare the two countries, and data collected from parents versus youth, physically violent methods do appear to be the least frequently used techniques. A comparison of Cuba and the Midwest sample, the sample consisting of only adolescent aged youth, suggests that U.S. parents are about twice as likely as Cuban parents to use hitting/beating.

CONCLUSION

Cuba has been masterful in overcoming the challenge resulting from the U.S. economic blockade and the collapse of the Soviet Union. The "special period," the time immediately following the Soviet Union's discontinuation of economic support, was hardest on those facing challenges (e.g., pregnant teens, single mothers, those with disabilities, school dropouts and unemployed youth–see Strug and Teague, 2002). The development of social work schools throughout the Island was the result of increases in problems faced by families and the need to provide a greater number of trained professionals to help.

Clearly there are major differences between Cuba and the United States in terms of economic systems, military power, world power, technology and medical advances. However, on major measures of educational achievement, Cuban youth are equal to or exceed that of youth in the U.S. Although medical technology and availability of pharmaceuticals developed in the U.S. are the leading edge and much admired throughout the world, Cuba also has made major advances in specific areas of medical technology and pharmaceutical development. Yet, despite Cuba's generally lower level of resources, health care is available for all youth, infant and child mortality rates are similar to those in the U.S., and the percentage of youth receiving immunizations is considerably higher than U.S. youth. Cuba also has provided resources so that major problems affecting poor families and youth in the U.S., including hunger, inadequate nutrition, and homelessness, do not appear to be problems any longer.

The fundamental observed difference is the concept held by Cubans, that children are their major resource–their future. Defining the young as Cuba's primary human capital is frequently identified by Fidel Castro and appears to shape most decision-making and allocation of resources. When children are considered to be the key to the country's future it appears that a greater flow of resources is allocated to benefit youth, and society as a whole views its role as protecting and nurturing them. It will be interesting to observe the changes in Cuba as reflected in the health and educational standards of youth during the next decade–a time most likely characterized by increasing differences in social status and values.

However, new challenges resulting from the growth of tourism based on U.S. dollars, an economic salvation, also has produced the first signs of class differentiation–those with access to dollars and those without. The tourist-based economy not only brought in an influx of tourists, it also resulted in changed behaviors (e.g., increases in prostitution, doctors and lawyers giving up their poorly paid state jobs for dollar-rich jobs such as cab drivers and waiters), as well as a weakening of the bonds and shared values that were Cuba's moral glue.

Was Marx wrong? It may be that fulfilling the goal of the *Communist Manifesto* may be critical for bringing the proletariat up to a uniformly high standard in terms of education (especially universal literacy) and health care and removing SES, gender or race-based differences. In fact, much of the communist ideology has been translated into real consequences for the parents, children, and youth of Cuba. However, once you have a highly educated, literate, and skilled population, it may be difficult to keep the population from desiring scarce nonessential or luxury items and developing mechanisms for obtaining them. Such changes in lifestyle are likely to have impact on cultural values, which in turn will alter how youth are socialized. It will be interesting to see how Cuba faces these new challenges and how such cultural transitions will have influence on the parents, youth, and the families of this unique Caribbean country.

NOTE

1. The United States data is part of a multi-nation project (Peterson, Bush, & Wilson, 1998), "Cross-national Research Project on Adolescent Social Competence," sample from Metropolitan Cincinnati, OH.

REFERENCES

Acosta, D. (Oct 30, 2000) Health-Cuba: Targeting women to promote safe sex. Inter Press Service. Retrieved Sept. 18, 2003 from http://ipsnews.net/caribbean.asp.
Aneki.com. (2003). Highest divorce rates in the world. Retrieved on Nov. 7, 2003 from *http://www.aneki.com/divorce.html*.

Applebee, A. N., Langer, J. A. & Mullis, I.V.S. (1986) The writing report card: Writing achievement in American schools. Princeton, N.J.: National Assessment of Educational Progress. Educational Testing Service.

Associated Press (July 1, 1998). Salsa declared a vegetable for school lunches. Retrieved on May 10, 2004 from *www.jsonline.com/alive/nutrition/0701salsa.stm.*

Bearman, P. & Bruckner, H. (March 9, 2004). Study: Teen abstinence no help to later STD rates. Retrieved on March 17, 2004 from http://www.cnn.com/2004/HEALTH/parenting/03/09/abstinence.study.ap/

Bureau of Western Hemisphere Affairs, (September, 2002) Cuba-Background Notes. U.S. Department of State, International Programs Information. Retrieved on August 2, 2003 from *http://usinfo.state.gov/regional/ar/us-cuba/*

Bush, G. W. (Jan. 8, 2002). Public Law print of PL 107-110, the No Child Left Behind Act of 2001 [1.8 MB. Retrieved on Feb 10, 2004 from http://www.ed.gov/policy/elsec/leg/edpicks.jhtml?src=az.

Castañeda, M. (Sept 9, 2003). Island Receives International Literacy Award. Digital Granma International. Retrieved on November 3, 2003 from http://granmai.cubaweb.com/ingles/2003/septiembre03/mar9/36premio-i.html.

Castro R.F. (May 26, 2003). The symbol of neoliberal globalization has received a colossal blow. Speech given by the President of the Republic of Cuba, Commander in Chief at the Law School of the University of Buenos Aires, Argentina. Digital Granma International. pp 1-32. Retrieved on June 19, 2003 from http://www.granma.cu/doumento/ingles/03/016.html).

Castro, R. F. (n.d.) Revolutionary Offensive. p. 217.

Castro, R. F. (n.d.) Fidel Castro on Chile, p. 134.

Centers for Disease Control (2002). STDs in Adolescents and young adults. Retrieved March 17, 2004 from http://www.cdc.gov/std/stats01/2001SFAdol&YAdults.htm.

Centers for Disease Control (2001). Surveillance Report. National Profile, Chlamydia Table 11, 21, 43. Retrieved on March 17, 2004 from http://www.cdc.gov/std/stats01/Tables/Table11.htm.

Chelala, C. (Feb. 24, 1998). Cuba shows health gains despite embargo. *British Medical Journal, 316* (Issue 7130), 497.

Cheng, Y. & Manning, P. (Sept., 2003). Revolution in education: China and Cuba in global context. *Journal of World History, 14,* 359-391.

Children's Defense Fund. (1995). *State of America's children yearbook.* Washington, DC.

Craighead, W.E. (1991). Cognitive Factors and classification issues in adolescent depression. *Journal of Youth and Adolescence, 20,* 311-315.

De La Osa, J. A. (Jan. 5, 2004). Infant mortality in 2003: Cuba has the lowest rate in Latin America. *Digital Granma.* Retrieved on Jan 6, 2004 from http://www.granma.cu/ingles/2004/enero/lun5/mortalidad.html.

Donahue, R. J., & Tuber, S. B. (1995). The impact of homelessness on children's level of aspiration. *Bulletin of the Menninger Clinic, 59* (2), 249-255.

Dowdy, Z. R. (Sept. 19, 2003). U.S. among nations high in child abuse deaths. *Indianapolis Star,* pg. A9.

Finn, J. D. (1989). Withdrawing from school. *Review of Educational Research, 59,* 117-142.

Figueroa, M., Prieto, A. & Gutierrez, R. G. (1974). Educational Department Center, Havana, Experiments and innovations in education; Study prepared for the International Bureau of Education, no. 7 (Paris: The UNESCO Press, p. 3).

Fried, B. J. & Gaydos, L. M (2002). *World health systems: Challenges and perspectives*. Chicago, Health Administration Press.

Gondar, A. D., Tenorio, M.D., Jiménez, Y. V., Córdova, A. G., & Hernnádez, A. C. (2003). Convivir en Familias sin Violencia." Una metodología para la intervención y prevención de la violencia intrafamiliar. (Living together in Families without Violence." A methodology for intervention and prevention of family violence). Department of Family Studies. Psychological and Sociological Research Center, Havana City. (With the collaboration of Save the Children Foundation UK.)

Grogg, P. (July 29, 1999). Vaccine may open window in U.S. Blockade. Retrieved on Feb 15, 2004 from http://www.cubasolidarity.net/vaccine.html.

Grogg, P. (Dec 3, 2003). Rural students benefit from computers and Solar panels. Retrieved on Feb. 15, 2004 from http://ipsnews.net/interna.asp?idnews=21394.

Helms-Burton (1996). H. R. 927. 140 Congress, 2nd session, January 3, 1996).

Henshaw S. K. (1998). Unintended pregnancy in the United States, *Family Planning Perspectives*, 30(1):24-29 & 46.

Horowitz, S.V., Springer, C. M., & Kose, G. (1988). Stress in hotel children: The effects of homelessness on attitudes towards school. *Children's Environments Quarterly*, 5, 34-36.

Jarjoura, G. R., Triplett, G. P., & Brinker, G. P. (2002) Growing up poor: Examining the link between persistent childhood poverty and delinquency, *Journal of Quantitative Criminology*, 18, 159-187.

Jacoby, J. (Jan 13, 2000). If Elian Returns to Cuba, Misery Awaits. *The Boston Globe*. Retrieved on March 23, 2004 from http://www.nocastro.com/archives/elian19.htm.

Krug, E. G., Dahlberg, L. L., Mercy, J. A., Zwi, A. B., & Lozano, R. (2002). World report on violence and health. Geneva: World Health Organization. Retrieved on September 10, 2003 from http://www.who.int/violence_injury_prevention/violence/world_report/wrvheng/en/ Tables A.7 and A.9.

Latin American Alliance. (1997). Cuba General Information. Retrieved on Nov 30, 2002 from http://www.latinsynergy.org/cuba.html.

Lerner, R. M. & Galambos, N. L. (1998). Adolescent development: Challenges and opportunities for research, programs, and policies. *Annual Review of Psychology*, 49, 413-446.

Lippman, W. (July 1, 2001). Two months in Cuba: Notes of a visiting Cuba solidarity activist. Retrieved on May 3, 2003 from http://www.blythe.org/2months.html.

Lloyd, D. (1978). Prediction on school failure from third-grade data. *Educational Psychological Measurement*, 38, 1193-1200.

Manlove, J., Ryan, S. & Franzetta, K. Patterns of contraceptive use within teenagers' first sexual relationships. Retrieved on Feb 10, 2004 from http://www.guttmacher.org/pubs/journals/3524603.html.

Marston, C. & Cleland, J. (March, 2003). Relationships between contraception and abortion: A review of the evidence. *International Family Planning Perspectives*, 29, 6-13.

Marx, K. & Engels, F. (1948). *The communist manifesto*. New York: International Publishers.

Marx, Karl (1936) *Capital*. New York: The Modern Library p. 526.

Marx, K. (1973) Compulsory education. In K. Padover (Ed.) *On the Third International* New York: McGraw-Hill p. 113.

McClam, E. (March, 2004). Abortion rates drop–except among poor. Retrieved on March 1, 2004 from http://www.kentucky.com/mld/kentucky/4238003.htm.

Medina, A. M. (2001). Family violence in relation with gender. Perception of a group of teenagers. Thesis for master candidacy in sexuality. National Center for Sexual Education, Havana, Cuba.

Mendez, M.A., Adair, L.S. (1999). Severity and timing of stunting in the first two years of life affect performance on cognitive tests in late childhood. *Journal of Nutrition*, 129 (8), 1555-1562.

National Institute for Literacy (2004). Adolescent literacy–Research informing practice: A series of workshops. Workshop 1: Adolescent Literacy Workshop: State of the Science and Research Needs (no date). Retrieved Feb. 8, 2004 from http://novel.nifl.gov/.

National Center for Education Statistics (Oct. 2001). Status dropout rates and number and percentage distribution of dropouts ages 16-24, by selected characteristics (Table 17-2). Retrieved on Feb. 12, 2003 from http://nces.ed.gov/programs/coe/2003/section3/tables/t17_2.asp

Nation's Health (April, 1997). Health status in Cuba declining under embargo. Vol 27, p.7.

Peterson, G.W., Bush, K.R., & Wilson, S.M. (1998). Cross-national Research Project on Adolescent Social Competence. Miami University, Oxford, Ohio. Sample from Metropolitan Cincinnati, OH.

Plisko, V. W. (July 10, 2003). The release of the National Assessment of Educational Progress (NAEP) The Nations' Report Card: Writing 2002. Retrieved on Feb. 16, 2004 from http://nces.ed.gov/commissioner/remarks2003/7_10_2003.asp.

Pollitt, E., Gorman, K.S., Engle, P.L., Rivera, J.A., & Martorell, R. (April 1995). Nutrition in early life and the fulfillment of intellectual potential. *Journal of Nutrition*, 125 (4S) 1111S-1118S.

Prescott-Allen, R. (2001) The well-being of nations, A country-by-country index of quality of Life and the Environment. IDRC/Island Press. Retrieved Jan. 2, 2004 from http://www.idrc.ca/acb/showdetl.cfm?&DS_ID=2&Product_ID=608&DID=6.

Public Health Ministry (n.d.). Características socio-culturales del aborto en Cuba: Investigación estadística. [Sociocultural characteristics of the abortion in Cuba: Statistical investigation]. Statistic National Direction.). FNUAP.

Riera, L. (Jan. 29, 2004). Cuban and U.S. psychiatrists meet in Havana: We have a lot to offer each other. Retrieved on February 2, 2004 from http://www.granma.cu/ingles/2004/enero/juev29/5psycho.html.

Robinson, R. (July, 1999). Why is Black Cuba suffering. *Essence*, *30*, p. 166+.

Rutter, M. (Ed.) (1995). *Psychosocial disturbances in young people: Challenges for prevention*. New York: Cambridge University Press.

Scrimshaw, N.S. (1998). Malnutrition, brain development, learning, and behavior. *Nutrition Research*, *18* (2), 351-379.

Sherman, A. (1994). *Wasting America's future: Children's Defense fund report on the costs of child poverty.* Boston: Beacon Press.

Singh, S. & Darroch, J.E. (2000)Adolescent pregnancy and childbearing: Levels and trends in developed countries. *Family Planning Perspectives, 32,* 14-23.

Snyder, T. D., Hoffman, C. M., & Geddes, C. M. (1996). *Digest of educational statistics* National Center for Educational Statistics. (GPO #065-000-00904-8). Washington, DC: Government Printing Office.

Steinmetz, S. K. (1999). Adolescence in contemporary families. In M. B. Sussman, S. K. Steinmetz & G. W. Peterson (Eds.) *Handbook of marriage and the family* (2nd Edition) New York: Plenum Press.

Straus, M. A. & Field, C. J (2003). Psychological aggression by American parents: National data on prevalence, chronicity, and severity. *Journal of Marriage and Family, 65:* 795-808.

Straus, M.A., Hamby, S.L., Finkelhor, D., Moore, David W., & Runyan, D. (1998). Identification of child maltreatment with the parent-child conflict tactics scales: Development and psychometric data for a national sample of American parents. *Child Abuse and Neglect, 22,* 249-270.

Strug, D. & Teague, W. (September 2, 2002). New Directions in Social Work Education. *Social Work Today,* pg 1-4.

Suárez, M. A., Reyes, I. R., Casañ, P. P. & Castañeda Marrero, A. V. (n.d.). Condition of childhood, adolescence, woman and family in Cuba. Center for Studies on Woman. UNICEF.

The State of the World's Children (2004). Official Summary. United Nations Children's Fund (UNICEF).

United States Cities Mayors (Dec.18, 2002). Press Release: Hunger, Homelessness on the Rise in Major U. S. Cities. Retrieved on Feb 10, 2004 from www.usmayors. org/uscm/news/press_releases/documents/hunger_121802.asp

U.S. Department of Health and Human Services. (March, 2003). Ending chronic homelessness: strategies for action. Executive Summary: Report from the Secretary's Work Group on Ending Chronic Homelessness. Retrieved Feb. 10, 2004 from http://aspe.hhs.gov/progsys/homeless/index.html.

U.S. Department of Justice (1990). *Missing, abducted, runaway, and thrownaway children in America, first report: Numbers and characteristics.* National Incidence Studies, Office of Juvenile Justice and Delinquency Prevention, Washington, DC.

U.S. Department of Justice (1996). Office of Elementary and Secondary Education, Safe and Drug Free Schools Program. *Manual to combat truancy.* Washington, DC: Government Printing Office.

U.S. Department of State, International Programs Information. Cuba–Background notes. Retrieved on Aug. 12, 2002 from *http://usinfo.state.gov/regional/ar/us-cuba/.*

Veeken, H. (Oct 7, 1995). Letters from Cuba-Cuba-Plenty of care, few condoms, no corruption. *British Medical Journal, 311,* 935-37.

Waitzkin, H., Wald, K., Kee, R., Danielson, R., & Robinson, L. (Sept. 1997). Primary care in Cuba: Low and high technology development pertinent to family medicine. *Journal of Family Práctice, 45,* 250-258. Retrieved on November 10, 2003 from http://www.cubasolidarity.net/waitzkin.html

White, R. (2002). Youth crime, community development, and social justice. In M. Tienda, & Wilson, W. J. (Eds.). *Youth in cities: A cross-national perspective* (pp. 138-164). New York: Cambridge University Press.

Willms, J.D., & Somers, M.A. (2001). Family, classroom, and school effects on children's educational outcomes in Latin America. *School Effectiveness and School Improvement,* 12 (4): 409-445.

Winborne, D. G., & Murray, G. J. (1992). Address unknown: An exploration of the educational and social attitudes of homeless adolescents. *High School Journal, 75,* (3), 144-149.

Wisconsin State Journal. (March 20, 1999). Cuban Health System Impresses UW group: Lack of Resources Overcome. Wisconsin State Journal; 03/20/99. Retrieved Nov. 25, 2003 from www.Jadecampus.com.

World Factbook (2003). Retrieved Feb. 2, 2004 from http://www.bartleby.com/151.

World Health Organization/ (Countries/Cuba) (2002). http://www.who.int/country/cub/en/. Retrieved Feb. 1, 2004.

World Bank (2002). Health Expenditures, Services and Use. Table 2.15. Retrieved on Nov. 1, 2003 from http://devdata.worldbank.org/hnpstats/files/Tab2_15.xls.

Zeitlin, A. G. (1993). Everyday stressors in the lives of Anglo and Hispanic learning handicapped adolescents. *Journal of Youth and Adolescence, 22,* 327-335

Persisting Issues in Cultural and Cross-Cultural Parent-Youth Relations

Gary W. Peterson
Suzanne K. Steinmetz
Stephan M. Wilson

The chapters in this collection illustrate the growing diversity of scholarship being conducted on parent-child/parent-adolescent relationships from different cultural and cross-cultural perspectives. Authors from many countries have raised important issues either directly in these chapters or indirectly through inferences about future work that is needed using the current scholarship as a springboard for thought. Among the multitude of possibilities, the issues of particular importance consist of: (1) the need for research based on more complex socialization models, (2) the need for scholarship that captures a more complex conception of culture, (3) dilemmas about cultural universals in the parent-child relationship, (4) An examination of problems with parental styles or typologies, (5) the need to expand beyond parental styles and behaviors as disproportionate preoccupations over other parental attributes and (6) the impact of shifting cultural, economic and political paradigms on values and attitudes regarding childrearing. The purpose of this concluding section to elaborate on these six issues.

THE NEED FOR RESEARCH BASED
ON MORE COMPLEX SOCIALIZATION MODELS

One of the issues in the current research on cultural and cross-cultural parent-youth relationships is the predominant and excessive use of social mold or deterministic perspectives. Partly as a means of demonstrating the influence of culture within the parent-youth relationship, much of the current research focuses on narrow avenues of socializing children within families and, most par-

http://www.haworthpress.com/web/MFR
© 2004 by The Haworth Press, Inc. All rights reserved.
Digital Object Identifier: 10.1300/J002v36n03_11

ticularly, cultural influence is viewed as proceeding from parent to child through primarily deterministic socialization processes. Given this preoccupation, more research is needed that captures the true complexity of how children and adolescents from diverse cultures become active participants in their socio-cultural environment. Part of this complexity involves examining the multi-directionality of socialization influences (Corsaro, 1997; Kuczinsky, 2003; Peterson & Hann, 1999). Part of this idea is concerned with how the family and other contexts of socialization operate either in conjunction with or in opposition to each other as influences on the development of youth. Such studies in this collection like that of Stolz et al. illustrate this idea by examining across cultures whether similar dimensions of socialization within both the family and the school can be examined for unique contributions and relative importance as predictors of developmental outcomes by adolescents. Moreover, increased research attention is needed across cultures on bi-directional influences that adolescents, their parents, and others experience within families (Kuczynski, 2003; Peterson & Hann, 1999; Peterson & Rollins, 1987). Some observers propose, for example, that children have greater influence on their parents in individualistic cultures such as European American cultures than is true for children in collectivistic cultures such as Asian or Latino cultures (Harkness & Super, 2002). This is an idea that requires careful empirical examination within many cultures before it becomes a principle we assume is true.

Studies in this collection by McClellan et al., Lu and Kao, Kaltenborn, and Xia et al. illustrate a bi-directional theme by focusing on such issues as process variables representing reciprocity between parents and adolescents (e.g., parent-adolescent conflict), how the birth of children impacts the lives of new parents (i.e., the transition to parenthood), and how children's beliefs and perspectives are important in shaping their own socialization. These chapters assist in providing a more complex view of socialization that supplements the strictly social mold or parental influence perspective.

THE NEED FOR SCHOLARSHIP THAT CAPTURES A MORE COMPLEX CONCEPTION OF CULTURE

Another issue raised by these studies is the need to view culture in more complex ways than simply a single category, often consisting of a racial, national, or ethnic designation (e.g., African, African-American, Mexican, Mexican-American, Latino) (Rogoff, 2003). This categorical or "social address" approach gives the false impression that there is greater homogeneity within such categories as "Asian," "Latino," and "Mexican" than is actually the case. For example, Esteinou, one of the authors in this collection, recognizes that the national designation "Mexican" clearly does not reduce to a unitary social address representing substantial homogeneity. Instead, she describes diverse parenting patterns within Mexican sub-populations ranging from urban middle-class to rural Mesoamerican families. Although national "cultures" may share some commonalities, we need to constantly remind ourselves that these national or social address categories are composed of subgroups that, in turn, may demonstrate even further heterogeneity within.

The influence of culture may be more aptly viewed in terms of the concept dynamic "cultural community," rather than as an entity defined by static membership in a homogeneous social group. Parent-youth relationships should be viewed in terms of individuals who co-construct a shared reality in one or more domains of life and who involve themselves in discourses and activities appropriate to some *approximately* agreed-upon level of commonality. From this perspective, a cultural community involves "contextualized individuals" who wish to accomplish some things together, but also are members of multiple communities, and contribute to a constantly changing social discourse. According to this view, a culture is an evolving array of social scripts that shapes individual's behavior but also requires a fluid and multi-dimensional definition of a person's cultural community membership (Strauss & Quinn, 1997). For one thing, parents and youth can be members of multiple cultural groups (e.g., peer groups, professions, subcultures, work groups, social class memberships, religious organizations, recreational endeavors, community and neighborhood settings), each with distinctive values, meanings, and priorities that influence the cultural identities of parents and children. Each parent-youth relationship, therefore, is a product of multiple group memberships as both parents and the young share discourses with others but interact based on somewhat different experiences and participations. Parent-youth discourses bring to bear the meanings assigned within each of the social associations that parents and youth experience in their everyday lives. Cultural influence within the parent-youth associations, therefore, is a product of multiple and differentially shared discourses by parents and children who engage in relationships with each other in terms of the multiple groups in which they participate. Simply looking for mean group differences in parent-child socialization across highly generalized cultures will not capture the diversity that actually exists within cultural groups (Rogoff, 2003).

DILEMMAS ABOUT CULTURAL UNIVERSALS WITHIN THE PARENT-CHILD RELATIONSHIP

Another issue addressed either explicitly or implicitly in these chapters is the extent to which cultural universals in parent-youth relations can be identified, particularly by conducting cross-national or cross-cultural research (see chapters by Bradford et al., Rohner et al., Stolz et al., and Vazsonyi in this collection). Much of this work provides useful information about the cross-cultural applicability of general dimensions of parental behavior such as connection, acceptance-rejection, regulation, and psychological autonomy. These dimensions of parental behavior are conceptually meaningful and tend to predict outcomes in youth in similar ways and with considerable regularity across cultures.

One should not, however, be too surprised by the apparent universal application of these dimensions of parental behavior, which are, after all, very generalized constructs that deal with fundamental issues within parent-child/adolescent relationships. These fundamental concerns of parents consist of how they communicate warmth and security, how they attempt to exercise influence over the young, and how much freedom from parental supervision they feel comfortable allowing. It does not seem too surprising, therefore, that parents from most, if not all, cultures use some means of communicating positive, affectionate feelings to the young, and when they do, this behavior has positive consequences for youthful development (Peterson & Hann, 1999; Rohner, 1986; Rollins & Thomas, 1979).

It would be unwise, however, to be lulled into premature satisfaction with such "universal" findings due to the fact that the "devil may be in the details." One obvious reason for identifying such universal patterns is that the commonly examined parental behavior dimensions in these studies are very general in nature. Consequently, although they operate in similar ways across culture, each of these "dimensions" is also composed of several more specific sub-dimensions that may not be interpreted in exactly the same way across cultures and may not have the same consequences for youthful dimensions. The concepts connection or acceptance-rejection, for example, are used to represent, in very general ways, the variety of means that parents use to convey warmth or support to their young. It is important to recognize, therefore, that these generalized conceptions of supportive behavior are composed of sub-dimensions including such behavior (among other dimensions) as giving praise for successful achievement by the young, communicating encouragement for future behavior (i.e., encouragement), spending positive time with the young (i.e., companionship), being physically affectionate (i.e., hugging and kissing), and seeking to maintain dependencies (i.e., dependency training) (Peterson & Hann, 1999).

Once we subdivide the general dimension of support, acceptance or warmth into its sub-dimensions, however, the meanings assigned across cultures to its specific components may not be as uniform as when the general dimension is considered in the abstract. Some cultures, for example, may be more physically demonstrative than others and gender differences may vary across cultures in the extent to which mothers and fathers are expected to convey physical affection to their sons versus their daughters. Cultures characterized as *individualistic* (i.e., value autonomy as a socialization outcome) versus *collectivistic* (i.e., emphasize the importance of maintaining family connections) may vary substantially in the meanings assigned to parental supportive behaviors that seek to foster dependent and compliant behavior in the young. Individualistic cultures may view very high amounts of supportiveness during adolescence as being efforts by parents to foster inappropriate levels of dependency, whereas some collectivistic cultures may view almost unconditional amounts of support as necessary to maintain strong familistic orientations (Arnett, 1995; Peterson, 1995). The point here is that greater cross-cultural variability may result, as we become more specific in defining our dimensions of parental behavior.

Parental regulation or a general form of control is another example of a concept composed of multiple dimensions including such parental attributes as having knowledge of children's activities (monitoring), establishing rules that regulate children's behaviors (consistent rule enforcement), the use of reasoning to convey expectations for behavior (induction), and placing demands on the young for achievement (achievement pressure). These behaviors, though components of what has been referred to as firm control (Baumrind, 1991; Peterson & Hann, 1999), may have somewhat similar implications for child and adolescent outcomes. However, it is unlikely that even these specific dimensions of parental control will have exactly the same meanings and consequences across cultures. Other forms of more coercive control, such as verbal hostility, physical coerciveness, and physical abuse often have been found to inhibit the development of many of the same youthful outcomes (e.g., self-esteem, school achievement, autonomy) that dimensions of regulation or firm control have been found to foster. The important point again, of course, is that control or regulation has long been found to be multidimensional, with each dimension communicating different meanings and having distinctive consequences for youthful outcomes (Maccoby & Martin, 1983; Peterson & Hann, 1999; Peterson & Rollins, 1987; Rollins & Thomas, 1979). Overall, we should expect that universal results will emerge less often to the extent that more specific strategies of parental socialization are defined and examined. More specific dimensions of parental behavior will vary in terms of their presence across cultures, in the meanings assigned to these socialization strategies, and in terms of their consequences for the development of youth.

PROBLEMS WITH PARENTAL STYLES OR TYPOLOGIES

Another related precaution addressed in these chapters is that scholars who are interested in studying parent-youth relationships from cultural perspectives have raised serious questions about the application of European American parental styles to non-Western cultures and to ethnic populations within the U.S. Styles or typologies refer to qualitatively different combinations of parental characteristics. Parental styles are supposed to provide ecological validity in the sense of being naturally occurring collections of parental attributes such as behaviors, attitudes, beliefs and values that make sense conceptually (Darling & Steinberg, 1997; Stewart & Bond, 2002). Such aggregated qualities create overall contexts of parenting that have been found empirically to have predictable consequences for the development of youth (Baumrind, 1991; Maccoby & Martin, 1983; Peterson & Hann, 1999).

A serious problem with parental styles, however, is the complexity and the difficulty that researchers face in understanding how specific aspects of a style contribute to adolescent development. Because parental styles provide a general context consisting of many parental qualities (Darling & Steinberg, 1993), it is difficult to identify precisely which aspect of a parent's child-rearing approach is the primary factor that truly influences a specific aspect of adolescent development. A related issue is that none of the parental styles incorporate either all the dimensions of parental practice currently identified in the research literature or the full range of variation in each of these dimensions. Consequently, the existing typologies fail to adequately represent the many parental styles that are conceptually possible in the overall population of parents (see Lim & Lim in this collection; Peterson & Hann, 1999; Peterson & Rollins, 1987).

Of particular concern for the cross-cultural study of parent-youth relations are tendencies to over-generalize about the specific effects of Western parental styles without recognizing cultural differences in the goals, conduct, and consequences of parenting (Chao, 2000, 2001; Kagitcibasi, 1996; see Lim & Lim, in this collection). Recent observers have proposed that the cultural roots of parenting styles are underestimated in the current research (Chao, 1994, 2000, 2001; Lim & Lim, in this collection; Peterson, Steinmetz, & Wilson, in this collection). An important point, for example, is that parental typologies, like the authoritative or authoritarian styles, are concepts based in European American cultural traditions and may not be consistent with non-Western cultural values. A possible consequence is that parenting practices used by ethnic minority parents may be studied "out of context," misunderstood, and misrepresented by models of parenting that are not reflective of native values and socialization goals.

Compared to European American cultures, for example, many non-Western cultures may place greater emphasis on collectivistic values consisting of group connections, family harmony, community interests over individual priorities, respect for authority, and the importance of tradition. This contrasts with basic European American values that underscore the importance of individuality, autonomy, democracy, and self-interest over the welfare of the group. Collectivistic values, therefore, may encourage very different meanings, even for behaviors that seem harsh or excessively rigid by European American standards. These behaviors may have a fundamentally different cultural basis within indigenous values and may be motivated by distinctive socialization goals from one culture to another. In other words, behavior that is viewed as harsh or intrusive in one culture might be viewed as an expression of concern to maintain group togetherness in another. Moreover, non-Western parents may express their own cultural values through the use of styles composed of disciplinary, controlling, nurturing, and rejecting behavior that differ either substantially or in nuance from western conceptions of parenting (i.e., authoritarian and authoritative styles as well as other identified or completely novel styles) (Chao, 1994, 2000, 2001; Kagitcibasi, 1996; Lim & Lim, in this collection). A reasonable amount of caution is required, therefore, when the substance, meaning and consequences of parental styles and behavior are examined across cultures. Because of their complexity, therefore, parental styles may carry a lot of culturally specific baggage that prevents their effective use across cultures.

As a result of such problems with parental styles, therefore, many researchers have preferred to study specific dimensions of parental behavior rather than deal with the many complexities of parental styles (cf. Bradford et al. in this collection; Darling & Steinberg, 1993; Lim & Lim, in this collection; Peterson, Cobas, Bush, & Wilson, in this collection; Stolz et al. in this collection). The most frequently studied child-rearing behaviors are parental warmth or support, autonomy-granting behavior, intrusive control, reasoning (induction), monitoring, and punitiveness. These socialization behaviors are examined as distinct dimensions and are less likely to be connected to and driven by the culturally based values and beliefs that are embedded in European American parental styles. However, such conclusions are, at best, tentative and must be addressed with systematic research in a wide variety of contests before firm generalizations can be made.

THE NEED TO EXPAND BEYOND PARENTAL BEHAVIORS

Another conclusion is that, although a great deal has been learned by studying parental styles and behaviors as predictors of adolescent development, it is time to expand beyond being so disproportionately preoccupied with these aspects of the parent-adolescent relationship (Steinberg, 2001). Preoccupation with parental styles and behaviors in parent-adolescent research may lead to underestimating how the sophisticated cognitive abilities of youth provide them with the capacity to be either responsive or nonresponsive to parents based on their interpretations or meaning of the long-term relationships they have with their elders. Both parental styles and behaviors seem best suited for examining parent-child relations with younger children and may have somewhat less utility with adolescents. Such is the case because, compared to younger children, adolescents have greater abstract thinking capacities, more extensive relationship memories, enhanced social perceptions, and greater experience with parents. These abilities allow adolescents to construct increasingly complex images or assessments of their parent's competence, wisdom, and authority. As a result, more complicated interpretations of the meaning of parent-adolescent relationships may be structured in ways that may be equally as influential for youth as reports of child-rearing behaviors of the moment.

Adolescents, with growing acuity in social perception, may be influenced extensively by whether or not they view their parents as being competent, as having wisdom, and as being recognized simply as authority figures (Peterson & Hann, 1999). Compared to momentary displays of childrearing behavior, these generalized *social constructions* of their parents are more abstract and summarized products of long-term relationships. Adolescents increasingly develop abilities to "size up" their parents' worthiness or unworthiness as social agents (i.e., their perception of parents' competence) and choose to accept or reject in complex ways the extent to which they will be influenced. It may also be true that perceptions of and the efficacy of such relationship concepts as parental authority, competence, and wisdom may have greater consequences for youthful development in cultures that emphasize collectivistic values, familistic bonds, or filial piety. Moreover, cultures that emphasize individualism may have greater tolerance for youthful efforts to engage in behavioral exchanges with parents that challenge (or seek to renegotiate) these non-behavioral sources of parental influence.

THE INFLUENCE OF SHIFTING POLITICAL
AND ECONOMIC PARADIGMS ON CHILDREARING

Bronfenbrenner (1979, 1986) has demonstrated the importance of examining the larger cultural, economic, and political context in understanding family interaction. Several other scholars (Elder, 1972; Elder, Eccles, Ardelt, & Lord, 1995; Kohn, 1969; Kohn & Schooler, 1983) have demonstrated the importance of macro-level social contexts such as social class in defining parent-child interaction and outcomes. Such influences on the parent-child socialization process by larger social contexts is based, in part, on the skills and values necessary for parents to achieve effectively in middle and working class employment settings. Consistent with this perspective, Steinmetz (1971) demonstrated that, rather than the social class per se, it was the specific skills associated with one's particular job that seemed to be most important in predicting childrearing techniques and outcomes.

It seems clear, therefore, that, in the U.S., a moderate relationship exists between one's occupation and how one raises his or her children in the United States (see Steinmetz, 1999). However, these same relationships may not hold within societies characterized by different economic and political environments. For example, in communist countries, the state controls access to education and occupations and defines how children should be raised and the values that are believed to be important for children to acquire (see Steinmetz in this collection). During the past few decades, a number of political and economic changes have occurred in different societies such as the fall of the U.S.S.R., the development of democracy in most of the emergent countries, and the rise to prominence of fundamentalist Islamic states. These shifts in political and economic systems have resulted in comparable changes in education, family patterns, gender roles, SES, and socialization processes that may deviate significantly from the paths of modern, westernized democracies.

Although it is anticipated that with the fall of communism will come a shift from the total control of all activities under the communist regime to an acceptance of the western ideals of individualism, freedom and equality, history has demonstrated that this is not necessarily true. Although a shift from communism to capitalism in some societies has resulted in a freeing-up of educational and occupational opportunities (e.g., in China and East Germany), it has also resulted in greater class differences and greater societal problems associated with the widening of the gap between the "haves" and "have nots" (see Walper, Kruse Noack, & Schwarz in this collection). In other societies such as Poland, the fall of communism has resulted in a return to the traditional ideas of Catholicism that glorify motherhood and favor male dominance in an ideological sense if not in practice. However, in other societies, the decline of communism, which severely limited religious freedom, was followed by the rise of Islamic fundamentalism and a reaffirmation of male dominance (see Wejnert & Djumabaeva in this collection). The shift to a fundamentalist Islamic leadership, such as the Taliban in Afghanistan, produced an extreme form of conservatism that denied education, employment and equality for women as well as removed a wide range of freedoms. Such socio-cultural transitions will have extensive consequences for the values and socialization strategies that become part of parent-youth relationships.

Communist countries have considerable impact on parent-child socialization values and strategies, many of which are mandated to an extent that socialization differences are expected to be minimal because the state's will is expected to be accepted. Consequently, these larger political and economic paradigms will have considerable influence on the values and attitudes that parents convey to their children. When socialist/communist countries such as Cuba carefully specify many aspects of childcare and provide for the welfare of all children regardless of their parents' economic and educational status, this may restrict some of the variability in children's outcomes that can possibly result from family influences.

Even in the United States, subtle paradigm shifts (perhaps less subtle in recent years) towards a more conservative, fundamentalist Christian value system fostered by our current political leadership may eventually result in corresponding childrearing attitudes, values and techniques. Indicators of this trend may be the growth of home schooling, charter schools, and parents' dissatisfaction with government financed public school systems that provide some support for separating the values of church and state. As a result, we may have experienced a recent trend for parents to foster beliefs in obedience, godliness, and the importance of following authority more than the recent past.

In conclusion, the scientific study of parent-youth relationships can only become more "scientific" to the extent that there are efforts to search for general patterns in the broadest range of cultural diversity. Treating a particular parent-child practice as a general developmental or relationship pattern without cross-cultural verification is a practice that is much too common but is becoming simply an indefensible example of poor social science. Current cross-cultural research provides general insights into patterns that parents, children, and youth may share, but it also teaches caution about making premature or excessive generalizations about the meaning of what occurs between the young and their parents.

REFERENCES

Arnett, J. J. (1995). Broad and narrow socialization: The family in the context of cultural theory. *Journal of Marriage and the Family, 54*, 339-373.

Baumrind, D. (1991). Effective parenting during the early adolescent transition. In P. A. Cowen & M. Hertheringron (Eds.) *Review of child development research* (vol 1, pp. 169-208). Chicago: University of Chicago Press.

Bronnfenbrenner, U. (1979). *The ecology of human development.* Cambridge, MA: Harvard University Press.

Bronnfenbrenner, U. (1986). Ecology of the family as a context for human development: Research perspectives. *Developmental Psychology, 22*, 723-742.

Chao, R. (1994). Beyond parental control and authoritarian parenting style: Understanding Chinese parenting through the cultural notion of training. *Child Development, 65*, 1111-1119.

Chao, R. K. (2000). Cultural explanations for the role of parenting in the school success of Asian-American Children. In R. Taylor & M. C. Wang (Ed.). *Resilience across contexts: Family, work, culture, and community* (pp. 333-363). Temple University: Center for Research in Human Development.

Chao, R. K. (2001). Extending research on the consequences of parenting style for Chinese Americans and European Americans. *Child Development, 72,* 1832-1843.

Corsaro, W. A. (1997). *The sociology of childhood.* Thousand Oaks, CA: Pine Forge Press.

Darling, N., & Steinberg, L. (1993). Parenting style as context: An integrative model. *Psychological Bulletin, 113,* 487-496.

Elder, G. H. (1972). *Children of the great depression.* Chicago: University of Chicago Press.

Elder, G. H., Jr., Eccles, J. S., Ardelt, M., & Lord, S. (1995). Inner-city parents under economic pressure: Perspectives of the strategies of parenting. *Journal of Marriage and the Family, 57,* 771-784.

Harkness, S., & Super, C. (2002). Culture and parenting. In M. H. Bornstein (Ed.). *Handbook of parenting* (2nd Ed.) (pp. 253-280). Mahwah, NJ: Lawrence Erlbaum Associates, Publishers.

Kagitcibasi, C. (1996). *Family and human development across cultures: A view from the other side.* Mahwah, NJ: Lawrence Erlbaum Associates.

Kuczynski, L. (2003). Beyond bidirectionality: Bilateral conceptual frameworks for understanding dynamics in parent-child relations. In L. Kuczinsky (Ed.). *Handbook of dynamics in parent-child relations* (pp.3-24). Thousand Oaks, CA: Sage Publications.

Kohn, M. L. (1969). *Class and conformity: A study in values.* Chicago: University of Chicago Press.

Kohn, M. L. & Schooler, C. (1983). *Work and personality: An inquiry into the impact of social stratification.* Norwood, NJ: Ablex.

Maccoby, E. E., & Martin, J. A. (1983). Socialization in the context of the family: Parent-child interaction. In P. H. Mussen (Series Ed.) and M. E. Hetherington (Ed.), *Handbook of child psychology: Vol. 4, Socialization, personality, and social development* (pp. 1-101). New York: Wiley.

Peterson, G. W. (1995). Autonomy and connectedness. In R. D. Day, K. R. Gilbert, B. H. Settles, & W. R. Burr (Eds.) *Research and theory in family science.* Pacific Grove, CA: Brooks/Cole.

Peterson, G. W., & Hann, D. (1999). Socializing parents and children in families. In M. B. Sussman, S. K. Steinmetz, & G. W. Peterson (Eds.). *Handbook of marriage and the family* (pp. 327-370). New York: Plenum Press.

Peterson, G. W., & Rollins, B. C. (1987). Parent-child socialization. In M. Sussman and S. K. Steinmetz (Eds.) *Handbook of marriage and the family* (pp.471-507). New York: Plenum Press.

Rogoff, B. (2003). *The cultural nature of human development.* New York: Oxford University Press.

Rohner, R. P. (1986). *The warmth dimension: Foundation of parental acceptance-rejection theory.* Beverly Hills, CA: Sage Publications.

Rollins, B. C., & Thomas, D. L. (1979). Parental support, power, and control techniques in the socialization of children. In W. R. Burr, R. Hill, F. I. Nye, & I. L. Reiss
(Eds.), *Contemporary theories about the family, Vol 1, Research based theories*
(pp. 317-364). New York: Free Press.

Steinberg, (2001). We know some things: adolescent-parent relationships in retrospect
and prospect. *Journal of Research on Adolescence, 11,* 1-20.

Steinmetz, S. K. (1971). Occupation and Physical Punishment: A Response to Straus.
Journal of Marriage and the Family. 33, 664-666.

Steinmetz, S. K. Adolescence in Contemporary Families. In M. B. Sussman, S. K. Steinmetz, &
G. W. Peterson (Eds.). *Handbook of marriage and the family* (pp. 327-370). New York:
Plenum Press.

Stewart, S. M., & Bond, M. H. (2002). A critical look at parenting research from the
mainstream: Problems uncovered while adapting Western cultures. *British Journal
of Developmental Psychology, 20,* 379-392.

Strauss, C., & Quinn, N. (1997). *A cognitive theory of cultural meaning.* New York:
Cambridge University Press.

Index

© 2005 by The Haworth Press, Inc. All rights reserved.

Family Systems and Inheritance Patterns, edited by Judith N. Cates and Marvin B. Sussman, PhD (Vol. 5, No. 3, 1983). *Specialists in economics, law, psychology, and sociology provide a comprehensive examination of the disposition of property following a death.*

Alternatives to Traditional Family Living, edited by Harriet Gross, PhD, and Marvin B. Sussman, PhD (Vol. 5, No. 2, 1982). *"Professionals interested in the lifestyles described will find well-written essays on these topics." (The American Journal of Family Therapy)*

Intermarriage in the United States, edited by Gary A. Crester, PhD, and Joseph J. Leon, PhD (Vol. 5, No. 1, 1982). *"A very good compendium of knowledge and of theoretical and technical issues in the study of intermarriage." (Journal of Comparative Family Studies)*

Cults and the Family, edited by Florence Kaslow, PhD, and Marvin B. Sussman, PhD (Vol. 4, No. 3/4, 1982). *"Enlightens not only the professional but the lay reader as well. It provides support and understanding for families . . . gives insight and . . . enables parents, friends, and loved ones to better understand what happens when one joins a cult." (The Family Psychologist)*

Family Medicine: A New Approach to Health Care, edited by Betty Cogswell and Marvin B. Sussman, PhD (Vol. 4, No. 1/2, 1982). *The history, rationale, and the continuing developments in this medical specialty all in one readable volume.*

Marriage and the Family: Current Critical Issues, edited by Marvin B. Sussman, PhD (Vol. 1, No. 1, 1979). *Covers pluralistic family forms, family violence, never married persons, dual career families, the "roleless" role (widowhood), and non-marital, heterosexual cohabitation.*

BOOK ORDER FORM!

Order a copy of this book with this form or online at:
http://www.haworthpress.com/store/product.asp?sku=5518

Parent-Youth Relations
Cultural and Cross-Cultural Perspectives

____ in softbound at $79.95 ISBN-13: 978-0-7890-2483-1. / ISBN-10: 0-7890-2483-7.
____ in hardbound at $109.95 ISBN-13: 978-0-7890-2482-4. / ISBN-10: 0-7890-2482-9.

COST OF BOOKS _____

POSTAGE & HANDLING _____
US: $4.00 for first book & $1.50
for each additional book
Outside US: $5.00 for first book
& $2.00 for each additional book.

SUBTOTAL _____

In Canada: add 7% GST. _____

STATE TAX _____
CA, IL, IN, MN, NJ, NY, OH, PA & SD residents
please add appropriate local sales tax.

FINAL TOTAL _____

If paying in Canadian funds, convert
using the current exchange rate,
UNESCO coupons welcome.

❏ BILL ME LATER:
Bill-me option is good on US/Canada/
Mexico orders only; not good to jobbers.
wholesalers, or subscription agencies.

❏ Signature _____

❏ Payment Enclosed: $ _____

❏ PLEASE CHARGE TO MY CREDIT CARD:

❏ Visa ❏ MasterCard ❏ AmEx ❏ Discover
❏ Diner's Club ❏ Eurocard ❏ JCB

Account # _____

Exp Date _____

Signature _____
(Prices in US dollars and subject to change without notice.)

PLEASE PRINT ALL INFORMATION OR ATTACH YOUR BUSINESS CARD
Name
Address
City   State/Province   Zip/Postal Code
Country
Tel   Fax
E-Mail

May we use your e-mail address for confirmations and other types of information? ❏ Yes ❏ No We appreciate receiving
your e-mail address. Haworth would like to e-mail special discount offers to you, as a preferred customer.
We will never share, rent, or exchange your e-mail address. We regard such actions as an invasion of your privacy.

Order from your **local bookstore** or directly from
The Haworth Press, Inc. 10 Alice Street, Binghamton, New York 13904-1580 • USA
Call our toll-free number (1-800-429-6784) / Outside US/Canada: (607) 722-5857
Fax: 1-800-895-0582 / Outside US/Canada: (607) 771-0012
E-mail your order to us: orders@haworthpress.com

For orders outside US and Canada, you may wish to order through your local
sales representative, distributor, or bookseller.
For information, see http://haworthpress.com/distributors

(Discounts are available for individual orders in US and Canada only, not booksellers/distributors.)

Please photocopy this form for your personal use.
www.HaworthPress.com

BOF05